AF411786

Current
Diagnosis *&* Treatment
A *Quick* Reference for the General Practitioner

Current
Diagnosis & Treatment

A *Quick* Reference for the General Practitioner

SECOND EDITION

Edited by

James O. Woolliscroft, MD

Professor of Internal Medicine
University of Michigan Medical School
Chief of Clinical Affairs
University of Michigan Hospitals
Ann Arbor, Michigan

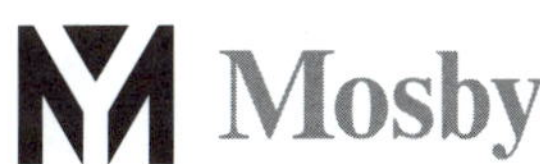

Mosby

St. Louis Baltimore Boston Carlsbad Chicago Naples New York Philadelphia Portland
London Madrid Mexico City Singapore Sydney Tokyo Toronto Wiesbaden

Developed by Current Medicine, Inc., Philadelphia

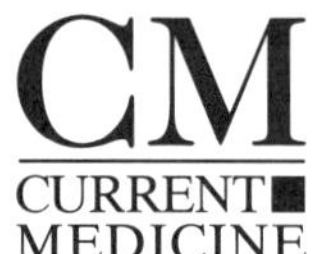 **Current Medicine, Inc.**
400 Market Street, Suite 700
Philadelphia, Pennsylvania 19106

Managing Editor: Lori J. Bainbridge
Developmental Editor: Lee Tevebaugh
Art Director: Paul Fennessy
Layout: Christine Keller-Quirk, Robert LeBrun, Patrick Whelan
Cover Design: Patrick Ward
Typesetting: Ryan Walsh
Illustration Director: Ann Saydlowski
Illustrators: Paul Bernson, Liz Carrozza, Stuart Molloy, Yaron Tracz
Production: Lori Holland, Sally Nicholson
Indexer: Maria Coughlin

Distribution rights for North America:
MOSBY-YEARBOOK, INC.
11830 Westline Industrial Drive
St. Louis, MO 63146

ISBN 1-57340-114-5
ISSN 1083-9666

Although every effort has been made to ensure that the drug doses and other information are
presented accurately in this publication, the ultimate responsibility rests with the prescribing
physician. Neither the publishers nor the authors can be held responsible for errors or for any
consequences arising from the use of the information contained herein. Products mentioned in this
publication should be used in accordance with the manufacturer's prescribing information. No
claims or endorsements are made for any drug or compound at present under clinical investigation.

Manufactured in the United States of America
Printed by Quebecor
5 4 3 2 1

Section Editors

AIDS & Infectious diseases

Powel H. Kazanjian, MD
Associate Professor
Department of Internal Medicine
University of Michigan Medical School
Director, HIV/AIDS Treatment Program
Ann Arbor, Michigan

Cardiology

Kim A. Eagle, MD
Associate Professor
Department of Internal Medicine
University of Michigan Medical School
Director, Clinical Cardiology
University of Michigan Medical Center
Ann Arbor, Michigan

Contributor
Michael Kim, MD
Fellow
Department of Internal Medicine
University of Michigan Medical School
Ann Arbor, Michigan

Dermatology

Bruce R. Nelson, MD
Associate Professor
Department of Dermatology
University of Texas Medical School
Houston, Texas

Denise C. Walker, MD
Resident
Department of Dermatology
University of Texas Medical School
Houston, Texas

Endocrinology & Metabolic disorders

Robert W. Lash, MD
Assistant Professor
Department of Internal Medicine
University of Michigan Medical School
Ann Arbor, Michigan

Gastroenterology & Hepatology

Joseph C. Kolars, MD
Associate Professor
Department of Internal Medicine
University of Michigan Medical School
Ann Arbor, Michigan

Contributor
W. Michael McDonnell, MD
Assistant Professor
Department of Internal Medicine
University of Michigan Medical School
Ann Arbor, Michigan

General medicine

Brent C. Williams, MD, MPH
Associate Professor
Department of Internal Medicine
University of Michigan Medical School
Ann Arbor, Michigan

Contributors
Robert D. Ernst, MD
Clinical Instructor
Department of Internal Medicine
University of Michigan Medical School
Ann Arbor, Michigan

Paul Fine, MD
Clinical Instructor
Department of Internal Medicine
University of Michigan Medical School
Ann Arbor, Michigan

Scott L. Furney, MD
Clinical Instructor
Department of Internal Medicine
University of Michigan Medical School
Ann Arbor, Michigan

Sean K. Kesterson, MD
Clinical Instructor
Department of Internal Medicine
University of Michigan Medical School
Ann Arbor, Michigan

Kym E. Orsetti, MD
Clinical Instructor
Department of Internal Medicine
University of Michigan Medical School
Ann Arbor, Michigan

Hematology & Oncology

Paula L. Bockenstedt, MD
Assistant Professor
Department of Internal Medicine
Director, Adult Hemophilia and Coagulation
    Disorders Clinic
University of Michigan Medical School
Ann Arbor, Michigan

Nephrology

Robert L. Schmouder, MD, MPH
Assistant Professor
Department of Internal Medicine
University of Michigan Medical School
Ann Arbor, Michigan

Neurology

Linda M. Selwa, MD
Clinical Assistant Professor
Department of Neurology
University of Michigan Medical School
Ann Arbor, Michigan

Contributor
John J. Wald, MD
Clinical Assistant Professor
Department of Neurology
University of Michigan Medical Center
Ann Arbor, Michigan

Pulmonary disorders

Cyril M. Grum, MD
Professor
Associate Chair, Undergraduate Education
Department of Internal Medicine
University of Michigan Medical School
Ann Arbor, Michigan

Contributor
Jeffrey E. Terrell, MD
Assistant Professor
Department of Otolaryngology
University of Michigan Medical Center
Ann Arbor, Michigan

Rheumatology & Musculoskeletal disorders

Mark A. McQuillan, MD
Clinical Assistant Professor
Department of Internal Medicine
University of Michigan Medical School
Ann Arbor, Michigan

Information management is arguably the most important challenge confronting busy clinicians. Maintaining an up-to-date knowledge base in diagnosis and disease management, especially for clinical problems encountered less frequently, can be a daunting task. *Current Diagnosis and Treatment*, second edition, is specifically structured to facilitate access to current information on a wide variety of diseases encountered in a general practice, emphasizing the adult patient. It is designed to remind clinicians who need to "brush up" on the diagnosis and management of a clinical entity, not to provide detailed information as is found in major medical texts.

Current Diagnosis and Treatment, second edition, follows a consistent layout throughout the book. This layout allows the clinician to rapidly access information on symptoms, signs, investigations, complications, differential diagnosis, etiology, and epidemiology on one page; and diet and lifestyle, pharmacological and other treatments, management issues, prognosis, and references on the next page. Our goal is to develop a user-friendly, clinically relevant reference for primary care physicians and other members of the health care team.

To maintain currency, the sections from the first edition have been extensively reviewed and revised based on new information and developments in the diagnosis and management of disease. For the second edition, approximately 40 new topics were introduced to make this edition even more comprehensive. This reflects our editors' commitment to currency and relevancy.

James O. Woolliscroft, MD
Ann Arbor, Michigan

Contents

Contents

AIDS

Cardiology

Dermatology

Endocrinology & Metabolic disorders

Gastroenterology

Contents by specialty

General medicine

Hematology & Oncology

Contents by specialty

Pulmonary disorders

Rheumatology & Muscular disorders

Figure acknowledgments

We gratefully acknowledge the publishers and individuals who allowed us to use the following figures and tables.

Page 4. Figure adapted with permission from Kokko JP: Disorders of fluid, volume, electrolyte, and acid-base balance. In *Cecil Textbook of Medicine.* Edited by Bennet JC, Plum F. Philadelphia: WB Saunders; 1996:543-551.

Page 22. Table adapted with permission from Ewing JA: Detecting alcoholism: the CAGE questionnaire. *JAMA* 1984, 252:1905-1907.

Page 22. Figure adapted with permission from Bradley KA: The primary care practitioner's role in the prevention and management of alcohol problems. *Alcohol Health Res World*, 1994 18:97-104.

Page 26. Figure adapted with permission from Hicks TC, Timmcke AE: Fissure in ano. In *Shackelford's Surgery of the Alimentary Tract*, edn. 3. Philadelphia: WB Saunders; 1991:286-293 and Barnett JL, Raper SE: Anorectal disease. In *Textbook of Gastroenterology*, edn. 2. Edited by Yamada T. Philadelphia: JB Lippincott; 1995:2036-2037.

Page 26. Figure reproduced from Barnett JL: Diseases of the anus. In *Gastroenterology and Hepatology: The Comprehensive Visual Reference: Colon, Rectum, and Anus*, vol. 2. Edited by Feldman M, Boland CR. Philadelphia: Current Medicine; 1996.

Page 54. Figure reproduced from Wong F, Blendis L: Cirrhosis: ascites and spontaneous bacterial peritonitis. In *Gastroenterology and Hepatology: The Comprehensive Visual Reference: The Liver*, vol. 1. Edited by Feldman M, Maddrey WC. Philadelphia: Current Medicine; 1996.

Page 68. Table adapted with permission from Barry WJ, *et al.*: The American Urologic Association Symptom Index for benign prostatic hyperplasia. *J Urol* 1992, 148:1549-1557.

Page 76. Figures reproduced with permission from Smith DE, *et al.*: Itraconazole versus ketoconazole in the treatment of oral and oesophageal candidosis in patients infected with HIV. *AIDS* 1991, 5:1367-1371.

Page 90. Figure adapted with permission from Ho-Yen DO: The epidemiology of post viral fatigue syndrome. *Scott Med J* 1988, 33:368-369.

Page 98. Figure adapted with permission form Swash M, Oxberry J (eds.): *Clinical Neurology*. Edinburgh: Churchill Livingstone; 1991:188-204.

Page 117. Figure adapted with permission from Kupfer DJ: Lessons to be learned from long-term treatment of affective disorder. *J Clin Psychiatry* 1991, 52(suppl):12-16.

Page 124. Figure adapted with permission from Besser GM, Bodansky HJ, Cudworth AG: *Clinical Diabetes: An Illustrated Text*. London: Mosby-Wolfe, an imprint of Times Mirror International Publishers; 1995.

Page 175. Figure adapted from Hoffman GS, *et al.*: Wegener granulomatosis: an analysis of 158 patients. *Ann Intern Med* 1992, 116:488-498.

Page 188. Figures courtesy of R. Burney, Ann Arbor, MI.

Page 214. Figure courtesy of Professor A. Grossman, Department of Endocrinology, St. Bartholomew's Hospital, London, UK.

Page 220. Figures reproduced with permission from Slade AKB, Saumarel RC, McKenna WJ: The arrhythmogenic substrate—diagnostic and therapeutic implications: hypertrophic cardiomyopathy. *Eur Heart J* 1993, 14:84-90.

Page 224. Figure adapted with permission from Frier BM, Fisher M (eds.): *Hypoglycaemia and Diabetes*. London: Edward Arnold; 1993.

Page 232. Figure courtesy of M. Scaglia, MD.

Page 238. Figure adapted with permission from Whitehead WE, Engel BT, Schuster MM: Irritable bowel syndrome: physiological and psychological differences between diarrhea-predominant and constipation-predominant patients. *Dig Dis Sci* 1980, 25:404-413.

Page 254. Figure courtesy of Dr. John Smith, Director, Essex Regional Immunology Service Tenovus Laboratory. Southampton General Hospital.

Page 256. Figure reproduced from Lee WM: Acute liver failure. In *Gastroenterology and Hepatology: The Comprehensive Visual Reference: The Liver*, vol. 1. Edited by Feldman M, Maddrey WC. Philadelphia: Current Medicine; 1996.

Page 270. Figures reproduced with permission from Ramsay M, *et al.*: The epidemiology of measles in England and Wales. *Commun Dis Rep* 1994, 4:R141-R145.

Page 292. Figure reproduced with permission from Scolar A, French P, Miller R: *Myobacterium avium intracellulare* infection in the acquired immunodeficiency syndrome. *Br J Hosp Med* 1991, 46:295-300.

Page 314. Figure adapted with permission from Wasnich RD: Epidemiology of osteoporosis. In *Primer on the Metabolic Bone Diseases and Disorders of Mineral Metabolism*, edn 3. Edited by Favus MJ. Philadelphia: Lippincott-Raven; 1996:250.

Page 319. Figure adapted with permission from Tsuchiya R: Resection of cancer of the pancreas—the Japanese experience. *Baillières Clin Gastroenterol* 1990, 4:431-434.

Page 334. Figure reproduced with permission from Gay NJ, *et al.*: Age specific antibody prevalence to parvovirus B19: how many women are infected in pregnancy? *Commun Dis Rep* 1994, 4:R104-R107.

Page 356. Table adapted with permission from Norton D, McLaren R, Exton-Smith AN: *An Investigation of Geriatric Nursing Problems in the Hospital*. London: National Corporation for the Care of Old People; 1962.

Page 370. Figure reproduced with permission from Stansby G, *et al.*: Atherosclerotic renal artery stenosis. *Br J Hosp Med* 1993, 49:388.

Page 398. Figures reproduced with permission from Miller E, *et al.*: Rubella surveillance to June 1994. *Commun Dis Rep* 1994, 4:R146-R152.

Page 426. Figure reproduced with permission from Franklyn JA, Sheppard MC: Thyroid nodules and thyroid cancer—diagnostic aspects. *Baillières Clin Endocrinol Metab* 1988, 2:767.

Page 410. Table adapted with permission from Cooper-Patrick L, Crum RM, Ford DE: Identifying suicidal ideation in general medical patients. *JAMA* 1994, 272:1757-1762.

Page 428. Table adapted with permission from Heatherton TF, Koziowski LT, Frecker RC, Fagerstrom KO: The Fagerstrom test for nicotine dependence: a revision of the Fagerstrom tolerance questionnaire. *Br J Addict* 1991, 86:1119-1127.

Page 440. Figure reproduced from *MMWR Morb Mortal Wkly Rep* 1992, 41:58.

Page 440. Figure reproduced from *MMWR Morb Mortal Wkly Rep* 1990, 39:421-423.

Page 444. Figure reproduced with permission from Kennedy DH: Extrapulmonary tuberculosis. *Update* 1983, 27:671-684.

Page 469. Table adapted with permission from U.S. Preventive Services Task Force: *Guide to Clinical Preventive Services*, edn 2, 1996: 74; and ACOG Committee Opinion Number 152, *Recommendations on Frequency of Pap Test Screening*. March 1995.

This book provides current expert recommendations on the diagnosis and treatment of all major disorders throughout medicine in the form of tabular summaries. Essential guidelines on each of the topics have been condensed into two pages of vital information, summarizing the main procedures in diagnosis and management of each disorder to provide a quick and easy reference.

Each disorder is presented as a "spread" of two facing pages: the main procedures in diagnosis on the left and treatment options on the right.

Listed in the main column of the **Diagnosis** page are the common symptoms, signs, and complications of the disorder, with brief notes explaining their significance and probability of occurrence, together with details of investigations that can be used to aid diagnosis.

The left shaded side column contains information to help the reader evaluate the probability that an individual patient has the disorder. It may also include other information that could be useful in making a diagnosis (*e.g.*, classification or grading systems, comparison of different diagnostic methods).

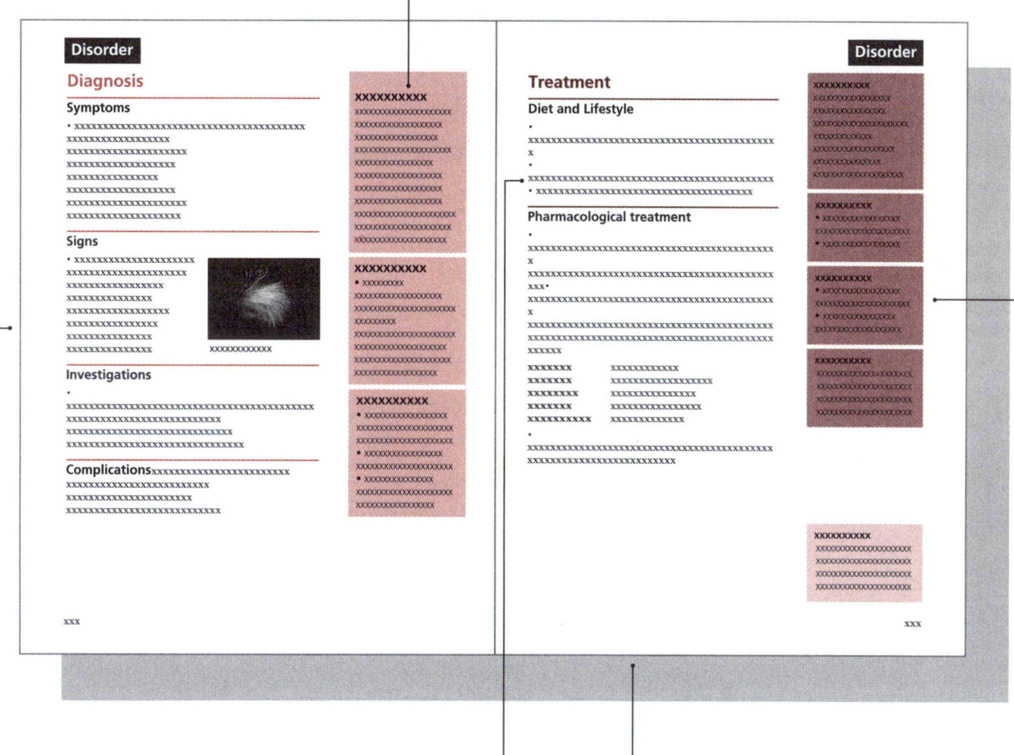

On the **Treatment** page, the main column contains information on lifestyle management and nonspecialist medical therapy of the disorder, with general information on specialist management when this is the main treatment.

Whenever possible under "Pharmacological treatment," guidelines are given on the standard dosage for commonly used drugs, with details of contraindications and precautions, main drug interactions, and main side effects. In each case, however, the manufacturer's drug data sheet should be consulted before any regimen is prescribed.

The main goals of treatment (*e.g.*, to cure, to palliate, to prevent), prognosis after treatment, precautions that the physician should take during and after treatment, and any other information that could help the clinician to make treatment decisions (*e.g.*, other nonpharmacological treatment options, special situations or groups of patients) are given in the right shaded side column. The key and general references at the end of this column provide the reader with further practical information.

Diagnosis

Symptoms

Dysphagia: usually perceived with both solid food and liquids [1].

Retrosternal chest pain: intermittent and variable duration, often related to eating.

Weight loss.

Regurgitation.

Nocturnal cough: related to regurgitation and aspiration.

Signs

• Usually no signs are manifest.

Evidence of weight loss.

Investigations

Radiography (plain film, erect): may show absence of air in gastric fundus or dilated esophagus with air-fluid level.

Radiography (barium swallow): shows delayed passage of contrast through cardia, absence of peristalsis (although "tertiary waves" may be prominent), or esophageal dilatation with "bird-beak" narrowing in the distal esophagus.

Upper gastrointestinal endoscopy: often normal; retained food or fluid may be encountered; increased resistance to passage of endoscope through cardia may be apparent.

Esophageal manometry: shows impaired relaxation of lower esophageal sphincter and absent peristalsis; may show prominent nonperistaltic (synchronous) contractions in esophageal body or elevated tonic pressure of lower esophageal sphincter [2].

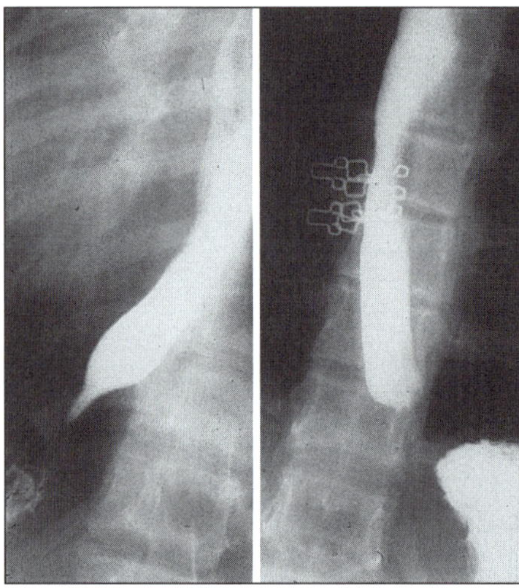

Classic "bird-beak" distal esophagus (*left*) and delay of barium swallow due to spasm (*right*).

Complications

Respiratory complications: *e.g.*, cough, aspiration pneumonitis, in 10% of patients.

Esophageal carcinoma: possibly a late complication; very unusual.

Malnutrition.

Treatment

Diet and lifestyle

• A mechanical soft diet with ingestion of meats and other solid food only if it has been ground into fine pieces.

Pharmacological treatment

• Nitrates and calcium antagonists (*e.g.*, nifedipine) reduce the lower esophageal sphincter pressure and may give short-term benefit before dilatation or surgery.

Nonpharmacological treatment

Dilatation of the cardia

• Endoscopic myotomy performed at the time of dilation using, for example, a Witzel balloon is the procedure of choice [3].

• Local injection therapy with botulinum toxin is also a consideration but may require repeat treatments.

• Dysphagia is relieved in about two-thirds of patients after one attempt; a second attempt is usually worthwhile if the first attempt was unsuccessful.

• Complications include esophageal perforation in 2%–10% of patients; surgical repair is not always needed.

Surgery

• Cardiomyotomy through the thorax or abdomen or as a "minimal-access" procedure should be pursued if the endoscopic approach is unsuccessful.

Treatment aims

To restore acceptable swallowing.

Prognosis

• Relief of dysphagia and retrosternal pain can be achieved in >80% of patients.

Follow-up and management

• Symptomatic gastroesophageal reflux occurs in 5%–10% of patients after successful dilatation or cardiomyotomy; treatment with an H_2 receptor antagonist or proton pump inhibitor is usually successful.

Key references

1. Howard PJ, *et al.*: Five year prospective study of the incidence, clinical features and diagnosis of achalasia in Edinburgh. *Gut* 1992, **33**:1011–1015.

2. Richter JE: Motility disorders of the esophagus. In *Textbook of Gastroenterology*. Edited by Yamada T. Philadelphia: JB Lippincott; 1995:1182–1194.

3. Parkman HP, *et al.*: Pneumatic dilatation or esophagomyotomy treatment for idiopathic achalasia: clinical outcomes and cost analysis. *Dig Dis Sci* 1993, **38**:75–85.

Diagnosis

Symptoms
• There are few symptoms associated with acid-base disorders.

Signs
• Signs are generally nonspecific and of limited help diagnostically.

Metabolic acidosis
Hyperventilation (including Kussmaul respiration).
Altered mental status, shock: in severe cases.

Metabolic alkalosis
Hypovolemia: may be associated with metabolic alkalosis.

Respiratory acidosis
Altered mental status (CO_2 narcosis): dilated retinal vessels, papilledema.

Respiratory alkalosis
Tingling of hands, feet, perioral area.
Tetany: in severe cases.

Investigations

All acid-base disorders
Electrolytes, blood urea nitrogen, creatinine, glucose.
Arterial blood gas: if clinically indicated.

Metabolic acidosis
Calculation of serum anion gap [Na - (Cl + HCO_3)].
Calculation of urinary anion gap [(Na + K) - Cl].
Serum ketones, lactate.
Toxicology: salicylates, methanol, ethylene glycol, paraldehyde.

Metabolic alkalosis
Urine chloride.

Respiratory acidosis
• *See* All acid-base disorders *above.*

Respiratory alkalosis
• *See* All acid-base disorders *above.*

Complications
• Most complications are secondary to the underlying disorder (*e.g.*, diabetic ketoacidosis, asthma exacerbation).

Metabolic acidosis
Diminished cardiac output leading to hypotension, decreased tissue perfusion, shock.

Metabolic alkalosis
Volume contraction, hypokalemia.

Respiratory acidosis
Hypoxemia, coma.

Respiratory alkalosis
Tetany, seizures: rare.

Differential diagnosis
Not applicable.

Etiology

Metabolic acidosis
Increased anion gap: diabetic ketoacidosis, alcoholic ketoacidosis, lactic acidosis, renal failure, salicylates, toxins (*see* Investigations).
Normal anion gap: gastrointestinal fluid losses (negative urinary anion gap)—diarrhea, small intestine losses, ureterosigmoidostomy.
Renal tubular acidoses (positive urinary anion gap).
Other causes: parenteral hyperalimentation, potassium sparing diuretics, rapid volume expansion, acetazolamide.

Metabolic alkalosis
U_{Cl} *<10 mmol/L*: these disorders are associated with hypovolemia and respond to saline infusion; etiologies include, vomiting, nasogastric suction, villous adenoma, diuretics, hypercapnia.
U_{Cl} *>20 mmol/L*: these disorders are unresponsive to saline infusion; etiologies include mineralocorticoid excess (various causes), severe hypokalemia (not diuretic induced), hypercalcemia, alkali ingestion.

Respiratory acidosis
Ventilatory failure (sedation, cardiac arrest, pulmonary disease, neuromuscular disease, CNS lesions).

Respiratory alkalosis
Hyperventilation (anxiety, CNS lesions, high altitudes, severe liver disease, febrile illnesses, salicylates, pregnancy).

Epidemiology
Not applicable.

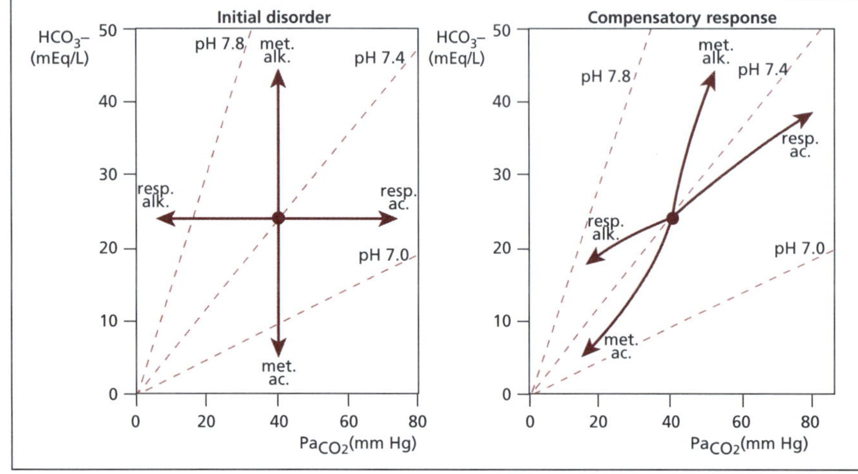

Acid-base disorders initially alter serum concentrations of either HCO_3 (in metabolic disorders) or Pa_{CO2} (respiratory disorders), leading to changes in arterial pH (*left*). Over time, compensatory mechanisms will shift serum pH back toward a pH of 7.4 (*right*).

Treatment

Diet and lifestyle

• Patients with chronic diseases such as type I diabetes and asthma should by encouraged to comply with medical regimens.

Pharmacological treatment

Metabolic acidosis

• Treatment of the underlying disorder (*e.g.*, diabetic ketoacidosis or sepsis) includes the following:

Alcoholic ketoacidosis: typically corrects with normal saline and glucose infusion.

Diarrhea/gastrointestinal losses: normal saline and electrolyte replacement (especially potassium).

Renal failure: HCO_3 >15 mEq/dL—no therapy required; HCO_3 <15 mEq/dL (without uremia)—oral alkali; severe acidosis with uremia—hemodialysis.

Toxins: supportive care for all patients; salicylates: hemodialysis for concentrations >100 mg/dL; methanol, ethylene glycol—usually requires hemodialysis.

Alkali therapy: most studies show no significant benefit; may be worthwhile in profound acidosis to keep arterial pH from falling below 7.1; do not use alkali to correct pH to normal.

Metabolic alkalosis

U_{Cl} <10 mmol/L: gastric losses—normal saline infusion; diuretic induced—normal saline infusion, potassium replacement.

U_{Cl} >20 mmol/L: treat underlying disorder (*e.g.*, adrenal disease); potassium replacement.

Respiratory acidosis

Ventilatory support; treat underlying disease; trial of naloxone if narcotic overdose is suspected.

Respiratory alkalosis

Treat underlying disorder; hyperventilation secondary to anxiety may be treated by breathing into a paper bag.

Treatment aims

To restore normal acid-base status.

To replace fluid and electrolytes.

To treat underlying disorder.

Prognosis

Generally good, but depends on underlying disorder.

Follow-up and management

Avoidance of precipitating events.

Ongoing treatment of underlying disorders.

Useful equations for calculating compensatory responses

Metabolic acidosis

For every 1.0 mEq/dL fall in HCO_3, Pa_{CO_2} will decrease 0.8 mm Hg.

Metabolic alkalosis

For every 1.0 mEq/dL rise in HCO_3, Pa_{CO_2} will increase 1.4–1.7 mm Hg.

Respiratory acidosis

Chronic: for every 10 mm Hg rise in Pa_{CO_2}, HCO_3 will increase 3.5–4.0 mEq/dL.

Respiratory alkalosis

Chronic: for every 10 mm Hg fall in Pa_{CO_2}, HCO_3 will decrease 4.0–5.0 mEq/dL.

• Simple compensatory mechanisms move pH back toward (but not all the way to) 7.4 (*see* figure). If this rule appears to be violated, look for a mixed disorder with two primary abnormalities.

General references

Haber RJ: A practical approach to acid-base disorders. *West J Med* 1991, **155**:146–151.

Kokko JP: Disorders of fluid, volume, electrolyte, and acid-base balance. In *Cecil Textbook of Medicine*. Edited by Bennet JC, Plum F: Philadelphia: WB Saunders; 1996:543–551.

Levinsky NG: Acidosis and alkalosis. In *Harrison's Principles of Internal Medicine*. Edited by Isselbacher KJ, Braunwald E, Wilson JD, *et al*. New York: McGraw-Hill; 1994:253–262.

Preuss JG: Fundamentals of clinical acid-base evaluation. *Clin Lab Med* 1993, **13**:103–116.

Diagnosis

Symptoms

Concern about appearance: even in cases that may be quite inconspicuous to the observer.

Social embarrassment.

Pain: from inflammatory papules, pustules, and cysts.

Signs

• Distribution is usually limited to the face, upper back, and chest, but acne can occur over the entire back and extend to the proximal arms in more severe cases.

• Lesions can be divided into inflammatory and noninflammatory.

Inflammatory
Papules.

Pustules.

Nodules and fluctuant cysts (nodulo-cystic acne).

Noninflammatory
Closed comedones (whiteheads).

Open comedones (blackheads).

Scars from resolved or treated areas of acne cysts.

Oily skin.

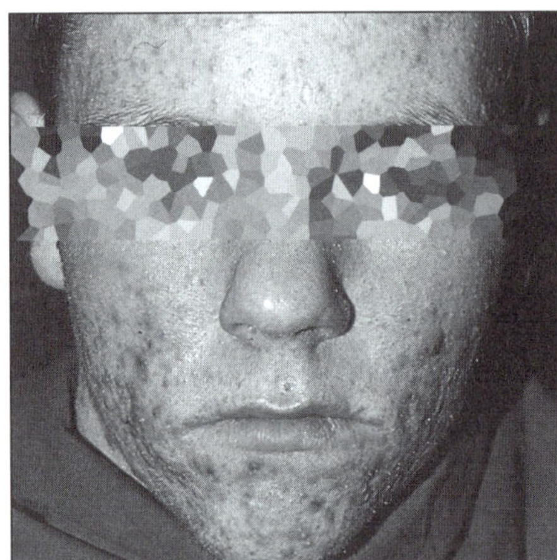
Moderate to severe facial acne. (*See* Color Plate.)

Investigations

• Acne is a clinical diagnosis.

Culture: may be helpful to identify gram-negative folliculitis unresponsive to conventional acne treatment.

Biopsy: may be used to rule out other diseases in cases with an atypical presentation.

• Women with severe acne resistant to standard therapy or with hirsutism or menstrual irregularities may have underlying endocrine abnormalities; often the work-up is normal, but polycystic ovaries and ovarian or adrenal tumors may be present and need to be excluded as part of the work-up [1].

Complications

Scarring: from resolving lesions; "ice-pick" scarring or depressed atrophic plaques.

Hyperpigmented macules: from resolving comedones especially in patients with pigmented skin.

Keloids: especially on anterior chest and back.

Solid persistent inflammatory edema unresponsive to conventional treatment for acne: as a sequela [2].

Osteolytic bone lesions with musculoskeletal pain and septic fever: in cases of acne fulminans, a rare ulcerative form of acne [3,4].

Vaginal yeast infections: in patients treated with systemic antibiotics.

Aggressive cutaneous basal cell carcinomas/thyroid carcinomas: prone to develop in patients who have had superficial x-ray irradiation for treatment of acne in the past; such patients should be closely followed and educated.

Differential diagnosis

Rosacea
Facial flushing with periorbital pallor; can be purely telangiectatic, spares the face; granulomatous, papular, pustular or any combination.

Perioral dermatitis
Combination of eczematous patches and inflammatory papules around the mouth, most commonly in women.

Steroid acne
Multiple monomorphous inflammatory papules or pustules. Can occur from application of fluorinated topical steroids especially on face or in patients on systemic steroids (on chest, back, and shoulders).

Drugs
Can cause acneiform eruption, especially phenytoin and lithium.

Halogenoderma
From iodide, bromide, or chloride.

Gram-negative folliculitis
Culture useful to differentiate from acne.

Excoriated acne
Can be incorrectly diagnosed as impetigo or factitial dermatitis.

Pyoderma faciale
Rapid development of indurated erythema and fluctuant abscesses on the face of young women.

Tumorous sclerosis
Angiofibromas often misdiagnosed as acne.

Acne fulminans
Severe sudden onset of painful inflammatory nodules mainly on the chest and back of adolescent boys common with associated leukocytosis, arthralgias, fever, and ulceration of the nodules.

Etiology

Defective keratinization that obstructs follicular outflow channels.

Increased sebum production (controlled by androgenic hormonal stimulation).

Inflammation: elevated population of *Propionibacterium acnes* within follicles behind obstructed follicular channels release lipases that act on triglycerides in sebum and release free fatty acids, which in turn causes inflammation; *P. acnes* also produces chemoattractants [5].

Epidemiology

• Acne is the most common skin disease in the United States.

• 85% of those between the ages of 12 and 25 years are affected.

• Peak incidence is between ages 16 and 18 years.

Treatment

Diet and lifestyle

• Diet appears to have little effect on acne.

• Long-term exposure to chlorinated hydrocarbons, coal tar, machine oils, greases, lubricating oils, and dioxin can cause acneiform lesions [6].

• Pomade oils and comedogenic cosmetics should be avoided [7].

Pharmacological treatment

• Most treatments take 4 to 6 weeks of therapy before clinical improvement occurs [8].

For mild acne: topical treatment

Standard dosage	Benzoyl peroxide, 2.5%–10%. Tretinoin, 0.025%, 0.05%, 0.1% cream; 0.01%, 0.025%, 0.025% gel; 0.05% liquid. Apply as tolerated; increase to twice daily.
Contraindications	None.
Special points	*Retinoic acid:* needs to be increased as tolerated; many patients experience an initial flare-up of their acne. Newly marketed topical retinoids include adapalene and tretinoin microsphere. Both possess the efficacy of a higher-strength retinoid with less skin irritation, are prescribed as a 0.1% gel, and can be used nightly as tolerated.
Main drug interactions	None.
Main side effects	Drying, irritation and stinging, excessive skin peeling.

For mild acne: topical antibiotics

Standard dosage	Clindamycin, 1% solution, gel, or lotion; erythromycin, 2% ointment, gel, or solution; meclocycline; tetracycline; benzamycin (3% erythromycin, 5% benzoyl peroxide); apply thin film to affected areas twice daily.
Contraindications	None.
Main drug interactions	None.
Main side effects	Local irritation and mild scaliness; gels tend to be drying, ointments make skin feel "oily."

For moderate acne: oral antibiotics

Standard dosage	Tetracycline, 1–2 g daily. Erythromycin, 1 g daily. Minocycline, 100–200 mg daily. Trimethoprim-sulfamethoxazole, 1–2 tablets daily.
Contraindications	*Tetracycline:* pregnancy and children <12 years of age. *Erythromycin:* patients taking terfenadine astemizole.
Special points	*Tetracycline, minocyline:* may cause pseudotumor cerebri. *Minocycline:* are acute hepatitis and liver failure, a Loffler-like syndrome, a lupus-like syndrome, and pustular folliculitis with eosinophilia (rare and often unrecognized side effects).
Main drug interactions	*Erythromycin:* interacts with cytochrome P450; reported to decrease the effectiveness of oral contraceptives.
Main side effects	*Tetracycline, minocycline:* nausea, vomiting, photosensitivity. *Erythromycin:* severe gastric irritation.

For moderate or severe acne

Standard dosage	Isotretinoin, 0.5–1 mg/kg daily in two doses with meals for 20 weeks.
Contraindications	Pregnancy; caution in pre-existing renal or hepatic disease.
Special points	Major fetal abnormalities have been reported; female patients in child-bearing years must use effective contraception during and at least 1 month after therapy. Liver function tests and serum lipoprotein levels should be monitored monthly.
Main drug interactions	Preparations containing high doses of vitamin A.
Main side effects	Cheilitis of the lips; drying of nasal mucosa with mild epistaxis and conjunctivitis; fetal death and malformation; arthralgias; elevated liver enzymes and triglycerides.

Key references

1. Lucky AW: Hormonal correlates of acne and hirsutism. *Am J Med* 1995, **98**:S89–S94.

2. Jungfer B, *et al.*: Solid persistent facial edema of acne: successful treatment with isotretinoin and ketotifen. *Dermatology* 1993, **187**:34–37.

3. Karvonen SL: Acne fulminans: report of clinical findings and treatment of twenty-four patients. *J Am Acad Dermatol* 1993, **28**:572–579.

4. Laasonen LS, *et al.*: Bone disease in adolescents with acne fulminans and severe cystic acne: radiologic and scintographic findings. *AJR Am J Roentgenol* 1994, **152**:1161–1165.

5. Pochi PE: The pathogenesis and treatment of acne. *Ann Rev Med* 1990, **41**:187–198.

6. Fischer AA: *Contact Dermatitis*, edn 3. Philadelphia: Lea & Febiger; 1989:368–393; 486–514.

7. Plewig G, *et al.*: Pomade acne. *Arch Dermatol* 1970, **101**:580–584.

8. Drake LA, *et al.*: Guidelines of care for acne vulgaris. *J Am Acad Dermatol* 1990, **22**:676–680.

Diagnosis

Symptoms

Episodic facial flushing.

Social embarrassment: concern about appearance.

Signs

Skin findings

• Distribution of skin findings is usually limited to the blush area of the face, including the nose, cheeks, chin, and central forehead; it may involve the neck and chest.

• The disease occurs in stages:

Erythema/edema.

Telangiectasias.

Papules/pustules.

Sebaceous gland hypertrophy.

Rhinophyma.

Ocular findings [1]

• In 20% of patients with rosacea, ocular findings are the presenting sign.

Pain/photophobia.

Blepharitis.

Recurrent chalazia.

Conjunctivitis.

Lid margin telangiectasias.

Punctate keratopathy.

Cornea infiltration and vascularization.

Episcleritis/scleritis.

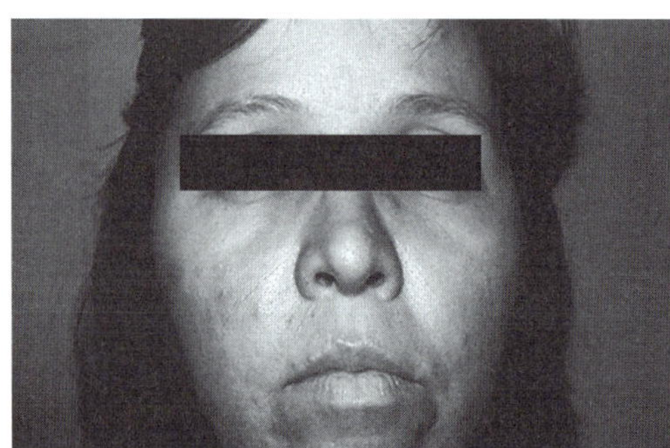

Classic acne rosacea. (*See Color Plate.*)

Investigations

Careful history: including drug history, relation to sun exposure, other systemic symptoms.

Culture: may be helpful to identify gram-negative or staphylococcus folliculitis, tinea faciei.

Biopsy: may be used to rule out other diseases (systemic lupus erythematosus, sarcoidosis) in patients with an atypical presentation.

Complications

Skin

Rhinophyma: disfiguring hypertrophy of the nose.

Peau d'orange skin: inflamed and thickened edematous skin with large pores, resembling the surface of an orange.

Leonine facies: massive tissue hypertrophy leads to facial folds and ridges; similar changes can be seen in leprosy and leukemia.

Ocular

Corneal scarring.

Corneal perforation.

Differential diagnosis [2]

Rebound rosacea

Seen in patients applying topical steroids. Involves much wider area of the face and sometimes also affects the neck, ears, and periocular or perioral areas.

Can see atrophy from steroid applications.

• SLE butterfly rash can mimic rosacea; other evidence of SLE includes oral mucosal involvement, hair loss, photosensitive dermatitis, arthritis, CNS or renal involvement.

Other photosensitive disorders

• Patients with drug-induced photosensitivity will usually have lesions in other sun-exposed sites, *e.g.*, folds of neck.

• Patients with polymorphous light eruption have an erythematous rash in sun-exposed areas, which appears 1–2 days after sun exposure and lasts <1 week.

Acne vulgaris: occurs in younger patients, often involves the neck, chest, and back in addition to the face and tends to scar more than rosacea. Comedones are the primary lesion of acne vulgaris but are typically absent in rosacea.

Acneogenic drugs: lithium, iodine, various neuroleptic agents, oral steroids.

Gram-negative or staphylococcus folliculitis: culture useful to differentiate from rosacea.

Tinea faciei: suspect in patients who have unilateral rosacea. KOH preparation of scale useful to make diagnosis.

Sarcoidosis: ask about arthritis, breathing problems, lesions on other body sites. Look for intranasal and periocular involvement; cystic changes of the distal fingers on radiography.

Etiology [2]

Unknown, possibly multifactorial.

Vascular disorder in which flushing leads to edema that produces papules, pustules, and eventual fibrosis.

• The following may also play a role:

Demodex infestation: produces folliculitis similar to rosacea; mites often found at the surface of the hair follicle.

Sun exposure: may act as a trigger factor via infrared heat.

Helicobacter pylori: prevalence is higher among rosacea patients.

Epidemiology [3]

• It affects 10%–20% of the adult population; 30%–50% of people >40 years of age.

• It may rarely be seen in children and blacks.

• Women are more likely to be affected than men, but disease often more severe in men.

• Ocular involvement occurs in >50% of patients and may be the presenting sign in 20%.

Treatment

Diet and lifestyle

• Patients should eliminate factors known to trigger flushing: hot drinks, hot baths, spicy foods, caffeine withdrawal, certain cosmetics, vasodilators.

Pharmacological treatment

For mild rosacea: topical treatment

Standard dosage	Metronidazole, 0.75% gel or cream [2]. Topical erythromycin or clindamycin, in concentrations from 0.5% to 2.0%; apply to affected areas twice daily. Sunscreens, preferably broad-spectrum UVA plus UVB with SPF of 15 or higher.
Contraindications	None.
Main side effects	Low irritation and mild scarring: gels tend to by drying, ointments tend to be oily.
Special points	Metronidazole has its greatest effect on papules and pustules. It does not alter telangiectasias, erythema, or flushing. Tetracycline has not proven to be an effective topical treatment. Topical steroids are contraindicated in the treatment of rosacea.

For moderate rosacea: oral antibiotics [4]

Standard dosage	Tetracycline, 1–2 g daily.
Alternatives	Erythromycin, 1 g daily. Ampicillin, 1–2 g daily.
Contraindications	*Tetracycline*: pregnancy and children <12 years of age. *Erythromycin*: patients taking terfenadine astemizole. *Ampicillin*: patients with penicillin allergy.
Special points	*Tetracycline*: also drug of choice for ocular rosacea [2].
Main drug interactions	*Erythromycin*: interacts with cytochrome P450; reported to decrease the effectiveness of oral contraceptives.
Main side effects	*Tetracycline*: nausea, vomiting, photosensitivity. *Erythromycin* and *ampicillin*: severe gastric irritation.

For moderate or severe rosacea

Standard dosage	Isotretinoin, 0.5 mg/kg/day.
Contraindications	Pregnancy; caution in preexisting renal or hepatic disease.
Special points	Major fetal anomalies have been reported; female patients in childbearing years must use effective contraception during and at least 1 month after therapy. Liver function tests, serum lipoprotein levels, and serum HCG levels should be monitored monthly. In patients with ocular rosacea, lower dosages of isotretinoin such as 0.1–0.2 mg/kg/day can be used to lessen the ocular dryness that may worsen symptoms.
Main drug interactions [5]	Preparations containing high doses of vitamin A. *Tetracycline, minocycline, trimethoprim-sulfamethoxazole*: in combination with isotretinoin may cause benign intracranial hypertension.
Main side effects	Cheilitis of the lips; dryness of nasal and ocular mucosa with mild epistaxis and conjunctivitis; fetal death and malformation; arthralgias/myalgias; elevated liver enzymes, triglycerides, and cholesterol.

Treatment aims

To reduce the number and severity of lesions.

To induce and/or maintain a remission.

Other treatments

For women flushing through menopause [1]: estrogen replacement therapy, clonidine.

For *H. pylori* in the stomach [2]: oral amoxicillin, metronidazole, and bismuth subsalicylate in combination.

For complicating *Demodex* on the face [1]: Y hexachlorocyclohexane (Lindane), crotamiton, or benzoyl benzoate; topical sulfur.

Vascular laser of telangiectatic vessels.

Carbon dioxide laser or rhinophyma [6].

Prognosis

Emphasize that rosacea is a condition that usually responds to therapy even though it cannot be cured.

Follow-up and management

• Patient education is key to success.

• All patients with progressive rosacea should be evaluated by an ophthalmologist.

References

1. Browning J, Proia A: Ocular rosacea. *Surv Ophthalmol* 1986, **31**:145–158.

2. Dahl MV (ed.): Perspectives. In *Current Concepts in Acne and Rosacea: A Symposium at the American Academy of Dermatology*. Orlando: Mark Dahl and Associates; 1996:8–14.

3. Wilkin JK: Rosacea: pathophysiology and treatment. *Arch Dermatol* 1994,**130**:1448.

4. Fitzpatrick TS, *et al.*: *Dermatology in General Medicine*, edn 4. New York: McGraw-Hill; 1993:727–735.

5. Katz HI: *Dermatologists' Guide to Adverse Therapeutic Interactions*. Philadelphia: Lippincott-Raven Publishers; 1997:82–84.

6. Milgraum SS, Glass AT: Recent advances in laser treatment of benign cutaneous lesions. *N J Med* 1993, **90**:744–748.

Diagnosis

Symptoms

• Symptoms are usually asymptomatic.

Mild local tenderness: occasionally.

Signs

Papules: 1–2-mm hyperkeratotic erythematous rough papules on the sun-exposed surfaces of the skin; can be >1 cm in diameter [1] and pigmented as well; occasionally can present as a "cutaneous horn" (*i.e.*, hypertrophic actinic keratoses); often more difficult to see clinically but are easily identified by touch.

Actinic keratoses of the lower lip (actinic cheilitis): presents as a diffuse, ill-defined scaling of the vermilion border of the lower lip that is more sensitive than usual, especially after sun exposure.

Fissuring and leukoplakia: may be present but ulceration is uncommon unless it has progressed to an invasive squamous cell carcinoma.

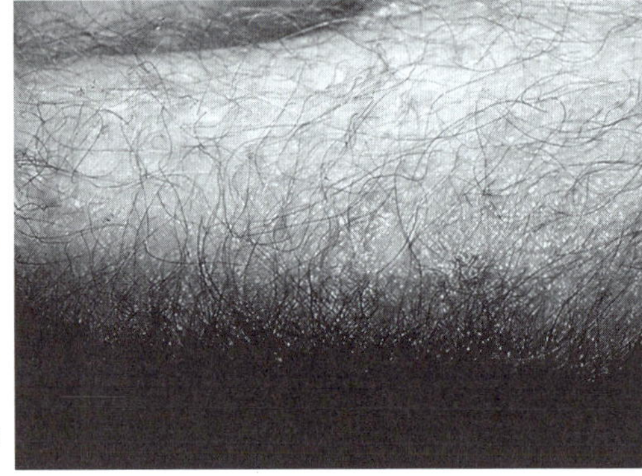

Actinic keratoses. (*See* Color Plate.)

Investigations

Asymptomatic actinic keratoses

• This clinical diagnosis is treated without biopsy confirmation; biopsy is indicated if condition does not respond to treatment.

Symptomatic or hypertrophic actinic keratoses

Skin biopsy: performed at the initial visit or empirical treatment with close follow-up. Biopsy is done if there is no response to treatment to rule out the possibility of an invasive squamous cell carcinoma. If ulceration or induration is present, then a biopsy is mandatory.

• Actinic keratoses are, in fact, squamous cell carcinomas in situ, and it follows that they evolve into squamous cell carcinomas, which in turn may become quite invasive and even metastasize; a high index of suspicion with sound clinical judgment is warranted when evaluating and treating these precancerous lesions.

• It is equally important that a well-experienced dermatopathologist interpret the biopsy specimens (*see* Differential diagnosis).

Complications

Squamous cell carcinoma: evolution of an actinic keratosis into an invasive squamous cell carcinoma is of special significance with regard to actinic cheilitis because squamous cell carcinomas of the lower lip have a high metastatic potential.

Differential diagnosis

Early seborrheic keratoses or macular seborrheic keratoses and verruca vulgaris [2]. Small lesions of chronic cutaneous lupus erythematosus, disseminated superficial actinic porokeratosis.

• When evaluating actinic cheilitis, the differential diagnosis should include squamous cell carcinoma, contact cheilitis, granulomatous cheilitis, necrotizing sialometaplasia, chronic "lip licking," and cheilitis from drugs such as isotretinoin and methotrexate.

• Histologically, actinic keratoses are, in fact, squamous cell carcinomas in situ; it is often necessary for the dermatopathologist to perform "levels" to rule out invasive squamous cell carcinomas.

• Inverted follicular keratoses are irritated seborrheic keratoses, and these look almost identical histologically to squamous cell carcinomas; trained dermatopathologists easily can distinguish the two, but pathologists without special dermatopathology training routinely miss the diagnosis, which results in the inappropriate treatment of a benign skin lesion as a malignant tumor.

• Large cell acanthomas may rarely histologically resemble an actinic keratosis; this holds true for benign lichenoid keratoses and photodamaged skin.

Etiology

• Causes include long-term UV light exposure, x-irradiation, artificial UV light from tanning booths, and polycyclic aromatic hydrocarbon exposure.

• Injury from UV light exposure can select for the clonal expansion of mutated chromosomal *P53* tumor suppressor oncogenes, which can give rise to both actinic keratoses and squamous cell carcinomas [3].

• Sunlight acts as both an initiator and promoter of nonmelanoma skin cancers.

Epidemiology

• Individuals with blonde hair and blue eyes and persons with a history of childhood freckling are at an increased risk to develop actinic keratoses [4].

• Actinic keratoses represent the most common epithelial precancerous lesions in light-complected individuals.

• Over 50% of elderly fair-skinned individuals in hot and sunny climates are affected [5].

• There is also an increased propensity to develop actinic keratoses as well as squamous cell carcinomas in renal transplant patients and other immunosuppressed patients [6].

Treatment

Diet and lifestyle

• Actinic keratoses develop on the exposed surfaces of the skin as a result of long-term sun exposure.

• Artificial UV light exposure in the form of tanning booths as well as x-irradiation and exposure to polycyclic aromatic hydrocarbons are causes as well.

Pharmacological treatment

Topical

Standard dosage	Topical 5-fluouracil [7], 1% or 5% cream applied twice daily for 3–4 weeks as tolerated. Masoprocol, apply cream twice daily to affected areas.
Contraindications	Previous sensitivity.
Main drug interactions	None.
Main side effects	Painful erosions and contact dermatitis (both).

Cryotherapy

Open spray technique with a freeze time of 5–10 seconds or alternatively the dipstick method.

Surgical

• Superficial dermabrasion, curettage, laser abrasion, and chemical peeling have been effective forms of treatment, especially when there is extensive involvement of the skin with actinic keratoses [8].

Treatment aims

To prevent the evolution of actinic keratoses into squamous cell carcinomas by early recognition and treatment and judicial biopsies when indicated.

Prognosis

• In a healthy immunocompetent person, actinic keratoses may spontaneously regress, remain unchanged, or may progress into a squamous cell carcinoma.

• It is difficult to ascertain the exact percentages of malignant transformation; two studies with a 1-year time course reported malignant conversion rates between 0.25% and 20% [9].

• It is nearly impossible to predict the life-time risk in patients with literally hundreds of actinic keratoses (*i.e.*, risk per lesion).

Follow-up and management

• Clinically suspected actinic keratoses that are unresponsive to treatment must undergo biopsy to rule out the possibility of invasive squamous cell carcinoma.

• Patients with multiple actinic keratoses are at an increased risk to develop melanoma and nonmelanoma skin cancers and should be monitored at 3–6-month intervals.

Key references

1. Dinehart SM, Sanchez RL: Spreading pigmented actinic keratosis: an electron micrographic study. *Arch Dermatol* 1988, **124**:680–683.

2. Schwartz RA, Still HL Jr.: Epithelial precancerous lesions. In *Dermatology in General Medicine*. New York: McGraw Hill; 1993:804–808.

3. Ziegler A, *et al.*: Sunburn and *p53* in the onset of skin cancer. *Nature* 1994, **372**:773–776.

4. Vitasa BC, *et al.*: Association of non-melanoma skin cancer and actinic keratosis with cumulative solar ultraviolet exposure in Maryland water-men. *Cancer* 1990, **65**:2811–2817.

5. Marks R: Solar keratoses. *Br J Dermatol* 1990, **122(suppl 35)**:49.

6. Lennard L, *et al.*: Skin cancer in renal transplant recipients is associated with increased concentrations of 6-thioguanine nucleotide in red blood cells. *Br J Dermatol* 1985, **113**:723–729.

7. Kulp-Shorten C, *et al.*: Comparative evaluation of the efficacy and safety of masoprocol and 5-fluorouracil cream for the treatment of multiple actinic keratoses of the head and neck. *J Geriatr Dermatol* 1993, **1**:161–168.

8. Drake LA, *et al.*: Guidelines of care for actinic keratoses. *J Am Acad Dermatol* 1995, **32**:95–98.

9. Callen JP, *et al.*: Actinic keratoses. *J Am Acad Dermatol* 1997, **36**:650–653.

Diagnosis

Symptoms

• Symptoms develop rapidly, often becoming maximal within 4–12 hours of onset.

• Usual sites are knee or wrist for pseudogout and first metatarsophalangeal joint, mid- or hindfoot, knee, or wrist for gout [1].

• Usually, only one or a few joints are involved; polyarticular attacks occur in <10%.

Severe pain: "worst ever."

Stiffness, tenderness, swelling.

Fever and systemic upset: particularly with large- or multiple-joint involvement.

Signs

Overlying erythema: later desquamation.

Red hot joint: *i.e.*, periarticular and articular inflammation; always suggests crystals or sepsis.

Tense effusion, increased warmth, marked joint-line and periarticular tenderness, restricted movement with stress pain: *i.e.*, florid synovitis.

Pyrexia: possible confusion, especially in elderly patients.

Turbid or blood-stained aspirated fluid: high cell count, >95% polymorphs.

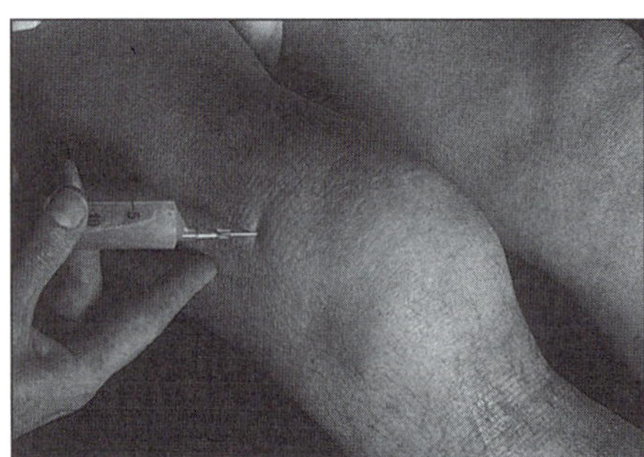
Turbid synovial fluid aspirated from acute knee synovitis due to gout. (*See* Color Plate.)

Investigations

Diagnostic: synovial fluid analysis
Compensated polarized light microscopy: usual method of crystal identification: monosodium urate crystals: strong (negative) birefringence, needle-shaped, 2–25 µm long, easily identified; calcium pyrophosphate dihydrate crystals: weak (positive) birefringence, rhomboid, 2–10 µm long, more difficult to identify; other crystals (cholesterol, oxalate, injected steroid) rare.

Gram stain and culture: essential to exclude sepsis.

Supportive but nondiagnostic
Radiography: to detect chondrocalcinosis (pseudogout); osteophyte, sclerosis, cysts, joint-space narrowing (pseudogout, gout); para-articular erosion (gout); although characteristic, such changes are not always present.

ESR, CRP measurement: usually raised.

Serum uric acid measurement: often but not always raised in gout.

Disease associations
• These should be considered after diagnosis and acute management.

Metabolic screening: calcium, alkaline phosphatase, ferritin, magnesium; if patient is aged <55 years or has polyarticular chondrocalcinosis (pseudogout).

Urea (blood urea nitrogen), creatinine measurement: for renal impairment in primary or secondary gout.

Lipoprotein measurement, liver function tests: in primary and alcohol-associated gout.

Complications

Cluster attacks: one attack triggers attacks at other sites.

Joint rupture: with associated soft-tissue inflammation.

Nerve entrapment: due to acute soft-tissue swelling (most often median nerve).

Differential diagnosis

Septic arthritis: sepsis usually superimposes on abnormal, previously symptomatic joint. Other crystal synovitis.

• Acute crystal synovitis and septic arthritis may coexist.

• More than one crystal type may be present ("mixed crystal deposition").

Etiology

Causes of primary gout
Inherited renal undersecretion of uric acid (in most patients).
Inherited overproduction of uric acid (rare).
Obesity, excess alcohol intake (mainly beer).
Inherited crystal nucleation or growth-promoting tissue factors.

Causes of secondary gout
Chronic diuretic treatment.
Chronic renal impairment.
Lead poisoning (in "moonshine" drinkers).

Causes of pseudogout
Sporadic isolated chondrocalcinosis, pyrophosphate arthropathy (osteoarthritis subset).
Familial predisposition (unusual).
Metabolic predisposition (rare): hemochromatosis, hypomagnesemia, hyperparathyroidism, hypophosphatasemia.

Triggering factors
Local trauma, intercurrent acute illness, surgery, initiation of drug treatment, *e.g.*, allopurinol (gout), thyroxine (pseudogout), parenteral fluids, joint lavage.

• "Shedding" of preformed (previously asymptomatic) crystals initiates acute attack (controversial).

Epidemiology

• Crystal synovitis is the most common cause of acute monoarthritis in middle-aged and elderly patients.

• Before the age of 65 years, more men than women present with gout (mainly primary).

• After the age of 65 years, as many men as women present with gout (mainly secondary).

• Patients with pseudogout are predominantly elderly, with as many men as women.

• Pseudogout is rare in patients aged <55 years (suggests familial or metabolic predisposition).

Treatment

Diet and lifestyle

- No special precautions are necessary in pseudogout.
- Avoidance of high-purine foods may be helpful in gout.

Pharmacological treatment

Oral NSAIDs
- Simple analgesics may be effective with other treatments, but quick-acting NSAIDs are generally preferred (*see* Gout *for further details*) [1,2].

Colchicine
- Colchicine is effective in any crystal synovitis, but it should be used only for very resistant attacks because of toxicity [1].

Standard dosage	Colchicine, 1 mg, then 0.5 mg orally every hour until pain controlled or side effects develop (maximum, 6 mg) in first 24 hours; then maximum dose of 0.6 mg 3 times daily.
Contraindications	Renal or hepatic impairment, dehydration.
Special points	Never given parenterally; not to be given again within 7 days. (Note: i.v. colchicine is hazardous.)
Main drug interactions	None.
Main side effects	Severe nausea, vomiting, watery diarrhea.

Intra-articular steroids
- Steroids are indicated for problematic attacks (large joints, polyarticular involvement, elderly ill patient) or if oral agents are contraindicated.
- They usually reduce synovitis within 24–48 hours.
- The dose should be varied according to joint size; doses listed here are for the knee [2].

Standard dosage	Methylprednisolone, 60 mg. Triamcinolone hexacetonide, 60 mg. Triamcinolone acetonide, 60 mg.
Contraindications	Coexistent sepsis.
Special points	Aseptic technique and single-dose vial should be used.
Main drug interactions	None.
Main side effects	Facial flushing, local skin or fat atrophy (mainly fluoridated steroids), exacerbation of pain (temporary), sepsis (rare).

Nonpharmacological treatment

Local physical measures
- The following are the first line of treatment and must be done early:

Aspiration: to reduce intracapsular hypertension (often temporary).

Local heat or cold: may ameliorate pain and swelling.

Resting support (possibly with splinting): to ease symptoms.

Elevation: to reduce edema.

Early rehabilitation (active movement, mobilization, graded exercise): to maintain muscle and range of movement.

- Prolonged immobilization should be avoided: regular passive movement should punctuate assisted rest.

Lavage
- Lavage is indicated for the following:

Coexistent sepsis.

Florid, large joint synovitis unresponsive after 48 hours to aspiration, steroid injection, and oral medications.

Large loculated effusion (inhibiting effective aspiration).

Treatment aims

To relieve pain.

To reduce intra-articular hypertension.

To avoid muscle wasting or capsular restriction.

Prognosis

- Acute attacks resolve spontaneously, even without treatment, within 1–3 weeks.
- Although prolonged florid synovitis is potentially detrimental, most episodes improve with no apparent lasting damage.
- Incomplete recovery of muscle strength or bulk is the most common problem.

Follow-up and management

- Long-term interventions should be instituted only after an acute attack of gout has settled.
- Metabolic screening for pseudogout should be undertaken if appropriate.
- Patients with associated chronic pyrophosphate arthropathy should be advised about alteration of adverse mechanical factors, reduction in obesity, appropriate exercise, and use of symptomatic agents.

Key references

1. Star VL, Hockberg MC: Prevention and management of gout. *Drugs* 1993, **45**:212–222.
2. Tan N, Lertratanakul W, Barr WG: Acute gouty arthritis: modern approaches to an ancient disease. *Postgrad Med* 1993, **94**:73–75;78;83–84.

Diagnosis

Symptoms

• Onset is usually insidious.

Dizziness and syncope.

Weakness, fatigue, weight loss: common.

Nausea, diarrhea: in ~50% of patients.

Increase in normal skin pigmentation: may appear well tanned (without tan lines).

Mental changes (especially depression).

Acute back pain: rare finding; limited to some patients with bilateral adrenal hemorrhage.

Signs

Postural hypotension: typically unresponsive to i.v. fluids.

Hypotension: usually systolic blood pressure <110 mm Hg.

Generalized pigmentation: common; extensor and exposed skin should be checked.

Buccal pigmentation: usually manifest with generalized pigmentation.

Scar pigmentation: only scars inflicted after onset of Addison's disease.

Signs of organ-specific autoimmune disease: *e.g.*, vitiligo, thyroid disease.

Hyponatremia: inability to excrete water due to raised antidiuretic hormone concentration and glucocorticoid effect on renal tubule (common).

Hyperkalemia: usually mild (normal in 40% of patients).

Family history of autoimmune endocrine diseases.

Hypercalcemia: in 10% of patients.

Hypoglycemia: sometimes seen in children or undernourished patients.

Investigations

Serum cortisol measurement: ideally should be done at 8 a.m. but valid results can also be obtained under stressful conditions. Values <7 µg/dL are most often associated with adrenal insufficiency. 7–18 µg/dL is indeterminate, and values >18 µg/dL are unlikely to represent Addison's disease. (Note: cortisol levels in the afternoon and evening are normally <7 in healthy individuals.)

Plasma corticotropic hormone (ACTH) measurement: concentration usually >80 ng/L in primary adrenal failure; low values for both cortisol and ACTH suggest pituitary disease (sample must be collected in the appropriate tube, put on ice, centrifuged, and frozen immediately).

Electrolytes.

Cosyntropin stimulation test: cosyntropin, 250 µg i.v.; cortisol measured at 0, 30, and 60 minutes (normal result: any value >20 µg/dL); the same test using 1 µg of cosyntropin may be more sensitive [1].

Blood count and film: eosinophilia, macrocytosis with coexistent vitamin B_{12} deficiency, normocytic anemia after volume replacement.

Chest radiography: to check for tuberculosis.

Insulin hypoglycemia test: can be used to differentiate primary from secondary adrenal failure. Potentially dangerous, and usually unnecessary. Under control conditions, 0.15 U/kg insulin is injected and serum glucose is monitored until <40 mg/dL. Samples for cortisol and ACTH measurement are drawn at baseline, during, and 30 and 60 minutes after hypoglycemia.

Complications

Death: if diagnosis missed, if patient not given extra steroids in stress situations, or if replacement steroids not taken; hydrocortisone *must* be given before thyroxine when hypothyroidism and Addison's disease coexist (Schmidt's syndrome) to prevent exacerbation of adrenal insufficiency by thyroid hormone.

Associated autoimmune endocrine failure: vitamin B_{12} deficiency, hypothyroidism, hypoparathyroidism.

Differential diagnosis

Secondary (pituitary) adrenal insufficiency: low ACTH and cortisol response to insulin-induced hypoglycemia.

Other causes of pigmentation: *e.g.*, hemochromotosis, ectopic ACTH.

Etiology

Autoimmune adrenalitis.

Tuberculosis (infrequently seen): whole-gland involvement, calcification on radiography or CT.

• Rare causes include the following, with 80%–90% of both adrenals affected:

Adrenal hemorrhage: usually in anticoagulated or septicemia patients.

Drugs: *e.g.*, ketoconazole, suramin.

HIV-related adrenalitis.

Metastases.

Sarcoidosis.

Hemochromatosis.

Adrenoleukodystrophy.

Amyloidosis.

Congenital adrenal hyperplasia.

Epidemiology

• The incidence of Addison's disease is estimated to be 40–60 in one million.

• The female:male ratio is 2:1.

Treatment

Diet and lifestyle

• Patients should always carry appropriate identification (*e.g.*, wallet card, bracelet, or necklace) and have access to an "emergency pack" (hydrocortisone, 100-mg ampule, with saline solution, needle, and 2-mL syringe).

• Patients and partners should be taught how to give an i.m. injection in case the patient is unable to take oral steroids.

• Patients should be educated about the need for extra hydrocortisone in case of illness or physical stress.

Pharmacological treatment

For acutely ill or hypotensive patients

• If the diagnosis is suspected, prompt diagnostic and therapeutic steps should be taken.

• In previously undiagnosed disease, blood should be drawn for cortisol, ACTH, and thyroid function tests.

Hydrocortisone, 100 mg i.v. bolus.

0.9% saline 1-L bolus initially in 1 hour followed by 0.9% saline infusion.

Glucose i.v. bolus to correct hypoglycemia.

• Inotropic agents are usually unnecessary and are rarely effective [2].

Continued treatment

Acute treatment	Hydrocortisone, 100 mg i.m. every 8 hours until clinical improvement; patients in intensive care units or on anti-coagulants can be treated by 100 mg in 50 mL saline solution at 2 mg/h i.v. infusion.
Contraindications	None.
Special points	When conscious and taking fluids orally, most patients can be converted to oral hydrocortisone; typical replacement dose is 20 mg every morning and 5 mg at bedtime. Prednisolone and dexamethasone sometimes used instead. Patients receiving large doses of hydrocortisone do not usually require mineralocorticoid replacement. Patients on standard oral replacements with hydrocortisone may need fludrocortisone for mineralocorticoid replacement (50–100 mg every day).
Main drug interactions	None.
Main side effects	Short-term treatment at these doses rarely has side effects, but glucose intolerance may occur.

Key references

1. Oelkers W, Diederich S, Bahr V: Diagnosis and therapy surveillance in Addison's disease: rapid adrenocorticotrophin (ACTH) test and measurement of plasma ACTH, renin activity, and aldosterone. *J Clin Endocrinol Metab* 1992, **75**:259–264.

2. Werbel SS, Ober, KP: Acute adrenal insufficiency. *Endocrinol Metab Clin North Am* 1993, **22**:303–328.

Diagnosis [1]

Symptoms

Dyspnea: variable severity, developing abruptly or gradual onset some days after initial insult.

Signs

Respiratory distress: labored breathing, intercostal retractions.

Tachypnea: rapid and shallow.

Warmth and peripheral vasodilatation.

Signs of pulmonary edema: on auscultation.

Other signs of underlying disease.

• Cyanosis may or may not be apparent.

Investigations

Chest radiography: for bilateral pulmonary infiltrates; to confirm pulmonary edema in presence of predisposing condition.

Pulmonary artery catheterization: to measure pulmonary capillary wedge pressure (normally <18 mm Hg) to exclude cardiogenic edema.

Arterial blood gas analysis: refractory hypoxemia unresponsive to increased inspired oxygen concentration (partial arterial oxygen pressure <70 mm Hg breathing 40% oxygen, arterial–alveolar oxygen tension ratio <0.25); low total respiratory compliance (<30 mL/cm H_2O).

Fiberoptic bronchoscopy and lavage or biopsy, upper respiratory tract cultures, CT and nuclear imaging, specialized blood tests (*e.g.*, plasma amylase): to establish underlying condition and assess presence of multisystem organ failure.

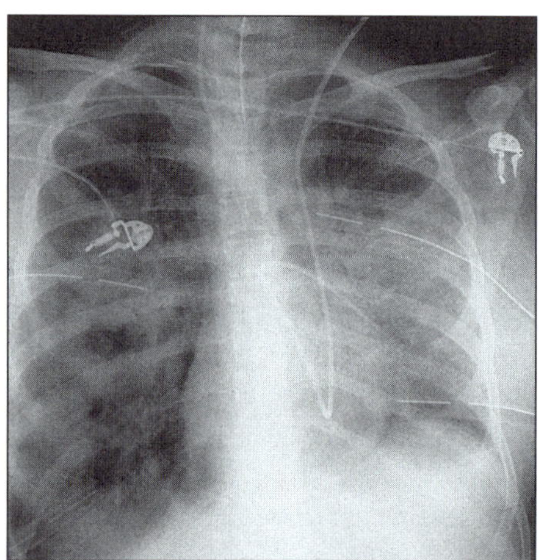

Typical chest radiograph appearance of established adult respiratory distress syndrome, showing pneumothoraces, position of endotracheal tube, intercostal chest drains, and pulmonary artery flotation catheter.

Complications [2]

Death.

Multisystem organ failure: especially renal failure.

Sepsis.

Shock.

Barotrauma: from mechanical ventilation (*e.g.*, pneumothorax).

Debilitation after intensive care: survivors usually recover fully within 12 months [3].

Differential diagnosis

• The diagnostic criteria exclude other diagnoses.

Etiology [4]

• The etiology follows severe systemic and pulmonary insults including:

Shock.

Sepsis.

Bacterial, viral, or drug-induced pneumonia.

Burns.

Aspiration of gastric contents.

Inhalation of toxic fumes.

Trauma.

Oxygen toxicity.

Disseminated intravascular coagulation.

Massive hemorrhage or multiple transfusion.

Pre-eclampsia.

Embolism: thrombotic, fat, or amniotic fluid.

Acute pancreatitis.

Head injury.

Various drugs and i.v. drug abuse.

Epidemiology

• Adult respiratory distress syndrome has an incidence of ~1.5 cases per 100 000 persons in the United States, although cases of acute lung injury not meeting the diagnostic criteria occur much more often.

• The prevalence varies according to the predisposing illness (2%–25%).

Pathophysiology

• Adult respiratory distress syndrome causes damage to capillary endothelial cells and alveolar epithelial cells resulting from the activation of many humoral and cellular events.

• It is uniformly characterized by increased permeability of the alveolar–capillary membrane, leading to pulmonary edema.

• Deranged cellular use of oxygen occurs as part of the syndrome and may result in widespread multiorgan failure of variable severity.

Treatment

Diet and lifestyle

• Patients need nutritional support by parenteral or enteral route while on the ventilator.

Pharmacological treatment [5–7]

• Underlying conditions should be fully investigated and steps taken to correct any reversible disorders.

• Nosocomial infection and sepsis should be managed aggressively.

• Vasopressor, inotropic, and chronotropic agents should be used to support circulation and urine output.

• Enteral nutrition should be given when possible.

Nonpharmacological treatment [5–7]

• The involvement of multiple organ systems in the disease process means that supportive measures are not confined to the respiratory system.

• All patients with severe lung injury and established adult respiratory distress syndrome should be managed in the intensive care unit.

• Full respiratory and invasive hemodynamic monitoring and urinary catheterization are often needed.

Respiratory support

• Endotracheal intubation and mechanical ventilation is almost always necessary; it should be instituted early in the course.

• The aim is to maintain oxygen saturation at ~90% using continuous positive airways pressure applied via a face mask or mechanical ventilation.

• New techniques (*e.g.*, pressure-controlled or inverse-ratio ventilation) are aimed at recruiting collapsed alveoli while reducing peak airway pressures (and therefore the risk of barotrauma) and raising mean airway pressures (thereby improving oxygenation).

• Oxygenation may be be improved by turning patients (supine/prone).

Cardiac and circulatory support

• The aim is to maximize oxygen delivery to tissues.

• Hemoglobin should be maintained at or above 10–12 g/dL, with a hematocrit >30%.

• Cardiac output and oxygen delivery may need to be optimized by the judicious manipulation of filling pressures and the use of inotropic drugs. The routine use of a pulmonary artery catheter however is discouraged.

Fluid balance

• The aim of manipulating fluid balance is to reduce circulating volume as much as possible in an effort to reduce further extravasation of edema into the alveoli.

• Pulmonary capillary wedge pressure should be maintained at 8–12 mm Hg.

• Diuretics may be needed to maintain urine output >0.5 mL/kg/h and to reduce intravascular volume.

Prevention

• No measures have been documented to prevent adult respiratory distress syndrome.

Key references

1. Bernard GR, *et al.*: The American-European Consensus Conference on ARDS: definitions, mechanisms, relevant outcomes, and clinical trial coordination. *Am J Respir Crit Care Med* 1994, **149**:818–824.

2. Bone RC, *et al.*: Adult respiratory distress syndrome: sequence and importance of multiple organ failure. *Chest* 1992, **101**:320–326.

3. McHugh LG, *et al.*: Recovery of function in survivors of the acute respiratory distress syndrome. *Am J Respir Crit Care Med* 1994, **150**:90–94.

4. Hudson LD, *et al.*: Clinical risks for development of the acute respiratory distress syndrome. *Am J Respir Crit Care Med* 1995, **151**:293–301.

5. Kollef MH, Schuster DP: The acute respiratory distress syndrome. *N Engl J Med* 1995, **332**:27–37.

6. Levy PC, Utell MJ, Sickel JZ, Apostolakos MJ: The acute respiratory distress syndrome: current trends in pathogenesis and management. *Compr Ther* 1995, **21**:438–444.

7. Hudson LD, New therapies for ARDS. *Chest* 1995, **108(suppl)**:79S–91S.

Diagnosis

Definition

• AIDS is defined by progressive immunodeficiency without another cause, manifest by various conditions, including the following:

Opportunistic infections

Viral: cytomegalovirus.

Bacterial: *Mycobacterium avium-intracellulare*, disseminated *M. tuberculosis*, recurrent *Salmonella* spp., pneumococcus.

Fungal: *Candida albicans, Cryptococcus neoformans, Histoplasma capsulatum, Aspergillus* spp.

Protozoan: *Pneumocystis carinii*, cryptosporidia, microsporidia, isospora, *Toxoplasma gondii*.

Unusual tumors

Kaposi's sarcoma.

Non–T-cell lymphoma.

Invasive cervical carcinoma.

Neurological manifestations

AIDS dementia complex.

Vacuolar myelopathy.

Progressive multifocal leukoencephalopathy.

Symptoms

• Skin rashes (persistent and severe herpes simplex or zoster infection) occur during the asymptomatic period of 10 years or more after seroconversion.

Skin rash, temperature, pharyngitis, lymphadenopathy (seroconversion illness): in 50% of patients.

Unexplained diarrhea, fever, dyspnea, focal neurological signs, minor opportunistic infections: particularly oral candidiasis and oral hairy leukoplakia; in "pre-AIDS."

Signs

Skin rash.

Lymphadenopathy.

Oral candidiasis, oral hairy leukoplakia: in pre-AIDS.

Opportunistic infection: in AIDS.

Investigations

• In the asymptomatic phase, the diagnosis can be made only by HIV testing.

HIV test: antibodies to HIV (usually occurring within 3 months of exposure) measured by enzyme-linked immunosorbent assay, confirmed by Western blot analysis.

CD4 lymphocyte count: used to assess immune function; normal value $\sim 800 \times 10^6$/L; patients with $<500 \times 10^6$/L have recurrent bacterial infections; patients with $<200 \times 10^6$/L at risk for developing opportunistic infections. Useful for determining prophylaxis against *P. carinii* and *M. avium*.

Direct measurement of viral load using polymerase chain reaction or B DNA assay: useful for predicting disease progression and monitoring antiviral therapy.

Complications

Not applicable.

Differential diagnosis

Congenital immunodeficiency.

Iatrogenic immunodeficiency: *e.g.*, after bone-marrow transplantation.

HIV-antibody–negative CD4 lymphopenia: rare; different epidemiology from HIV infection.

Etiology

• AIDS is caused by infection by HIV.

• HIV leads to a progressive fall in T-helper (CD4) cells and a failure of T-cell proliferation after antigenic stimulation, even by T cells uninfected by HIV.

Epidemiology

• Geographically, three patterns of disease are seen:

North America and Western Europe

• Transmission is among men having sex with men, among intravenous drug users, heterosexual transmission, and transmission vertically or among recipients of blood products (patients with hemophilia who received blood products between 1975 and 1984).

• In the United States and United Kingdom, transmission among men having sex with men is declining and the number of heterosexual people and intravenous drug users is increasing.

Sub-Saharan Africa

• The disease is predominantly a heterosexual epidemic, with major transmission vertically and through blood products.

Asia

• An explosive increase in numbers is occurring, mainly by heterosexual transmission.

Treatment

Diet and lifestyle

• No special precautions are necessary.

Pharmacological treatment

• Combination antiviral therapy using two nucleoside agents prolongs life. A triple-drug regimen is indicated for patients with AIDS or earlier in infection in those with a significant HIV viral load.

Nucleoside agents

Standard dosage	AZT, 200 mg 3 times daily.
Contraindications	Bone-marrow suppression.
Special points	Use as part of multidrug regimen.
Main drug interactions	Drugs with similar toxic profile.
Main side effects	Bone-marrow suppression, headache, insomnia, occasionally myopathy.

Didanosine (ddl)

Standard dosage	Didanosine, 200 mg twice daily.
Contraindications	Previous pancreatitis, peripheral neuropathy.
Special points	Part of multidrug regimen.
Main drug interactions	Given in alkaline buffer, which may reduce absorption of compounds needing acidification in the stomach.
Main side effects	Pancreatitis, peripheral neuropathy.

Stavudine

Standard dosage	Stavudine, 40 mg twice daily.
Contraindications	Pre-existing peripheral neuropathy.
Special points	Part of multidrug regimen.
Main drug interactions	None known.
Main side effects	Peripheral neuropathy.

Lamivudine (3TC)

Standard dosage	150 mg twice daily.
Contraindications	None.
Special points	Use with AZT or D4T.
Main side effects	Bone-marrow suppression.

Protease inhibitors

Standard dosage	Inbinavir, 800 mg 3 times daily.
	Ritonavir, 600 mg twice daily.
	Saguinavir, 600 mg 3 times daily.
	Nelfinavir, 750 mg 3 times daily.
Contraindications	Terfenedine, multiple drug interactions.
Special points	Use with nucleoside agents.
Main side effects	Nephrolithiasis, gastrointestinal toxicity.

Prognosis

• 60% of patients progress to AIDS within 10 years of seroconversion in the absence of antiviral therapy.

• 5% remain well, with no evidence of immunological deterioration at this time.

• The median survival from AIDS diagnosis is 2 years; this is prolonged in patients receiving antiviral therapy.

Follow-up and management

• Patients should have CD4 counts measured 4 times a year to determine antiviral load.

• Patients with CD4 counts $<200 \times 10^6$/L should receive *P. carinii* pneumonia prophylaxis; those with CD4 counts $<75 \times 10^6$/L should receive *M. avium* complex prophylaxis.

General references

Deeks SG, Smith M, Holodney M, Kahn JO: HIV-1 protease inhibitors: a review for clinicians. *JAMA* 1997, **277**:145–153.

Doran CM: New approaches to using antiretroviral therapy for the management of HIV infection. *Ann Pharmacother* 1997, **31**:228–236.

Emmons W: Accuracy of oral specimen testing for human immunodeficiency virus. *Am J Med* 1997, **102**:15–20.

Lewis JS II, Terieff CM, Coulston DR, Garrison MW: Protease inhibitors: a therapeutic breakthrough for the treatment of patients with human immunodeficiency virus. *Clin Ther* 1997, **19**:187–214.

Sheppard HW, Ascher MS: The natural history and pathogenesis of HIV infection. *Annu Rev Microbiol* 1992, **460**:533–564.

Weissman IL: AIDS: the whole body view. *Curr Biol* 1993, **30**:766–769.

Diagnosis

Symptoms

• Lymphoma B symptoms may be difficult to differentiate from other symptoms of HIV infection and AIDS.

Persistent, unilateral, and enlarging nodes: <50% of patients.

Cough, shortness of breath.

Abdominal pain.

Headaches, focal neurological deficits.

Painful and ulcerated mucosal lesions.

Localized indurated skin nodule.

Weakness, weight loss, night sweats, fever.

Signs

Enlarged discrete rubbery nodes in neck, axillae, or groins.

Hepatosplenomegaly.

Enlarged retroperitoneal adenopathy.

Increased intracranial pressure, papilledema, focal neurological signs.

Mass involving unusual site: *e.g.*, pericardium, testicle, oral mucosa.

Anemia, pyrexia, petechiae.

Investigations

Biopsy: to type lymphoma.

Complete blood count: baseline for treatment.

CT of chest, abdomen, and pelvis.

Lumbar puncture: high incidence of CSF involvement.

MRI, CT, CT-guided biopsy: of solitary brain lesion to detect cerebral lymphoma.

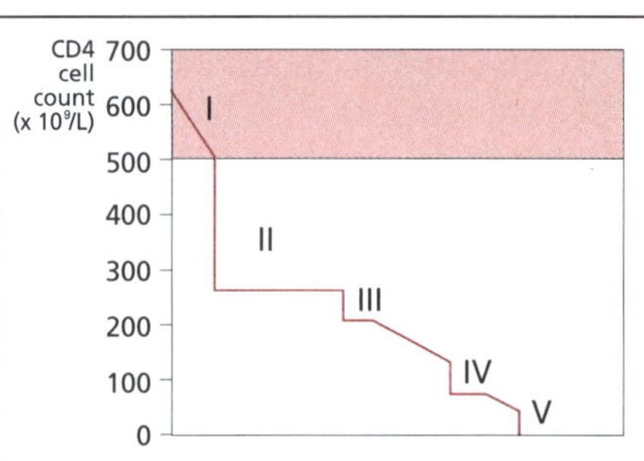

Relationship of CD4 cell count to clinical condition.

Complications

Poor bone-marrow reserve: because of infections or drugs.

Many opportunistic infections.

Treatment

Diet and lifestyle

- No special precautions are necessary.

Pharmacological treatment

- Specialist supervision is needed.

- Discussion of treatment options with the patient is vital.

- Patients with good performance status and high CD4 counts are treated by conventional CHOP chemotherapy (cyclophosphamide, vincristine, adriamycin, prednisolone) or short-course high-dose multiple-agent regimens; traditional non-AIDS regimens may cause worsening of prognosis in poor-risk AIDS patients.

- Patients with poor performance status, low CD4 counts ($<100 \times 10^6$/L), and previous AIDS-defining diagnoses can receive low-dose CHOP or vincristine and bleomycin with steroids.

- CNS prophylaxis with intrathecal methotrexate is important because CNS involvement is frequent.

- All chemotherapy is immunosuppressive, depresses bone-marrow function, and may precipitate infection.

Treatment aims

To avoid overwhelming infection in good-risk patients receiving high-dose chemotherapy. To maintain quality of life.

Other treatments

Radiotherapy

- This is useful in palliative treatment of nodal masses unresponsive to chemotherapy or when chemotherapy is not possible.

External beam radiotherapy for localized extranodal sites: *e.g.*, lymphoma of tonsil. Whole-brain radiotherapy for cerebral lymphoma.

Bone-marrow support

With colony-stimulating factors.

Prognosis

- The median survival is <6 months (worse than for non–HIV-related non-Hodgkin's lymphoma, stage for stage).

- Factors associated with poor prognosis include having AIDS before diagnosis of lymphoma, poor performance status (<70% Karnofsky), having a CD4 count $<100 \times 10^6$/L.

- 50% of patients die of non-Hodgkin's lymphoma, 50% of AIDS-related problems.

- Burkitt's lymphoma responds better to chemotherapy than immunoblastic lymphoma does.

- The median survival for cerebral lymphoma is 4–8 weeks.

Follow-up and management

- Patients should be provided with psychological support and continuing care.

General references

Ioachim HL, *et al.*: Acquired immunodeficiency syndrome associated lymphomas. Clinical, pathologic, immunologic, and viral characteristics of 111 cases. *Hum Pathol* 1991, **22**:659–673.

Sandler AS, Kaplan L: AIDS lymphomas. *Curr Opin Oncol* 1996, **8**:377–385.

Straus DJ: Human immunodeficiency virus–associated lymphomas. *Med Clin North Am* 1997, **81**:495–570.

Diagnosis

Classification

• Alcohol problems may be classified into several types of decreasing severity: dependence, abuse, and hazardous drinking (*see* Figure) [1].

Alcohol dependence: presence of physical tolerance; history of withdrawal symptoms; persistent desire or lack of success in efforts to cut down; reduction in social, occupational, or recreational activities attributable to alcohol; or continued use despite knowledge or experience of undesirable effects.

Alcohol abuse: recurrent alcohol use resulting in a failure to fulfill major role obligations (work, family, school) in potentially hazardous situations (*e.g.*, driving) or resulting in legal difficulties.

Hazardous drinking: drinking pattern that places patient at increased risk but has not yet resulted in problems. Patients who regularly drink three or more drinks daily (one or more drinks daily if elderly), or who drink five or more drinks per occasion (three or more if elderly) should be considered at risk [1].

Symptoms

A "yes" response to one or more questions from the following alcoholism evaluation (CAGE) identifies patients who are likely to be abusing or dependent on alcohol.

CAGE questionnaire

1. Have you ever felt you should *Cut* down on your drinking?
2. Have people *Annoyed* you by criticizing your drinking?
3. Have you ever felt bad or *Guilty* about drinking?
4. Have you ever taken a drink first thing in the morning (*Eye*-opener) to steady your nerves or get rid of a hangover?

• Patients with one or more positive responses should be further evaluated with a detailed alcohol history.

Signs

Unexplained elevation of hepatic transaminase levels or macrocytosis.

• Cardiac, neurological (including cognitive) systems should be evaluated through history and physical examination.

Investigations

• A detailed alcohol history is essential for all new patients and periodically thereafter, and among patients in whom an alcohol problem is suspected; areas to be included are:

Family history of alcohol problems.

Age of onset of drinking.

Amount and frequency of alcohol use.

Changes in role functioning (occupational, social, familial).

Concomitant substance abuse.

Laboratory studies: none are routine. In patients suspected of a chronic moderate or severe alcohol problem, hepatic and renal chemistry tests, complete blood count, and folate and magnesium levels should be obtained.

Complications

Social morbidity: disruption of family relationships and occupational and social functioning.

Trauma, including motor vehicle accidents, physical fights, and drowning.

Physical illness: such as hypertension, acute and chronic liver disease, cardiovascular disease, cancer, and morbidity from withdrawal syndromes.

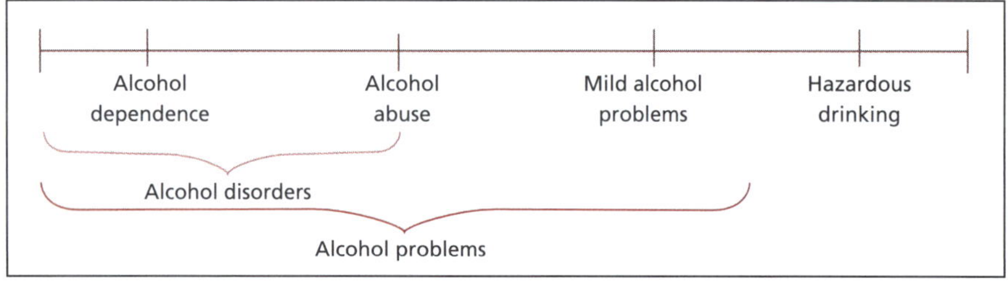

Differential diagnosis

• Complications or consequences of alcohol problems are often mistaken for primary rather than secondary problems (*e.g.*, trauma from motor vehicle accidents), or viewed as outside the purview of primary care physicians and therefore not mentioned by the patient, or not investigated by the practitioner (*e.g.*, job loss, marital difficulties).

• Psychiatric complaints such as depression, insomnia, and anxiety are often clues to underlying alcohol problems.

Etiology

• Risk factors for alcohol problems include:

Male gender.

Heavy drinking in teenage years.

Drinking regularly before age 16 years.

Psychiatric illness.

History of antisocial behavior.

Alcoholic relatives.

Northern European ethnicity.

Some Native American groups.

Epidemiology

Alcohol abuse and dependence

11%–20% of patients in general medicine practice.

20% of emergency room patients.

Hazardous drinking

20% of people who drink.

20% of women in gynecology practices.

Alcohol problems among the elderly [3]

Largely unrecognized problem.

5% of community-dwelling elderly.

20% of medically hospitalized patients.

• Due to polypharmacy, the elderly are at particular risk for adverse drug–alcohol interactions (*e.g.*, benzodiazepines, antidepressants, NSAIDs, oral hypoglycemics).

1989 alcohol-related health care costs among the elderly: $233 million.

Spectrum of problems related to alcohol use.

Treatment

Diet and lifestyle

Alcohol abuse and dependence

• Referral to alcoholism treatment programs or self-help groups (*e.g.*, Alcoholics Anonymous) is a mainstay of therapy; practitioners should identify a colleague (social worker, alcoholism treatment specialist, counselor) who can recommend the most appropriate programs for individual patients based on availability, patient preferences, insurance coverage, and cost.

• Letters, phone calls, and follow-up appointments from primary care practitioners may help motivate patients to remain in treatment.

Hazardous drinking

• Effective, brief, office-based interventions include the following:

Recommending decreasing drinking to moderate levels (rather than complete abstinence), which may improve compliance, for patients who are not abusers or dependent.

Setting specific drinking goals (amount, frequency) mutually with the patient.

Associating physical problems (macrocytosis, transaminase elevation) with alcohol use.

Motivated patients may benefit from programs aimed at developing controlled drinking habits (*e.g.*, DrinkWise, Moderation Management).

Pharmacological treatment

Indicated in chronic alcohol abuse or dependence, usually after acute withdrawal and detoxification, to maintain sobriety; usually reserved for recurrent, severe problem drinkers or for impulsive drinkers who drink on the spur of the moment, then drink to excess.

Disulfiram

Standard dosage	250–500 mg daily for 1–2 weeks, then 250 mg daily, for several months to years; tablets are crushed in water with a water "chaser," at least 12 hours after the last drink.
Contraindications	Heart disease, psychosis, chronic liver disease, pregnancy, inability to comprehend or comply with therapy; use with caution in diabetes, hypothyroidism, seizure disorders, and nephritis.
Special points	Attendance in treatment program or self-help group (*e.g*, Alcoholics Anonymous) is mandatory; monitor liver transaminases after 1–2 weeks of therapy, then every 2–4 weeks thereafter; monitor complete blood count and "SMA-12" chemistries every 6 months. Treatment of disulfiram-ethanol reaction (flushing, headache, dyspnea, nausea, vomiting; cardiovascular collapse in severe cases) is largely symptomatic and supportive.
Main drug interactions	Phenytoin levels increase in patients on disulfiram. Reduce disulfiram dose to 250 mg three times per week and monitor phenytoin levels. Disulfiram increases levels of coumarin anticoagulants and barbiturates.
Main side effects	Severe side effects (other than the disulfiram-ethanol reaction) are rare; most common side effect is somnolence, usually improved after 10–14 days of therapy; other reported side effects include rash and hepatitis.

Naltrexone [4]

Pure opiate antagonist demonstrated in short-term trials to enhance abstinence from alcohol.

Standard dosage	50 mg daily, usually for 12 weeks. First dose after 7–10 days abstinence from opiates; to assure opiate abstinence, naloxone challenge test should be given prior to first dose.
Contraindications	Demonstrated or suspected opiate use; liver disease (transaminases > 4 times normal or elevated bilirubin, acute hepatitis, liver failure).
Special points	Simultaneous participation in treatment program or self-help group is mandatory; monitor liver function tests monthly; can precipitate severe opiate withdrawal.
Main drug interactions	Opiate agonists (including medications for cough and cold, diarrhea, and pain).
Main side effects	Nausea and/or vomiting, headache; hepatotoxic at high doses.

Key references

1. Bradley KA: The primary care practitioner's role in the prevention and management of alcohol problems. *Alcohol Health Res World* 1994, **18**:97–104.

2. Ewing JA: Detecting alcoholism: the CAGE questionnaire. *JAMA* 1984, **252**:1905–1907.

3. Fink A, Hays RD, Moore AA, Beck J: Alcohol-related problems in older persons. *Arch Intern Med* 1996, **156**:1150–1156.

4. O'Brien CP, Volpicelli LA, Volpicelli JR: Naltrexone in the treatment of alcoholism: a clinical review. *Alcohol* 1996, **13**:35–39.

Diagnosis

Symptoms and signs
• Alopecia is a clinical sign and needs to be classified as either scarring or nonscarring before an accurate diagnosis can be made.

Scarring (cicatricial alopecia)
Lichen planopilaris, kerion (fungal), dissecting cellulitis of the scalp, sarcoidosis, trauma (burns, chemical, direct trauma), localized secondary to fetal scalp monitor, aplasia cutis congenita.
Alopecia neoplastica: secondary to metastatic breast carcinoma.
Linear scleroderma, chronic cutaneous lupus (discoid lupus erythematosus).

Nonscarring (noncicatricial alopecia)
Alopecia areata, trichotillomania, telogen effluvium, anagen effluvium, tinea capitis ("ringworm").

Androgenetic alopecia [1]
• Males present with a receding anterior hair line, especially in the parietal regions, which results in an M-shaped recession. A bald spot subsequently may appear on the posterior crown. In contrast, females usually experience a more diffuse pattern of hair loss, which often begins at the part line. In young women with androgenetic alopecia, signs of virilization such as clitoral hypertrophy, acne, and facial hirsutism should be sought to rule out endocrine dysfunction.

Alopecia areata, with deficient melanin in area of regrowth. (*See* Color Plate.)

Alopecia areata [2]
Localized "ring shaped" area of diffuse or complete nonscarring alopecia: hallmarked by short, tapered "exclamation point" hairs.
Pitted or onychodystrophic nails: may be present.
Alopecia totalis (entire scalp) or alopecia universalis (entire body surface): may occur in rare instances.
Gray or depigmented hair: often regrows.

Trichotillomania (traumatic alopecia)
Incomplete nonscarring hair loss: hairs of unequal length in alopecic areas; most patients deny (or are unconscious of) pulling out hairs.

Spared pony tail growth in trichotillomania. (*See* Color Plate.)

Lichen planopilaris
Lichen planus of the scalp: often no lichen planus elsewhere; cicatricial alopecia and follicular erythema within the alopecic areas.

Chronic cutaneous lupus erythematosus
Cicatricial alopecia with follicular prominence and plugging: frequent cutaneous involvement of the external pinnae (especially conchal bowl of the ears); may or may not be associated with systemic disease.

Fungal infection
Kerion.
Tinea capitis.

Investigations
Skin biopsy: diagnostic in cases of alopecia areata in which the clinical presentation is not classic; reveals follicular hemorrhage and empty follicles in trichotillomania.
Scalp biopsy: in lichen planopilaris; diagnostic in chronic cutaneous lupus erythematosus.
Fungal scrapings: often negative in kerion; can be helpful in tinea capitis along with culture.
Hormone studies: in women with hair loss and evidence of increased androgens.

Complications
Severe scarring: in kerions.
Squamous cell carcinomas: in areas of cicatricial alopecia from lupus (rare).

Differential diagnosis

Alopecia areata
Androgenetic alopecia (diffuse in alopecia areata); trichotillomania; alopecia neoplastica.

Androgenetic alopecia
Thyroid disorders, systemic lupus erythematosus, telogen effluvium, seborrheic dermatitis.

Trichotillomania
Tinea capitis; alopecia areata; hair shaft disorders.

Lichen planopilaris
Pseudopelade; sarcoid; folliculitis decalvans.

Chronic cutaneous lupus
Necrobiosis lipoidica diabeticorum; sarcoid.

Kerion
Dissecting cellulitis of the scalp; folliculitis decalvans.

Tinea capitis
Alopecia areata; hair shaft disorders.

Etiology

Alopecia areata
Autoimmune [3,4]; rarely may be associated with thyroid disease, pernicious anemia, or vitiligo.

Androgenetic alopecia
Increased expression of androgen receptors and/or changes in androgen metabolism of the scalp hair follicles. Heredity in males is polygenic or autosomal dominant; autosomal recessive in females.

Trichotillomania
Psychological stresses.

Lichen planopilaris
Unknown.

Chronic cutaneous lupus
Autoimmune.

Epidemiology

Alopecia areata
• 75% of patients present before age 25 years.
• Patients with Down syndrome, positive family history of alopecia areata, or atopy appear to be more prone; no consistent HLA genotypes have been identified.

Androgenetic alopecia
• May begin any time after puberty in males; often fully expressed by the forties. Females are affected later; approximately 40% present in the sixth decade.

Trichotillomania
• Patients are predominantly female.

Chronic cutaneous lupus
• Appears to be more common in black women.

Fungal infections
• *Microsporum* spp. infection is associated with animal contact and usually affects children.
• *Trichophyton tonsurans* is the most common cause of tinea capitis in the United States and usually occurs in school-age children.

Treatment

Diet and lifestyle

• Other than alteration of the underlying behavior of trichotillomania, there does not appear to be any role of diet and lifestyle.

Pharmacological treatment

Alopecia areata

• Alopecia areata usually resolves with no treatment but may be resistant to treatment.

• Potent topical steroids, intralesional steroids, topical irritants or allergens, and topical minoxidil have all been used successfully.

• Systemic steroids or cyclosporine have been effective but are often not used because of side effects.

Standard dosage	Clobetasol propionate, 0.05% cream or ointment applied twice daily. Triamcinolone acetonide, 10 mg/mL intralesionally every 2–4 weeks.
Contraindications	Local infection, atrophy.
Special points	Potent topical steroids: used over a large area can result in systemic absorption.
Main drug interaction	None.
Main side effects	Local steroid atrophy, steroid acne, systemic steroid absorption.

Androgenetic alopecia

• There is no highly effectice therapy to prevent the progression of androgenetic alopecia.

Standard dosage	Topical minoxidil 2% topical solution; apply twice a day for >32 weeks.
Contraindications	None.
Special points	Helpful in reducing rate of hair loss or partially restoring hair in some patients. Frontal-bitemporal recession often fails to respond. Therapy must be continued or hair loss recurs. If response poor or absent, can be mixed 50:50 with 0.01% tretinoin and applied twice daily.
Main drug interaction	None.
Main side effects	None.

Trichotillomania

Psychiatric counseling.

Lichen planopilaris

• Treatment is the same as for alopecia areata except irritants and allogens should be avoided.

Chronic cutaneous lupus

• After the condition is under control, alternative treatment should be substituted, *e.g.*, systemic antimalarial therapy, given by a specialist, and sunscreens and protective wear.

Standard dosage	Intralesional triamcinolone, 10 mg/mL.
Contraindications	None.
Special points	Intralesional triamcinolone is only a local treatment; it does not affect systemic disease.
Main drug interaction	None.
Main side effects	Atrophy, hypopigmentation, systemic absorption.

Treatment aims
To arrest and reverse pathological hair loss.

Other treatments [5]
• Several antiandrogens (spironolactone, cyproterone acetate, flutamide, and cimetidine) have been reported to be useful in the treatment of androgenetic alopecia.
• Finasteride is an oral 5α-reductase type II inhibitor currently undergoing testing. Preliminary results suggest a higher success rate than minoxidil in the treatment of androgenetic alopecia.

Prognosis
Alopecia areata
• 50% of patients will have complete regrowth of localized areas in 1 year; one-third of patients never regrow hair.
• Scarring alopecia usually results even if treated. Poor prognostic indicators as follows: early onset, severe initial involvement, total alopecia for >1 year, nail dystrophy, ophiasis pattern (alopecia around periphery of scalp).
Androgenetic alopecia
Usually gradual progression of hair loss over years to decades.
Trichotillomania
Good with appropriate psychological counseling.
Lichen planopilaris
Poor even with treatment except androgenetic alopecia patients, who can be followed up every 6–12 months or more frequently depending on medication regimen.
Chronic cutaneous lupus
Poor response in this chronic disease requiring long-term follow-up; antinuclear antibody (ANA)-negative patients can develop ANA-positive symptomatic systemic disease.

Follow-up and management
Every month at least in all diseases mentioned except androgenetic alopecia patients, who can be followed up every 6–12 months or more frequently depending on medication regimen.

Key references
1. Fitzpatrick TE: *Color Atlas and Synopsis of Clincial Dermatology*. New York: McGraw-Hill; 1997:22–27.
2. Nielson TA, Reichel M: Alopecia: diagnosis and management. *Am Fam Phys* 1995, **51**:1513–1522; 1527–1528.
3. Tobin DJ, Bystryn JC: Immunity to hair follicles in alopecia areata. *J Invest Dermatol* 1995, **104(suppl 5)**:135–145.
4. McDonagh AJ, Messenger AG: The etiology and pathogenesis of alopecia areata. *J Dermatol Sci* 1994, **7(suppl)**:S125–S135.
5. Sawaya ME: Clinical updates in hair. *Dermatol Clin* 1997, **15**:37–43.

Diagnosis

Symptoms

Burning or tearing perianal pain: while defecating, often accompanied by small amounts of bright red blood on the tissue paper or surface of the stool.

Signs

Linear ulcer: in the distal portion of the anus; most typically located in the posterior midline. Fissures may also occur in the anterior midline, particularly in women. These are best seen by direct visualization of the distal anus after spreading the buttocks. Linear ulcers in the lateral quadrants are atypical for simple fissures, and other diseases such as Crohn's disease, rectal trauma, or sexually transmitted disease should be considered.

A hood of granulation tissue (*i.e.*, a sentinel tag): often seen at the distal margin of fissures, outside the anus; should prompt closer examination for a linear ulcer.

A hypertrophied anal papilla: often palpable as a large grain of rice on digital examination just proximal to the ulcer.

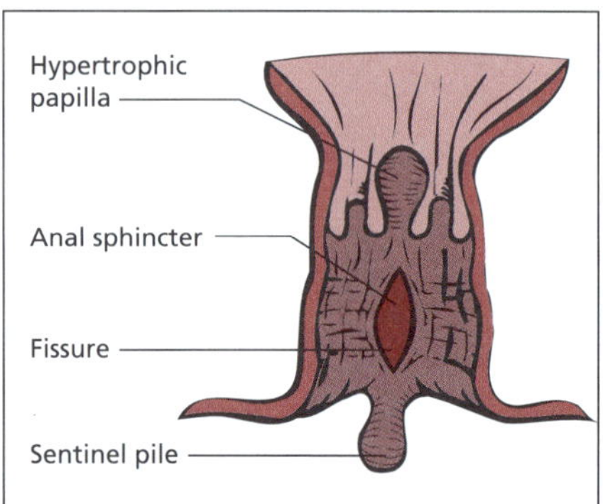

The classic chronic anal fissure triad includes the hypertrophic anal papilla, anal fissure, and sentinel skin tag. The fissure margins may appear fibrotic and slightly undermined, and exposed internal sphincter muscle fibers may be visible.

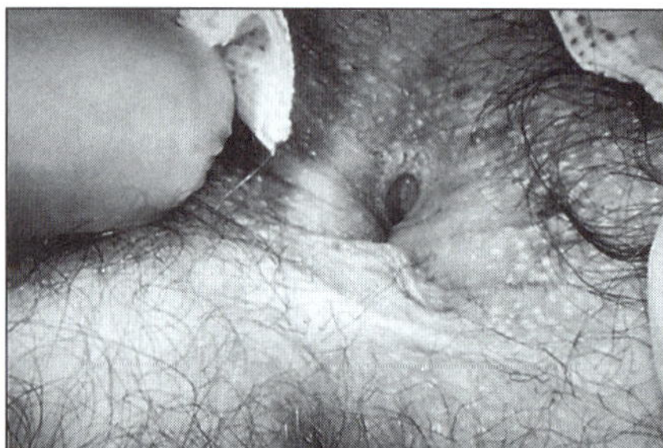

Typical fissure in ano located in the posterior midline. (*See* Color Plate.)

Investigations

Direct inspection: best method to see anal fissure.

Anoscopy: often painful and may traumatize the area of ulceration.

• Atypical or nonhealing ulcers should be carefully examined for associated disease such as inflammatory bowel disease, malignancy, or infection; sigmoidoscopy with careful visualization of the proximal mucosa and biopsy of the ulcer should be considered in these situations.

Complications

Chronic ulcer.

Constipation.

Persistent bleeding.

Differential diagnosis

Inflammatory bowel disease (Crohn's disease more than ulcerative colitis).

Hidradenitis suppurativa.

Carcinoma.

Syphilis.

Tuberculosis.

Hemorrhoid.

Perianal abscess.

Anal trauma.

Etiology

• Higher resting anal sphincter pressure with an abnormally brisk contraction following defecation is found in patients prone to anal fissures; the fissure is often initiated by passage of a large, hard stool and then perpetuated by the increased tone and contraction reflex following defecation.

Epidemiology

Common, particularly in young and middle-aged adults.

• Fissures occur equally in women and men.

Treatment

Diet and lifestyle

- Patients should be placed on a high-fiber diet to achieve soft stools.
- Patients should take sitz baths twice daily to promote healing.

Pharmacological treatment

• Stool softening agents (*e.g.*, synthetic mucilloids or psyllium preparations) should be titrated at a dose that will minimize straining and achieve 1–2 soft bowel movements each day. A typical starting dose consists of one heaping tablespoon (*e.g.*, Metamucil) in 8 oz of water once or twice each day with advancement in the dose frequency every 3–4 days until the desired effect is realized. The patient should be instructed to drink the preparation immediately after mixing and informed that a few days of increased flatus or bloating is commonly experienced at the start of therapy.

• Topical emollients with local anesthetics (*e.g.*, benzocaine, witch hazel) may be used to provide symptom relief; patients should be instructed to apply these preparations locally twice daily as needed for symptom control.

Treatment aims

To reduce pain and bleeding.

Other treatment options

• Chronic fissures that are refractory to the approaches previously mentioned often require a surgical procedure to reduce the internal sphincter tone; this is best achieved by a lateral subcutaneous internal anal sphincterotomy, which is typically performed as a outpatient procedure; manual dilation is an alternative approach.

Prognosis

• Anal fissures often require 4–6 weeks of medical therapy before complete healing is achieved; surgery, when required, has a cure rate in excess of 90%.

Follow-up and management

• The accurate diagnosis of a benign anal fissure is ultimately confirmed by the response to treatment; patients should be seen in clinic until the problem is resolved and to monitor for other possible diagnoses (*see* Differential diagnosis).

General reference

Barnett JL, Raper SE: Anorectal disease. In *Textbook of Gastroenterology*, edn 2. Edited by Yamada T. Philadelphia: JB Lippincott; 1995:2036–2037.

Diagnosis

Symptoms

• Symptoms and signs are due to and relate to the severity of the peripheral blood pancytopenia.

Fatigue, shortness of breath on exertion, headache, palpitation: symptoms of anemia.

Easy bruising and petechiae, gum bleeding, buccal hemorrhage, visual disturbance due to retinal hemorrhage: symptoms of thrombocytopenia.

Mouth and tongue ulcers: symptoms of infection due to leukopenia.

History of jaundice: may indicate posthepatitic aplasia or associated paroxysmal nocturnal hemoglobulinuria.

Signs

• Bleeding manifestations are usually more common than infection.

Pallor.

Ecchymoses, petechiae of skin and mouth, retinal hemorrhage.

Fever.

Mouth and tongue ulceration.

Pharyngitis, pneumonia.

Skin and perianal sepsis.

Skeletal, skin, and nail anomalies; short stature: may occur in congenital aplastic anemia.

• Spleen, liver, and lymph nodes are not enlarged.

Investigations

Complete blood count and examination of blood film: show pancytopenia (isolated cytopenias may occur in early stages), macrocytosis, toxic granulation of neutrophils.

Reticulocyte count: shows absolute reticulocytopenia.

Bone-marrow aspiration and biopsy: shows hypocellular bone marrow, no abnormal infiltration, no increase in reticulin, colony-forming cells low or absent; cytogenetic studies to exclude preleukemia; in Fanconi's anemia, cultured peripheral blood lymphocytes show increased chromosomal breaks with DNA cross-linking agent (*e.g.*, diepoxybutane).

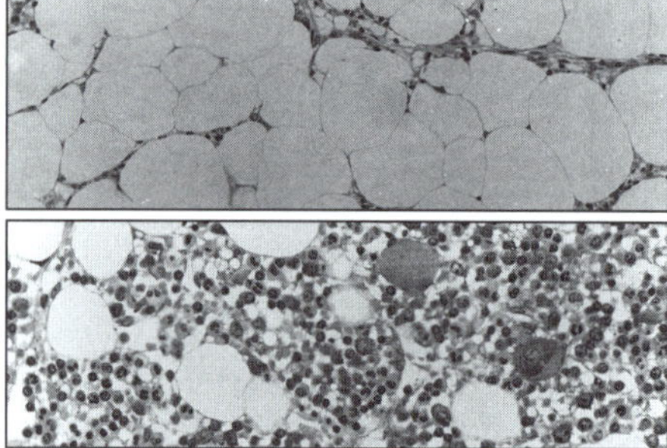

Aplastic anemia bone marrow (*top*), normal bone marrow (*bottom*).

Ham's test and urine hemosiderin analysis: classically negative in aplastic anemia and positive in paroxysmal nocturnal hemoglobulinuria (PNH), but a small proportion of PNH cells can be detected in up to 30% of patients with aplastic anemia.

Liver function tests and viral studies: to detect antecedent hepatitis; test for hepatitis A, B, and non-A, non-B (hepatitis C); Epstein–Barr virus; cytomegalovirus; and parvovirus B19 (parvovirus classically causes pure erythrocyte aplasia and can also cause pancytopenia associated with hemophagocytosis).

Chest and sinus radiography.

Hand and forearm radiography: may be abnormal in congenital aplastic anemia.

Abdominal ultrasonography: to exclude splenomegaly; anatomically displaced or abnormal kidneys in Fanconi's anemia.

Complications

Failure of random donor platelet transfusions to increase recipient's platelet count, increased bone-marrow graft rejection potential: due to sensitization to non-HLA antigens from multiple blood transfusions.

Late clonal evolution to myelodysplastic syndrome or acute myeloid leukemia in 10% of patients with aplastic anemia or paroxysmal nocturnal hemoglobulinuria in 10% of untransplanted patients.

Differential diagnosis

Hypoplastic myelodysplastic syndrome or hypoplastic acute myeloid leukemia in adults.

Hypoplastic acute lymphoblastic leukemia in children.

Hairy cell leukemia.

Other bone-marrow infiltration: *e.g.*, lymphoma, carcinoma, myelofibrosis.

Anorexia nervosa.

Severe infection: *e.g.*, tuberculosis, overwhelming gram-negative or gram-positive sepsis.

Systemic lupus erythematosus.

Etiology

Congenital causes

E.g., Fanconi's anemia, dyskeratosis congenita.

Acquired causes

Idiopathic: in 75% of patients.

Drugs: *e.g.*, NSAIDs, gold, chloramphenicol, sulfonamides.

Chemicals: benzene, organic solvents, aniline dyes.

Viruses: hepatitis A, B, or non-A, non-B (hepatitis C), and other as yet unidentified viruses; Epstein–Barr virus.

Paroxysmal nocturnal hemoglobinuria: 25% of patients later develop aplastic anemia.

Rare causes

SLE, pregnancy.

Epidemiology

• The annual incidence in the United States is 2–8 per million.

• The male:female ratio is equal.

• Two peaks are seen in the age incidence for men: 15–25 years and >60 years; one peak for women: >60 years.

Treatment

Diet and lifestyle

• If neutrophils are <0.5×10^9/L, food should be well cooked and fresh fruit washed before consumption.

Pharmacological treatment [1]

• Drugs are indicated for patients ineligible for bone-marrow transplantation.

• High-dose corticosteroids should be avoided because of toxicity (infection, hypertension, diabetes, avascular necrosis of bone) and lack of convincing benefit in aplastic anemia.

• Drugs that affect platelet function (aspirin, NSAIDs) or that may cause aplastic anemia must be avoided.

Antilymphocyte globulin (ALG) or antithymocyte globulin (ATG)

• Horse ATG should be used initially.

Standard dosage	ATG, 10–20 mg/kg daily for 8–14 consecutive days followed by alternate day therapy for another 14 days, or 40 mg/kg/day for 4 days equally effective.
Contraindications	Hypersensitivity or severe systemic reaction to test dose, active infection, hemolytic paroxysmal nocturnal hemoglobinuria, SLE.
Special points	Central line infusion to prevent thrombophlebitis; platelet transfusion before each dose; low-dose prednisone to prevent serum sickness.
Main drug interactions	None.
Main side effects	Anaphylaxis or allergic reactions (during infusion); serum sickness (7–14 days after starting treatment).

Cyclosporine

• Cyclosporine can be used after ALG, in combination with ALG, or as a single agent.

Standard dosage	Cyclosporine, 12 mg/kg/day orally for 3–6 months.
Contraindications	Renal or liver impairment, breast-feeding.
Special points	Drug blood concentration, blood pressure, renal and liver function must be monitored regularly.
Main drug interactions	Erythromycin, ketoconazole, aminoglycosides, vancomycin, amphotericin B, rifampin, phenytoin.
Main side effects	Nephrotoxicity, nausea, tremor, hypertension, hypertrichosis, gum hypertrophy, hepatotoxicity.

Oxymetholone

• Oxymetholone is now used after ALG and cyclosporine rather than as a single agent.

Standard dosage	Oxymetholone, 2.5 mg/kg orally daily (0.5–1 mg/kg daily for Fanconi's anemia).
Contraindications	Liver impairment, breast and prostate cancer, pregnancy; caution in children (behavioral problems) and elderly men (prostatic hypertrophy).
Special points	Serum cholesterol concentration must be monitored.
Main drug interactions	Other potentially hepatotoxic drugs, *e.g.*, erythromycin, rifampin, ketoconazole, cyclosporine.
Main side effects	Reversible cholestatic jaundice, liver tumors, and peliosis hepatitis with long-term use, virilization in females, acne.

Key references

1. Young NS, Barrett AJ: The treatment of severe acquired aplastic anemia. *Blood* 1995, **85**: 3367–3377.

2. Soutar RL, King DJ: Bone marrow transplantation. *BMJ* 1995, **310**:31–36.

3. Tsai TW, Freytes CO: Allogenic bone marrow transplantation for leukemias and aplastic anemia. *Adv Intern Med* 1997, **42**:423–451.

4. Marsh JCW, *et al.*: Haemopoietic growth factors in aplastic anemia: a cautionary note. *Lancet* 1994, **344**:172–173.

Diagnosis

Symptoms

• Many patients have no symptoms; the disease is suspected on routine blood count.

Dyspnea on exertion, tiredness, headache.

Painful tongue.

Paraesthesias in feet, difficulty walking: vitamin B_{12} deficiency only.

Infertility.

Signs

Pallor of mucous membranes: if hemoglobin concentration <9 g/dL.

Mild jaundice.

"Beefy red" glossitis.

Signs of vitamin B_{12} neuropathy: if present.

Investigations [1,2]

General

Blood count: raised mean cell volume (>100 fL), reduced erythrocyte count, hemoglobin, and hematocrit, low reticulocyte count, reduced leukocyte and platelet counts (in severely anemic patients).

Blood film: shows oval macrocytes, hypersegmented neutrophils (>5 nuclear lobes).

Bone-marrow analysis: in severely anemic patients the bone marrow is hypercellular with increased proportion of early cells, many dying cells, megaloblastic erythroblasts, giant and abnormally shaped metamyelocytes, and hypersegmented megakaryocytes.

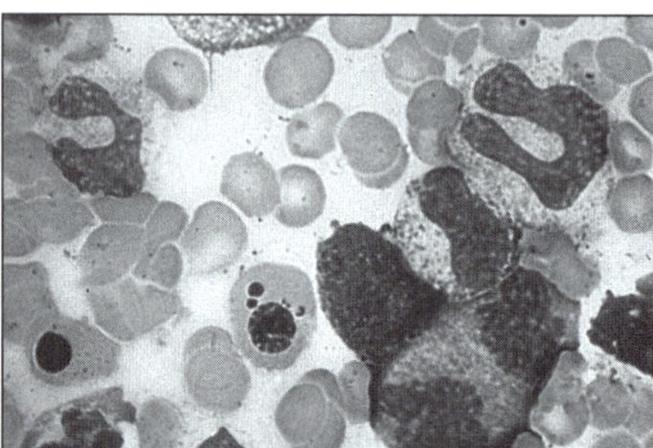

Bone marrow with megaloblastic anemia. (*See* Color Plate.)

Serum indirect bilirubin and lactic dehydrogenase measurement: concentrations raised.

Direct Coombs test: complement only, positive in some patients.

Tests for disseminated intravascular coagulation or intravascular hemolysis: positive in some patients.

Tests for vitamin B_{12} (B_{12}) or folate deficiency: serum B_{12} low in B_{12} deficiency, normal or slightly low in folate deficiency; serum folate normal or raised in B_{12} deficiency, low in folate deficiency; erythrocyte folate normal or low in B_{12} deficiency, low in folate deficiency.

Deoxyuridine suppression, serum homocysteine and methylmalonic acid measurement: additional tests performed in some laboratories for B_{12} or folate deficiency [3].

Special

Diet history: to exclude veganism, low folate intake.

Schilling test: for B_{12} absorption.

Serum analysis: for intrinsic factor and parietal cell antibodies.

Fiberoptic endoscopy: for gastric biopsy, exclusion of gastric polyps, carcinoma in pernicious anemia.

Contrast radiography: to detect gastric atrophy, neoplasm (pernicious anemia), or small intestinal lesions.

Endoscopy and jejunal biopsy: if gluten-induced enteropathy is suspected in patients with folate deficiency.

Complications

Neuropathy: due to B_{12} deficiency.

Neural tube defects in fetus: risk reduced by folate treatment.

Carcinoma of stomach: in pernicious anemia.

Treatment

Diet and lifestyle

• The quality of the diet must be increased in patients with dietary folate deficiency.

Pharmacological treatment [1,2]

For vitamin B_{12} deficiency

Standard dosage	Hydroxocobalamin, 1 mg i.m. 6 times in 2–3 weeks, then 1 mg every 3 months or 100–200 µg i.m. monthly.
Contraindications	Rare hypersensitivity.
Special points	No evidence suggests that more frequent doses are needed for B_{12} neuropathy.
Main drug interactions	None.
Main side effects	Gout and significant hypokalemia a few days after commencing treatment.

For folate deficiency

Standard dosage	Folic acid, 5 mg orally daily for 4 months, then 5 mg daily or weekly as needed.
Contraindications	B_{12} deficiency, malignancy (unless deficiency is clinically important).
Special points	B_{12} deficiency must be excluded because B_{12} neuropathy could be precipitated or aggravated.
Main drug interactions	None.
Main side effects	None.

• Folic acid should be used as prophylaxis in pregnancy (300–400 µg daily; 5 mg daily if previous neural defect in fetus), and also in renal dialysis.

• In women of childbearing age, folate intake should be increased to at least 400 µg daily by diet or folate supplement.

• For premature babies (birth weight <1500 g), folic acid, 1 mg daily, is indicated.

Treatment aims

To correct anemia by replenishing body stores of vitamin.

To correct underlying disease.

To restore normal neurological status (vitamin B_{12} deficiency).

Other treatments

• Packed erythrocyte transfusion should be used only if essential: removal of equivalent volume of plasma in patients with congestive heart failure.

Prognosis

• Prognosis depends mainly on the underlying cause.

• Life expectancy is reduced slightly in patients with pernicious anemia because of the risk of carcinoma of the stomach.

Follow-up and management

• Patients with pernicious anemia should have annual clinical review and blood count.

• Routine endoscopy is not recommended.

• Patients having total gastrectomy or ileal resection need prophylactic hydroxocobalamin, 1 mg every 3 months, from the time of surgery for life.

Key references

1. Anthony AC: Megaloblastic anaemias. In *Hematology. Basic Principles and Practice*. Edited by Hoffman R, *et al.* New York: Churchill Livingstone; 1991:392–422.

2. Savage DG, Lindenbaum J: Folate–cobalamin interactions. In *Folate in Health & Disease*. Edited by Baily L. New York: Marcel Dekker; 1994:237–285.

3. Hoffbrand AV, Jackson BFA: The deoxyuridine suppression test and cobalamin–folate interrelations. *Br J Haematol* 1993, **85**:232–237.

Diagnosis

Definition

Malabsorption of vitamin B_{12} (cobalamin) due to lack of normal intrinsic factor production by the stomach.

Symptoms

• Symptoms often not apparent (vitamin B_{12} deficiency or atrophic gastritis may be an incidental finding).

• When present, symptoms are usually due to anemia or complications of vitamin B_{12} deficiency.

Shortness of breath, lethargy.

Sore tongue: glossitis in 50% of patients.

Parasthesias: due to peripheral neuropathy; classic "stocking-glove" distribution.

Gait disturbance: due to myelopathy (subacute combined degeneration of spinal cord).

Depression, impaired memory.

Loss of taste.

Signs

Mucosal pallor: reflecting anemia.

Glossitis.

Mild splenomegaly.

Signs of other organ-specific autoimmune disease: *e.g.*, hypothyroidism.

Peripheral sensory neuropathy with absent reflexes.

Pyramidal or long-tract neurological signs; loss of joint position sense.

Investigations

Hematology: for macrocytic anemia (mean corpuscular volume >100 fL), leukopenia or thrombocytopenia, hypersegmented neutrophils on blood film.

Bone-marrow analysis: megaloblastic changes with maturation arrest.

Liver function test: increased bilirubin due to ineffective erythropoiesis.

Serum vitamin B_{12} measurement: to detect low concentrations (normal, >160 ng/L).

Schilling test: abnormal part I test using ^{58}Co-labeled vitamin B_{12} (<10% urinary excretion); part II corrects to normal after administration of intrinsic factor.

Serum gastrin measurement: raised concentration in pernicious anemia (normal <100 pmol/L).

Gastric analysis: shows achlorhydria.

Endoscopy and biopsy: for atrophic gastritis on endoscopy and histological assessment of stage of gastritis.

Complications

Gastric carcinoid and enterochromaffin cell hyperplasia: associated with reflex rise in serum gastrin due to reduced gastric acid; 2%-9% prevalence of gastric carcinoid in patients with pernicious anemia [1].

Gastric carcinoma: 1%-7% increased risk in patients with pernicious anemia [2].

Peripheral sensory neuropathy, subacute combined degeneration of spinal cord: affects pyramidal tracts, causing spastic paraparesis and bladder involvement, and dorsal columns, causing sensory ataxia and impaired joint position sense.

High-output cardiac failure, myocardial ischemia: in severe anemia.

Dementia.

Differential diagnosis

Type B chronic gastritis related to *Helicobacter pylori* infection.

Other causes of vitamin B_{12} deficiency: *e.g.*, dietary deficiency in vegans, terminal ileitis (Crohn's disease), terminal ileal resection, blind loop syndromes, small bowel diverticula or bacterial overgrowth, postgastrectomy states, pelvic irradiation.

Etiology

• Pernicious anemia is an organ-specific autoimmune disease, with a strong association with other organ-specific autoimmune diseases, especially thyroid disease.

Epidemiology

• Pernicious anemia occurs more often in female patients than in male.

• Pernicious anemia is common in all races and countries.

Immunology

• Antigastric parietal-cell antibodies (probably involved in pathogenesis) occur in 70%–90% of patients, anti-intrinsic factor antibodies in 50%–70%.

• Antibodies have been shown to be directed against membrane-bound hydrogen/potassium ATPase pump, resulting in blockade of hydrochloric acid secretion and correlating with concentrations of gastric parietal-cell antibodies.

Treatment

Diet and lifestyle

• No special precautions are necessary for uncomplicated disease except for avoidance of extreme isometric exercise.

Pharmacological treatment

Standard dosage Hydroxocobalamin, 1 mg i.m. 6 times in 2–3 weeks, then 1 mg every 3 months.

Contraindications None.

Special points Can cause initial hypokalemia and folate deficiency in patients with marked vitamin B_{12} deficiency; chloride and folic acid supplements are advisable.

Main drug interactions None.

Main side effects None.

Treatment aims

To prevent neurological complications.
To correct anemia.

Prognosis

• Despite the small risk of gastric carcinoid or carcinoma, life expectancy is little altered in patients with uncomplicated disease [1,2].

• Gastric carcinoids have a good prognosis, with no reported cases of carcinoid syndrome in these patients and a low reported incidence of local or regional spread.

Follow-up and management

• The cost of endoscopic surveillance has been shown to outweigh the benefit of screening for the few patients who are found to have unsuspected malignancy; it should probably be reserved for patients who develop symptoms.

• Regular vitamin B_{12} supplementation in outpatients must be ensured.

Key references

1. Born K, *et al.*: Gastric endocrine cell hyperplasia and carcinoid tumors in pernicious anemia. *Gastroenterology* 1985, **88**:638–648.

2. Lechago J, Correa P: Prolonged achlorhydria and gastric neoplasia: is there a causal relationship? *Gastroenterology* 1993, **104**:1554–1557.

Diagnosis

Symptoms

Seizures.

Headache: dull frontal or sudden and severe thunderclap headaches.

Visual field deficits.

Diplopia.

Hemiparesis.

Cognitive dysfunction.

Lethargy or coma (*see* Intracranial hemorrhage).

Signs

Third nerve compression with pupillary dilatation and ptosis (internal carotid artery or posterior communicating artery aneurysm).

Fourth cranial nerve palsy (anterior communicating artery compression).

Cavernous sinus syndrome with ophthalmoparesis and facial numbness.

Reduced visual acuity or visual field deficits.

Hemiparesis.

Bruit.

Dysphasia.

Investigations

CT: can identify large arteriovenous malformations (AVMs), especially when calcified.

MRI and MR angiography: can identify large (≥1.5 cm) aneurysms easily and is very useful for AVMs, but four-vessel cerebral angiography is most definitive diagnostically and helpful therapeutically.

• Make sure to evaluate for second aneurysm, present in 20%–30% of cases.

Lumbar puncture: for evaluation for subarachnoid hemorrhage if headache is present.

Complications

Intracerebral hemorrhage.

Progressive seizures, weakness, or neural compression.

Differential diagnosis

Cerebral neoplasm, especially vascular meningiomas.

Cerebral abscess.

CNS sarcoidosis.

Venous angioma or cavernous hemangioma.

Etiology

• Most AVMs are congenital.

• Aneurysms may be defects in the media of vessels at bifurcations or posttraumatic.

• Aneurysms can also be mycotic (subacute bacterial endocarditis), fungal, or neoplastic.

Epidemiology

• 7%–20% of patients with subarachnoid hemorrhage due to aneurysm rupture have a first-degree relative with an aneurysm.

• 20%–30% of patients with one aneurysm have multiple aneurysms.

• Rebleed rate is 3.5% per year for untreated aneurysms.

• Aneurysms found in association with polycystic kidney disease, Ehlers-Danlos syndrome, Marfan syndrome, and neurofibromatosis type 1.

• AVM incidence is one-seventh that of aneurysms.

Treatment

Diet and lifestyle

- Limit sports or activities that can cause head trauma.
- Pregnancy increases the likelihood of rupture.

Pharmacological treatment

Anticonvulsant agents for seizures as required.

Control hypertension aggressively.

Treatment aims

To prevent cerebral hemorrhage.
To treat sinuses.

Other treatments

Embolization, radiosurgery, and resection of accessible AVMs.

Clipping and/or endovascular thrombosis of aneurysms (endovascular coil thrombosis especially effective in lesions with small necks).

Prognosis

Aneurysm rebleed rate 3.5% per year.

AVM morbidity/mortality 3%–4% per year.

- Posterior fossa AVMs have a particularly poor prognosis.
- Larger AVMs may be less likely to rupture.
- CNS steal syndromes may lead to ischemic deficits.

Follow-up and management

Follow-up seizures and neurological examination every 6–12 months and refer to neurosurgery for definitive management.

General references

Gobin YP, Laurent A, Merienne L, *et al*.: Treatment of brain arteriovenous malformations by embolization and radiosurgery. *J Neurosurg* 1996, **85**:19–28.

Scheinevink WI: Intracranial aneurysms. *N Engl J Med* 1997, **336**:28–40.

Sinson G, Phillips MF, Flamm ES: Intraoperative endovascular surgery for cerebral aneurysms. *J Neurosurg* 1996, **84**:63–70.

Diagnosis

Symptoms

Chest discomfort: brought on by physical exertion or emotions, *e.g.*, anger, excitement; repeatable in onset, rapid resolution with rest, worse in cold weather and after meals; heavy, constricting, crushing, not sharp, often described as unpleasant rather than painful; may radiate down inner aspects of arms or into neck or jaw, rarely radiates into epigastrium or back. May cause effort dyspnea only, particularly in the elderly.

Signs

• Typically no signs are manifest, but patients should be examined for evidence of the following:

Hyperlipidemia.

Hypertension.

Left ventricular outflow obstruction: *i.e.*, aortic stenosis, hypertrophic cardiomyopathy.

Diabetes.

Previous myocardial damage.

Investigations

Complete blood count: anemia aggravates angina.

Resting ECG: to detect left ventricular hypertrophy or past myocardial infarction.

Chest radiography: to check heart size and pulmonary vasculature.

Exercise stress test: to precipitate symptoms, to document workload at onset, and to record any associated ECG abnormality (planar ST segment depression or arrhythmia).

Thallium myocardial perfusion imaging: mainly used when conventional exercise stress test cannot be done or when ECG cannot be interpreted (*e.g.*, left bundle branch block); thallium administered during exercise or pharmacological stress test delineates an area of myocardial hypoperfusion; re-imaging after rest shows redistribution unless infarction has occurred. Alternative is exercise-stress or pharmacological-stress echocardiography. Ischemia manifest as wall motion abnormality such as hypokinesis, akinesis, or dyskinesis in region that is normal or mildly hypokinetic at rest.

Coronary angiography: gold standard; provides detailed anatomical information about site and severity of luminal narrowing but does not show atherosclerosis itself or functional importance of anatomical occlusive disease; prerequisite for consideration of angioplasty or surgery.

Complications

Unstable angina.

Acute myocardial infarction.

Arrhythmias.

Death.

Differential diagnosis

Cardiac
Pericarditis.
Myocardial infarction.
Aortic dissection.

Noncardiac
Esophageal spasm.
Reflux esophagitis.
Peptic ulceration.
Musculoskeletal pain.
Cervical spondylosis.
Da Costa's syndrome.

Etiology

Causes
Coronary atherosclerosis in 99% of patients.
Aortic stenosis.
Hypertrophic cardiomyopathy.
Arteritis.

Risk factors
Family history.
Smoking.
Diabetes.
Hypertension.
Hyperlipidemia.
Obesity.
Post menopause

Epidemiology

• Coronary atherosclerosis is endemic in industrialized countries, but the incidence is decreasing.

• In the United States, >500 000 myocardial infarctions are reported per year.

• No accurate figures are available for the prevalence of angina pectoris, but, in people aged >30 years, it is >2.6%.

Treatment

Diet and lifestyle

• Exercise should be encouraged, obesity corrected, and cigarette smoking stopped.

• Diet low in fat and cholesterol is critical.

Pharmacological treatment

• All patients should be screened for hyperlipidemia and treated as appropriate, including dietary and drug treatment as indicated.

• For patients with LDL cholesterol levels exceeding 100–130 mg/dL, therapy with an HMG-CoA reductase inhibitor is indicated [1].

• Hypertension and diabetes should be managed aggressively.

• An individual patient may, at different stages, need medical treatment, percutaneous transluminal coronary angioplasty, and coronary artery bypass grafting.

Nitrates

• For patients with mild symptoms, short-acting sublingual nitrates may be sufficient (including prophylactic use).

• With long-acting oral nitrates, tolerance is common, so a nitrate-free period should be provided.

Standard dosage	Sublingual or oral nitrates or nitrate patches, dose depends on agent.
Contraindications	Hypotension.
Special points	Glyceryl trinitrate tablets have a limited shelf life.
Main drug interactions	Reduced effect of sublingual preparations with drugs causing dry mouth (*e.g.*, disopyramide, tricyclic antidepressants, atropine); hypotension with other vasodilators; reduced heparin effect with glyceryl trinitrate.
Main side effects	Headache, postural hypotension.

Beta-blockers

• Beta-blockers are the mainstay of regular antianginal treatment.

Standard dosage	Depends on agent.
Contraindications	Atrioventricular conduction defects, heart failure, asthma; caution in diabetes (masks symptoms of hypoglycemia), peripheral vascular disease.
Special points	May be usefully combined with short- and long-acting nitrates and calcium antagonists.
Main drug interactions	Increased risk of hypotension, bradycardia, and atrioventricular block with many agents.
Main side effects	Lethargy, impotence, bronchospasm, cold extremities.

Calcium antagonists

• Calcium antagonists are useful in patients in whom beta-blockers are contraindicated or who cannot tolerate beta-blockers; in such cases, a calcium antagonist with negative chronotropic action should be prescribed (*e.g.*, diltiazem, verapamil).

• If used in the setting of an impaired ventricle, a calcium antagonist without negative inotropic activity should be prescribed (*e.g.*, amlodipine).

Standard dosage	Depends on agent. Once-a-day preparations preferred.
Contraindications	Depend on chronotropic and inotropic effect.
Main drug interactions	Increased hypotensive effect with many agents; increased risk of atrioventricular block when negatively chronotropic agents combined with many agents (*e.g.*, beta-blockers); increased effect of some antiepileptics (*e.g.*, phenytoin, carbamazepine).
Main side effects	Headache, edema, flushing.

Antiplatelet agents

• Aspirin has a controversial role in primary prevention, but all patients with obstructive arterial disease benefit from long-term medium doses, so aspirin should be omitted only if strongly contraindicated [2].

Treatment aims

To control symptoms and restore normal exercise tolerance.

To prevent disease progression (myocardial infarction and death).

To improve prognosis.

Other treatments

Percutaneous transluminal coronary angioplasty (with or without coronary stent) Complementary to drug treatment and surgery; no improvement in survival.

• Best results are achieved in discrete single-vessel coronary artery disease.

• The restenosis rate is ~30% at 6 months; for balloon angioplasty with stenting, restenosis rate is lower, ~20% [3].

Coronary artery bypass grafting

• This has prognostic value in patients with left main-stem coronary stenosis or three-vessel coronary artery disease and impaired left ventricular function.

• The risk of surgery is related to the degree of impairment of left ventricular function.

Prognosis

• 14% of patients with newly diagnosed angina pectoris progress to unstable angina, myocardial infarction, or death within 1 year.

• Mortality at coronary artery bypass grafting with normal ventricular function is 1%.

Follow-up and management

• Atherosclerosis is a progressive disease with no cure, so follow-up is important.

• Risk factor modification is essential.

Key references

1. Scandanavian Simvastatin Survival Study Group: Randomised trial of cholesterol lowering in 4444 patients with coronary heart disease (4s). *Lancet* 1994, **344**:383–389.

2. Antiplatelet Trialists' Collaboration: Collaborative overview of randomised trials of antiplatelet therapy. I: Prevention of death, myocardial infarction, and stroke by prolonged antiplatelet therapy in various categories of patients. *BMJ* 1994, **308**:81–106.

3. Sirnes PA, *et al.*: Stenting in chronic coronary occlusion: a randomized, controlled trial of adding stent implantation after successful angioplasty. *J Am Coll Cardiol* 1996, **28**:1444–1451.

Diagnosis

Symptoms

Angina occurring at rest or on trivial provocation.

Signs

• During pain, autonomic manifestations may occur, *e.g.*, the following:

Sweating.

Pallor.

Tachycardia.

Investigations

Complete blood count: anemia aggravates angina; leukocytosis suggests infarction.

Cardiac enzyme measurement: to exclude infarction, creatine kinase MB preferable.

Cardiac troponin measurement: elevation of troponin I or T in unstable angina identifies patients with higher risk of infarction.

ECG: at rest and during pain to document phasic change, typically ST segment depression.

Chest radiography: to assess heart size and pulmonary vasculature.

Echocardiography: to assess ventricular function and to exclude differential diagnosis, *e.g.*, aortic stenosis, aortic regurgitation, hypertrophic cardiomyopathy with obstruction.

Coronary angiography: if pain does not settle with bed rest, to assess for further treatment (coronary artery bypass grafting or percutaneous transluminal coronary angiography); usually identifies "culprit" lesion [1].

Complications

Myocardial infarction.

Ventricular tachycardia, ventricular fibrillation.

Differential diagnosis

Cardiac
Myocardial infarction.
Aortic dissection.
Pericarditis.
Acute myocarditis.

Noncardiac
Pulmonary embolism.

Etiology

• Unstable angina is caused by rupture of a lipid-laden, macrophage-rich, atherosclerotic plaque; rupture occurs when circumferential tension exceeds the tensile strength of the fibrous cap [2].

• Exposure of blood to the ruptured plaque leads to activation of platelets and coagulation system, with consequent thrombosis and coronary artery spasm; in the setting of unstable angina, vessel occlusion is either transient or incomplete.

Epidemiology

• 14% of patients with newly diagnosed stable angina progress to unstable angina, myocardial infarction, or death within 1 year.

Treatment

Diet and lifestyle
• Patients should be hospitalized, with strict bed rest, possibly with sedation.

Pharmacological treatment
• Patients should be admitted to a high-dependency or coronary care unit and have continuous ECG monitoring.

Antiplatelet agents
Standard dosage	Aspirin, 300 mg initially, 75 mg daily maintenance. Ticlopidine, 250 mg twice daily.
Contraindications	*Aspirin:* hypersensitivity.
Special points	*Aspirin:* dipyridamole should be used if patient is allergic to aspirin.
Main drug interactions	*Aspirin:* warfarin.
Main side effects	*Aspirin:* gastric erosion. *Ticlopidine:* agranulocytosis in small fraction of patients.

Anticoagulants
Standard dosage	Heparin i.v. continuous infusion, dose adjusted according to activated partial thromboplastin time.
Contraindications	Gastrointestinal bleeding, recent major surgery, hemorrhagic stroke.
Main drug interactions	Reduced effect with glyceryl trinitrate.
Main side effects	Bleeding, rarely thrombocytopenia.

Nitrates
• Nitrates are used to reduce coronary artery spasm at the site of plaque rupture and enhance collateral blood flow.

Standard dosage	Nitroglycerine or isosorbide i.v. infusion, starting at 20–30 µg/min, adjusted according to symptoms.
Contraindications	Severe symptomatic hypotension.
Special points	Patients may develop drug tolerance.
Main drug interactions	Reduced heparin effect.
Main side effects	Hypotension, headache.

Beta-blockers
Standard dosage	Depends on agent.
Contraindications	Atrioventricular conduction defects, heart failure, asthma; caution in diabetes (masks symptoms of hypoglycemia), peripheral vascular disease.
Special points	May be usefully combined with short- and long-acting nitrates.
Main drug interactions	Increased risk of hypotension, bradycardia, and atrioventricular block with many agents.
Main side effects	Lethargy, impotence, bronchospasm, cold extremities.

HMG-CoA reductase inhibitors
• In patients with established coronary artery disease and elevated LDL cholesterol, statins reduce the incidence of myocardial infarction, coronary death, and need for revascularization by 25%–40% [3].

Calcium antagonists
• Calcium antagonists are useful in patients in whom beta-blockers are contraindicated or who cannot tolerate beta-blockers; in such cases, a calcium antagonist with negative chronotropic action should be prescribed (*e.g.*, diltiazem).

• If used in the setting of an impaired ventricle, a calcium antagonist without negative inotropic activity should be prescribed (*e.g.*, amlodipine).

Standard dosage	Depends on agent. Once-a-day agents preferred.
Contraindications	Depend on chronotropic and inotropic effect.
Main drug interactions	Increased hypotensive effect with many agents; increased risk of atrioventricular block when negatively chronotropic agents combined with many agents (*e.g.*, beta-blockers); increased effect of some antiepileptics (*e.g.*, phenytoin, carbamazepine).
Main side effects	Headache, edema, flushing; may increase mortality in ischemic syndrome complicated by congestive heart failure.

Other treatments
• Unstable angina is a medical emergency: patients whose symptoms do not resolve rapidly on full medical treatment should be transferred to a cardiothoracic center for coronary angiography with a view to revascularization.

• The choice between percutaneous transluminal coronary angiography and coronary artery bypass surgery depends on the anatomical substrate of the unstable plaque and the presence or absence of additional disease. Both procedures carry an increased risk if performed in the setting of unstable symptoms. In patients with level 2 or 3 vessel disease and diabetes, bypass surgery is preferred [4].

Prognosis
• In hospital, the mortality is 1%; nonfatal myocardial infarction is 8%.

Follow-up and management
• After the ruptured plaque has healed, the patient's symptoms depend on the degree of fixed luminal obstruction; the patient should be investigated and managed as for angina pectoris [5].

Key references

1. McMurray J, Rankin A: Treatment of myocardial infarction, unstable angina and angina pectoris. *BMJ* 1994, **309**:1343–1350.

2. MacIsaac IA, Thomas JD, Topol EJ: Toward the quiescent coronary plaque. *J Am Coll Cardiol* 1993, **22**:1228–1241.

3. Scandanavian Simvastatin Survival Study Group: Randomised trial of cholesterol lowering in 4444 patients with coronary artery disease (4s). *Lancet* 1994, **344**:383–389.

4. The Writing Group for the Bypass Angioplasty Revascularization Investigation (BARI) Investigators: Five-year clinical and functional outcome comparing bypass surgery and angioplasty in patients with multivessel coronary disease. *JAMA* 1997, **277**:715–721.

5. Braunwald E, *et al.*: Unstable angina: diagnosis and management. In *Clinical Practice Guideline*, Number 10. Rockville, MD: US Dept of Health and Human Services; 1994. [Agency for Health Care Policy and Research Publication 94–0602.]

Diagnosis

Symptoms

• Symptoms usually begin during the third decade, although some patients present in their teens and a few in their 30s [1].

• Onset is insidious, not associated with trauma.

Back pain and stiffness: worse in morning, improving with exercise, deteriorating with rest.

Peripheral joint symptoms: in 40%; affecting particularly shoulders, hips, knees.

Fatigue.

Uveitis and other stigmata of the spondylarthropathies: *e.g.*, related to psoriatic spondylitis, reactive arthropathy, enteropathic arthritis.

Signs

• Signs may be nonexistent or minimal.

Decreased mobility of lumbar spine, reduced chest expansion, poor mobility of cervical spine.

Decreased mobility of hips and shoulders, knee synovitis, Achilles tendinitis, dactylitis, psoriasis, psoriatic nail change.

Evidence of uveitis: during active attack.

Increasing "stoop": with disease progression.

Anemia of chronic disease: particularly in patients with peripheral joint involvement.

Investigations

Radiography of pelvis: reveals sacroiliitis (sacroiliac change may be minimal, moderate, or severe), juxta-articular sclerosis and erosions, lumbar spine changes, calcification, cervical spine involvement.

ESR, plasma viscosity, CRP measurement: raised values in 50% of patients, but laboratory changes may be absent even in severely ill patients.

Complications

Hip deterioration: ~20% of patients who develop the disease in their teens or early 20s need one or two new hips within 15 years of disease onset.

Knee involvement: occasionally results in need for total knee replacement.

Deteriorating vision: resulting from persistent uveitis.

Spinal fracture: can occur as a result of osteoporotic changes associated with spinal fusion; resulting spinal-cord injury can be catastrophic.

Cauda equina syndrome: rare.

Pulmonary apical fibrosis: may be worse in smokers.

Differential diagnosis

Reactive arthropathy (Reiter's syndrome) [2], psoriatic arthropathy, inflammatory bowel disease.

Nonspecific back pain (much more common): radiography differentiates the two.

Other causes of peripheral joint disease with coincidental back pain [3].

Etiology [1]

• Ankylosing spondylitis is the result of interplay between HLA B27 and other genes and environmental triggers.

• Environmental triggers probably include agents recognized in other forms of reactive arthropathy (*e.g.*, *Chlamydia* spp.; ureaplasma; *Campylobacter*, *Shigella*, *Yersinia*, and *Salmonella* spp.; and other gram-negative organisms) [2].

Epidemiology

• Ankylosing spondylitis occurs in 0.5% of the population in communities where HLA B27 is prevalent (northern Europe, United States, Asia, Central America).

• The male:female ratio is 2.5:1 overall, 3:1 in teenagers, and 1.5:1 with onset in the late 20s.

Treatment

Diet and lifestyle

• Exercise is of paramount importance [4].

• Attention to posture throughout the day and night is essential.

• Hydrotherapy and physical therapy are needed as an initial introduction to a lifelong exercise program.

• Patients and family members must understand the concept of treatment, and literature should be available describing the precise exercise program needed.

• Patients should avoid smoking.

Pharmacological treatment

• NSAIDs are needed by 80% of patients [4].

Standard dosage	Indomethacin, 75 mg slow release once or twice daily; dose and frequency titrated against patient's needs.
Contraindications	Active peptic ulcer disease, indomethacin intolerance (alternative NSAID should be tried); caution in elderly patients, those on anticoagulants, and those with past history of gastrointestinal bleed or perforation.
Main drug interactions	Warfarin and other anticoagulants.
Main side effects	CNS disturbance, gastrointestinal problems.

• Sulfasalazine may be useful in patients with peripheral joint involvement but may have little effect on spinal disease [4–6].

Treatment aims

To allow a good night's sleep.

To decrease morning stiffness (pharmacological treatment).

To enable patient to follow the important exercise program.

To maintain good function and posture.

Prognosis

• Outcome is determined by genetic and environmental factors.

• Although the disease does not burn out, most patients can follow a normal social, family, and professional life.

• Up to 10% of patients have relentless progression, with deteriorating posture and spinal fusion, perhaps requiring surgery.

• Patients with early age of onset and lower educational or social status may be at most risk of severe disease.

Follow-up and management

• After the patient has become stable, visits every 6–12 months to the rheumatologist suffice.

• For patients with severe disease, specialist inpatient management may be appropriate.

Patient support

Spondylitis Association of America
PO Box 5872
Sherman Oaks, CA 91413

Key references

1. Gran JT, Husby G: The epidemiology of ankylosing spondylitis. *Semin Arthritis Rheum* 1993, **22**:319–334.

2. Hughes RA, Keat AC: Reiter's syndrome and reactive arthritis: a current view. *Semin Arthritis Rheum* 1994, **24**:190–210.

3. Leirisalo-Repo M: Enteropathic arthritis, Whipple's disease juvenile spondyloarthropathy and uveitis. *Curr Opin Rheumatol* 1994, **6**:385–390.

4. Creemers MC, *et al.*: Treatment of seronegative spondyloarthropathies. *Semin Arthritis Rheum* 1994, **24**:71–81.

5. Dougados M, *et al.*: Sulfasalazine in the treatment of spondyloarthropathy. A randomized multi-center double-blind placebo controlled study. *Arthritis Rheum* 1995, **38**:618–627.

6. Cuellar ML, Espinoza LR: Management of spondyloarthropathies. *Curr Opin Rheumatol* 1996, **8**:288–295.

Diagnosis

Symptoms

Severe back or chest pain: tearing quality; sudden onset; back pain associated with dissection of descending thoracic aorta [1].

Neck or jaw pain: may indicate involvement of aortic arch.

Nausea, vomiting, sweating.

Syncope.

Dyspnea: resulting from pulmonary edema.

Paraplegia.

Abdominal pain.

Signs

General
Hypertension.
Mild pyrexia.

Proximal dissection
Loss of upper limb pulses or differential limb blood pressure.
Aortic regurgitation.
Cardiac tamponade.
Neurological deficit.
Hypotension: often associated with cardiac tamponade.

Distal dissection
Lower limb ischemia.
Hypertension.
Oliguria or anuria.

• The distinction between proximal and distal dissection should not be based solely on clinical criteria.

Investigations

ECG: to detect acute myocardial infarction and hypertensive changes.

Chest radiography: for widening of mediastinum, pleural effusion, pericardial effusion.

Echocardiography: to detect flap in ascending aorta, presence of aortic regurgitation, and pericardial effusion.

Transesophageal echocardiography: to detect true and false channel, presence and extent of intimal flap in thoracic aorta, relationship to coronary ostia, pericardial effusion, presence of aortic regurgitation.
Advantages: rapid diagnosis; can be performed in intensive care unit.
Disadvantages: needs sedation; may precipitate hypertensive reaction; proximal aortic arch not well visualized [2-4].

CT or MRI: to detect presence and extent of intimal flap, true and false channel, pericardial effusion, extension of dissection to abdominal aorta [2-4].
Advantages: visualization of entire aorta; identification of visceral jeopardy; noninvasive.
Disadvantages: time-consuming; unsuitable for unstable patients who must be moved from intensive care.

Contrast angiography: largely superseded by above investigations, although some centers still prefer coronary angiography before surgical intervention.

Complications

Death.
Aortic rupture.
Stroke.
Paraplegia.
Ischemic bowel.
Renal infarction.
Limb ischemia.
Acute myocardial infarction.

Differential diagnosis

Acute myocardial infarction.

Acute myocardial ischemia.

Acute aortic regurgitation.

Thoracic aortic aneurysm.

Musculoskeletal chest pain.

Pulmonary embolism.

Pericarditis.

Etiology

• The underlying disease process is cystic medial necrosis of the aorta.

• Related processes include the following:

Hypertension (in most patients).

Marfan syndrome.

Atheroma.

Pregnancy.

Epidemiology

• The annual incidence of acute aortic dissection is ~5–10 in one million population.

• 80%–90% of patients are aged >60 years.

Classification

DeBakey classification

Type I: tear in ascending aorta, with dissection extending into arch and descending aorta.
Type II: tear and dissection localized to ascending aorta.
Type III: originates in descending aorta, usually propagating distally for a variable distance.

Stanford classification

Type A: includes all proximal dissections and distal dissections that extend proximally to involve the arch and ascending aorta.
Type B: all other distal dissections without proximal extension.

Acute versus chronic

Acute: symptom onset within 2 weeks.

Chronic: symptom onset longer than 2 weeks.

Treatment

Diet and lifestyle

• After surgical repair, patients are generally advised to avoid circumstances that cause an acute rise in blood pressure, *e.g.*, lifting or carrying heavy objects or weights.

Pharmacological treatment

• Treatment for patients with acute type A dissections is primarily surgical.

• Pharmacological treatment is usually reserved for patients with type B dissections.

• All patients require chronic medical therapy to control hypertension, particularly beta-blocking drugs.

Emergency treatment

• In addition to bed rest and arterial blood pressure monitoring, patients should be treated by oral beta-blockade to reduce the rate of blood pressure rise and sodium nitroprusside to maintain systolic blood pressure at 100–120 mm Hg.

Subsequent treatment

• Long-term management of hypertension is necessary, with medication (oral beta-blockade, calcium antagonism, angiotensin-converting enzyme inhibition) to reduce blood pressure and the rate of rise of blood pressure; systolic blood pressure of 130–140 mm Hg or less is the aim. *See* Hypertension *for details.*

Nonpharmacological treatment

Indications for surgery

Type A dissection.

Type B dissection: limb ischemia, renal compromise, aortic rupture, extension of dissection to proximal aorta.

Types of surgery

Excision of intimal tear.

Obliteration of proximal false lumen.

Resuturing of aorta, possibly with interposition graft.

Resuspension of aortic valve in patients with aortic regurgitation secondary to proximal extent of dissection.

Aortic valve replacement.

Composite aortic graft (with attached mechanical aortic valve replacement) and reimplantation of coronary arteries; operation of choice in patients with Marfan syndrome.

Interposition aortic graft to descending aorta (vital organ perfusion may arise from false lumen, which may need to be left open at its proximal or distal end).

Complications of surgery

Death.

Bleeding.

Infection.

Renal failure.

Spinal-cord ischemia with paraplegia.

Progressive aortic regurgitation.

Aneurysm formation.

Redissection.

Acute myocardial infarction.

Treatment aims

To provide analgesia and sedation.

To stabilize dissection flap.

To treat underlying condition, usually systemic hypertension.

Prognosis

• Prognostic data from patients with untreated aortic dissection are sparse.

• In patients with type A dissection, mortality is ~60% after nonsurgical treatment (inpatient: 1 month) and 15%–30% after surgical treatment.

• In patients with type B dissection, 1-month mortality is <10% after non-surgical treatment.

Follow-up and management

• Follow-up should be under the supervision of a cardiologist.

• Regular MRI, spriral CT, or transesophageal echocardiography is advised to screen for aneurysm formation. These tests are usually performed twice yearly to identify aneurysm of the dissected false channel and/or to detect new aneurysm formation in previously unaffected aortic segments.

Key references

1. Guilmet D, *et al.*: Aortic dissection: anatomic types and surgical approaches. *J Cardiovasc Surg (Torino)* 1993, **34**:23–32.

2. Nienaber CA, *et al.*: The diagnosis of thoracic aortic dissection by noninvasive imaging procedures. *N Engl J Med* 1993, **328**:1–9.

3. Cigarroa JE, *et al.*: Diagnostic imaging in the evaluation of suspected aortic dissection. *N Engl J Med* 1993, **328**:35–43.

4. Sommer T, *et al.*: Aortic dissection: a comparative study of diagnosis with spiral CT, multiplanar transesophageal echocardiography, and MR imaging. *Radiology* 1996, **199**:347–352.

Diagnosis

Symptoms

• Many patients are asymptomatic.

Dyspnea and fatigue: due to left ventricular impairment and low cardiac output initially on exertion.

Symptoms of left ventricular failure: later.

Angina: less common than in aortic stenosis; usually indicates coronary artery disease.

Signs

Pulse

Large volume, rapid fall with low diastolic pressure: "collapsing."

Head nodding in time with pulse: Musset's sign.

Visible pulsation in neck: Corrigan's sign.

Capillary pulsation in fingernails: Quincke's sign.

A booming sound heard over femorals: "pistol-shot femorals."

Systolic and diastolic murmur: produced by compression of femorals by stethoscope; Duroziez's sign.

Heart

• Heart sounds are usually normal.

Forceful, displaced, "heaving" apex: may be seen and felt.

Ejection click: in early systole with bicuspid valve.

Third heart sound: in early diastole with left ventricular failure.

High-frequency early diastolic murmur: maximal at left sternal edge in expiration.

Ejection systolic murmur: resulting from increased flow across valve.

Low-frequency mid-diastolic murmur (Austin Flint): at apex, similar to murmur of mitral stenosis but without preceding opening snap.

Pulmonary hypertension, loud pulmonary component of second heart sound: in advanced cases.

Investigations

Chest radiography: usually normal in mild aortic regurgitation; possibly valvular calcification; cardiomegaly almost always in severe aortic regurgitation; possibly pulmonary venous congestion after left ventricular failure.

ECG: signs of left ventricular hypertrophy and strain (increased QRS amplitude and ST/T wave changes in precordial leads) and left atrial hypertrophy (wide P wave in lead II and biphasic P in lead V_1).

Echocardiography: for left ventricular size and function; valve may appear normal; fluttering on anterior leaflet of mitral valve and early closure of mitral valve in diastole indicate important aortic regurgitation; may also give useful information on state of aortic root. Transesophageal echo will help delineate pathologic lesion (*e.g.*, aortic dissection) and may be used to help plan valve replacement or repair.

Doppler ultrasonography: best method of detecting aortic regurgitation.

Cardiac catheterization: essential when coronary artery disease suspected (*e.g.*, in patients >40 years) and when severity of aortic regurgitation doubted; injection of contrast into aortic root gives information on degree of regurgitation and state of aortic root (presence of dilatation, dissection, root abscesses).

MRI or spiral CT: for assessment of aortic root.

Complications

Cardiac failure: most important cause of disability and death.

Infective endocarditis: should be considered in patients with unexplained illness; may lead to sudden and catastrophic aortic regurgitation.

Arrhythmias: ventricular tachycardia, usually indicating left ventricular failure.

Differential diagnosis

Pulmonary regurgitation: usually accompanying signs of pulmonary hypertension; echo-Doppler examination should resolve the issue.

Patent ductus arteriosus: continuous murmur heard well to the left of sternum; again, echo-Doppler is definitive investigation.

Etiology

Rheumatic disorder in 30% of patients: *e.g.*, coexistent mitral valve disease.

Aortic root dilatation in 20%: *e.g.*, aortic dissection (frequently leads to aortic regurgitation, an indication for urgent surgery) or degeneration of aortic media (frequently idiopathic but may underlie more generalized conditions, *e.g.*, Marfan syndrome, Ehler–Danlos syndrome, osteogenesis imperfecta).

Inflammations in 10%: *e.g.*, rheumatoid arthritis, syphilis, ankylosing spondylitis, Reiter's syndrome.

Bicuspid valve in 15%: usually causes stenosis, can become regurgitant (bicuspid valves present in 1% of population).

Infective endocarditis in 20%: may occur on a bicuspid valve, leading to rupture of a valve cusp.

Epidemiology

• Aortic regurgitation is one of the most common valve lesions.

Treatment

Diet and lifestyle

• Competitive sports should be discouraged.

Pharmacological treatment

Antibiotic prophylaxis

• Prophylaxis is needed against infective endocarditis in asymptomatic patients with known aortic regurgitation; it is particularly important before dental procedures. *See* Endocarditis *for specific details.*

Vasodilatation [1,2]

• Surgery is the main treatment, but angiotensin-converting enzyme (ACE) inhibitors have a role in reducing systemic vascular resistance and decreasing aortic regurgitation. For patients unable to take ACE inhibitors, nifedipine, a calcium channel blocker, is a reasonable alternative [1].

Standard dosage	Captopril, 6.25-mg test dose, then 25–50 mg three times daily.
Contraindications	Hypotension, severe left ventricular impairment, renal failure; extreme caution with coexistent aortic stenosis.
Main drug interactions	Increased hypotensive effect with beta-blockers, diuretics, calcium antagonists.
Main side effects	Hypotension, renal failure.

Nonpharmacological treatment

• Surgery is the main form of treatment for aortic regurgitation [3].

• Aortic valve with or without root replacement is indicated for onset of symptoms, increased heart size, and change in ECG, all of which indicate onset of left ventricular dysfunction. By echocardiography, end-systolic left ventricular diameter >55 mm may be used to determine operative timing in patients with no or minimal symptoms.

Treatment aims

To prevent or delay deterioration of left ventricular function and relieve symptoms of dyspnea and fatigue.

Prognosis

• Prognosis depends mainly on the underlying condition and left ventricular function.

• Rheumatic aortic regurgitation, if detected early, has an excellent prognosis.

• Acute aortic regurgitation due to a dissection or endocarditis is fatal unless treated promptly.

• Patients with an underlying collagen disorder, *e.g.*, Marfan syndrome, have a poor prognosis.

Follow-up and management

• Patients with aortic regurgitation should be seen at regular intervals in a cardiology clinic; signs of deteriorating left ventricular function should be vigorously sought by follow-up echocardiography.

• Patients who have had valve replacement should also be seen regularly and monitored for signs of failure of the aortic valve prosthesis (particularly in patients with biological valves) and endocarditis.

Key references

1. Scognamiglio R, *et al.*: Long-term nifedipine unloading therapy in asymptomatic patients with chronic severe aortic regurgitation. *J Am Coll Cardiol* 1990, **16**:424–429.

2. Greenberg B, *et al.*: Long-term vasodilator therapy of chronic aortic insufficiency. A randomized double-blinded, placebo-controlled clinical trial. *Circulation* 1988, **78**:92–103.

3. Bonow RO, *et al.*: Survival and functional results after valve replacement for aortic regurgitation 1976 to 1983: impact of preoperative left ventricular function. *Circulation* 1985, **72**:1244–1256.

Diagnosis

Symptoms [1,2]

• Many patients are asymptomatic.

Angina: in ~70% of adult patients.

Syncope: in ~25% of patients, during or immediately after exercise.

Dyspnea: common presenting symptom; severe dyspnea, paroxysmal nocturnal dyspnea, and orthopnea late manifestations indicating left ventricular dysfunction.

Signs [1,2]

Pulse

• The pulse is normal in mild aortic stenosis (gradient <50 mm Hg).

Slow rise with diminished "volume," sometimes with "notch" on upstroke ("anacrotic"): indicating severe aortic stenosis; with associated aortic regurgitation, double pulse may be felt ("bisferious").

Heart

Undisplaced, "thrusting" apex beat: thrill may be palpable at base of heart.

Delayed or absent aortic component in second heart sound: in severe aortic stenosis and calcified valves, respectively.

Added sounds: ejection click may be heard at apex in bicuspid aortic valve; fourth heart sound may be heard in severe aortic stenosis; third sound implies impaired left ventricular function.

Murmurs: midsystolic, rough; best heard at base of heart in second right interspace but often heard anywhere over precordium, almost always radiating to neck in severe aortic stenosis, increased in expiration; may be very soft with poor left ventricular function and low cardiac output.

Investigations

ECG: usually shows left ventricular hypertrophy, possibly left axis deviation, later left atrial hypertrophy (negative P wave in V_1), conduction abnormalities due to calcification of conducting tissues (first-degree heart block, left bundle branch block).

Chest radiography: may show cardiac enlargement, poststenotic dilatation of aorta, calcification of aortic valve (particularly in older patients).

Echocardiography: normal valve appearance excludes significant aortic stenosis in adults; also helps to define level of obstruction (*i.e.*, valvar, supravalvar, subvalvar); left ventricular function can also be assessed; Doppler examination permits determination of peak gradient across the valve.

Cardiac catheterization: necessary if coronary artery disease suspected or diagnosis doubted; aortography useful in presence of concomitant aortic regurgitation; retrograde crossing of valve indicated only if echocardiography inadequate; gradient obtained using this method is peak-to-peak, 10–15 mm Hg less than peak instantaneous gradient measured by Doppler examination.

Complications

Sudden death: in 10%–20% of adults and 1% of children.

Cardiac failure: indicates poor prognosis unless valve replaced.

Arrhythmias and conduction abnormalities: ventricular arrhythmias more common than supraventricular arrhythmias; heart block may occur because of calcification of conducting tissues.

Systemic embolization: caused by deposits breaking off valve apparatus or by concomitant aortic atheroma.

Infective endocarditis: should be considered in patients with aortic stenosis who present with unexplained illness.

Differential diagnosis

Aortic sclerosis: old age, normal pulse character, echocardiogram with mild thickening of leaflets without restricted motion or gradient.

Flow murmur (pregnancy, anemia, thyrotoxicosis): large-volume pulse, normal echocardiogram, no gradient.

Mitral regurgitation: pansystolic murmur, no radiation to neck, mitral valve abnormality on echo-Doppler examination.

Hypertrophic cardiomyopathy: late systolic murmur, jerky pulse, echocardiogram showing left ventricular hypertrophy, asymmetric septal hypertrophy, systolic anterior motion of mitral valve.

Ventricular septal defect: pansystolic murmur at left sternal edge with thrill, jet detected on Doppler examination.

Etiology

Congenital: bicuspid or unicuspid valve

• The disease is usually manifest in early childhood or adolescence.

• It may be associated with other congenital abnormalities (coarctation of aorta and patent ductus arteriosus).

• Subvalvar stenosis is more common in boys and accounts for 10% of congenital cases.

• Supravalvar aortic stenosis is rare, usually a component of Williams syndrome.

Acquired

• The disease can be calcific (calcified bicuspid or tricuspid aortic valves manifest in adults) or rheumatic (rarely isolated; usually accompanies rheumatic mitral valve disease).

Epidemiology

• Valvar aortic stenosis is the most common valve lesion in adults in industrialized countries.

• 70% of patients suffer from calcific stenosis (60% bicuspid, 10% tricuspid), 15% rheumatic, and 15% other forms.

Treatment

Diet and lifestyle

• Patients must avoid strenuous exercise and competitive sports.

Pharmacological treatment

• Drug treatment has no place in the treatment of aortic stenosis, but patients should be given antibiotic prophylaxis against infective endocarditis (*see* Endocarditis *for details*).

Nonpharmacological treatment

Surgery

• Surgery is mandatory for symptomatic patients.

• It should be considered in asymptomatic patients objectively with severe aortic stenosis (peak-to-peak gradient >50 mm Hg) [3]. Efforts to objectively exclude symptoms in sedentary patients who report no symptoms may be useful, *e.g.*, gentle treadmill test.

• Age alone is not a contraindication.

• Patients with severe aortic stenosis should have valve replacement early to avoid deterioration in left ventricular function.

Balloon valvuloplasty

• This is useful in infants (in whom the results of surgery are poor) and in children and young adults (in whom the valve apparatus is not calcified).

• It should only be considered in adults when surgery is contraindicated [4].

Treatment aims

To replace valve before left ventricular dysfunction occurs.

Prognosis

• Up to 20% of patients with severe congestive aortic stenosis die during childhood, mainly because of progressive heart failure.

• In adults, the 5-year survival rate is 40%.

• The prognosis after surgery depends on age and left ventricular function.

Follow-up and management

• Patients with mild to moderate aortic stenosis should be monitored for increasing severity.

• Patients who have had valve replacement should be monitored for failure of the valve prosthesis (particularly biological valves) and endocarditis.

Key references

1. Braunwald E: Valvular heart disease. In *Heart Disease,* edn 4. Edited by Braunwald E. Philadelphia: WB Saunders; 1992:1007–1077.

2. Selzer A: Changing aspects of the natural history of valvular aortic stenosis. *N Engl J Med* 1987, **317**:91–98.

3. Kennedy KD, *et al.*: Natural history of moderate aortic stenosis. *J Am Coll Cardiol* 1991, **17**:13–19.

4. Bernard Y, *et al.*: Long-term results of percutaneous aortic valvuloplasty compared with aortic valve replacement in patients more than 75 years old. *J Am Coll Cardiol* 1992, **20**:796–801.

Diagnosis

Symptoms and signs

Any form of psoriasis or a history compatible with psoriasis.

Skin lesions: possibly years after arthritis (family history of psoriasis may be suggestive).

Peripheral polyarthritis: frequently symmetrical; may be indistinguishable from rheumatoid arthritis, involving small joints of hands and feet, wrists, ankles, knees, and elbows.

Inflammatory oligoarthritis: mainly lower limbs, asymmetrical.

Inflammatory involvement of distal interphalangeal joints: nearly always with psoriatic nail changes.

Asymmetrical spondylitis and sacroiliitis, insertion enthesopathy, *e.g.*, **of Achilles tendon, plantar fascia, musculotendinous insertions around pelvis.**

Mutilating arthritis: with telescoping of fingers and toes (rare).

Dactylitis: "sausage" digits.

• Rheumatoid nodules and other extra-articular features are absent.

Investigations

Blood tests: rheumatoid factor absent; biochemical response to active disease similar to rheumatoid arthritis; ESR or plasma viscosity may be best guide to activity.

Radiography: shows asymmetrical small joint changes, tendency to ankylosis, osteolysis with pencil-in-cup deformity, whittling terminal phalanges (especially hallux); enthesitis; asymmetrical sacroiliitis and syndesmophytes.

Complications

Amyloidosis, exfoliation of skin: rare.

Differential diagnosis

Rheumatoid arthritis.

Reactive (Reiter's syndrome).

Etiology

• Psoriatic arthritis has a genetic component: HLA B27 positive in 71% of patients with psoriatic spondylitis, 32% in distal joint group.

• It may be triggered by trauma.

Epidemiology

• 5%–8% of patients with psoriasis have psoriatic arthritis.

• The male:female ratio is equal, but more men have the distal-joint and spondylitic forms.

• Juvenile psoriatic arthritis is rare; it is found in groups similar to those of adult disease.

Classification

Classic psoriatic arthritis: involving predominantly distal interphalangeal joints of hands and feet, in 5% of patients.

Arthritis mutilans: with sacroiliitis, in 5%.

Symmetrical polyarthritis: resembling rheumatoid arthritis but with negative serum rheumatoid factor, in 15%.

Asymmetrical, pauci-articular, small joint involvement: with "sausage" digits, in 70%.

Ankylosing spondylitis: with or without peripheral arthritis, in 5%.

Associated features

Palmar-plantar pustulosis: sternoclavicular hyperostosis, chronic sterile multifocal osteomyelitis, hyperostosis of spine and peripheral arthritis.

Eye lesions: conjunctivitis in 20% of patients; iritis in 7%.

Edema: unilateral.

HIV infection: exacerbates psoriatic but not rheumatoid arthritis.

Keratoderma blenorrhagica of Reiter's syndrome: may develop into psoriasis vulgaris.

Treatment

Diet and lifestyle

- Activity should be encouraged.
- No special diet is necessary.

Pharmacological treatment

Principles

For psoriasis (simple cases): topical steroids, coal tar (*see* Psoriasis *for further details*).

For arthritis (simple cases): NSAIDs, analgesics [1].

For severe cases: second-line treatment according to severity of each system.

Second line for arthritis alone

Standard dosage	Sulfasalazine, 1g twice daily. Sodium aurothiomalate, 10-mg i.m. test dose, then 50 mg increase weekly to 1g, then spaced out to monthly maintenance.
Contraindications	*Sulfasalazine:* hypersensitivity to sulfonamides or salicylates. *Sodium aurothiomalate:* pregnancy, lactation, renal or hepatic disease, history of blood dyscrasias, exfoliative dermatitis, or SLE; caution in elderly patients, urticaria, eczema, colitis.
Special points	*Sulfasalazine:* complete blood count initially and monthly for first 3 months, liver function tests also monthly for first 3 months. *Sodium aurothiomalate:* urine test for protein before injection, skin inspection for rash; complete blood count and urine checks monthly. Antimalarials, *e.g.*, chloroquine, hydroxychloroquine, can also be used.
Main drug interactions	*Sodium aurothiomalate:* aspirin.
Main side effects	*Sulfasalazine:* nausea (dose must be reduced), reversible azoospermia, bone-marrow suppression. *Sodium aurothiomalate:* proteinuria, bone-marrow suppression, dermatitis.

Second line for arthritis and skin involvement

- Treatment should be given under specialist supervision [1].

Standard dosage	Methotrexate, azathioprine, possibly etretinate, or possibly cyclosporine.
Contraindications	*Methotrexate:* liver damage, excess alcohol intake, pregnancy. *Azathioprine:* pregnancy. *Etretinate:* hepatic and renal impairment, pregnancy. *Cyclosporine:* renal impairment.
Special points	*Methotrexate:* regular blood tests (complete blood count, liver function).
Main drug interactions	*Methotrexate:* NSAIDs, co-trimoxazole, phenytoin, retinoids, diuretics. *Azathioprine:* allopurinol, rifampin. *Etretinate:* anticoagulants, methotrexate. *Cyclosporine:* angiotensin-converting enzyme inhibitors, NSAIDs.
Main side effects	*Methotrexate:* bone-marrow suppression, liver damage, nausea and vomiting, stomatitis. *Azathioprine:* bone-marrow suppression. *Etretinate:* fetal malformation, cheilosis, hypercholesterolemia. *Cyclosporine:* impaired renal function, nausea.

Treatment aims

To relieve pain and stiffness.
To achieve full functional capacity.
To prevent progression of arthritis.
To minimize skin lesions.

Prognosis

- Prognosis is usually good.
- A few patients are disabled.

Follow-up and management

- A few patients need regular review.
- Second-line drugs need blood monitoring.

Orthopedic guidelines

- Psoriatic arthritis has the same indications as other arthropathies.
- It has no more infective complications than other diseases.
- Physicians should consult with medical, physical therapy, and occupational therapy staff.
- Early postoperative mobilization is advised.

Key reference

1. Pioro MH, Cash JM: Treatment of refractory psoriatic arthritis. *Rheum Dis Clin North Am* 1995, **21**:129–149.

Diagnosis

Symptoms

Painful, swollen, warm joints, with morning stiffness and impaired function: onset usually insidious, sometimes rapid; characteristically in hands or feet, occasionally monoarticular (most often in a knee); often accompanied by tiredness.

Signs

Articular

Warm, tender, swollen joints: decreased range of movement; peripheral joints most often affected; characteristic symmetry of involvement; proximal interphalangeal, metacarpophalangeal, wrist, and metatarsophalangeal joints usually affected.

Extra-articular

Bursitis: *e.g.*, olecranon.

Tenosynovitis.

Nodules: extensor surfaces.

Serositis: *e.g.*, pleurisy.

Keratoconjunctivitis sicca: secondary Sjögren's syndrome.

Vasculitis, scleritis.

Fibrosing alveolitis.

Investigations

• No single diagnostic test is available; the diagnosis relies on some or all of the following:

ESR, CRP, plasma viscosity measurement: for evidence of inflammation.

Immunology: rheumatoid factor positivity (not essential for diagnosis); present in up to 80%.

Radiography: initially shows periarticular osteoporosis, followed by erosions around affected joint.

Blood count: for anemia of chronic disease, thrombocytosis.

Serum immunoglobulin measurement: for polyclonal gammopathy.

• In addition, the duration of morning stiffness, level of functional impairment, and number of inflamed joints must be monitored in established disease.

Complications

• The following occur in patients with established disease and global decline in function or severe systemic malaise.

Widespread active synovitis.

Septic arthritis.

Systemic rheumatoid disease.

Iatrogenic problems: *e.g.*, NSAIDs and anemia, gold and renal impairment.

Atlantoaxial subluxation.

Non-Hodgkin's lymphoma: possible.

Amyloidosis.

Incapacitation: patient may become bedridden.

Differential diagnosis

Seronegative spondyloarthritis.

Reactive arthritis: gastrointestinal or sexually acquired.

Viral arthritis: *e.g.*, rubella, hepatitis B virus infection.

Septic polyarthritis: *e.g.*, staphylococcal or gonococcal infections.

Crystal polyarthritis: *e.g.*, gout.

Generalized nodal osteoarthritis: may have inflammatory component in 10%.

SLE.

Etiology

• The cause of rheumatoid arthritis is unknown, but the following have a role:

Genetic factors: subtypes of HLA DR4 and DR1.

Hormonal factors: remission during pregnancy; contraceptive pill protects from disease.

Epidemiology

• Rheumatoid arthritis is a significant disease that affects 1%–2% of the population.

• It is a chronic disease, with high prevalence and low incidence.

• It is a modern disease, with little evidence to indicate its presence >400 years ago.

• The female:male ratio is 3:1.

Treatment

Diet and lifestyle

- Activity should be encouraged, but heavy work intensifies joint inflammation.
- Physical therapy, taught exercise, and "joint protection" are helpful to maintain strength and function.
- Omega-3 fatty acids may reduce inflammation [1].

Pharmacological treatment

NSAIDs

- The response is variable and idiosyncratic; if one drug fails, another from a different group may be worth trying.
- The most commonly used drugs are diclofenac, ibuprofen, indomethacin, naproxen, and salicylate.

Standard dosage	Depends on drug used.
Contraindications	Caution in peptic ulceration, asthma, renal impairment, pregnancy, and elderly patients.
Special points	No influence on disease progression.
Main drug interactions	Diuretics, warfarin.
Main side effects	Dyspepsia, renal impairment, fluid retention.

Second-line agents

- These are increasingly started early in the disease process, particularly in patients who do not respond to NSAIDs or who respond partially but have evidence of active disease [2–4].

Standard dosage	Sulfasalazine, 2–3 g daily, with gradual build-up over 4 weeks. Methotrexate, 2.5–15 mg orally once weekly (not daily) [4,5].
Contraindications	*Sulfasalazine:* sulfonamide and salicylate hypersensitivity. *Methotrexate:* pregnancy, liver disease.
Special points	*Sulfasalazine:* complete blood count every 4 weeks for 2 months, monthly for 2–3 months, then 3-monthly; liver function test at onset, monthly for 3 months, then 3-monthly. *Methotrexate:* complete blood count monthly, liver function test 3-monthly; close monitoring in renal impairment; alcohol use should be avoided; NSAIDs must be used cautiously.
Main drug interactions	*Sulfasalazine:* warfarin, co-trimoxazole. *Methotrexate:* co-trimoxazole, trimethoprim, phenytoin.
Main side effects	*Sulfasalazine:* nausea, vomiting, rashes, reversible azoospermia. *Methotrexate:* nausea, diarrhea, rash, pulmonary hypersensitivity, blood dyscrasias.

Other options [2,4,6,7]

Gold (oral or i.m.) [4].

Hydroxychloroquine.

Penicillamine.

Local steroids.

Systemic steroids: either induction before or adjunctive to second-line agents in poorly controlled disease [3].

Immunosuppressants: for severe articular or extra-articular disease.

Minocycline [6].

Nonpharmacological treatment

Physical therapy: during active disease.

Occupational therapy.

Surgery: synovectomies, arthroplasty, arthrodesis, tendon repair; for painful joints (particularly at night), functionally restricted joints, and joints that do not respond to other treatments.

Treatment aims

To decrease pain and symptoms and signs of inflammation.

To prevent progression of irreversible joint damage.

To monitor for and treat extra-articular manifestations.

To restrict disability and handicap.

Prognosis

- The prognosis is variable.
- Poor prognostic markers include female sex, insidious onset, high-titer rheumatoid factor, low educational achievement, persistently raised ESR or CRP, and extra-articular manifestations [8].

Follow-up and management

- Second-line treatment must be monitored regularly.
- Stable disease needs occasional assessment for progressive functional decline.
- Active disease needs regular follow-up so that modifying the various treatment options can be considered.
- Care should be shared between primary care and musculoskeletal specialists (rheumatologist, orthopedic surgeon, physiatrist).

Key references

1. Geusens P, *et al.*: Long term effect of omega 3 fatty acid supplementation in active rheumatoid arthritis; a 12 month double blind controlled study. *Arthritis Rheum* 1994, **37**:824–829.

2. Anonymous: Slow-acting antirheumatic drugs. *Drug Ther Bull* 1993, **31**:17–20.

3. Harris ED: Rheumatoid arthritis. Pathophysiology and implications for treatment. *N Engl J Med* 1990, **332**:1277–1289.

4. Wilke WS, *et al.*: Early aggressive therapy for rheumatoid arthritis concerns, descriptions and estimates of outcome. *Semin Arthritis Rheum* 1993, **23**:26–41.

5. Weinblatt ME, *et al.*: Methotrexate in rheumatoid arthritis. A five year prospective multi-center study. *Arthritis Rheum* 1994, **37**:1492–1498.

6. Kloppenburg M, *et al.*: Minocycline in active rheumatoid arthritis: a double blind placebo controlled trial. *Arthritis Rheum* 1994, **37**:629–636.

7. Jain R, Lipsky PE: Treatment of rheumatoid arthritis. *Med Clin North Am* 1997, **81**:57–84.

8. Tugwell P, *et al.*: End points in rheumatoid arthritis. *J Rheumatol* 1994, **42(suppl)**:2–8; 20–24.

Diagnosis

Symptoms

• Symptoms and signs are more difficult to interpret in the presence of pre-existing joint disease and may be muted in immunosuppressed or elderly patients [1].

• Polyarticular infection occurs in 10%–15% of patients [1–3].

Pain: most consistent feature; typically progressive; may be worse at night; with pre-existing joint disease, change or exacerbation of pain is an important warning sign [3].

Loss of function, limp: possibly presenting feature in children [2].

Fever: possibly only manifestation, particularly in elderly patients [3].

Signs

Swelling and local tenderness, pain and restriction of movement: most marked in previously fit younger patients [2].

Local erythema: possibly but often less marked than in crystal synovitis.

Fever: although temperature normal in up to one-third of patients.

Confusion: possibly prominent feature in elderly patients [3].

Investigations

• Most investigations are nonspecific, and results may be normal; a high index of suspicion is necessary to make the diagnosis [4].

• Adequate specimens must be obtained for microbiological examination before antimicrobial treatment is started.

Synovial fluid analysis: Gram stain positive in 50% of patients; culture positive in 75%; presence of leukocytes not diagnostic; crystals may coexist with sepsis.

Blood cultures: positive in 50% (may be presenting feature of subacute bacterial endocarditis).

Urogenital swabs: should be obtained if gonococcal infection suspected.

Plain radiography: usually unhelpful in early stages of infection [4].

Complications

Death: in up to 15%, especially elderly, immunosuppressed, and rheumatoid arthritis patients.

Loss of function of joint.

Loss of prosthesis.

Osteomyelitis: from direct spread.

Bacterial endocarditis, disseminated intravascular coagulation.

Differential diagnosis

Acute flare of inflammatory joint disease.
Crystal synovitis.
Hemarthrosis.
Bacterial endocarditis.

Etiology

• Pathogens depend on age and predisposing factors; most infections are due to *Staphylococcus aureus* and streptococci; in children aged <5 years, *Haemophilus influenzae* type b has been an important pathogen; gonococcal infection appears to be in decline but should be considered in sexually active patients.

• Spread is usually hematogenous; joint disease or blunt trauma may act to localize blood-borne pathogens.

• Direct inoculation during surgery, injection, or trauma occurs but is unusual.

• Risk factors include extremes of age, previous joint disease, diabetes mellitus, immunosuppression, prosthetic joint material, and corticosteroids.

Epidemiology

• The incidence of septic arthritis is unknown but is estimated to be 3–10 in 100 000 population.

Treatment

Diet and lifestyle

• No special precautions are necessary.

Pharmacological treatment

General principles

• A possible septic arthritis is a medical emergency and should be urgently referred to a specialist (rheumatologist or orthopedic surgeon).

• High-dose antibiotics are given i.v. for at least 2 weeks, then orally for at least a further 2–4 weeks, depending on the clinical response and presence of prosthesis.

• Antibiotics should be started only after appropriate specimens for culture have been obtained.

• Initially, a "best guess" choice of antibiotics is used, based on the most probable pathogen, patient's age, and sensitivities of pathogen; treatment is later tailored by the results of the Gram stain and culture.

Possible "best-guess" regimen

Child aged <5 years: cefotaxime and nafcillin [2].

Child aged >5 years: nafcillin (with penicillin G if gonococcal infection likely) [1–3,5,6].

Adult, immunosuppressed, prosthetic-joint patient: cefotaxime and floxacillin. Vancomycin i.v. for methicillin-resistant *S. aureus*.

Specific drugs

Standard dosage	Nafcillin, 2 g i.v. every 4 hours.
	Penicillin G, 4.8–9.6 g i.v. daily.
	Cefotaxime 3–6 g i.v. daily.
	Vancomycin, 1 g i.v. every 12 hours.
Contraindications	Hypersensitivity.
Special points	Complete blood count needed twice weekly.
	Aminopenicillin can be used instead of penicillin V for oral treatment.
Main drug interactions	None.
Main side effects	Rash, hypersensitivity reaction (rare), neutropenia (after prolonged treatment), diarrhea.

Treatment aims

To prevent septicemia or osteomyelitis.
To preserve joint function.
To resolve infection.

Other treatments

• Repeated medical aspiration with adequate drainage may be associated with better outcome than surgical drainage [7].

• Surgery is indicated for the following [8]:
Inability to drain medically.
Failure to improve on antibiotic or medical management.
Osteomyelitis.
Prosthetic joints (surgical drainage, debridement, or removal).

Prognosis

• The overall mortality is 15%.

• The prognosis is worse if treatment is delayed, in elderly patients with gram-positive infection, and in patients with predisposing joint or systemic disease.

• Infection of prosthetic material carries a particularly poor prognosis; revision or removal of the prosthesis is a common outcome.

Follow-up and management

• Patients with infected prostheses may need long-term suppressive antibiotic treatment, although, in most, revision surgery is delayed rather than prevented.

Key references

1. Goldenberg DL: Bacterial arthritis. *Curr Opin Rheumatol* 1994, **6**:394–400.

2. Shaw BA, Kasser JL: Acute septic arthritis in infancy and childhood. *Clin Orthop* 1990, **257**:212–225.

3. Esterhai JL Jr, Gelb I: Adult septic arthritis. *Orthop Clin North Am* 1991, **3**:503–514.

4. Hendrix RW, Fisher MR: Imaging of septic arthritis. *Clin Rheum Dis* 1986, **12**:459–487.

5. Norden C, *et al.*: Evaluation of new anti-infective drugs for the treatment of infectious arthritis in adults. Clin Infect Dis 1992, **15(suppl)**:S167–S171.

6. Steere AC: Diagnosis and treatment of Lyme arthritis. *Med Clin North Am* 1997, **81**:179–194.

7. Broy SB, Schmid FR: A comparison of medical drainage (needle aspiration) and surgical drainage (arthrotomy or arthroscopy) in the initial treatment of infected joints. *Clin Rheum Dis* 1986, **12**:501–522.

8. Parisien JS, Shaffer R: Arthroscopic management of pyarthrosis. *Clin Orthop* 1992, **275**:243–247.

Diagnosis

Symptoms

Uncomplicated ascites
Abdominal distension and discomfort.

Dyspnea: due to splinting of diaphragm.

Fatigue, encephalopathy, and other symptoms of chronic liver disease: present to variable degrees.

Spontaneous bacterial peritonitis
Pain, fever: in <50% of patients.

Deterioration in liver function, renal impairment, gastrointestinal hemorrhage, encephalopathy: present to variable degrees.

Signs

Uncomplicated ascites
Physical examination often insensitive.

Distension.

Shifting dullness on percussion of flanks, fluid wave.

Ballotable liver.

Spontaneous bacterial peritonitis
• Often no additional clinical signs are manifest.

Fever, encephalopathy: more common than tenderness, rebound, rigidity.

Investigations

In all cases
Measurement of serum and ascitic albumin: to allow calculation of concentration gradient (*i.e.*, serum albumin in g/dL–ascites albumin in g/dL) [1].

Cell count using ascites: >250 polymorphonuclear neutrophils/mL suggests peritonitis; lymphocyte predominance suggests tuberculosis or malignancy.

Cytological study: of fluid to evaluate for malignancy.

Gram stain and culture of ascites: blood culture bottle inoculation; polymicrobial infections suggest perforation of the gastrointestinal tract.

Urine electrolytes analysis.

Serum electrolytes, blood urea nitrogen, creatinine.

Specific tests for selected presentations
Amylase measurement: concentration raised in pancreatic ascites.

Cholesterol or triglyceride measurement: concentration raised in chylous ascites.

Total protein: high in malignancy, tuberculosis, cardiac ascites.

Laparoscopy and biopsy: for tuberculosis.

Abdominal ultrasonography or CT: for malignant ascites.

Complications

Spontaneous bacterial peritonitis: most common in patients with high serum-ascites albumin gradients or low ascites protein.

Pleural effusion: may occur without ascites.

Inguinal, femoral, or umbilical hernias.

Mesenteric venous thrombosis.

Renal failure, hepatorenal syndrome.

Umbilical rupture.

Empyema.

Differential diagnosis

High serum-ascites albumin gradient (*i.e.*, ≥1.1 g/dL)
Portal hypertension.
Cirrhosis.
Cardiac ascites.
Fulminant hepatitis.
Budd-Chiari/veno-occlusive disease.
Myxedema.

Low serum-ascites albumin gradient (*i.e.*, <1.1 g/dL)
Peritoneal carcinomatosis.
Tuberculosis.
Pancreatic ascites.
Biliary ascites.
Nephrotic syndrome.

Chylous
Trauma and surgery, abdominal tuberculosis, lymphoma or other malignancy, filariasis.

Etiology

High serum-ascites albumin gradient
Overflow hypothesis: primary increase in renal sensitivity to aldosterone, causing sodium retention or volume expansion, ascites forming in abdomen because of portal hypertension and hypoalbuminemia.
Underfill hypothesis: fluid sequestration in abdomen, causing renal hypoperfusion and secondary hyperaldosteronism, renal retention of sodium to maintain circulating volume.
Vasodilatation hypothesis: overflow factors initiating and underfill factors perpetuating ascites.

Low serum-ascites albumin gradient
Increased capillary permeability.

Chylous
Lymphatic leakage.

Epidemiology

• 80% of patients with cirrhosis develop ascites during their course (spontaneous bacterial peritonitis in 10%).

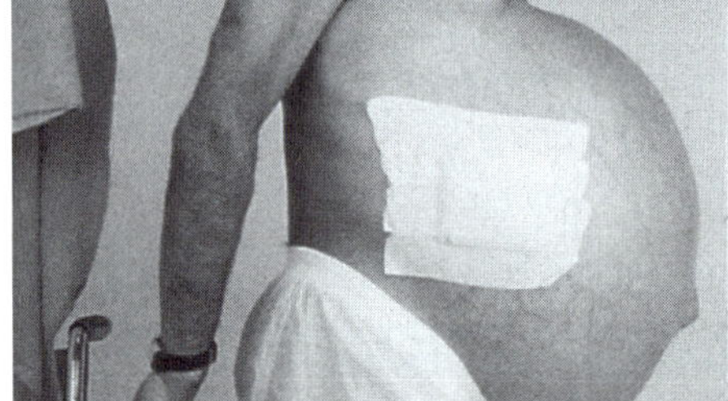

Distended abdomen with protuberant umbilicus in a patient with massive ascites. (*See* Color Plate.)

Treatment

Diet and lifestyle

• Patients should have a low-salt diet (<2 g daily) and maintain an adequate intake of calories.

• Bed rest during mobilization of ascites may be of benefit by lowering renin–angiotensin concentrations.

Pharmacological treatment

For uncomplicated ascites [2]

• Initially, treatment should involve spironolactone, with high-volume paracentesis reserved for patients with respiratory compromise or those with disease that is refractory to diuretic management.

• Furosemide can be added if no response is seen after 3 days and is more effective in patients with peripheral edema.

Standard dosage	Spironolactone, 100 mg daily, or furosemide, 40 mg daily, aiming for 1.0 kg of weight loss per day if pedal edema present and 0.5 kg per day if there is no pedal edema; dosage is increased slowly depending on diuresis to maximum spironolactone, 400 mg, or furosemide, 160 mg daily.
Contraindications	Renal failure.
Special points	Renal function should be watched carefully and diuretics decreased or witheld for any increase in creatinine of 0.5 mg/dL over baseline. Hyponatremia <122 mEq/L should be treated with fluid restriction. Hyperkalemia should be managed by a decrease in spironolactone or an increase in furosemide.
Main drug interactions	Diuretics and aminoglycosides may have increased nephrotoxicity in this context; NSAIDs should be avoided.
Main side effects	Hyponatremia, impaired renal function with raised creatinine, hyperkalemia [3]. For patients with gynecomastia from spironolactone, amiloride is an alternative (5–10 mg daily).

Nonpharmacological treatment [3,4]

• High-volume paracentesis (removal of >6 L of ascites) should be done in cases refractory to diuretic management. Caution should be exercised in patients with renal dysfunction (creatinine >2.0 mg/dL). Intravenous albumin (10 g/L of ascites removed) administered to patients with elevated creatinine or those without pedal edema may protect against progressive renal dysfunction [3].

For functional renal failure: renal failure is often precipitated by infection, hemorrhage, hypotension, or overaggressive diuretic treatment; it may reverse after orthotopic liver transplantation. Treatment involves central venous monitoring, volume expansion, and treatment of precipitating factors; renal vasodilators are of no proven benefit.

For resistant ascites: juguloperitoneal shunt, transhepatic intravascular portal systemic stent shunt, or orthotopic liver transplantation.

For spontaneous bacterial peritonitis [4]

• 80% of organisms are aerobic gram-negative bacilli; 20% are nonenteric organisms.

• Cefotaxime or ceftizoxime is effective in up to 85%; ciprofloxacin and amoxicillin may be as effective, but gentamicin is potentially more toxic.

• Treatment should last 5–7 days.

• Antibiotic treatment is influenced by hospital sensitivities.

• Clearance of ascitic leukocytes should be checked after 3 days, and renal function should be monitored daily.

• Long-term antibiotic prophylaxis with antibiotics (*e.g.*, norfloxacin) may prevent recurrence; consider in patients with previous episodes of spontaneous bacterial peritonitis or patients with ascites fluid protein <1.0 g/dL.

Treatment aims

To reduce ascitic volume.

Prognosis

• 1-year and 5-year survival rates after development of ascites without renal impairment are 50% and 20%, respectively.

• 80% of patients respond to medical treatment.

• 30% develop functional renal failure within 24 months.

• When urine sodium is <5 mmol/L or diuretic-resistant ascites has developed, 1-year survival is <50%.

• Spontaneous bacterial peritonitis has a hospital mortality of up to 50%.

• >50% of survivors have a recurrence in the following year.

Follow-up and management

• Patients with uncomplicated ascites must be monitored using weight and daily fluid input and output charts.

• If no response is seen at maximum tolerated dose of diuretic, the development of hepatoma, portal-vein thrombosis, or spontaneous bacterial peritonitis must be excluded.

Key references

1. Runyon BA, Montano AA, Akriviadis EA, *et al.*: The serum-ascites albumin gradient is superior to the exudate-transudate concept in the differential diagnosis of ascites. *Ann Intern Med* 1992, **117**:215–220.

2. Strauss RM, Boyer TD: Diagnosis and management of cirrhotic ascites. In *Hepatology: A Textbook of Liver Disease.* Edited by Zakim D, Boyer TD. Philadelphia: WB Saunders; 1996:764–788.

3. Runyon BA: Patient selection is important in studying the impact of large-volume paracentesis on intravascular volume. *Am J Gastroenterol* 1997, **92**:371–373.

4. Runyon BA: Care of patients with ascites. *N Engl J Med* 1994, **330**:337–342.

Diagnosis

Symptoms

Wheezing.

Breathlessness.

Chest tightness: not pain.

Cough: with or without sputum; may be the only symptom, especially in children.

Exercise-induced cough or wheezing.

• Symptom severity shows considerable temporal variation; they are often worse at night or in early morning.

Signs

Tachypnea.

Diffuse wheezing.

Use of accessory muscles of respiration: in severe attack, due to high negative intrapleural pressure or rapid respiratory rate.

Tachycardia: in severe attack.

Pulsus paradoxus: in severe attack.

Cyanosis or confusion: signs of impending respiratory arrest; wheezing may be absent.

Rhinitis, nasal polyps, atopic dermatitis: often associated with asthma.

Investigations

On presentation

Spirometry: forced expiratory volume in 1 second (FEV_1) and forced vital capacity; response to beta-2 agonist (>15% improvement in FEV_1 confirms reversible airflow obstruction; failure to improve does not exclude asthma).

Serial peak flow monitoring: early peak flow often low in asthma; >15% diurnal variation strongly suggests asthma, peak flow reduced after work or exposure to sensitizing agent.

Airways hyperresponsiveness test: increased sensitivity to methacholine, shown by 20% fall in FEV_1 to abnormally small doses of nebulized methacholine.

For acute episodes

Spirometry or peak flow rate measurement: to assess severity.

Arterial blood gas analysis: partial oxygen pressure reduced; partial carbon dioxide pressure usually low in acute episode; rising or raised partial carbon dioxide pressure suggests exhaustion and impending respiratory arrest; different patterns in acute exacerbations of chronic obstructive pulmonary disease (*see* Chronic obstructive pulmonary disease *for details*).

Chest radiography: to check for pneumothorax or pneumonia and to exclude heart failure.

ECG: if cause of breathlessness unclear.

Sputum culture: good samples often difficult to obtain; most exacerbations due to viral not bacterial infection.

Complications [1]

Respiratory arrest and death.

Pneumothorax.

Recurrent bronchial infection.

Irreversible airflow limitation.

Differential diagnosis

Acute or chronic bronchitis.

Irreversible airway obstruction (chronic obstructive pulmonary disease).

Rhinitis with postnasal drip.

Left ventricular failure.

Pulmonary embolism.

Etiology

• Asthma has an important genetic component, which is inherited separately from the genetic tendency to atopy.

• ~50% of patients have associated atopic allergy, especially children.

• All grades of asthma show airway inflammation, with eosinophils, mononuclear cells, and epithelial desquamation.

• Viral infections are clearly linked to exacerbations of asthma and may be responsible for initiating asthma in patients with adult-onset disease.

• Exposure to environmental chemicals and pollution is blamed for the current increase in prevalence: clear evidence of a causal relationship is awaited.

Epidemiology

• The prevalence of asthma appears to be increasing in the United States; an estimated 5%–10% of the population is asthmatic.

• Asthma is more common in children, and may remit as they grow.

Treatment

Diet and lifestyle

• Special diets are not usually needed; patients with salicylate or sulfite sensitivity should avoid foods containing salicylates or sulfites.

• Exercise is encouraged; swimming is often better tolerated than outdoor sports (exercise-induced asthma is triggered by cold dry air).

• Patients should be educated to develop a partnership in asthma management; this is a critical component.

Pharmacological treatment [2–8]

Corticosteroids [5,6]

Standard dosage *Inhaled corticosteroids:* starting dose varies according to severity and corticosteroid formulation (*e.g.*, beclomethasone, 200–400 µg twice daily).
Oral corticosteroids: prednisone, 30 mg daily for 5 days; longer courses may be needed if improvement is slow; dose need not be tapered if course lasts <14 days.

Contraindications None.

Special points Rinsing mouth after inhaling steroids reduces risk of oropharyngeal side effects.
Spacer device should be used.

Main drug interactions None.

Main side effects *Inhaled steroids:* hoarse voice, oropharyngeal candidiasis.
Oral steroids: cushingoid features, especially osteoporosis, bruising, weight gain.

Short-acting beta-2 agonists [3]

Standard dosage Depends on agent and device, *e.g.*, albuterol, terbutaline, 1–2 puffs as needed.

Contraindications None.

Special points Frequent use of short-acting beta-2 agonists suggests suboptimal control.

Main drug interactions Beta-blockers must be avoided.

Main side effects Tremor.

Leukotriene inhibitors [2]

Standard dosage Zafirlukast, 20 mg twice daily.

Zileutin, 600 mg four times daily.

Main side effects *Zileutin:* elevation of hepatic enzymes.

Xanthines [8]

Standard dosage Theophylline, dose adjusted to give blood concentrations of 10–15 mg/L.

Contraindications Liver disease, heart disease, epilepsy, porphyria.

Special points Narrow therapeutic margin, so dose should be low initially and adjusted with aid of plasma drug concentrations.

Main drug interactions Plasma concentration increased with many other drugs, *e.g.*, antibiotics (ciprofloxacin, erythromycin), cimetidine, antidepressants, diltiazem, verapamil, fluconazole.

Main side effects Nausea, reflux esophagitis, tremor.

For severe attacks [1]

Hospital admission.

Severity assessment (especially spirometry and blood gases).

Oxygen administration as needed.

Maximal bronchodilatation (nebulizer).

Intravenous prednisone administration.

Ventilation if patient is tired or weakening or if blood gases show rising arterial blood pressure.

Treatment aims

To find minimum level of treatment to suppress symptoms.
To enable patients to take responsibility for day-to-day management of the condition.
To enable patients to avoid days off work or school.
To reduce the frequency of exacerbations and to avoid hospital admissions.

Prognosis

• Many children with asthma experience spontaneous remission in their second decade of life.
• Adult-onset asthma rarely remits.
• Most asthmatic patients cope well with their disease and have a normal life expectancy.
• A few severely ill or unstable asthmatic patients are at risk of respiratory arrest; often, these patients need large doses of oral corticosteroids to control the disease.

Follow-up and management

• Exacerbations should be treated by the following:
Increased dose of inhaled corticosteroid.
Oral prednisone, 30 mg daily for 5–7 days.
Antibiotics if patient is febrile or sputum discoloured.
Increased dose of bronchodilators.

Key references

1. Corbridge TC, Hall JB: The assessment and management of adults with status asthmaticus. *Am J Respir Crit Care Med* 1995, **151**:1292–1316.
2. Holgate ST, Bradding P, Sampson AP: Leukotriene antagonists and synthesis inhibitors: new directions in asthma therapy. *J Allergy Clin Immunol* 1996, **98**:1–13.
3. Nelson HS: Beta-adrenergic bronchodilators. *N Engl J Med* 1995, **333**:499–506.
4. National Asthma Education and Prevention Program—Expert Panel Report 2: *Guidelines for the Diagnosis and Management of Asthma*. Washington, D.C.: U.S. Department of Health and Human Services, Public Health Service, National Institutes of Health; 1997.
5. Chapman K, *et al.*: Effect of a short course of prednisone in the prevention of early relapse after the emergency room treatment of acute asthma. *N Engl J Med* 1991, **324**:788–794.
6. McFadden E Jr: Dosages of corticosteroids in asthma. *Am Rev Respir Dis* 1993, **147**:1306–1310.
7. Barnes PJ: Inhaled glucocorticoids for asthma. *N Engl J Med* 1995, **332**:868–875.
8. Weinberger M, Hendeles L: Theophylline in asthma. *N Engl J Med* 1996, **334**:1380–1388.

Diagnosis

Symptoms

Breathlessness at rest or on exertion, wheezing, worsening after work, improvement at weekends or during holidays.

Signs

Diffuse wheezing.

Use of accessory muscles of respiration: due to high negative intrapleural pressure or rapid respiratory rate.

Tachycardia: in severe attack.

Pulsus paradoxus: in severe attack.

Rhinitis.

Cough.

Investigations [1,2]

Baseline spirometry: response to beta-2 agonist.

Bronchial hyper-responsiveness test: using methacholine PC_{20} (>20% fall in forced expiratory volume in 1 second, with no such change on control day).

Serial measure of airway responsiveness.

Detailed peak flow monitoring: at work and on days off or vacations.

Detailed list of materials encountered in the workplace.

Specific challenge tests: to confirm role of new agent in causing asthma or to determine responsible agent when several agents are present in the workplace (available only in very specialized centers).

Complications

Interstitial fibrosis.

Respiratory failure.

Chronic breathlessness.

Treatment

Diet and lifestyle

• Exposure should be reduced (to zero if possible) by moving to low-exposure zone, provision of personal respirator, or leaving employment.

Pharmacological treatment [4,5]

• Treatment is the same as for other forms of asthma (*see* Asthma *for details*).

• All cases of occupational lung disease need specialist assessment to ensure that the correct diagnosis is reached and appropriate treatment instituted.

• Most patients need inhaled corticosteroids and bronchodilators.

Standard dosage	Beclomethasone, 400–800 µg daily.
Contraindications	None.
Special points	Rinsing of mouth after inhaling steroids reduces risk of oropharyngeal side effects. Spacer device should be used.
Main drug interactions	None.
Main side effects	Hoarse voice, oropharyngeal candidiasis.

Treatment aims

To control symptoms of asthma and restore normal levels of activity.

To reduce risk of developing chronic asthma.

Prognosis

• Most patients improve when withdrawn from exposure.

• >40% should have no residual signs or symptoms of asthma, but up to 30% have chronic persistent symptoms, despite full withdrawal from exposure.

• Persistent asthma is especially frequent with low molecular weight sensitizers but can also occur with high molecular weight (protein) antigens.

Follow-up and management

• Patients should be followed carefully to check whether asthma resolves with time.

• Regular radiographic monitoring is necessary for patients with interstitial fibrosis.

Key references

1. Chan-Yeung M, Malo JL: Occupational asthma. *N Engl J Med* 1995, **333**:107–112.

2. Bright P, Burge PS: Occupational lung disease: 8. The diagnosis of occupational asthma from serial measurements of lung function at and away from work. *Thorax* 1996, **51**:857–863.

3. Bernstein IL, *et al.* (eds.): *Asthma in the Workplace.* New York: Marcel Dekker; 1993.

4. Newman LS: Occupational asthma: diagnosis, management, ocent, and prevention. *Clin Chest Med* 1995, **16**:621–636.

5. Garshick E, Schenker MB, Dosman JA: Occupationally induced airway obstruction. *Med Clin North Am* 1996, **80**:851–878.

Diagnosis

Symptoms

Gait imbalance: including the following:

Wide-based gait, falls.

Tremor.

Difficulty with fine coordinated movements, clumsiness.

Rotated or tilted head postures.

Signs

Wide-based gait.

Titubation.

Dysmetria, dysdiadochokinesis.

Dysarthria.

Rotated or tilted head postures.

Hypotonia.

Investigations

Family history evaluation.

TSH, T3, T4.

MRI, PET.

CSF examination or angiography if relevant illness suspected.

Check for drug toxicity, heavy metal toxicity.

Vitamin levels.

Ceruloplasmin.

Lipid and fatty acid and aryl sulfatase levels.

Complications

Inability to walk.

Falls, hip fracture.

Differential diagnosis

Acute intoxication.

Hysteria and malingering.

Miller-Fisher variant of Guillain–Barré syndrome.

Etiology

• Degenerative disorders are most common:

Alcoholic degeneration, olivopontocerebellar atrophy, Friedreich's ataxia, multiple system atrophy.

Vascular hemorrhage or infarction.

Multiple sclerosis.

Neoplastic or paraneoplastic syndrome.

Drug toxicity.

Inherited malformations (Dandy–Walker syndrome, Arnold–Chiari deformity).

Viral infections in children.

Myxedema.

Epidemiology

• Chronic alcoholism is probably the most common cause of chronic progressive ataxia in adults.

Treatment

Diet and lifestyle

• Patients should abstain from alcohol.

Pharmacological treatment

Clonazepan, 0.5–2 mg twice daily may be helpful symptomatically.

Treatment of underlying disorder (*e.g.,* immunosuppression for multiple sclerosis, thyroid replacement, thiamine for alcoholic degeneration).

Treatment aims

To maintain safety.
To treat tremor.

Other treatments

Physical therapy for gait retraining and adaptation.
Posterior fossa decompression for some malformations with progressive compression of cerebellar structures.
Address safety issues in patient's home.

Prognosis

• Depending on illness, degenerative disorders usually progress gradually over a decade.

Follow-up and management

Neurological examinations and discussion of function and safety every 6 months.

General references

Gilman S: Cerebellar disorders: clinical features and treatment. In *Movement Disorders: Neurologic Principles and Practice.* Edited by Watts RL, Koller WE. New York: McGraw Hill; 1997: in press.

Harding S: Ataxic disorders. In *Neurology in Clinical Practice,* vol 1. Edited by Bradley WG, Daroff RB, Fenichel GM, Marsden CD. Boston: Butterworth Heinemann; 1991:337–346.

Diagnosis

Symptoms

Ostium secundum defect [1–3]
- Patients are often asymptomatic in early life.
- Children may have increased incidence of chest infections.
- Symptoms increase with age: >70% of adults are symptomatic by 40 years.

Palpitation: indicating atrial arrythmias.
Dyspnea.
Productive cough: indicating recurrent chest infections.
Fatigue, ankle swelling: indicating right-sided congestive heart failure.
Symptoms of paradoxical emboli.

Ostium primum defect
- Patients may develop symptoms and heart failure in childhood.

Failure to thrive.
Chest infections.
Poor development.

- In adults, in addition to the same symptoms as for secundum defect, the following occur:

Syncope: indicating heart block.
Symptoms of infective endocarditis.

Signs [1–3]

Ostium primum and secundum defects
- The following signs of pulmonary hypertension may be manifest:

Right ventricular hypertrophy, palpable pulmonary closure, pulmonary ejection click, early diastolic murmur of pulmonary regurgitation.

Normal or small-volume pulse.
Normal or raised venous pressure: raised pressure with pulmonary hypertension and right ventricular enlargement.
Prominent right ventricular impulse.
Widely split second sound in inspiration and expiration (fixed).
Ejection systolic flow murmur in pulmonary area and mid-diastolic tricuspid flow murmur: increased right-sided flows, louder on inspiration.

Ostium primum defect only
Pansystolic murmur at apex: indicating mitral regurgitation (mitral valve abnormal).

Investigations

ECG: for ostium secundum defect, shows right axis deviation, right bundle branch block; for ostium primum defect, shows left axis deviation, right bundle branch block, prolonged PR interval.
Chest radiography: for secundum and primum defects, shows moderate cardiac enlargement, small aortic knuckle, large pulmonary artery, pulmonary plethora.
Two-dimensional echocardiography: identifies precise anatomy in most patients; contrast studies may reveal site of shunting.
Cardiac catheterization: often unnecessary in diagnosis but may be used to assess shunt with saturation samples taken from right and left heart, right heart pressures, and pulmonary vascular resistance.

Complications

Atrial arrhythmias: atrial fibrillation is most common.
Pulmonary hypertension and development of right ventricular disease.
Eisenmenger's syndrome with reversal of shunt.
Paradoxical embolus.
Infective endocarditis: in patients with ostium primum defect only.

Differential diagnosis

Uncomplicated ostium secundum defect
Mild pulmonary stenosis.

Atrial septal defect with pulmonary hypertension
Rheumatic mitral and tricuspid valve disease.
Mitral valve prolapse.
Primary pulmonary hypertension.
Cor pulmonale.

Etiology
- The cause is unknown.

Epidemiology
- Atrial septal defect constitutes 7% of all congenital heart disease and 30% of congenital heart disease in adults.
- The female:male ratio is 2:1.

Types

Ostium secundum
Defect of fossa ovalis (most common; 70% of all defects).

Ostium primum
Defect in septum inferior to fossa ovalis; may occur in isolation or as atrial component of atrioventricular septal defect.

Sinus venosus
Defect at base of superior vena cava/upper part of interatrial septum; often associated with anomalous pulmonary venous drainage.

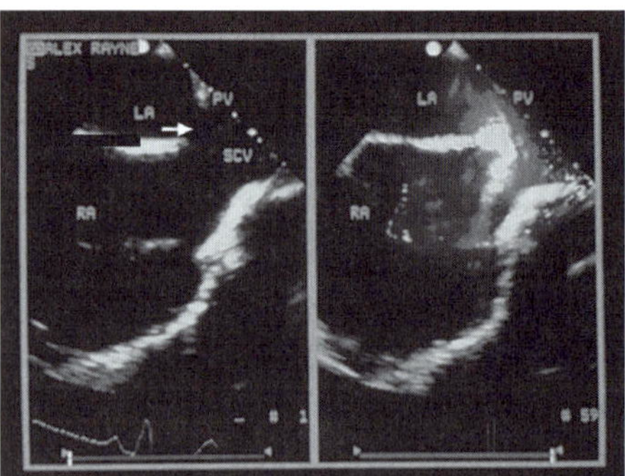

Sinus venosus atrial septal defect (*arrow*). (*See* Color Plate.)

Treatment

Diet and lifestyle

• No special precautions are necessary.

Pharmacological treatment

• Drug treatment has a role only in the management of complications of the defect such as atrial fibrillation (antiarrhythmic agents), right ventricular failure (diuretics), and infective endocarditis of a primum defect (antibiotics).

Nonpharmacological treatment

• Treatment of the defect itself involves surgical closure or transcatheter delivery of an umbrella or clamshell device across the defect [4].

Ostium secundum defect

• Asymptomatic infants and children are usually followed, with closure advocated before the age of 10 years, if the pulmonary : systemic flow ratio is >1.5 : 1; the feasibility of device closure is determined on transthoracic and transesophageal echocardiography.

• If the child is unsuitable for transcatheter closure, surgical placement of pericardial or Dacron patch should be used.

• For adults, the debate continues on whether closure is worthwhile, but, if symptomatic with shunt >2 : 1, most experts advocate closure; transcatheter device closure may be feasible [5].

• Contraindications to closure are pulmonary vascular resistance >6 Woods units, and age >65 years with small shunt [5].

Ostium primum defect

• All patients with significant shunt, unless complicated by severe pulmonary vascular disease, should have surgical closure, with repair of associated mitral valve abnormalities.

Treatment aims

To prevent late-onset pulmonary hypertension.

To avoid right ventricular failure.

To reduce or delay incidence of atrial arrhythmias.

Prognosis

• In patients with ostium secundum defect, mortality of repair in an uncomplicated case is <1%; in older patients with rise in pulmonary vascular resistance, mortality is higher.

• Most patients with unoperated ostium primum defect die by the age of 30 years; operative mortality varies with the complexity of the defect but is usually 5%–10%.

Follow-up and management

• Patients must be observed for symptoms of atrial arrhythmias, developing pulmonary hypertension, and right ventricular failure.

• After repair of an ostium primum defect, heart block is possible.

Key references

1. Dexter L: Atrial septal defect. *Br Heart J* 1956, **18**:209–225.

2. Perloff JK: Atrial septal defect. In *The Clinical Recognition of Congenital Heart Disease*, edn 3. Edited by Perloff JK. Philadelphia: WB Saunders, 1987:272–349.

3. Liberthson RR: Atrial septal defect. In *Congenital Heart Disease: Diagnosis and Management in Children and Adults*. Boston: Little Brown; 1989:45–60.

4. Murphy JG: Long-term outcome after surgical repair of isolated atrial septal defect. *N Engl J Med* 1990, **323**:1645–1650.

5. Sutton MGS, Tajik AJ, McGoon DC: Atrial septal defect in patients aged 60 years or older: operative results and long-term postoperative follow-up. *Circulation* 1981, **64**:402–409.

Diagnosis

Definition

• Normally, the microflora of the small intestine consists of a small number of aerobic, gram-positive organisms derived from the upper gastrointestinal tract. In bacterial overgrowth, these are replaced by anaerobic, facultative gram-negative organisms, especially *Escherichia, Bacteroides,* and *Clostridium* spp. at $>10^5$ colony-forming units/mL on culture [1]. Bacterial overgrowth may also occur in segments of the intestinal tract excluded surgically (*e.g.*, by a Billroth II procedure) or due to fistualizations (*e.g.*, Crohn's disease).

Symptoms

• Many patients are asymptomatic and suffer no adverse effects.

• Bacterial overgrowth of the proximal small intestine tends to produce more marked symptoms than overgrowth of the distal small bowel.

Diarrhea: watery, without blood.

Abdominal pain, weight loss, nausea, and vomiting.

Signs

Steatorrhea: bulky, oily stools.

Anemia: megaloblastic, secondary to vitamin B_{12} deficiency.

Ataxia, neuropathy: due to vitamin B_{12} deficiency.

Fevers, peritoneal signs of bleeding: suggest an alternative diagnosis.

Ecchymosis: vitamin K deficiency.

Investigations

• Diagnosis is often rendered solely on symptoms and signs in susceptible patients in whom other competing diagnoses have been eliminated.

Complete blood count: macrocytic anemia present in those with long-standing disease.

Vitamin B_{12} measurement: concentration low or normal.

Serum or erythrocyte folate measurement: concentration high or normal; "inverted" profile (*i.e.*, elevated folate with low B_{12}), suggestive but nonspecific marker.

Schilling test with intrinsic factor: absorption not corrected; also found in terminal ileal disease.

Qualitative (*i.e.*, spot) fecal fat analysis with Sudan red: marker for neutral stool fat.

3-day fecal fat collection: useful but unpopular test to quantify steatorrhea.

Barium follow-through: for jejunal diverticulosis, strictures, and fistulas; delayed transit of barium through small intestine indirect evidence of impaired motility.

Duodenal aspiration: gold standard for culture and species identification; presence of detectable concentrations of unconjugated bile acids and short chain fatty acids can provide useful adjunct, although these tests are not widely available; false-negative results do not exclude bacterial overgrowth distal to ligament of Treitz.

Duodenal biopsy: to assess villous architecture and exclude parasitic infestation (*i.e.*, giardiasis, Whipple's disease, celiac sprue).

Breath tests: simple, noninvasive, and increasingly available; early rise of breath hydrogen after lactulose or glucose, ^{14}C D-xylose or ^{14}C glycocholic acid.

Complications

• In patients with long-standing symptoms, complications result in chronic malnutrition and debility.

Secondary weight loss: if food exacerbates abdominal pain.

Subacute combined degeneration of spinal cord: after profound vitamin B_{12} deficiency (rare).

Dehydration.

Treatment

Diet and lifestyle

• A high-protein, high-energy, high-fat diet is recommended.

• Vitamin supplementation, especially injections of vitamin B_{12} and fat-soluble vitamins (A, E, D, K), or oral iron may be beneficial.

• Total parenteral nutrition is rarely necessary.

• Lactose is poorly tolerated during periods of bacterial overgrowth.

Pharmacological treatment

• Treatment is often empirical, the diagnosis being made by observing improvement in symptoms and biochemical abnormalities after treatment.

Antibiotics

Standard dosage
Trimethoprim, 160 mg/sulfamethoxazole, 800 mg twice daily.
Metronidazole, 500 mg 3 times daily.
Tetracycline, 250 mg 4 times daily.
Ciprofloxacin, 500 mg twice daily (1-week course usually adequate).
2-week course may be adequate, but maintenance with alternating courses of two agents may be needed.

Contraindications
Trimethoprim/sulfamethoxazole: sensitivity to sulfa.
Metronidazole: pregnancy, lactation.
Tetracycline: renal insufficiency, children aged <12 years, lactation.
Ciprofloxacin: children or adolescents, glucose 6-phosphate dehydrogenase deficiency, epilepsy, lactation.

Special points
Metronidazole: Antabuse (disulfiram-like) effect with alcohol.
Tetracycline: permanent tooth discoloration if used during dental development.
Ciprofloxacin: causes arthropathy in immature animals.

Main drug interactions
Trimethoprim/sulfamethoxazole: potentiates anticoagulant effect of warfarin, prolongs half-life of phenytoin and sulfonylureas.
Metronidazole: potentiates warfarin.
Tetracyclines: calcium, magnesium, iron, and aluminum salts (*e.g.*, milk, antacids) impair absorption.
Ciprofloxacin: magnesium, aluminium salts inhibit absorption; theophylline levels raised; anticoagulants potentiated.

Main side effects
Metronidazole: metallic taste (meteorism), furred tongue, peripheral neuropathy with prolonged use.
Tetracyclines: gastrointestinal disturbances, photosensitive rash, hypersensitivity (rare).
Ciprofloxacin: gastrointestinal symptoms, rashes, restlessness, dizziness, pruritis, tremor, convulsions.

Treatment aims

To clear and prevent recurrence of bacterial overgrowth.
To reduce diarrhea.
To correct hematological abnormalities and secondary nutritional deficiencies.

Other treatments

Surgery to correct underlying anatomical abnormality; may cause prolonged post-operative ileus.

Prognosis

• The prognosis depends on the underlying disease: motility disorders have the worst prognosis.

Follow-up and management

• Regular infrequent outpatient follow-up may be needed to monitor for symptoms and to detect relapses early.

• Long-term maintenance antibiotic treatment is only rarely needed, and surgical treatment is a consideration for patients refractory to medical management.

Key references

1. Kirsch M: Bacterial overgrowth. *Am J Gastroenterol* 1990, **85**:231–237.

2. Cook GC: Hypochlorhydria and vulnerability to intestinal infection. *Eur J Gastroenterol Hepatol* 1994, **6**:693–695.

3. Fried M, *et al.*: Duodenal bacterial overgrowth during treatment in outpatients with omeprazole. *Gut* 1994, **35**:23–26.

4. Larner AJ, Hamilton MIR: Infective complications of therapeutic gastric inhibition. *Aliment Pharmacol Ther* 1994, **8**:579–584.

Diagnosis

Symptoms

Patient concern regarding clinical appearance and/or progressive growth of a suspicious lesion.

Signs

Skin findings

Papules: typically pink- to flesh-colored with a translucent surface and overlying telangiectatic vessels; may have a rolled border and central ulceration; may bleed intermittently; occur on sun-exposed areas of the head, neck, and upper trunk; most common location is the face, especially the nose.

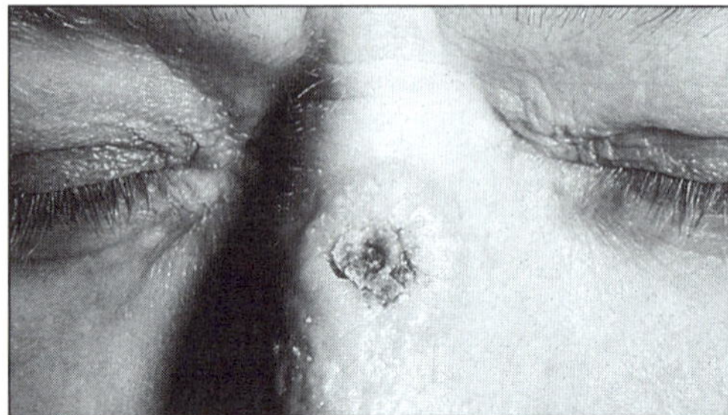

Classic basal cell carcinoma. (*See* Color Plate.)

Clinical variants

Superficial basal cell carcinoma (BCC): frequently occurs as a dry, scaly psoriasis-like lesion on the covered portions of the trunk; edge of lesion shows a thread-like raised border; may show central atrophy.

Pigmented BCC: shows brown or black pigmentation in addition to typical features; seen more frequently in Latin Americans, Asians.

Morpheaform (sclerosing) BCC: waxy white plaque most commonly found on the head and neck; characteristically lacks a rolled border, so edges are ill-defined; resembles a small scar.

Basal cell nevus syndrome (BCNS): rare, autosomal dominant disorder of the skin and internal organs; develops before the age of 20 years; associated signs are "pitting" of the palms and soles, mandibular cysts, partial agenesis of the corpus collosum, bifid ribs, and hypertelorism; patients are also predisposed to other neoplasms, including ovarian fibroma and medulloblastoma.

Investigations

Diagnosis generally made clinically, aided by an accurate history of the duration and behavior of the lesion; predisposing etiologic factors.

• Biopsy is required for diagnosis and accurate histological classification, which may be important in choosing the method of treatment.

Complications

• A neglected BCC that slowly progresses over many years may become a large, gnawed-out mutilating lesion known as a "rodent ulcer."

• The incidence of metastases for BCC has been reported to be slightly <0.1%.

• An increased incidence of metastatic BCC has been noted in AIDS patients.

Differential diagnosis

Typical BCC
Nevus, fibrous papule, seborrheic keratosis, amelanotic melanoma.

Superficial BCC
Psoriasis, nummular eczema, Bowen's disease, extramammary Paget's disease.

Pigmented BCC
Pigmented seborrheic keratosis, malignant melanoma.

Morpheaform BCC
Scar.

Etiology [1]

Ultraviolet radiation (sunshine) most common.

Trauma.

Chronic arsenic exposure.

Genodermatoses (BCNS, albinism, xeroderma pigmentosum).

Radiation therapy (used in the treatment of acne vulgaris until 1950).

Immunosuppression (secondary to organ transplantation, chemotherapy, or AIDS).

Long-standing dermatoses (linear epidermal nevi, nevus sebaceous and porokeratosis of Mibelli may develop into BCC).

Chronic venous stasis dermatitis and stasis ulcers.

• BCNS [2]: the gene responsible for BCNS has recently been discovered to be the *PATCHED* gene, located on chromosome 9. In normal embryonic development, the *PATCHED* gene, which represses growth, works in counterbalance with the *HEDGEHOG* gene, which stimulates growth. It appears that a mutation in the *PATCHED* gene allows for the cutaneous and extracutaneous overgrowth found in the BCNS.

Epidemiology

• BCC is the most common of all human cancers.

• It affects 750 000 people yearly in the United States alone.

• It is most common in light-skinned people aged >40 years with a history or UV exposure.

• BCNS affects 1 in 56 000 individuals.

Treatment

Diet and lifestyle
• No special diet is necessary.
• Emphasize the importance of sun avoidance and sun protection. Sun protection includes the use of protective clothing (hats, long-sleeved shirts) and daily sunscreens, preferably of broad-spectrum UVA plus UVB with SPF of 15 or higher.

Surgical treatment
For high-risk BCCs [1]
• Mohs' microscopic surgery (a very precise staged method of excision) is the treatment of choice. Indications for Mohs' surgery include: location in the canthi, nasolabial folds, or postauricular folds; size >2 cm; aggressive histological growth pattern including morpheaform and keratinizing BCCs; recurrent tumors after any treatment modality; tumors arising in areas of previous radiation exposure; incompletely excised tumors; tumors with clinically ill-defined borders; tumors with perineural invasion.
Advantages: achieves the highest cure rate available (99% for primary BCCs, 94% for recurrent BCCs).
Disadvantages: cost.

For low-risk BCCs
Treatment of choice:
For lesions 5 mm–2 cm in diameter, simple elliptical excision with 2–5-mm margins.
For lesions <5 mm: punch biopsy or tangential (shave) excision with curettage and/or electrodessication of the lesion base.
Advantages: cure rate of 90%–93% for primary BCCs; less expensive than Mohs' surgery.
Disadvantages: recurrence rate up to 40% for high-risk BCCs.

For prophylaxis
• For patients with severely sun-damaged skin who are experiencing frequent precancerous and cancerous lesion, prophylaxis may be obtained with 5% 5-fluorouracil cream and low-dose isotretinoin.

Standard dosage	5-fluorouracil, topically to affected area twice daily for 2–4 weeks; may be repeated twice yearly. Low-dose isotretinoin, 10 mg/day.
Contraindications	*5-fluorouracil*: unavoidable sun exposure. *Low-dose isotretinoin*: pregnancy; use caution in pre-existing renal or hepatic disease.
Special points	*Low-dose isotretinoin*: liver function tests and serum lipoprotein levels should be monitored monthly.
Main drug interactions	*5-fluorouracil*: none. *Low-dose isotretinoin*: preparations containing high doses of vitamin A; tetracycline, minocycline, trimethoprim-sulfamethoxazole in combination with isotretinoin may cause benign intracranial hypertension.
Main side effects	*5-fluorouracil*: extensive swelling, erosions, and pain 3–5 days after the start of treatment; may require analgesics, topical steroids, oral and/or topical antibiotics; ideally treatment should be carried out in the winter; patients usually cannot tolerate the use of sunscreen on areas undergoing 5-fluorouracil therapy until they heal; contact dermatitis may develop with repeated courses of 5-fluorouracil; diagnostic clues include development of pruritis and extension of the erythema and crusts beyond the treated areas. *Low-dose isotretinoin*: fetal death and malformation, elevated liver enzymes, triglycerides, and cholesterol; however, side effects are significantly less common with lower dosages.

For patients with BCNS
• A team approach is required [3].
• Current management recommendations include regular visits to a dermatologist every 2–3 months beginning in adolescence or earlier as necessary with simple excision or Mohs' microscopic surgery for developing BCCs.
• Patients should have yearly panoramic radiographs of the jaws with referral to an oral surgeon for excision if odontogenic cysts are found.
• Infants at risk should have an annual MRI to exclude medulloblastoma and periodic radiographs to rule out skeletal anomalies and cardiac fibromas.
• Photodynamic therapy is a relatively new form of cancer treatment that may be effective in adults with BCNS.
• Management should always include appropriate genetic counseling because each affected individual carries a 50% risk of transmitting the disease to his/her children.

Key references
1. Carter D, Lin A: Basal cell carcinoma. In *Dermatology in General Medicine*, edn 4, vol 1. New York: McGraw-Hill; 1993:840–847.
2. Nelson B: Malignant cutaneous tumors. *Dermatol Focus* 1996, 15:1–7.
3. Walker D, Tschen J: Basal cell carcinoma: predisposing genetic syndromes and clinical association. In *Cutaneous Oncology*. Hartford, CT: Andover Publishing Service; in press.

Diagnosis

Symptoms [1]

Obstructive
Sensation of incomplete bladder emptying, decreased force of urine stream, straining to urinate, dribbling.

Irritative
Urgency, frequency, nocturia, dysuria.

• Self-administered questionnaire to evaluate symptom severity and response to therapy is shown in the table [2].

American Urological Association Symptom Index

Over the past month or so, how often have you:	Possible answers for questions 1–6:
1. Had the sensation of not emptying your bladder completely after you finished urinating?	0=Not at all.
2. Had to urinate again less than 2 hours after you finished urinating?	1=Less than one time in 5.
	2=Less than half the time.
3. Found you stopped and started again several times when you urinated?	3=About half the time.
4. Found it difficult to postpone urination?	4=More than half the time.
5. Had a weak urinary stream?	5=Almost always.
6. Had to push or strain to begin urination?	
7. Over the past month, how many times did you typically get up to urinate from the time you went to bed at night to the time you got up in the morning?	Possible answers: 0,1,2,3,4, ≥5 times

Symptom score (sum of all the answers): Mild symptoms: 0–7 points; Moderate symptoms: 8–19 points; Severe symptoms: 20–35 points

---

Signs

• None; size of prostate on physical examination does not correlate with symptoms.

Investigations [1]

For all patients
Comprehensive history and physical examination.

Detailed urinary history: with focus on symptom severity using American Urological Association (AUA) symptom index.

Digital rectal examination and focused neurological examination: perineal sensation, rectal tone, presence of diabetic neuropathy.

Urinalysis and sediment examination: to rule out infection or hematuria.

Serum creatinine: to assess renal function

Additional studies if clinically indicated
Postvoid residual (PVR) urine volume if concern for large retained urine volumes: palpable bladder, overflow incontinence.

Pressure-flow studies: if there is concern for primary bladder dysfunction from neurological disease.

Urethrocystoscopy: if surgical therapy is planned.

• Prostate-specific antigen (PSA) testing is optional, because benign prostatic hypertrophy (BPH) may raise PSA levels; therefore PSA does not discriminate well between BPH and early prostate cancer.

Complications

Acute urinary obstruction: may be precipitated by alcohol, sedatives, sympathomimetics, or anticholinergics.

Obstructive uropathy with chronic renal insufficiency: rare.

Urinary tract infections and bladder decompensation: rare.

Bladder stones: 1%–2% found at time of prostate surgery.

Differential diagnosis

Dysuria: urinary tract infection.

Urgency, frequency: infection, excessive caffeine intake.

Polyuria: diabetes mellitus, diabetes insipidus, hypercalcemia.

Bladder tumor.

Detrusor muscle instability.

Neurological bladder dysfunction, such as neurogenic bladder with diabetes or spasticity with prior cerebrovascular accident.

Etiology

Hyperplasia of prostatic tissue, both stromal and epithelial components.

Risk factors are advancing age and presence of androgens.

Epidemiology

• Histologic evidence of BPH is evident in 10% of men at age 30 years, >50% at age 60, >90% at age 85.

• Only 50% of patients with histological evidence of BPH have clinical symptoms.

• 10% of men with BPH will require transurethral resection of prostate (TURP) for urinary obstruction.

• 400 000 surgical procedures are performed per year in the United States.

Treatment

Diet and lifestyle
- Avoidance of caffeine may improve frequency, urgency.
- Avoid fluid intake after dinner to decrease nocturia.

Decision making
- For mild symptoms (AUA scores 0–7) watchful waiting is appropriate.
- For moderate to severe symptoms (AUA scores 8–35), risks and benefits of surgery vs. watchful waiting vs. medical therapy should be discussed.

Pharmacological treatment [1]

Alpha-blockers
Standard dosage	Prazosin, doxazosin, or terazosin decrease symptoms; terazosin doses titrated from 1 to 5–10 mg every night.
Contraindications	Known hypersensitivity, hypotension, or postural hypotension.
Special points	First-dose hypotension (1%–2%), orthostasis best prevented by nightly dosing, caution in the elderly.
Main drug interactions	Caution with other antihypertensive medications.
Main side effects	Aesthenia (6%–10%), postural hypotension (6%–8%), dizziness (5%–10%), rhinitis (6%–8%).

Finasteride
Standard dosage	5–10 mg daily.
Contraindications	Known hypersensitivity.
Special points	Only beneficial in patients with enlarged prostates and moderate to severe symptoms.
Main drug interactions	None.
Main side effects	Sexual dysfunction, loss of libido (3%–5%)

Intermittent straight-catheterization
Treatment of choice for patient with high PVR on maximal medical therapy who declines or is not a surgical candidate.

Indications for referral to urologist
If diagnosis uncertain, especially if neurological bladder dysfunction is suspected secondary to CVA or diabetes.

Refractory urinary retention on maximal medical therapy.

Recurrent urinary tract infections.

Recurrent gross hematuria.

Bladder stones.

Renal insufficiency secondary to BPH.

Refractory symptoms despite maximal medical therapy.

Treatment aims

To relieve symptoms.
To improve quality of life.
To prevent infections and renal insufficiency.

Surgical therapy with TURP

Effective for symptoms in 80%–90%.
Postoperative mortality 0.2%–1.5%.
Retrograde ejaculation (75%).
Impotence (13%).
Urethral stricture (3%–5%).
Partial to complete incontinence (2%–5%).

Prognosis

- Disease progresses slowly and is quite variable among patients.
- Spontaneous improvement in symptoms common (30%–50%).

Follow-up and management

Regular review of symptoms and response to therapy.

Key references

1. McConnell JD, *et al.*: Benign prostatic hyperplasia: diagnosis and treatment. In *Clinical Practice Guideline*, no 8. Rockville, MD: Agency for Health Care Policy and Research (AHCPR), Public Health Service, U.S. Department of Health and Human Services. [AHCPR publication no 94-0582.]

2. Barry MJ, *et al.*: The American Urologic Association Symptom Index for benign prostatic hyperplasia. *J Urol* 1992, **148**:1549–1557.

Diagnosis

Symptoms
•Symptoms of breast cancer are few. Some patients may note a mildly tender lump under the arm or in the breast.

Signs
•Signs are not always manifest.

Breast lump.

Abnormal skin over breast: dimpling, ulceration, edema, erythema.

Fixation of mass to chest wall.

Nipple changes: retraction, discoloration, erosion, discharge.

Adenopathy: axillary, cervical, supraclavicular, infraclavicular.

Investigations

For diagnosis
Bilateral mammography.

Needle aspiration of breast mass with cytological examination: 95% sensitivity; rapid, inexpensive, and painless; will not distinguish carcinoma in situ from invasive carcinoma.

Stereotactic core biopsy: more painful, but has lower false-negative rate than needle aspiration.

Excisional biopsy: provides optimum pathological specimen, but is more painful and has cosmetic effects.

For staging
Axillary node dissection with pathological examination of 10–20 nodes.

Chest radiography.

Complete blood, differential, and platelet counts: persistently abnormal complete blood count may be an indicator of bone-marrow involvement; bone-marrow biopsy should be performed.

Liver function tests: may indicate liver metastasis.

Bone scan for suspected stage III disease.

Head CT scan or MRI: if neurological symptoms are present.

Special investigations
Tumor estrogen and progesterone receptor status: useful in determining response to hormonal therapy with tamoxifen.

Breast cancer antigen (CA 15-3) tumor marker level: useful more as a marker during follow-up examination of disease progression in patients with breast cancer.

BRCA1 and *BRCA2* **mutation analysis:** useful in familial breast cancer analysis.

Complications
Pain.

Pleural or pericardial effusion.

Metastases to bone, brain, liver.

Recurrent venous thrombosis.

Pathological fracture.

Differential diagnosis
Fibrocystic disease.

Mastitis.

Other tumors: lymphoma, sarcoma, melanoma, phyllodes tumors.

Etiology
• The cause of breast cancer is unknown but is presumed to be due to genetic mutations, the risk of which is increased by DNA damage.

• Patients who carry the *BRCA1* mutation have a 50% risk of developing breast cancer by age 45 years and an 85% lifetime risk of breast cancer. Increased risk is also conferred by the presence of the *BRCA2* mutation.

Epidemiology
• Breast cancer tumors are the most common tumors in women in the United States and account for 25% of all cancers in women.

• An association exists between breast cancer and a high-fat diet, chronic alcohol ingestion, age of menarche and menopause, and age at birth of first full-term child. There is a more controversial association with estrogen supplementation and high-fat diet.

• Women with a first-degree relative with breast cancer have a 2–3-fold increased risk for breast cancer.

Treatment

Diet and lifestyle
• Weight loss is not generally significant unless it is related to complications of chemotherapy.

• Patients should be encouraged to be active.

Treatment
• Treatment is dependent on disease stage, age, and tumor histology.

• Treatment should be given under specialist supervision.

Surgery
• Surgery is the mainstay of therapy, with procedures ranging from partial mastectomy to modified radical mastectomy available.

• Breast conserving surgeries with or without radiation are possible when the tumor is small, but are contraindicated when the disease is multifocal or associated with diffuse indeterminate calcifications on mammogram.

• Axillary lymph node resection with removal of 10–20 nodes is performed at the time of definitive surgery, but may not be done in patients who are aged >65 years with no palpable nodes.

Radiation therapy
• Radiation therapy is used to prevent local recurrence following surgery.

• Some studies suggest radiation therapy can be omitted in postmenopausal women if the tumor is <2.5 cm and a quadrantectomy is performed.

Chemotherapy
• Complex decision making is based on disease stage, but chemotherapy may be administered in node-negative patients who are considered high risk.

• Adjuvant chemotherapy generally consists of a combination of two or more of the following agents: cyclophosphamide, methotrexate, vincristine, doxorubicin, 5-fluorouracil, or prednisone.

• Chemotherapy is the mainstay of stage IV disease and may include paclitaxel or mitomycin C.

Hormonal therapy
• Adjuvant tamoxifen hormonal therapy is used in postmenopausal women of all stages and may also be used in premenopausal patients with breast cancer that is estrogen receptor–positive.

• Luteinizing hormone–releasing analogs, aminoglutethimide, and progestins are additional agents used in stage IV disease.

Complications of therapy
Lymphedema after axillary node dissection, accelerated coronary artery disease after radiation to chest, osteoporosis, bladder dysfunction, hot flashes, vaginal dryness, emotional lability on antiestrogen therapy.

• Hypercalcemia and accelerated bone pain is sometimes seen with tamoxifen therapy.

Treatment aims
To identify patients with surgically resectable disease at the earliest stage.

To identify patients with more indolent disease histologies who do not require aggressive surgical management or adjuvant chemotherapy.

To prevent distant metastasis through adjuvant therapy.

To provide emotional support.

Prognosis
• Prognosis is directly related to the number of positive axillary nodes, tumor size, tumor histology and nuclear grade, and estrogen receptor status.

• Ductal carcinoma in situ has a 98% cure rate with local and regional therapy alone.

• Five-year survival for stages I–IIIB are 90%, 80%, 65%, 50%, and 40%, respectively.

Follow-up and management
Patients must be followed up regularly for local and distant recurrence and side effects of therapy.

Relapsed disease
• Chemotherapy is palliative in stage IV disease with a median duration of response of 9–12 months.

• High-dose chemotherapy with autologous bone-marrow transplant shows promise with 30% of patients who achieve complete cancer-free remission at 3 years.

General references

Donegan WL: Tumor-related prognostic factors for breast cancer. *Cancer* 1997, **47**:28–51.

Feig SA: Mammographic screening of women aged 40–49 years: benefit, risk and cost considerations. *Cancer* 1995, **76(suppl 10)**:2097–2106.

Phillips DM, Balducci L: Current management of breast cancer. *Am Fam Physician* 1996, **53**:657–665.

Veronesi U, Luini A, Del Vecchio M, *et al.*: Radiotherapy after breast preserving surgery in women with localized cancer of the breast. *N Engl J Med* 1993, **328**:1587–1591.

Diagnosis

Symptoms

Cough, purulent, large-volume sputum, episodic fever or malaise, night sweats, nasal discharge, possibly with purulent sinusitis, dyspnea, recurrent hemoptysis, pleuritic chest pain, recurrent pneumonia.

Weight loss, anemia: often seen.

Signs

Clubbing, rhonchi, coarse crackles, tachypnea, hyperinflation, signs of weight loss.

Foul-smelling plegm: classically separates into three layers.

Investigations [1]

Sputum culture: for *Staphylococcus aureus*, *Haemophilus influenzae*, and *Pseudomonas* spp. and to exclude active tuberculosis.

Sputum cytology: to exclude malignancy.

Serum immunoglobulin measurement.

Chest radiography: shows hyperinflation, crowded lung markings, and ring shadows.

High-resolution CT: shows ring and cystic lesions and bronchial wall thickening.

Respiratory function tests: for obstructive or mixed ventilatory defect.

Aspergillus skin and precipitin tests.

Complications

Infective exacerbations: viral or bacterial.

Pneumothorax.

Respiratory failure.

Cor pulmonale.

Empyema.

Chest pain: usually pleuritic, associated with an area of bronchiectasis.

Hemoptysis.

Metastatic spread of infection: now rare; brain abscess was classic complication.

Arthropathy: rheumatoid arthritis and nonspecific seronegative arthritis related to activity of disease.

Amyloidosis.

Differential diagnosis

Asthma.
Interstitial fibrosis.
Chronic bronchitis.
Lung carcinoma.
Sinusitis with chronic cough.

Etiology [2,3]

• Bronchiectasis is caused by recurrent inflammation or infection. Congenital causes include cystic fibrosis, immunodeficiency states and alpha$_1$ antitrypsin deficiency.

• Acquired causes include defective mucociliary clearance, bronchial obstruction, inflammatory pneumonitis, fibrotic or granulomatous lung disease, previous severe infection, allergic aspergillosis, and acquired immunodeficiency (*e.g.*, AIDS, chemotherapy).

Epidemiology

• The estimated prevalence of bronchiectasis is declining with the advent of modern antibiotics.

Associated diseases

Rheumatoid arthritis.
Purulent sinusitis.
Allergic bronchopulmonary aspergillosis.
Malignancy.
Connective tissue disorders.
Vasculitis.
Infertility.
Primary ciliary dyskinesia.
Immune deficiency syndromes.

Treatment

Diet and lifestyle

• Adequate nutrition is important.

Pharmacological treatment [3,4]

General guidelines

• Treatment specific to the underlying cause includes the following:

Removal of foreign body or inspissated mucus.

Replacement of immunoglobulins: for panhypogammaglobulinemia, selective IgM and IgG, and possibly IgG_2 deficiency, but not for selective IgA deficiency (risk of anaphylaxis).

Treatment of associated conditions, *e.g.*, rheumatoid arthritis.

Antibiotics: drug choice based on sputum culture; given either for exacerbations or at regular intervals; courses should last 2–3 weeks, and antimicrobial agents should be given in high doses; for patients colonized with *Pseudomonas* spp., specific antipseudomonal antibiotics should be given, including nebulized antibiotics, *e.g.*, gentamycin, for maintenance treatment between courses.

Bronchodilators: for patients with demonstrable airflow obstruction.

Steroids: improved morbidity in short term, but effects on prognosis not known; inhaled steroids recommended for patients with prominent or reversible airflow obstruction.

Nonpharmacological treatment

Physical therapy

• Physical therapy is the main form of nonpharmacological treatment.

• Methods include postural drainage, deep cough, and forced expiratory maneuvers twice daily.

Other options

For hemoptysis: bed rest and antibiotics, selective embolization, intubation and balloon tamponade, or local resection.

For pneumothorax: aspiration, intercostal drainage, pleurodesis or partial pleurectomy (if recurrent or unresponsive).

For respiratory failure: supplemental oxygen therapy, nasal ventilation.

For severe localized disease: surgery.

Lung transplantation.

Treatment aims

To minimize lung damage by limiting pulmonary infection and increasing clearance of pulmonary secretion.

Prognosis

• The prognosis of bronchiectasis depends on the severity of the disease.

Follow-up and management

• All patients with moderate to severe bronchiectasis need regular care from a respiratory physician.

Patient support

Counselling regarding lung transplantation, fears of dying, reproduction, etc.

Key references

1. Smith IE, Flower CD: Review article: imaging in bronchiectasis. *Br J Radiol* 1996, **69**:589–593.

2. Barker AF, Bardana EJ: Bronchiectasis: update of an orphan disease. *Am Rev Respir Dis* 1988, **137**:969–978.

3. Weg J: Bronchiectasis. *Semin Respir Med* 1992, **13**:177–189.

4. Nicotra MD: Bronchiectasis. *Semin Respir Infect* 1994: **9**:31–40.

Diagnosis

Symptoms

Pemphigus vulgaris
Painful oral ulcers; erosions of mucous membranes; weeping, uncomfortable skin erosions.

Bullous pemphigoid
Large, tense blisters on the skin: gradually expanding and uncomfortable.
Oral symptoms: occur rarely.

Dermatitis herpetiformis
Intense, severe, pruritis: seemingly out of proportion to the sparse clinical signs.

Signs [1,2]

Pemphigus vulgaris
Oral ulcerations and gingivitis: often sole manifestation of disease and precede skin involvement.
Flaccid blisters: rupture easily.

Bullous pemphigoid
Large, tense blisters: often on urticarial or erythematous bases in elderly patients.
Oral involvement: only in one-third of patients.

Dermatitis herpetiformis
Groups of papules and vesicles: on an erythematous base; often excoriated with a predilection for the extensor surfaces of the extremities and buttocks.

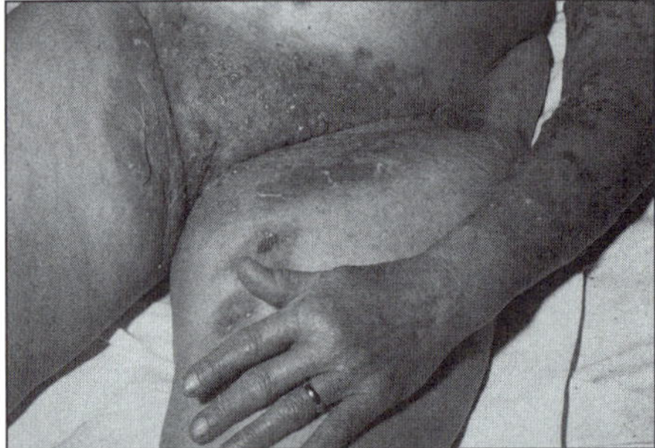

Bullous pemphigoid. (*See* Color Plate.)

Investigations

Pemphigus vulgaris
Biopsy: of perilesional skin to detect directed acantholysis (intraepidermal blister).
Direct immunofluorescence: to detect IgG and C3 directed at keratinocyte cell membranes (intraepidermal band).
Indirect immunofluorescence: to detect circulating intercellular antibodies. Initially the titers are monitored weekly and give an indication of disease activity. Following clinical remission, titers may be monitored monthly and generally parallel disease activity.

Bullous pemphigoid
Biopsy: of perilesional skin to detect subepidermal split; many eosinophils.
Direct immunofluorescence: IgG and C3 directed at the dermoepidermal junction (linear band at base of epidermis).

Dermatitis herpetiformis
Biopsy: of perilesional skin to detect papillary dermal neutrophilic abscesses (subepidermal).
Direct immunofluorescence: to detect granular deposits of IgA and C3 in the dermal papillary tips.

Complications

Pemphigus vulgaris
Secondary bacterial infection: in denuded areas.
Fluid and electrolyte imbalance: in severe cases.
Sepsis: in severe cases (especially immunosuppressed patients).
Thymoma and myasthenia gravis (unusual).

Bullous pemphigoid
Underlying occult malignancy: controversial association.
Pemphigus vulgaris, lichen planus, psoriasis: associated.

Dermatitis herpetiformis
Gluten sensitive enteropathy: in approximately 90% of cases.
Lymphoma: possible increased incidence, especially in jejunum.

Differential diagnosis
Infections: *e.g.,* varicella zoster, herpes simplex, zosteriform herpes simplex, bullous impetigo.
Bullous bite reaction (insect bites).
Drug-induced pemphigus.
Epidermolysis bullosa.
Porphyria cutanea tarda.
Pseudo–porphyria cutanea tarda.
Sweat gland necrosis.
Diabetic bullosis.
Bullous cellulitis.
Pompholyx.
Cicatricial pemphigoid.
Urticaria pigmentosa.
Bullous fixed drug reaction.

Etiology [3–5]
Pemphigus vulgaris

Molecular immunopathogenesis: autoantibody against transmembrane cadherin family of intercellular adhesion molecules (desmoglein desmosomal component).

Involves interaction of endogenous (genetic and autoimmune) and exogenous (inducing) factors. The list of factors includes drugs (especially thiols), physical injury (especially burns), neoplasms, pregnancy, contact dermatitis, nutritional factors, emotional stress, herpesvirus infections.

Bullous pemphigoid

Molecular immunopathogenesis: auto-antibody against proteins on the basilar keratinocyte that anchor keratin intermediate filaments to the basement membrane by a hemidesmosone (bullous pemphigoid antigen 1, a 230-kD intracellular protein, and bullous pemphigoid antigen 2, a 180-kD transmembrane protein).

Dermatitis herpetiformis

Molecular immunopathogenesis plus HLA-B8 and DW3-associated autoimmune disorder; also associated with gluten-sensitive enteropathy.

Epidemiology
Pemphigus vulgaris

More common in patients with Jewish or Mediterranean heritage.

Bullous pemphigoid

Most common in patients 60–70 years of age (less common variant can occur in children).

• 75% of treated patients have remission after ~5 years.

Dermatitis herpetiformis

Onset between 2–4 decades of life.

Annual incidence of 1:100 000 in Scandinavian patients.

Usually chronic when untreated.

Treatment

Diet and lifestyle

• Dietary measures applicable only in dermatitis herpetiformis, in which a gluten-free diet may be curative.

• Wound care of open erosions is essential to prevent secondary infection in all bullous diseases.

Pharmacological treatment

• Treatment should be administered by a specialist with experience in treating bullous disorders.

Gold: bone-marrow suppression, renal toxicity, cutaneous allergic reactions.

• Systemic steroids are the mainstay of therapy for moderate to severe pemphigus vulgaris and bullous pemphigoid.

• Other drugs listed may be used as steroid-sparing agents, adjunctive or maintenance therapy.

• Dapsone is the treatment of choice for dermatitis herpetiformis.

Standard dosage	Prednisone, 80–160 mg orally, daily initially to control; then 40–60 mg daily; then, taper as tolerated to a maintenance dose of 5–10 mg daily. Cyclophosphamide, 100–200 mg orally daily. Azathioprine, 100–200 mg orally daily. Gold sodium thiomalate, 10 mg i.m. initial test dose; followed by 25 mg at weeks 2 and 3; then 25–50 mg i.m. every week. Dapsone, 100 mg orally, daily; may have to increase dose up to 400 mg daily; can often lower the dose in patients on gluten-free diet [6,7].
Contraindications	*Prednisone*: gastric ulcers, underlying infections, hypertension, diabetes, history of tuberculosis. *Cyclophosphamide, azathioprine*: pregnancy. *Gold*: pregnancy. *Dapsone*: pregnancy.
Special points	Only those physicians with experience and training to monitor these diseases and the drugs used to treat them should follow-up these patients.
Main drug interactions	*Azathioprine*: allopurinol enhances effect and increases toxicity.
Main side effects	*Prednisone*: weight gain, hypertension, diabetes, fragile skin, decreased wound healing, adrenal suppression. *Cyclophosphamide, azathioprine*: bone-marrow suppression, hemorrhagic cystitis, potential for malignancy. *Dapsone*: gastrointestinal upset (common), hemolytic anemia in patients with glucose-6-phosphate dehydrogenase deficiency, agranulocytosis, methemoglobinemia; peripheral neuropathy.

Other treatments

Plasmapheresis.

Extracorporeal immunoabsorption of autoantibodies.

Intravenous gammaglobulin.

Prognosis

Pemphigus vulgaris
• Mortality rate is <10% today.
• Patients do very well with close control and monitoring of this chronic disease.

Bullous pemphigoid
• It is usually self-limited, with remission in 75% of patients in 3–6 years.
• Mortality rate of 10%–20% is related to systemic steroid treatment.

Dermatitis herpetiformis
• It has a chronic course when untreated, with temporary remission.
• It appears to be a risk of bowel lymphoma.
• Response to dapsone is dramatic; pruritis and skin lesions resolve within the first week of therapy.

Follow-up and management
• Long-term follow-up by a specialist is advised.

Key references

1. Crosby DL, Diaz LA: Introduction. *Dermatol Clin* 1993, **2**:373–378.

2. Guidice GJ, Diaz LA: New laboratory methods in the investigation of bullous diseases. *Dermatol Clin* 1993, **2**:419–427.

3. Giudice GJ, *et al.*: Development of an ELISA to detect anti-BP180 autoantibodies in bullous pemphigoid and herpes gestationis. *J Invest Dermatol* 1994, **102**:878–881.

4. Klatte DH, Jones JC: Purification of the 230kD bullous pemphigoid antigen (BP230) from bovine tongue mucosa: structural analyses and assessment of BP230 tissue distribution using a monoclonal antibody. *J Invest Dermatol* 1994, **102**:39–44.

5. Beutner EH, Jordon RE: Demonstration of skin antibodies in sera of pemphigus vulgaris patients by indirect immunofluorescent staining. *Proc Soc Exp Biol Med* 1964, **117**:505–510.

6. Zuidema J, *et al.*: Clinical pharmacokinetics of dapsone. *Clin Pharmacokinet* 1986, **11**:299–315.

7. Stern RS: Systemic dapsone. *Arch Dermatol* 1993, **129**:301–303.

Diagnosis

Symptoms

- 30% of patients are asymptomatic.

Altered taste sensation.

Oral discomfort or pain.

Coated mouth or tongue.

Dysphagia.

Odynophagia.

Loss of appetite.

Signs

Angular cheilitis.

Intraoral removable white plaques, with erythematous underlying mucosa.

Intraoral mucosal ulceration or erythema with or without whitish plaques.

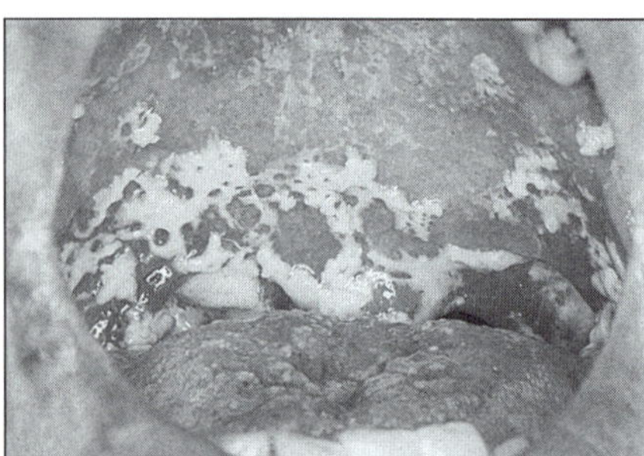 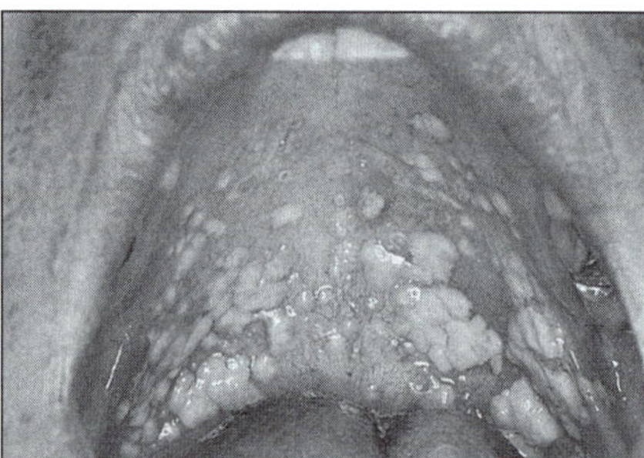

Curdish white plaques of pseudomembranous candidiasis. (*See* Color Plates.)

Investigations

Buccal candidiasis

- The diagnosis is usually obvious without further investigation.

Direct microscopy: direct staining of mouth scraping with hydrogen peroxide or Gram stain rapidly confirms presence of fungal hyphae.

Mouth swab or washings: to determine sensitivity of *Candida* spp.

Esophageal candidiasis

Fiberoptic endoscopy: allows direct visualization of esophageal involvement, with biopsy confirming diagnosis; should be considered gold standard.

Barium-swallow radiography: can highlight linear filling defects.

Complications

Oral ulceration.

Weight loss: secondary to depressed appetite.

Esophageal obstruction: rarely, secondary to overgrowth of *Candida* spp. (systemic dissemination unusual).

Differential diagnosis

Oral hairy leukoplakia.

HIV-related gingivitis, periodontitis, herpes simplex, or giant aphthous ulcers.

Cytomegalovirus ulceration, Kaposi's sarcoma, or lymphoma.

Etiology

- Candidiasis is the overgrowth and invasion of mucosal surfaces by *Candida albicans* or occasionally other *Candida* spp. The emergence of clinical disease is related to the loss of cell-mediated immunity and not to the presence of more virulent *Candida* strains.

- In HIV infection, buccal candidiasis is often seen when the number of circulating CD4 lymphocytes is $<350 \times 10^6$/L , and esophageal candidiasis is seen when CD4 cells are $<250 \times 10^6$/L .

Epidemiology

- *C. albicans* is a normal commensal of the mouth and can be cultured from 30% of the population.

- Although both buccal and esophageal candidiasis have been described during acute primary infection with HIV, they are generally associated with moderate to severe immunodeficiency 4–10 years after initial infection.

- 90% of HIV-infected patients develop candidiasis at some stage of their illness.

- Esophageal, bronchopulmonary, or invasive candidiasis is classified as an AIDS-defining opportunistic infection.

Treatment

Diet and lifestyle

No special precautions are necessary.

Pharmacological treatment

Topical antifungals

• Nystatin and clotrimazole are of benefit in cases of buccal candidiasis; however, they do not treat any esophageal involvement.

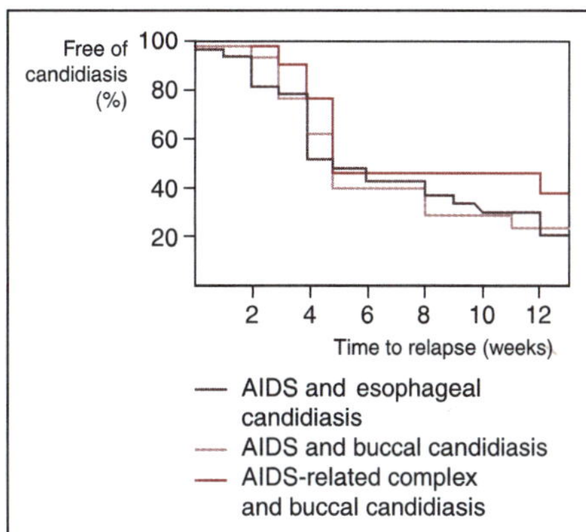

Patients free of relapse after clinical and myco-logical clearance.

Fluconazole

• Fluconazole is effective for all esophageal candidiasis and oral candidiasis unresponsive to topical agents. Improvement results in 3–5 days. It is predominantly renally excreted so the patient does not suffer from hepatic metabolism problems.

Standard dosage	Fluconazole, 100 mg daily for 1 week for oral candidiasis, 3 weeks for esophageal candidiasis.
Contraindications	Azole hypersensitivity.
Special points	Reduced dose in patients with renal impairment.
Main drug interactions	Pentamidine, amphotericin-induced nephrotoxicity may impair renal excretion.
Main side effects	Abnormalities in liver function (higher doses), rashes.

Itraconazole

• Itraconazole is used in patients who cannot tolerate fluconazole (70% response rates at 1 week and 90% at 1 month) and is less hepatotoxic than ketoconazole.

Standard dosage	Itraconazole, 200 mg daily for 1–4 weeks.
Contraindications	Azole hypersensitivity.
Special points	An oral suspension is available with better absorption features.
Main drug interactions	Decreased absorption with antacids, cimetidine, or omeprazole; increased metabolism with rifampicin, rifabutin, or phenytoin.
Main side effects	Rash, nausea.

General references

Klein RS, et al.: Oral candidiasis in high risk patients as the initial manifestation of the acquired immunodeficiency syndrome. *N Engl J Med* 1984, **311**:354-358.

Barbara G, Barbiremi G, Di Lorenzo G: Fluconazole vs. itraconazole-flucytosine association in the treatment of esophageal candidiasis in AIDS patients: a double-blind multicenter, placebo-controlled study. *Chest* 1996, **110**:1507–1514.

Greenspan D, Greenspan JS: HIV-related oral disease. *Lancet* 1996, **348**:729–733.

Diagnosis

Symptoms

- Dilated cardiomyopathy starts as asymptomatic left ventricular dysfunction.
- Cardiac failure is defined as symptomatic left ventricular dysfunction.

Exertional fatigue, dyspnea, ankle edema: major symptoms.

Nocturia, urinary frequency, chest discomfort: less common symptoms.

Signs

Cardiac failure

- Cardiac failure can be free of objective signs.

Edema, raised jugular venous pressure, lung crepitations: signs of fluid retention.

Cold clammy skin, low blood pressure: signs of impaired perfusion.

Displaced left ventricular apex, right ventricular heave, third or fourth heart sound, functional mitral or tricuspid regurgitation, tachycardia: signs of ventricular dysfunction.

Underlying disorder

Valvular disease.

Atherosclerotic vascular disease.

Severe hypertension.

Severe anemia or volume overload: *e.g.*, arteriovenous shunt.

Pathological arrhythmia.

Evidence of generalized myopathy or poisoning.

Investigations

Chest radiography, echocardiography, cardiopulmonary exercise testing: to confirm diagnosis.

ECG: to look for underlying cause, *e.g.*, ischemia or infarction, left ventricular hypertrophy, arrhythmia, other causes of pathological Q waves.

Echocardiography: to look for valvular disease; differentiates globally impaired left ventricle (*e.g.*, dilated cardiomyopathy) from segmental dysfunction (*e.g.*, ischemic heart disease).

Blood tests: for rare causes, *e.g.*, hypocalcemic cardiomyopathy, thyroid heart disease, iron-storage diseases, anemia, heavy metal poisons, amyloid (serum electrophoresis, rectal biopsy), sarcoid (serum angiotensin-converting enzyme); for associated disease; renal, liver, and electrolyte disturbances common.

Coronary angiography: occasionally, to identify ischemic heart failure.

Ventricular biopsy: rarely, for specific myocarditis, especially viral.

Radionuclide ventriculography or echocardiography: for ejection fraction, to quantitate severity of systolic dysfunction.

24-hour Holter ECG monitoring: for ventricular arrhythmias.

Complications

Atrial and ventricular brady- and tachyarrhythmias: especially atrial fibrillation and ventricular tachycardia.

Peripheral emboli, postural hypotension.

Renal failure.

Hepatic congestion and dysfunction.

Poor gastrointestinal absorption.

Muscle wasting, tissue abnormalities, oxidative enzyme depletion, early fatigue.

Pulmonary congestion, nonasthmatic bronchial constriction, respiratory muscle weakness.

Pulmonary hypertension and right ventricular failure: rare.

Differential diagnosis

Chronic lung disease.

Psychogenic dyspnea.

Etiology

Ischemic heart disease: in 40%–70% of patients.

Hypertension: in 10%–30%.

Idiopathic, alcoholic, puerperal, or familial dilated cardiomyopathy: in 10%–20%.

Valvular heart disease: in 5%–10%.

Postviral myocarditis: possibly in 1%–10% (but presumed cause for many idiopathic).

HIV-related.

Epidemiology

- 1% of the general adult population suffers from cardiac failure or dilated cardiomyopathy.

- The incidence increases with age (>10% in people aged ≥ 80 years).

Treatment

Diet and lifestyle

• Patients should be encouraged to restrict sodium and alcohol intake and to maintain ideal weight. Advanced disease may require fluid restriction.

• Patients with stable moderate cardiac failure should undertake exercise training; patients with unstable cardiac failure or intercurrent illness should rest.

Pharmacological treatment

Diuretics

• Patients with fluid retention should be given thiazides for mild disease, loop diuretics for moderate disease, or combinations of loop, thiazide, and potassium-sparing agents for severe cardiac failure; metolazone is particularly effective with loop diuretics.

Standard dosage	Depends on degree of fluid retention.
Contraindications	Renal failure, hypokalemia (both relative).
Main drug interactions	Low potassium with digoxin.
Main side effects	Hypokalemia, renal impairment.

Angiotensin-converting enzyme inhibitors

• These are used for symptomatic heart failure without contraindications and asymptomatic left ventricular dysfunction in some patients (*e.g.*, after myocardial infarction).

Standard dosage	Higher doses, *e.g.*, captopril 25–50 mg 3 times daily, or enalapril, 10 mg twice daily.
Contraindications	Worsening renal function, allergy, severe cough.
Main drug interactions	Hyperkalemia with potassium-sparing agents.
Main side effects	Cough, renal failure.

• For patients with intractable cough, angiotensin-2 inhibitors such as losartan hold promise for similar benefits on symptoms and survival [1].

Digoxin

• Digoxin is used to control ventricular response rate in atrial fibrillation; its role in sinus rhythm is controversial.

Standard dosage	Digoxin, 0.0625–0.25 mg daily.
Contraindications	Renal failure.
Special points	Serum concentrations must be monitored.
Main drug interactions	Diuretic-induced low potassium.
Main side effects	Arrhythmias, nausea, visual disturbances.

Beta-blockers and partial beta-agonists

• These are generally used only cautiously by heart failure specialists. Newer agents such as carvedilol hold promise over and above older beta-blockers [2].

Standard dosage	Slow-dose increments.
Contraindications	Worsening cardiac failure, heart block, asthma.
Main drug interactions	Other bradycardic agents (digoxin, some calcium antagonists).
Main side effects	Worsening cardiac failure, heart block.

Sympathomimetics and phosphodiesterase inhibitors

• Such agents are indicated only for acute short-term support, not for chronic oral administration.

• No beneficial effect has been found in ambulatory patients.

• They interact with monoamine oxidase inhibitors.

• They can cause ventricular arrhythmias.

Antiarrhythmics

• With the exception of digoxin, antiarrythmics are advisable only in symptomatic life-threatening arrhythmias. Amiodarone is probably the best choice (implantable defibrillators are an expensive alternative).

Standard dosage	Amiodarone, 100–200 mg daily.
Contraindications	Severe heart failure, heart block.
Main drug interactions	Digoxin, warfarin doses must be reduced.
Main side effects	Proarrhythmic effects, worsening heart failure, liver and lung toxicity, thyroid dysfunction.

Treatment aims

To alleviate symptoms.

To delay disease progression.

To reduce mortality.

Other treatments

Coronary bypass grafting: in selected patients with severe coronary disease.

Heart transplantation: for younger patients with severe left ventricular disease; organ supply remains inadequate for demand.

Anticoagulants: indicated for the prevention of stroke in patients with atrial fibrillation, prior embolus, or demonstrated thrombus on noninvasive imaging.

Prognosis

• Adverse prognostic features include the following:

Old age, low ejection fraction, poor exercise tolerance, ischemic origin, ventricular arrhythmias, reduced heart rate variability, high plasma noradrenaline concentration, low serum sodium concentration.

• The annual mortality is 50% in patients with severe heart failure and 10%–20% in patients with mild to moderate heart failure.

Follow-up and management

• Life-long regular review is needed.

Key references

1. Pitt B, *et al.*: Randomised trial of losartan versus captopril in patients over 65 with heart failure. *Lancet* 1997, **349**:747–752.

2. Australia/New Zealand Heart Failure Research Collaborative Group: Randomised, placebo-controlled trial of carvedilol in patients with congestive heart failure due to ischaemic heart disease. *Lancet* 1997, **349**:375–380.

General references

Cohn JN, *et al.*: A comparison of enalapril with hydralazine-isosorbide dinitrate in the treatment of chronic congestive heart failure. *N Engl J Med* 1991, **325**:303–310.

CONSENSUS Trial Study Group: Effects of enalapril on mortality in severe congestive heart failure: results of the Co-operative North Scandinavian Enalapril Survival Study. *N Engl J Med* 1987, **316**:1429–1435.

SOLVD Investigators: Effect of enalapril on survival in patients with reduced left ventricular ejection fractions and congestive heart failure. *N Engl J Med* 1991, **325**:293–302.

Basic life support

Definition

• The term "basic life support" refers to maintaining an airway and supporting breathing and the circulation without equipment [1].

• This is a practical skill, and training must be sought.

• Health care professionals should also have more complex skills, including the use of airway adjuncts, *e.g.*, Guedel airway plus face-mask (with or without a nonreturn valve) or bag-mask ventilation and two-rescuer resuscitation.

Assessment [1]

Approach

• Safety for the rescuer and the patient must be assessed.

Responsiveness

• The rescuer should gently shake the patient's shoulders and ask loudly, "Are you all right?"

• If the patient is unresponsive, the rescuer should call for help.

• The airway is opened by the combined maneuver of head tilt and chin lift; in most cases, this alone lifts the tongue from the back of the throat.

• If neck injury is likely, a chin lift or jaw thrust must be performed without moving the head or neck to open the airway.

• Any obvious obstruction should be removed from the mouth.

• Well-fitting dentures should be left in place because these help to maintain a mouth seal during ventilation.

Breathing

• After opening the airway, the rescuer should look for chest movements, listen for breath sounds at the mouth, and feel for exhaled air with the cheek.

• These must be done for 5 seconds before deciding that breathing is absent.

Pulse

• The best pulse to feel in any emergency is the carotid.

• This should be palpated for 5 seconds to ensure that circulation is absent.

Action

For respiratory arrest

• If the patient is not breathing but a pulse is present, 10 breaths/min expired-air ventilation must be given.

• The pulse must be checked again after every 10 breaths, and full cardiopulmonary resuscitation instituted if the pulse disappears.

For cardiorespiratory arrest

• If the patient is unconscious and not breathing and the pulse is absent, ventilation and initiation of chest compression are needed at a rate of 2 breaths : 15 compressions, with 80 compressions/min (single rescuer).

• Chances are remote that effective spontaneous cardiac action will be restored without other techniques of advanced life support (including defibrillation), so time should not be wasted by further checks for the presence of a pulse [2].

• If, however, the patient makes a movement or takes a spontaneous breath, the carotid pulse should be checked to establish whether the heart is beating, taking no more than 5 seconds, and breathing should be checked.

• Otherwise, resuscitation must not be interrupted [3].

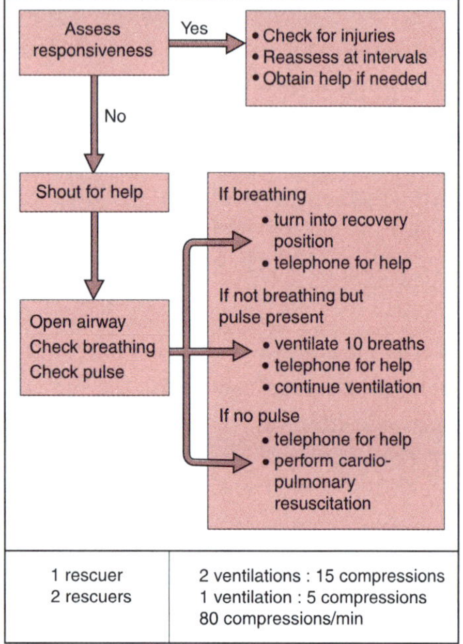

Basic life support.

Advanced life support

Defibrillation

• Electrical defibrillation is the only effective method of terminating ventricular fibrillation, a lethal rhythm disturbance, and of restoring a perfusing cardiac rhythm.

• The success of electrical defibrillation depends on time and the metabolic state of the myocardium.

• The delay in the administration of defibrillating shocks should be minimal.

• If the first three shocks, at 200 J, 200 J, and 360 J, can be delivered quickly (within 30–45 seconds), the sequence should not be interrupted by basic life support.

• If the time to charge a manual defibrillator or to confirm that the rhythm is still ventricular fibrillation is likely to be unduly prolonged, one or two sequences of basic life support should be administered between shocks.

• The prospects of success decrease relatively rapidly over a few minutes after cardiac arrest.

• Basic life support is unlikely to improve the odds of successful defibrillation; its value is in maintaining some cerebral perfusion and in slowing myocardial deterioration.

• After repeating the loops 3 times, different paddle position, a different defibrillator, and other antiarrythmic drugs (*e.g.*, amiodarone, lidocaine, bretylium tosylate) are still worth considering for refractory ventricular fibrillation.

• The position of the defibrillation paddles influences current flow through the myocardium; one electrode should be placed below the second intercostal space midclavicular line on the right and the other just outside the usual position of the cardiac apex (V_4–V_5).

Precordial thump

• The precordial thump is recommended for patients in ventricular fibrillation, pulseless ventricular tachycardia, or asystole.

• The application of a precordial thump takes only 2–3 seconds and should not cause a significant delay in the application of electric defibrillation; it should be used only when advanced life support is available.

Pharmacological treatment

Indications

For ventricular fibrillation and pulseless ventricular tachycardia: epinephrine.

For asystole: adrenaline, atropine.

For electromechanical dissociation: treatment of cause (*e.g.*, hypovolemia, tension pneumothorax, cardiac tamponade, pulmonary embolism, drug overdose or intoxication, hypothermia, electrolyte imbalance); consideration of routine pressor agents, calcium chloride, alkalizing agents, or high-dose adrenaline (one or more of these may be of value in some circumstances).

For prolonged resuscitation or according to blood gas analysis: sodium bicarbonate.

Specific drugs

Adrenaline, 1 mg i.v. (10 mL 1:10 000 solution); should be followed by 10 sequences of 5 compressions:1 ventilation; high-dose epinephrine (5 mg) should be considered in asystole and electromechanical dissociation, although value unproven if no response after 3 cycles.

Atropine, 3 mg.

Sodium bicarbonate, 50 mmol (50 mL 8.4% solution).

Calcium chloride, 1 g (10 mL 10% solution).

• A large peripheral or central vein should be the standard route, with rapid infusion.

• The endotracheal route should be used only if an i.v. line cannot be established, in which case, double or triple doses of adrenaline or atropine should be given through an endotracheal tube.

Key references

1. Emergency Cardiac Care Committee and Subcommittees, American Heart Association: Guidelines for cardiopulmonary resuscitation and emergency cardiac care. *JAMA* 1992, **268**:2172–2298.

2. O'Nunain S, Ruskin J: Cardiac arrest. *Lancet* 1993, **341**:1631–1647.

3. Cohen TJ: A comparison of active compression-decompression CPR with standard CPR for cardiac arrests in the hospital. *N Engl J Med* 1993, **329**:1918–1921.

4. Lombardi G: Outcome of out of hospital cardiac arrest in New York City. *JAMA* 1994, **271**:678–683.

Diagnosis

Symptoms

Numbness, tingling, pain, burning in distribution of median nerve.

Weakness, loss of grip strength.

Incoordination: dropping objects.

Awakening from sleep, shaking hand and wrist to relieve tingling sensation: cardinal symptom.

Proximal upper extremity pain: uncommon.

Signs

Numbness.

Diminished pin-prick sensation.

Diminished grip strength.

Muscular atrophy of thenar eminence.

Phalen's test and reverse Phanlen's test: "praying hands" position recreates neuropathic symptoms.

Tinel's sign: percussion over median nerve at volar aspect of wrist with reflex hammer reproduces symptoms; nonspecific.

Investigations

Electromyography.

Complications

Numbness.

Decrease in grip strength.

Work impairment.

Atrophy of thenar eminence.

Differential diagnosis

Cervical radiculopathy.

• Other causes of localized wrist pain include:

Osteoarthritis.

Rheumatoid arthritis.

Etiology

Osteoarthritis.

Diabetes mellitus.

Pregnancy.

Hypothyroidism.

Rheumatoid arthritis.

Acromegaly.

Dysproteinemia (*e.g.*, multiple myeloma).

Amyloidosis.

Epidemiology

• Carpal tunnel syndrome has become the second most common cause of work impairment (after back pain).

Pathophysiology

Repetitive trauma (*e.g.*, jack hammer operators, meat cutters).

Infiltration (amyloidosis, hypothyroidism, diabetes).

Edema: osteoarthritis, pregnancy.

Idiopathic: 20% of cases are of unknown cause.

Treatment

Diet and lifestyle

• Patients should implement dietary changes such as those used to control diabetes.

• Wrists should be splinted.

Pharmacological treatment

• NSAIDs are of limited value.

• Corticosteroid injection into carpal tunnel volar sheath has a very limited role. It should be performed by an orthopedic surgeon or rheumatologist (if at all).

Nonpharmacological treatment

Splinting: symptomatic improvement may occur with inexpensive cock-up wrist splints. Custom-molded fabricated splints offer no additional advantage.

Rehabilitation.

Treatment aims

To eliminate symptoms of pain and numbness.

To improve function.

To improve sleep.

To restore grip strength.

Prognosis

• Carpal tunnel release surgery has variable results.

• Traditionally, cure rates exceeding 90% were routinely reported, however, postsurgical recurrences of carpal tunnel syndrome after return to repetitive stress work environments may approach 80%.

• Careful patient selection prior to surgery is crucial, along with rehabilitation for possible job modifications prior to return to work.

General reference

von Schroeder HP, Botte MI: Carpal tunnel syndrome. *Hand Clin* 1996, **12**:643–655.

Diagnosis

Symptoms

• Only 50% of patients present with the classic symptoms of diarrhea associated with malabsorption. Many are detected because of anemia (especially iron or folate deficiency) [1].

Symptoms of steatorrhea: foul-smelling stools, oil residue or undigested food particles in toilet bowl.

Weight loss: common, as is amenorrhea.

Skin rashes, easy bruising.

Signs

Evidence of weight loss [2].

Pallor: anemia due to iron or folic acid deficiency.

Ecchymosis.

Calcium deficiency: with possible tetany.

Chelosis.

Papulovesicular rash of dermatitis herpetiformis on extensor surfaces.

Investigations

Initial

Complete blood count, serum iron, ferritin, or folate, and erythrocyte folate measurement: to identify microcytic (iron deficiency) or macrocytic (folic acid deficiency) anemia or a dimorphic pattern of anemia due to both.

Vitamin B_{12} measurement: concentration frequently low but rarely abnormal.

Serum calcium and magnesium measurement: concentration possibly depressed.

Protime: prolonged in patients with vitamin K deficiency.

Specific

Upper gastrointestinal endoscopy with biopsy of duodenum or proximal jejunum: reveals short (or absent) villi, intraepithelial lymphocytes, and crypt hyperplasia; for unequivocal diagnosis, at least six biopsy specimens should be obtained; celiac disease is confirmed when subsequent biopsy results are normal on a gluten-free diet.

Circulating antibody (antigliadin, antiendomysial) measurement: concentrations always raised; may be used as a screening test, particularly in children.

Fecal fat estimation: 3-day fecal fat excretion >7 g/day in patients ingesting at least 100 g fat daily (sensitive for malabsorption but not specific for celiac disease).

Contrast radiography: small bowel follow-through to assess small intestine; poor sensitivity, luminal dilation, and altered mucosal folds often observed.

Complications

Anemia: due to iron or folic acid deficiency.

Osteomalacia, osteoporosis: due to hypocalcemia (tetany and seizures due to exacerbation by magnesium deficiency).

Ulcerative jejunitis: rare, possibly early manifestation of malignancy.

Small-intestinal lymphoma: T-cell lymphoma complicating 5%–10% of cases; may be manifest as unexplained small intestinal perforation.

Wernicke's encephalopathy or Korsakoff's psychosis: due to acute or prolonged vitamin B_1 (thiamine) deficiency.

Differential diagnosis

Infectious diarrhea.

Chronic pancreatitis.

Inflammatory bowel disease.

Giardiasis.

Tropical sprue.

Lactose intolerance.

Small bowel bacterial overgrowth.

Laxative abuse.

Whipple's disease.

Irritable bowel syndrome.

Etiology

• In northern Europeans, 98% of cases of celiac disease are associated with the extended haplotype HLA B8, DR3, DQ2, although, in southern Europeans, HLA DR5/7, DQ2 accounts for one-third of cases.

• 10%–20% of first-degree relatives of probands are similarly affected.

• Family history often reveals a Celtic ancestry [3].

Epidemiology

• Accurate data relating to the incidence and prevalence of celiac sprue in the United States are lacking.

• The prevalence of celiac disease in the United Kingdom is particularly high (1 in 1200 people, rising to 1 in 300 around Galway Bay in Ireland).

• Slightly more women than men suffer from celiac disease; an association with anemia due to menstruation and pregnancy is possible.

• The incidence of presentation has three peaks:
infancy (9–36 months), on introduction of foods containing gluten;
third decade, frequently manifest as severe anemia of pregnancy;
fifth decade, normally manifest with a specific nutritional deficiency *e.g.*, iron, folic acid, or calcium.

Treatment

Diet and lifestyle

• A gluten-free diet is the mainstay of treatment and involves avoiding products containing wheat, rye, barley, or oats. Care should be taken to avoid any food contaminated by these cereals or their partial hydrolysates, including beer. Women of childbearing age who experienced amenorrhea due to nutritional deficiencies will probably have a return of regular menstruation. Men who have had long-standing disease may complain of impotence and infertility. These problems normally resolve within 2 years of starting a gluten-free diet.

• Specific nutritional deficiencies should be treated by replacement: iron, calcium, vitamin B_{12}, folic acid, or magnesium.

Pharmacological treatment

• For most patients, a gluten-free diet is sufficient; patients with refractory disease or severe malnutrition may benefit from steroid therapy.

Standard dosage	Prednisone, 20–40 mg daily initially, usually rapidly reduced to 5–10 mg daily. Hydrocortisone, 50–100 mg i.v. every 6 hours in patients who need i.v. fluid replacement.
Contraindications	Caution in diabetes mellitus, or pregnancy.
Special points	Care should be taken to avoid high-dose (prednisone >10 mg/day), long-term steroid treatment because of side effects.
Main drug interactions	Mild antagonism to thiazide diuretics.
Main side effects	Weight gain, fluid retention, osteoporosis, cushingoid facies, diabetes mellitus.

Treatment aims

To improve general well-being, small intestinal mucosal structure, and associated nutritional deficiencies.

To reduce the risk of development of small intestinal lymphoma.

Prognosis

• With a gluten-free diet, general health is improved within a few weeks.

• Untreated patients are at a 5%–10% risk of developing a small intestinal T-cell lymphoma, the incidence of which probably falls if they maintain a strict diet.

• Failure to improve suggests incorrect initial diagnosis, failure to adhere strictly to a gluten-free diet, or concurrent disorder (*i.e.*, malignancy) [4].

Follow-up and management

• Outpatients must be reassessed 6–8 weeks and 3–4 months after starting a gluten-free diet, when repeat biopsy should be done.

• A further biopsy should be done 1 year after starting treatment, when continued improvement in the structure of the small-intestinal mucosa should be expected.

• Annual hematological screening is recommended to exclude development of specific nutritional deficiencies.

• When the diagnosis is doubtful, a gluten challenge, with 40 g gluten or 4 slices of normal bread daily for 2 weeks (adults) or 6 weeks (children), may be followed by a repeat jejunal biopsy.

Key references

1. Ciclitira PJ: Coeliac disease and related disorders and the malignant complications of coeliac disease. In *Gastroenterology: Clinical Science and Practice.* Edited by Bouchier I, Hodgson H. London: Baillière Tindall; 1993.

2. Ferguson A, Arranz E, O'Mahony S: Clinical and pathological spectrum of coeliac disease: active, silent, latent, potential. *Gut* 1993, **34**:150–155.

3. Kagnoff MF: Celiac disease: a gastrointestinal disease with environmental, genetic, and immunologic components. *Gastroenterol Clin North Am* 1992, **21**:405–425.

4. Trier JS: Celiac sprue. *N Engl J Med* 1991, **325**:1709–1719.

Diagnosis

Symptoms

• Symptoms generally include the following, alone or in combination:

Epilepsy: in >50% of patients by presentation; associated focal features may suggest localization of brain tumor; simple partial seizures particularly common.

Dysphasia, hemiparesis, intellectual failure, personality change, cranial nerve abnormalities.

Headache, papilledema, visual failure, vomiting: alone or in combination indicate raised intracranial pressure due to intracranial mass lesions.

Signs

Papilledema, impaired visual acuity, visual field defects.

Diplopia: with or without clear III or VI nerve palsy.

Facial weakness.

Dysphasia.

Hemiparesis, hyperreflexia, extensor plantar response, hemisensory loss.

Signs of primary malignancy in secondary brain tumors: *e.g.*, site of previous melanoma excision visible in skin.

Investigations

Neuroradiography: primarily CT and MRI of brain; more invasive procedures (*e.g.*, angiography or PET) sometimes needed for management.

Chest radiography: important as part of general screening for extracerebral primary or metastatic tumor in lungs.

EEG: possibly needed as secondary investigation to elucidate epileptic manifestations.

Blood tests: possibly needed to clarify differential diagnosis, *e.g.*, blood cultures when metastatic brain abscess suspected.

Lumbar puncture: to identify meningeal spread of malignancy.

Complications

Blindness: papilledema due to progressive raised intracranial pressure leads to blindness if unrelieved.

Herniation: brain shift due to increasing mass of cerebral tumor can lead to central or transtentorial brain herniation, with irreversible ischemic brain damage and fatal apnea due to failure of brain stem function.

Differential diagnosis

Cerebrovascular disease.

Other organic brain disease (*e.g.*, encephalitis or demyelination).

Other extradural intracranial tumors (*e.g.*, meningioma).

Cerebral abscess: an important differential diagnosis; often no signs of acute infection in patients, despite relevant history of middle ear disease, bronchiectasis, or valvular heart disease.

Etiology

• The cause of most cerebral tumors remains unknown, although the incidence is increased after exposure to radiation, in patients with neurofibromatosis, and in some rare inherited immunodeficiency diseases.

• Increasing evidence indicates that cerebral astrocytomas are associated with loss of tumor suppressor gene function from chromosomes 17 and 10 and with amplification of epidermal growth factor receptor.

Epidemiology

• Primary cerebral tumors account for ~55% of intracranial tumors in adults and are the tenth most common tumors in men.

• The annual incidence of cerebral tumor is ~10 in 100 000 population.

• The peak incidence is in the fifth decade, with a small male preponderance (55%).

• Secondary brain tumors are common and account for 15%–20% of intracranial tumors in neurological series.

Treatment

Diet and lifestyle

- No special diet is necessary for patients with primary brain tumors.
- Impaired cognitive function and fatigue may limit employment.

Pharmacological treatment

For epilepsy

- Anticonvulsant drug treatment is usually started for supratentorial tumors in both epileptic and nonepileptic patients.

Standard dosage	Phenytoin, 300–400 mg daily, or carbamazepine, 600–1000 mg daily.
Contraindications	Hepatic impairment, severe cytopenia.
Main drug interactions	Analgesics, antibiotics, antidepressants.
Main side effects	Confusion, skin eruptions, gum swelling, diplopia, ataxia.

For raised intracranial pressure and stabilization of brain function

Standard dosage	Dexamethasone, 4 mg every 6 hours (adult) initially; up to 20 mg every 6 hours may be useful for a few weeks as palliative terminal treatment.
Contraindications	Peptic ulcers.
Special points	When surgical decompression and adjuvant radiotherapy have been completed, steroids may be gradually withdrawn or reduced to a minimum level that keeps the patient asymptomatic. While the patient is taking dexamethasone, the risk of peptic ulcers is increased; H_2 antagonists such as ranitidine, 150 mg twice daily, are usually also prescribed.
Main drug interactions	Hypoglycemia agents, diuretics.
Main side effects	Peptic ulcers, weight gain, demineralization.

For acutely raised intracranial pressure

- In patients who are unconscious as a result of raised intracranial pressure from cerebral tumor or in those who have herniated, with respiratory arrest, artificial ventilation, mannitol as an osmotic diuretic, and i.v. dexamethasone may be needed in an emergency department or intensive care unit setting.

Chemotherapy

- After surgery and adjuvant radiotherapy, antitumor chemotherapy may be indicated for malignant glioma, either as an adjuvant or at the time of relapse.
- Nitrosoureas and procarbazine are the agents chiefly used.

Treatment aims

To relieve symptoms; curing malignant primary or secondary brain tumors is generally not possible.

Other treatments

Surgery: almost always indicated to establish histological diagnosis and grading and, where possible, to reduce tumor bulk.
Radiotherapy: localized to tumor and surrounding area, usually given for malignant primary cerebral tumors; secondary metastatic cerebral tumors treated by whole-brain radiation.

Prognosis

- Prognosis is related to tumor type and histological grade, patient age, and functional performance at the time of treatment.
- The median survival with grade 4 astrocytomas is ~9 months and with grade 2 astrocytomas ~6 years.

Follow-up and management

- Clinical assessment of neurological and performance status, with follow-up brain scanning at intervals of 3–6 months, is used to monitor progress.
- At disease progression, further surgery is considered in 10%–15% of patients, as are novel treatments, *e.g.*, focused radiation or immunotherapy.
- The terminal phase is usually short, from a few days to 6 weeks, and patients may often be managed in the home, although hospice care may sometimes be preferable.

General references

Apuzzo MLJ (ed.): *Malignant Cerebral Glioma*. Illinois: American Association of Neurological Surgeons, 1990.

Fernandez PM, Brem S: Malignant brain tumors in the elderly. *Clin Geriatr Med* 1997, **13**:327–338.

Mahaley MS: Neuro-oncology index and review (adult primary brain tumors). *J Neurooncol* 1991, **11**:85–147.

Thomas DGT (ed.): *Neuro-Oncology*. London: Arnold; 1990.

Diagnosis

Symptoms

Pruritis, fatigue: >50% of patients.

Right upper quandrant pain: intermittent.

• Patients may present with symptoms of end-stage liver disease (variceal bleeding, encephalopathy, ascites).

• 25% of patients are asymptomatic; diagnosis is made after discovery of abnormal liver function tests, particularly in patients with ulcerative colitis.

Jaundice: intermittent.

Weight loss.

Fever: unusual unless previous intervention, *e.g.*, endoscopic retrograde cholangio-pancreatography, surgery.

Bleeding esophageal varices, edema, ascites: late features.

Signs

• Signs are not always manifest [1–2].

Right-upper quandrant tenderness, fevers: during episodes of cholangitis.

Hepatomegaly: >50%.

Splenomegaly: ~30%.

Jaundice: in more advanced cases.

Spider nevi, palmar erythema, ascites: late.

Investigations

Liver chemistries: cholestatic pattern with raised alkaline phosphatase, gamma-glutamyl transpeptidase, bilirubin (late); low albumin, prolonged prothrombin time (late); antimitochondrial antibody usually negative.

Cholangiography: the diagnostic test; endoscopic retrograde cholangiography first choice, percutaneous route only if endoscopic route fails; bile-duct stricturing interspersed with dilatation (beading); intra- and extrahepatic duct changes in most patients.

Liver biopsy: changes suggestive (portal edema, fibrosis, duct proliferation) rather than diagnostic; biopsy staging: 1, portal changes; 2, periportal extension; 3, septum formation; 4, cirrhosis.

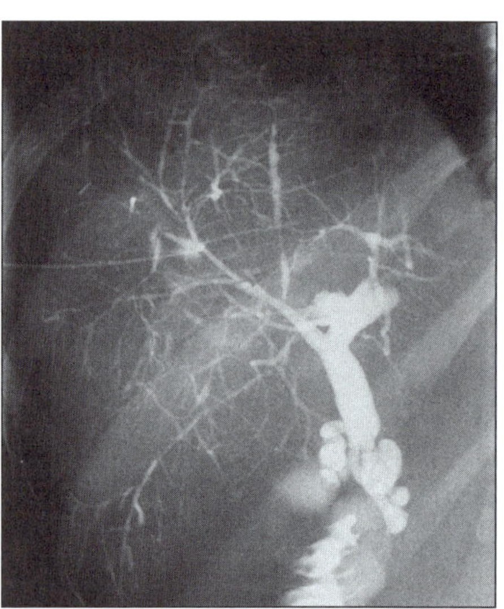

Classic intrahepatic changes of primary sclerosing cholangitis (bleeding and stricturing) on percutaneous cholangiography. The common bile duct is dilated because of involvement of the lower end by primary sclerosing cholangitis. Endoscopic cholangiography was unsuccessful.

Complications

Recurrent cholangitis.

Cholangiocarcinoma: in 10%–15% of patients.

Metabolic bone disease.

Portal hypertension, variceal hemorrhage, edema, ascites, encephalopathy: late.

Differential diagnosis

Bile duct stones.

Cholangiocarcinoma.

Drug-induced cholestasis.

Primary biliary cirrhosis.

Surgical stricture.

Secondary sclerosing cholangitis.

Metastatic tumor.

Granulomatous liver disease (*e.g.*, sarcoid).

AIDS cholangiopathy.

• Distinction of benign primary sclerosing cholangitis stricture from cholangiocarcinoma is very difficult; brush or bile cytology is only 50%–60% sensitive.

Etiology

• Primary sclerosing cholangitis has a known strong association with inflammatory bowel disease (ulcerative colitis) and HLA B8 and DR3.

• The pathogenetic mechanism is unknown.

• The current hypothesis is that infection, or absorption of bacterial products or both occur in predisposed (HLA DR) individuals.

Epidemiology

• 70% of patients with primary sclerosing cholangitis have ulcerative colitis; 4% of patients with ulcerative colitis have primary sclerosing cholangitis.

• The prevalence of primary sclerosing cholangitis is 2–7 in 100 000.

• The male:female ratio is 2:1.

• The most common age of presentation is 25–45 years.

Treatment

Diet and lifestyle

- Careful attention to adequate nutrition is recommended.
- If steatorrhea is problematic, fat intake may be reduced.

Pharmacological treatment

Symptomatic

- Drugs are indicated to relieve pruritus.

Standard dosage	Cholestyramine, 4–12 g daily.
Contraindications	Complete biliary obstruction.
Special points	May interfere with absorption of fat-soluble vitamins, so supplementation may be needed.
Main drug interactions	Delayed or reduced absorption of digitalis, tetracycline, chlorothiazide, warfarin, thyroxine.
Main side effects	Increased bleeding tendency, constipation, diarrhea.

Prophylactic

- For proven fat-soluble vitamin deficiency or jaundice, the following are indicated:

Vitamin K, 10 mg i.m. monthly.

Vitamin D, 100 000 U i.m. monthly.

Vitamin A, 100 000 U i.m. 3-monthly.

- Adequate calcium intake must be ensured.

Therapeutic

- No medical treatment has been definitively shown to delay progression or reverse changes of primary sclerosing cholangitis [3].

- Ursodeoxycholic acid, 10–15 mg/kg orally daily, improves liver function tests, but benefit for liver histology, cholangiography, or survival has not been established.

- The choice of antibiotics for cholangitis (when no remediable dominant stricture) depends on bile or blood culture; empiric considerations include ciprofloxacin, ampicillin, or a cephalosporin.

Treatment aims

To relieve symptoms.

To prevent recurrence of cholangitis.

Other treatments

Endoscopic or radiographical balloon dilation/stent placement: for symptomatic dominant strictures (cholangitis, itching) [4].

Surgical palliation: appropriate for dominant stricture only if transplantation is not an option and an endoscopic or a percutaneous approach has failed.

Orthotopic liver transplantation: for refractory cases; ~70% 1-year survival; unexpected cholangiocarcinoma often found [5].

Prognosis

- Prognosis varies greatly.

- Factors at presentation related to prognosis (Mayo model) include serum bilirubin concentration, histological stage on liver biopsy, age, and presence of splenomegaly [3,6,7].

Follow-up and management

- Patients should be monitored clinically for signs and symptoms of cholangitis.

- Patients should be reviewed monthly if they have symptomatic or biochemical deterioration and are approaching transplantation.

Key references

1. Wiesner RH: Current concepts in primary sclerosing cholangitis. *Mayo Clin Proc* 1994, **69**:969–982.

2. Broome U, Olsson R, Loof L, *et al.*: Natural history and prognostic factors in 305 Swedish patients with primary sclerosing cholangitis. *Gut* 1996, **38**:610–615.

3. Lindor KD: Ursodiol for primary sclerosing cholangitis. *N Engl J Med* 1997, **336**:691–695.

4. Gaing AA, Geders JM, Cohen SA, Siegel JH: Endoscopic management of primary sclerosing cholangitis: review, and report of an open series. *Am J Gastroenterol* 1993, **88**:2000–2008.

5. Narumi S, Roberts JP, Emond JC, *et al.*: Liver transplantation for sclerosing cholangitis. *Hepatology* 1995, **22**:451–457.

6. Dickerson ER, *et al.*: Primary sclerosing cholangitis: refinement and validation of survival models. *Gastroenterology* 1992, **103**:1893–1901.

7. Shetty K, Rybicki L, Carey WD: The Child-Pugh classification as a prognostic indicator for survival in primary sclerosing cholangitis. *Hepatology* 1997, **25**:1049–1053.

Diagnosis

Symptoms

Major

Fatigue: lasting >3–6 months, with 50% reduction in activity; worsened by physical or mental stress; relapsing, with good and bad days.

Prominent disturbance of concentration or short-term memory.

Minor

Initiating viral-like illness, with pyrexia and malaise, common.

Myalgia: especially limb and chest pain; worse after activity.

Joint pain: especially in large joints.

Abdominal pain or bloatedness, nausea, alternating constipation and diarrhea.

Headaches, dizziness, tinnitus, paresthesias.

Sleep disturbance: initially more sleep, followed by disturbed sleep or vivid dreams.

Sensitivity to heat or cold, inappropriate sweating.

Adverse effects of alcohol.

Signs

• Most patients have been previously well; few clinical signs are manifest.

Localized areas of tender muscle: about 1 cm diameter in affected muscle groups.

Enlarged lymph nodes, glands, or inflamed throat: in periods of relapse.

Muscle weakness: in patients who have been ill for many years.

Investigations

• Diagnosis must not be made on the presence of fatigue alone; the two major symptoms and at least four minor items from symptoms, clinical signs, or positive laboratory investigations must be present.

• No diagnostic test exists; investigations are designed to exclude other causes of a similar clinical syndrome.

Initial investigations

• All of the results should be normal, if other illnesses are to be excluded.

Hemoglobin measurement: to exclude anemia.

Leukocyte count: to identify infection or a hematological condition.

Thyroid function tests: to exclude thyroid disease.

Plasma viscosity or ESR and CRP measurement: nonspecific indicator of an underlying disorder.

Further investigations

• Other conditions suggested by the patient's history or examination must be excluded, especially infection, *e.g.*, tick bites (Lyme disease) or consumption of raw meat (toxoplasmosis).

Complications

Psychiatric disorder: especially depression and anxiety.

Irritable bowel syndrome.

Severe disability: patient may become bedridden.

Differential diagnosis

Infections, especially Epstein–Barr virus, Lyme disease, toxoplasmosis, hepatitis A, brucellosis.

Endocrine disease, especially hypothyroidism.

Psychiatric disease, especially if patient has been ill for many years.

Malignancy.

Autoimmune disease, sarcoidosis.

Drugs or toxins.

Etiology

• The cause is unknown; probably several conditions are involved, including continuing infection and immune response to infection.

Epidemiology

• Chronic fatigue syndrome occurs throughout the world.

• ~1.3 in 1000 population are affected.

• Both sexes and all ages are affected; women are more likely to have prolonged illness.

Nomenclature

• Chronic fatigue syndrome is also known as the following:

Postviral fatigue syndrome.

Myalgic encephalomyelitis.

Effort syndrome.

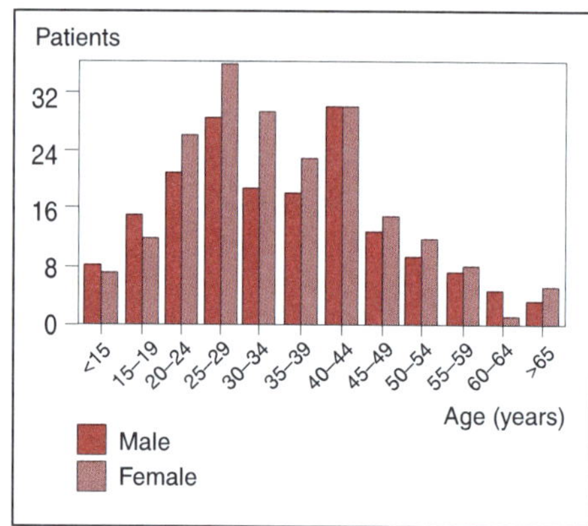

Patients affected by chronic fatigue syndrome, according to age and sex (204 females, 177 males; ratio, 1.2:1).

Treatment

Diet and lifestyle

• If patients have a normal diet, vitamins or mineral supplements are unnecessary.

• Patients should remain within their energy limits; sleep should not be resisted (at least 10 h/day); sleep and relaxation techniques increase energy levels; energy is lost through physical activities and mental exertion (such as concern about jobs, finances, and relationships).

Pharmacological treatment

• Although moderating activity is the best method of controlling symptoms, many patients need additional supportive treatment.

• Several drugs may have to be tried before the most appropriate is found.

Analgesics

• Mild analgesics, *e.g.*, acetaminophen or aspirin, should be tried initially; if they are unsuccessful, dihydrocodeine or ibuprofen may help.

Benzodiazepines

• Because of their hypnotic, sedative, anxiolytic, and muscle-relaxant actions, these drugs are useful in patients who have difficulty sleeping.

• Intermediate-acting compounds are best (temazepam, lormetazepam).

Standard dosage	Temazepam, 10 mg orally at night for 3–4 weeks.
Contraindications	Respiratory depression, phobic or obsessional states.
Main drug interactions	Alcohol.
Main side effects	Drowsiness, dizziness.

Antidepressants

• The most useful agents are amitriptyline, doxepin, dothiepin, and fluoxetine.

Standard dosage	Amitriptyline, 10 mg orally at night.
Contraindications	Heart disease.
Special points	Patients should be given low doses initially, with gradual increase if necessary.
Main drug interactions	Alcohol.
Main side effects	Dry mouth, blurred vision, nausea, constipation.

Treatment aims

To reduce fatigue and prevent relapses.
To relieve other symptoms.
To allow patient to resume normal activity, *e.g.*, to return to work or school.

Prognosis

• Patients may recover after a fluctuating illness, usually in the first 4 years, achieve stability at a lower energy level, or deteriorate and become chronically disabled.

Follow-up and management

• Patients should keep a daily diary, monitoring activities and energy levels.

• Activities may be increased and a return to work or school encouraged when energy levels are 70%–80% of normal.

Causes of treatment failure

Overoptimistic reassurance of recovery.
Patient's inability to change lifestyle.
Too much energy being spent pursuing alternative cures.

General references

Buchwald D: Fibromyalgia and chronic fatigue syndrome: similarities and differences. *Rheum Dis Clin North Am* 1996, **22**:219–243.

Thomas PK: The chronic fatigue syndrome: what do we know? *BMJ* 1993, **306**:1557–1558.

Tirelli U, *et al.*: Clinical and immunologic study of 205 patients with chronic fatigue syndrome. *Arch Intern Med* 1993, **153**:116–120.

Wallace DJ: The fibromyalgia syndrome. *Ann Int Med* 1997, **29**:9–21.

Diagnosis [1]

Symptoms

Cough: chronic bronchitis is defined as a cough productive of sputum on most days for at least 3 consecutive months in 2 successive years.

Productive sputum.

Increasing dyspnea: especially with exertion.

Weight loss.

History of smoking: present in the great majority of cases.

Signs

Onset usually in the 5th or 6th decade.

Barrel-shaped chest, decreased cardiac dullness and reduced breath sounds, palpable liver due to hepatic displacement, signs of hyperexpansion.

Increased respiratory rate, use of accessory muscles of respiration, "pursed lip" breathing, reduced breath sounds: signs of airflow obstruction.

Cyanosis.

Right ventricular heave, raised jugular venous pressure, peripheral edema: signs of pulmonary hypertension.

Fine inspiratory crackles: frequently found in chronic obstructive airway disease and do not necessarily imply coexistent heart failure.

Hyperresonance with percussion.

Investigations

Complete blood count: polycythemia found in some patients.

ECG: to detect right axis deviation or signs of right-sided strain.

Chest radiography: to detect signs of chronic obstructive pulmonary disease (low flat diaphragms, long thin heart), emphysema (hypodense bullae, large retrosternal airspace on lateral radiography), or pulmonary hypertension (prominent hilum, with reduced peripheral vascular shadows).

Pulmonary function testing: to confirm obstructive picture and to show degree of reversibility to therapeutic agents; diffusing capacity estimates gas transfer.

Arterial blood gas measurement: to check for hypoxia and carbon dioxide retention; high bicarbonate concentration suggests more chronic carbon dioxide retention.

Chest CT scan: may confirm emphysema.

Complications

Infective exacerbations: acute bronchitis, pneumonia.

Pulmonary hypertension, cor pulmonale.

Pulmonary embolism.

Respiratory failure, death.

Pneumothorax.

Lung cancer: when smoking is cause of chronic obstructive pulmonary disease (COPD).

Hemoptysis.

Differential diagnosis

Asthma.
Left ventricular failure.
Large airway obstruction, *e.g.*, proximal tumor.
Allergic bronchopulmonary aspergillosis.
Aspiration.
Bronchiectasis.
Cystic fibrosis.

Etiology

Cigarette smoking: most important cause.
Atmospheric pollution: much less important than smoking.
Airway infections/inflammation.
Alpha, antitrypsin deficiency: rare; homozygous form present in 1 in 5000 people, and not all of these develop chest disease; causes basal emphysema [2].
Intravenous drug abuse.

Epidemiology

• Estimates indicate that ~15 million Americans have COPD.

• Chronic obstructive airway disease is estimated to cause >90 000 deaths per year.

Treatment

Diet and lifestyle

- Stopping smoking reduces the rate of deterioration of lung function to that of non-smokers and, at an early stage, may improve symptoms.
- Loss of weight improves functional capacity.
- Patients' homes can be assessed for the need for aids to daily living.

Pharmacological treatment [1,3–5]

- Inadequate inhaler technique is one of the main reasons for treatment failure; inhaler technique must always be checked before treatment is initiated or changed.

Inhaled anticholinergics

Standard dosage	Ipratropium bromide inhaler, 20–40 µg 4 times daily.
Contraindications	Hypersensitivity; caution in glaucoma (nebulized solutions).
Main drug interactions	None.
Main side effects	Dry mouth (rare).

Inhaled beta-2 agonists (*e.g.,* albuterol, metaproterenol, terbutaline)

Standard dosage	Two puffs up to 4 times daily (dosage varies with formulation).
Contraindications	Hypersensitivity.
Special points	Patient responses vary; clinical improvement may occur but may not be detected on spirometric assessment.
Main drug interactions	None.
Main side effects	Tremor, palpitations.

Inhaled steroids

- Inhaled steroids are indicated for patients who have shown an objective response.

Standard dosage	Dosage varies with formulation.
Contraindications	Hypersensitivity.
Special points	Systemic absorption can be reduced with a spacer device.
Main drug interactions	None.
Main side effects	Oral candidiasis.

Oral steroids

- Oral steroids are indicated for exacerbations of chronic obstructive pulmonary disease and for maintenance treatment in severely ill steroid-responsive patients.

Standard dosage	Prednisone, 30–60 mg in the morning for exacerbations; lowest possible dose for maintenance treatment.
Contraindications	None.
Special points	Steroid responsiveness should be shown by >10% improvement in forced expiratory volume in 1 second after 3 weeks of prednisone.
Main drug interactions	None.
Main side effects	Osteoporosis, diabetes, steroid psychosis.

Theophyllines

- Use is controversial.

Standard dosage	Theophylline, 300–900 mg daily.
Contraindications	None.
Special points	Plasma concentrations must be monitored; they should be maintained at 10–20 µg/L.
Main drug interactions	Cimetidine, erythromycin, ciprofloxacin, and oral contraceptives reduce metabolism; cigarettes, alcohol, phenytoin, and rifampin increase metabolism.
Main side effects	Tachycardia, arrythmias.

Treatment aims

To maximize functional capacity.
To reduce decline in lung function.

Other treatments [3,6]

Long-term oxygen therapy (>16 hours daily): indications include the following:
Partial pressure of oxygen <55 mm Hg on two successive occasions when patient is stable.
Increasing hypoxemia with sleep or exercise.
Nonsmoking patient.
Failure to show carbon dioxide retention after a trial of oxygen.
At least one episode of peripheral edema.
Lung volume reduction surgery: an experimental procedure with promising results.
Lung transplantation: an option in selected patients, particularly younger patients with alpha, antitrypsin.
Nasal intermittent positive pressure ventilation: may be suitable in patients who retain carbon dioxide with oxygen therapy.
Smoking cessation.
Chest percussion and postural drainage.
Aerobic exercise programs.

Prognosis

- The 5-year survival rate after the initial episode of respiratory failure averages 15%–20%.

Follow-up and management

- Forced expiratory volume in 1 second must be monitored.
- Response to treatment must be assessed.

Key references

1. American Thoracic Society: Standards for the diagnosis and care of patients with chronic obstructive pulmonary disease. *Am J Respir Crit Care Med* 1995, **152(52 Pt 2)**:S77–S121.

2. American Thoracic Society: Guidelines for the approach to the patient with severe hereditary alpha 1-antitrypsin deficiency. *Am Rev Respir Dis* 1989, **140**:1494–1497.

3. Ferguson GT, Cherniak RM: Management of chronic obstructive pulmonary disease. *N Engl J Med* 1993, **328**:1017–1022.

4. McEvoy CE, Niewoehner DE: Adverse effects of corticosteroid therapy for COPD: a critical review. *Chest* 1997, **111**:732–743.

5. Celli BR: Current thoughts regarding treatment of chronic obstructive pulmonary disease. *Med Clin North Am* 1996, **80**:589–609.

6. Tarpy SP, Celli BR: Long-term oxygen therapy. *N Engl J Med* 1995, **333**:710–714.

Diagnosis

Symptoms

• Disease may be an incidental finding (abnormal liver tests on routine screening for other conditions) or manifest in one of the following ways:

Lethargy and pruritus: in middle-aged women (classic).

Right-sided abdominal pain: uncommon.

Ascites or variceal hemorrhage: indicating portal hypertension.

Signs

Jaundice: in later stages.

Xanthoma and xanthelasma.

Hepatomegaly.

Splenomegaly.

Ascites: may be present in late stage.

Spider nevi: often absent.

Investigations

Complete blood count: usually normal, but mean cell volume possibly raised.

Liver tests: show cholestasis; in early stage, raised serum alkaline phosphatase, gamma-glutamyl transpeptidase, serum bilirubin concentrations; raised cholesterol concentration.

Immunological tests: raised serum IgM and IgG concentrations (IgG less marked); antimitochondrial antibodies (AMA M_2 subclass) almost diagnostic; other autoantibodies, *e.g.*, antinuclear antibodies, occasionally manifest [1].

Liver histology: shows nonsuppurative destructive cholangitis or hepatitis involving portal tracts, which may also contain granulomas.

Complications

• Complications are the same as for end-stage liver disease.

Variceal hemorrhage.

Ascites.

Osteoporosis: hepatic osteopenia.

Liver failure.

Hepatocellular carcinoma.

Encephalopathy.

Differential diagnosis [1]

Primary sclerosing cholangitis.

Autoimmune hepatitis.

Drug-induced jaundice.

Sarcoidosis.

Chronic viral hepatitis.

Etiology

• The cause is unknown, although the following may have a role:

Infectious agents: bacterial or viral.

Autoimmune disorders.

Drugs: benoxaprofen, chlorpromazine.

Epidemiology

• In the United Kingdom, estimates of point prevalence of primary biliary cirrhosis are 2.3–14.4 in 100 000 people.

• The disease is less common in Africa and India.

Associated syndromes

Common

Arthralgia.

Hyperlipidemia.

Osteoporosis

Rare

Thyroid disease.

Sicca syndrome.

Glomerulonephritis.

Pulmonary fibrosis.

Sclerodactyly (CREST syndrome).

SLE.

Addison's disease.

Celiac disease.

Raynaud's phenomenon.

Histology [2]

Stage 1

Florid duct lesions, septal duct damage surrounded by dense inflammatory infiltrate, lymphoid aggregates; granulomas.

Stage 2

Ductular proliferation, fibrosis, fewer ducts.

Stage 3

Scarring (less inflammation), fibrous septa expanding from portal tracts; periportal cholestatis.

Stage 4

True cirrhosis; few or no bile ducts.

Treatment

Diet and lifestyle

• Patients must avoid regular alcohol intake.

• Careful attention must be paid to adequate nutrition.

• Prolonged cholestasis may result in vitamin K deficiency as manifest by a prolonged prothrombin time.

• Calcium and vitamin D supplementation should be considered early.

Pharmacological treatment

Symptomatic

• Drugs are indicated to relieve pruritus.

Standard dosage	Cholestyramine, 4–16 g daily, or colestipol.
Contraindications	Complete biliary obstruction.
Special points	May interfere with absorption of fat-soluble vitamins, so supplementation may be needed.
Main drug interactions	Delayed or reduced absorption of digitalis, tetracycline, chlorothiazide, warfarin, thyroxine.
Main side effects	Increased bleeding tendency, constipation, diarrhea.

• Treatment to prevent osteoporosis and supportive treatment for associated symptoms should also be provided.

Definitive

• Treatment should be done under specialist supervision.

• No drug has been shown to arrest disease; anti-inflammatories and antifibrotics (corticosteroids, azathioprine, cyclosporine, colchicine, methotrexate, penicillamine) have been used with no major clinical benefit [3].

• Ursodeoxycholic acid may help; biochemistry is improved, but data on long-term survival are controversial [4].

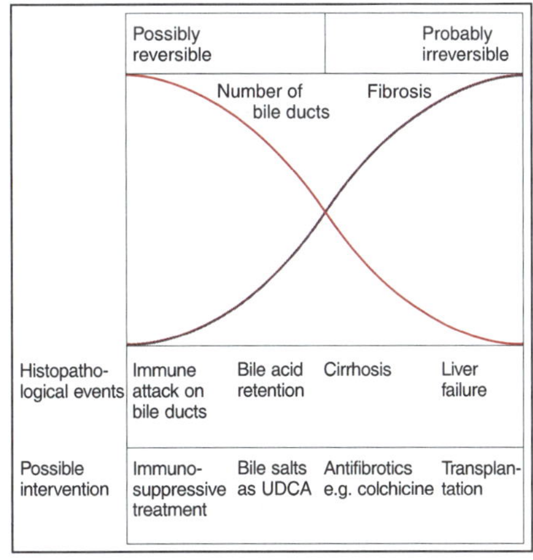

Progression of primary biliary cirrhosis and possible interventions. UDCA, ursodeoxycholic acid.

Treatment aims

To prevent progression.

To reverse symptoms.

Other treatments

Liver transplantation for end-stage disease or intractable symptoms [5].

Prognosis [6]

• Prognosis depends on serum bilirubin concentration: >10 mg/dL implies an 18-month survival.

• The median time from diagnosis to death is 10 years.

Follow-up and management

• Progression must be monitored.

• Complications must be prevented or treated.

Key references

1. Laurin JM, Lindor KD: Primary biliary cirrhosis. *Dig Dis Sci* 1994, **12**:331–350.

2. Locke GR III, Therneau TM, Ludwig J, *et al.*: Time course of histological progression in primary biliary cirrhosis. *Hepatology* 1996, **23**:52–56.

3. Lindor KD: Primary biliary cirrhosis: questions and promises. *Ann Intern Med* 1997, **126**:733–735.

4. Lindor KD, Therneau TM, Jorgensen RA, *et al.*: Effects of ursodeoxycholic acid on survival in patients with primary biliary cirrhosis. *Gastroenterology* 1996, **110**:1515–1518.

5. Ricci P, Therneau TM, Malinchoc M, *et al.*: A prognostic model for the outcome of liver transplantation in patients with cholestatic liver disease. *Hepatology* 1997, **25**:672–677.

6. Metcalf JV, Mitchison HC, Palmer JM, *et al.*: Natural history of early primary biliary cirrhosis. *Lancet* 1996, **348**:1399–1402.

Diagnosis

Symptoms

Change of bowel habit.

Blood in stools: often occult.

Loss of weight.

Tenesmus: rectal lesions.

Abdominal pain or swelling: not a common presentation for colorectal cancer.

Signs

Pallor: in patients with anemia.

Abdominal mass or distension.

Mass or blood on digital rectal examination.

Peritonitis: perforation.

Mechanical bowel obstruction.

Hepatomegaly: metastatic disease.

Cachexia, clinical evidence of weight loss.

Hematochezia: melena occasionally occurs with right-sided lesions.

Investigations

• Lesions identified during screening flexible sigmoidoscopy should undergo biopsy; patients with multiple or large (>1 cm) adenomas should be referred for colonoscopy.

Assessment of primary tumor

Colonoscopy: of patients with symptoms or signs of colorectal cancer; any polyps in these patients should be removed for histological examination; malignancy confined to the mucosa or Dukes' stage A (*see* Pathology) do not require surgery or chemotherapy if the lesion can be completely resected via the colonoscope (*i.e.*, the resection margins are free of disease [1].

Air contrast barium enema: highly competent radiologists can detect significant lesions at a sensitivity that approximates colonoscopy at a lower cost. However, the frequency of colonic lesions in older patients and inability to assess histology by this technique commonly favors colonoscopy.

Assessment of disseminated disease

Liver chemistry tests: metastatic disease often presents with an elevated alkaline phosphatase level.

Chest radiography: may detect solitary or multiple peripheral lung nodules.

Abdominal CT: to assess tumor burden in pelvis and to look for evidence of adenopathy or hepatic disease.

Liver ultrasonography: in absence of CT; inexpensive but lower sensitivity than CT.

Screening for prevention

Fecal occult blood testing: yearly in asymptomatic patients >50 years of age will reduce mortality but requires extensive resources to pursue the large number of false-positive tests [2,3].

Flexible sigmoidoscopy: every 5 years in asymptomatic patients >50 years of age [2].

Colonoscopy: for high-risk groups, *e.g.*, patients with two or more first-degree relatives with colon cancer or one first-degree relative <50 years of age with colon cancer; patients with a family history of familial polyposis or hereditary nonpolyposis colorectal cancer require surveillance colonoscopy beginning at an early age [2].

Complications

Obstruction: usually left-sided lesions.

Perforation, sepsis.

Acute hemorrhage or iron-deficiency anemia.

Fistula formation.

Differential diagnosis

Diverticular disease.
Inflammatory bowel disease.
Irritable bowel syndrome.
Adhesions.
Arteriovenous malformations.
Solitary rectal ulcer.
Mesenteric ischemia.

Risk factors

High-fat, low-fiber diet.
Chronic ulcerative colitis (>10 years).
Genetic: hereditary nonpolyposis colorectal cancer, familial polyposis coli.
Colorectal adenomas.

Epidemiology

• An asymptomatic average adult individual in the United States has a lifetime risk of 6% of developing colorectal cancer.

• The peak incidence is at 60–69 years of age.

• Colon cancer is the second most frequent cause of death due to malignancy in developed countries.

Pathology

Microscopic: adenocarcinoma.
Macroscopic: polypoidal, ulcerative, annular, diffuse or colloidial lesions.

Site
Rectum: 30%.
Cecum and ascending colon: 25%.
Sigmoid colon: 20%.
Descending colon: 15%.
Transverse colon: 10%.

Spread
Direct, lymphatic, venous.

Stage (Dukes' classification)
A: confined to mucosa/submucosa.
B: invasion of muscularis propria.
C: local node involvement.
D: distant metastases.

Treatment

Diet and lifestyle

• For primary prevention, fat intake should be reduced to 30% of energy intake. Unrefined fiber, fruit, and vegetable consumption should be increased. Regular aspirin intake has also been associated with a lower risk of colonic adenocarcinoma.

Pharmacological treatment

• Postoperative chemotherapy is of benefit in patients with Dukes' stage C disease. 5-Fluorouracil appears to be the most important component coupled with either leucovorin (6 months) or levamisole (12 months). There is no evidence of benefit in disseminated disease [4-6].

Nonpharmacological treatment

Elective surgery

Curative resection: right hemicolectomy, left hemicolectomy, anterior resection, or abdominoperineal excision, depending on site and extent of lesion.

Palliative resection or bypass.

Local treatment for rectal lesions: local transanal resection (open or endoscopic), laser therapy, or intracavity radiation.

Emergency surgery

• 20% of patients present with obstruction, possibly with perforation.

Adjuvant radiotherapy

• For rectal carcinoma, radiotherapy may be used preoperatively to reduce tumor burden.

Management of recurrence

• Management depends on the site, size, and number of metastases.

• Serial carcinoembryonic antigen estimation can predict recurrence and may be followed if the patient is a candidate for aggressive surgical management of extracolonic lesions (*e.g.*, solitary hepatic mestastases).

• Fewer than 20% of patients with recurrence after a "curative" resection are suitable for another resection.

Site of recurrence: local (20%; related to Dukes' stage), hepatic (30%), abdominal (20%), pulmonary (20%), retroperitoneal (10%).

For local disease: 50% amenable to further ablative surgery, with potential cure in 25%; radiotherapy effective palliation for rectal recurrence but limited by myelotoxicity.

For hepatic metastases: <20% (solitary or unilobar) amenable to curative resection; possible short-term benefit from hepatic artery infusion of 5-fluorodeoxyuridine; possible symptomatic relief for capsular distension with fractionated radiotherapy.

Treatment aims

To remove primary tumor and regional nodes, including mesorectum for rectal lesions (curative resection).

To remove or bypass the primary lesion with advanced local or metastatic disease, in order to ameliorate symptoms (palliative resection or bypass).

To control local disease in patients unfit for resection.

Prognosis

• 25% of patients have metastases at the time of presentation.

• In-hospital postoperative mortality (5%–7%) is related to intra-abdominal sepsis, obstruction, age, or cardiopulmonary complications.

• Overall 5-year survival rates are 80%–90% for Dukes' stage A, 50%–60% for stage B, 30% for stage C, and 5% for stage D.

Follow-up and management

• Patients resected for cure should undergo surveillance colonscopy within 6–12 months of resection to exclude missed lesions, and every 3–5 years in the absence of symptoms.

Key references

1. Bond JH, *et al.*: Polyp guideline: diagnosis, treatment, and surveillance for patients with nonfamilial colorectal polyps. *Ann Intern Med* 1993, **119**:836–843.

2. Winawer SJ, *et al.*: Colorectal cancer screening: clinical guidelines and rationale. *Gastroenterology* 1997, **112**:594–642.

3. Mandel JS, *et al.*: Reducing mortality from colorectal cancer by screening for fecal occult blood. *N Engl J Med* 1993, **328**:1365–1371.

4. Fuchs CS, Mayer RJ: Adjuvant chemotherapy for colon and rectal cancer. *Semin Oncol* 1995, **22**:472–487.

5. Moertal CC: Drug therapy: chemotherapy for colorectal cancer. *N Engl J Med* 1994, **330**:1136–1142.

6. O'Connell MJ, *et al.*: Controlled trial of fluorouracil and low dose leucovorin given for 6 months as postoperative adjuvant therapy for colon cancer. *J Clin Oncol* 1997, **15**:246–250.

Diagnosis

Definition

• Coma is a state of unresponsiveness to external stimuli in which the patient lies with eyes closed.

• In practice, the condition may usefully be defined as a patient with a Glasgow coma scale of 2:4:2 or less (*see box*).

Symptoms

• Coma is a symptom.

Signs

Fever: indicating infection (meningitis, encephalitis, systemic).

Hypothermia: may be cause or effect.

Neck stiffness, Kernig's sign, papilledema.

Cardiac abnormalities: can indicate subacute bacterial endocarditis or emboli.

Hypertension or hypotension.

Slow, shallow respiration: suggesting drug intoxication.

Rapid respiration: suggesting infection or acidosis.

Anemia, jaundice, rash.

Intoxication, diabetes, hepatic failure.

Organomegaly, polycystic kidneys, subarachnoid hemorrhage.

Meningitis, subarachnoid hemorrhage, raised intracranial pressure.

Investigations

History from a witness: for evolution of coma, circumstances of patient's discovery, trauma, seizure, drugs, previous medical history.

Glasgow coma scale: for level of consciousness [1].

Brain stem function tests: pupillary response, spontaneous eye movements, oculovestibular responses.

Motor function tests: for lateralizing features.

Fundal examination: for papilledema, hemorrhage, emboli.

Blood analysis: for biochemistry, *e.g.*, glucose, electrolytes; hepatic, renal, and thyroid function; toxin exposure; etc.

CT or MRI: for coma with focal signs or if the diagnosis is uncertain.

Lumbar puncture: for coma without focal signs but with stiff neck.

Hematological assays, chest radiography, EEG: for coma without focal signs or stiff neck (raised intracranial pressure must be excluded first).

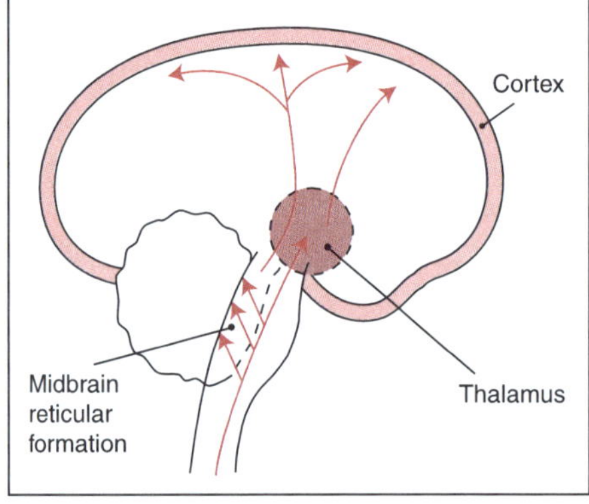

The anatomy of consciousness.

Complications

Infections: particularly respiratory or renal, *e.g.*, aspiration pneumonia.

Metabolic abnormalities.

Disseminated intravascular coagulation.

Decubitus ulcers.

Contractures.

Deep venous thromboses.

Corneal abrasion.

Death.

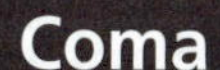

Treatment

Diet and lifestyle

• No special precautions are necessary.

Pharmacological treatment [3]

• Patients may need treatment for causative or concurrent disorders: antibiotics and antiviral agents, antifungal agents, correction of metabolic abnormalities, removal of toxic substances, treatment of mass lesions, s.c. heparin to prevent thrombotic complications.

• Steroids or mannitol should not be given routinely in comatose patients but may help in specific instances when raised intracranial pressure, due to edema, can be corrected.

Treatment aims

To correct cause.

To maintain hydration and nutrition.

To reverse coma and return normal physiological and psychological function.

Prognosis

• Sedative drugs or alcohol overdoses are not usually lethal, and the prognosis is good if the circulation and respiration are protected.

• The prognosis of other causes of non-traumatic coma depends on the cause (metabolic coma has better prognosis than hypoxic ischemic coma), the depth (the deeper the coma, the worse the prognosis), the duration (the longer the coma, the worse the prognosis), and clinical signs, *e.g.*, brain stem reflexes.

• Overall, only 15% of patients in non-traumatic coma for >6 hours make a good or moderate recovery.

Follow-up and management

• The airway must be maintained.

• The patient must be given adequate nutrition.

• Skin, chest, bladder, and bowel must be protected.

• Progress must be monitored.

Key references

1. Plumer F, Posner JB: *Stupor and Coma*, edn 3. Philadelphia: FA Davis; 1982.

2. Giacino JT: Disorders of consciousness: differential diagnosis and neuro-pathologic features. *Semin Neurol* 1997, **17**:105–111.

3. Bates D: The management of medical coma. *J Neurol Neurosurg Psychiatry* 1993, **56**:589–598.

Diagnosis

Symptoms

• Cor pulmonale is the enlargement of the right ventricle due to pulmonary hypertension that occurs in diseases of the lung, the chest wall, or the pulmonary circulation. By definition, primary diseases of the left side of the heart and congenital heart diseases are excluded.

• Although overt right ventricular failure is often present, right ventricular failure is not necessary for cor pulmonale.

Pedal edema, right upper quadrant pain, distended neck veins: symptoms related to right ventricular failure.

Exertional dyspnea, easy fatiguability, weakness: nonspecific findings.

Symptoms of chronic obstructive pulmonary disease (COPD), arthritic symptoms of connective tissue diseases: symptoms of the underlying pulmonary disorder may often predominate.

Signs

Right ventricular heave, right ventricular gallop, distended neck veins, tender and enlarged liver, pedal edema, severe limitation to exercise, cyanosis, clubbing, and orthostatic syncope: signs of right-sided cardiac failure.

Polycythemia, arterial hypoxemia: oxygen saturation is often <85%.

Chronic obstructive lung disease, cystic fibrosis, severe restrictive lung disease: signs of the underlying disorder may predominate.

Investigations

Arterial blood gases: should be done to assess the degree of arterial oxygen desaturation as well as the level of PCO_2 because COPD is the major cause of cor pulmonale.

Chest radiography: needed to assess the degree of pulmonary interstitial or parenchymal disease, to assess the size of the pulmonary arteries, and to document the enlarged right ventricle. Often the central pulmonary artery is enlarged, but distal pulmonary vessels are severely reduced, giving the patient the "pruned tree" appearance.

Pulmonary function tests: needed to assess the degree of underlying lung disease; will distinguish between obstructive and restrictive causes of pulmonary impairment.

ECG: may show a right axis deviation with right ventricular hypertrophy and right atrial enlargement (*i.e.*, P pulmonale). Deep S-waves are often present in lead V-6; low voltage is often seen in the presence of chronic obstructive lung disease. Arrhythmias, especially atrial tachyarrhythmias, are common.

Echocardiography: helpful in ruling out left ventricular disease; it is less helpful in pure right ventricular failure because air in the distended lungs makes it technically difficult to assess the right ventricle.

Ventilation perfusion scans: in the presence of right ventricular failure, these are not as helpful to assess vascular disease. Pulmonary angiography is the preferred method for diagnosis and assessment of pulmonary embolization.

Catheterization of the right side of the heart: will establish the ventricular and pulmonary artery pressures as well as determine cardiac output. Catheterization is often useful to exclude left ventricular failure.

Complications

Atrial tachyarrhythmias, particularly atrial fibrillation and supraventricular tachycardia: common.

Acute or chronic respiratory failure: often present due to the underlying lung disease in combination with the right ventricular failure. Emergency hospital admissions are often necessary due to respiratory infection.

• Complications of the underlying lung disease will often predominate (*e.g.*, in COPD, these would include infective exacerbations, respiratory failure and death, pneumothorax and lung cancer).

Treatment

Diet and lifestyle

• Patients should be encouraged to restrict sodium and maintain ideal weight.

• The use of alcohol and sedatives should be minimized to prevent episodes of respiratory failure.

Pharmacological treatment

Oxygen

• The mainstay of therapy is treatment of hypoxia by the administration of oxygen. The oxygen is most often given via nasal cannula, but in chronic situations may also be given through a transtrachael catheter.

Diuretics

• Patients with cor pulmonale generally will need diuretics to minimize fluid retention. The smallest amount of diuretic necessary to achieve the desired effect should be used. Over-aggressive use of a loop diuretic may precipitously decrease cardiac output, causing orthostatic hypotension and syncope.

Standard dosage	Depends on the degree of fluid retention. Patients with mild fluid retention may be managed with thiazide diuretics. Progression to loop diuretics is needed for most moderate to severe disease; combination of loop and thiazide diuretics or calcium channel blocker may be needed in the very severe cases. Fluid restriction may be needed in advanced disease.
Contraindications	Severe hypotension, renal failure, and hypokalemia (relative).
Main drug interactions	Potent diuresis seen occasionally with combination diuretic therapy.
Main side effects	Hypokalemia, renal impairment, orthostatic hypotension.

For underlying lung disorders

• Aggressive treatment of the underlying lung disorders is necessary. In most patients, this will be treatment of COPD, which would include bronchodilators, both inhaled beta-2 agonists and inhaled cholinergics, and inhaled steroids. Oral steroids would be indicated for acute exacerbations. (*See* Chronic obstructive pulmonary disease.)

• Antibiotics are appropriate for managing infective exacerbations of the pulmonary disorder, which often can contribute to worsening cor pulmonale.

• Digoxin is not used for right-sided failure unless the patient is in atrial fibrillation.

Treatment aims

To minimize alveolar hypoxia.

To minimize pedal edema.

To maximize respiratory function.

Other treatments

• Heart/lung transplantation should be considered, especially in younger patients with cor pulmonale.

Prognosis

• Prognosis in patients with cor pulmonale usually depends on the underlying pulmonary disease.

• The underlying pulmonary disease is a better predictor of survival than the severity of right ventricular failure.

• An average life expectancy in a patient after the development of cor pulmonale may be 2–5 years; however, this can vary widely.

General references

Klinger JR, Hill NS: Right ventricular dysfunction in chronic obstructive pulmonary disease: evaluation and management. *Chest* 1991, **99**:715.

MacNee W: Pathophysiology of cor pulmonale in chronic obstructive pulmonary disease. *Am J Respir Crit Care Med* 1994, **150**:833–1158.

Diagnosis

Symptoms [1–3]

Headache: present in 75% of patients; at any site, often throbbing, unilateral or asymmetrical, worse at night; scalp soreness and tenderness frequent.

Polymyalgia: proximal limb pain and stiffness in 58%.

Malaise, fatigue, weight loss: in 56%.

Jaw pain and fatigue: masticatory "claudication" in 40%.

Fever: in 35%.

Cough: in 17%.

Amaurosis fugax: in 10%.

Permanent visual loss: in 8%.

Limb claudication: in 8%.

Transient ischemic attack or stroke: in 7%.

Depression or confusional state: in 3%.

Diplopia: in 2%.

Signs

Abnormal temporal artery: tenderness, nodularity, thickening or reduced pulsation in 49% of patients.

Scalp tenderness elsewhere.

Tenderness of common carotid arteries.

Diminished carotid or limb pulses.

Ischemic optic neuropathy: pale, swollen disc in a recently blinded eye.

Ophthalmoplegia: due to cranial nerve or brain stem lesion.

Confusional state or encephalopathy.

Investigations

ESR measurement: substantially raised in most patients; mean, 85 ± 32 mm/h (<30 mm/h in 3% of patients).

Complete blood count: mild anemia, thrombocytosis, and raised leukocyte count common.

Liver function tests: raised gamma glutamyltransferase, alkaline phosphatase, or aspartate transaminase in 15% of patients.

Lumbar puncture: necessary only if low-grade meningitis or cortical thrombophlebitis considered in differential diagnosis.

Temporal artery biopsy: essential when diagnosis not absolutely clear cut on clinical grounds; at least 2–3 cm length biopsy (longer segment more likely to yield positive result); occipital artery biopsy alternative in selected patients.

Angiography: necessary only to exclude arterial dissection or other arteritides in selected patients; may show abnormalities in all major branches of aortic arch in cranial arteritis; lacks sensitivity and specificity as diagnostic test.

Complications

Permanent blindness: in 8% of patients.

Brain stem or carotid territory infarction: in <5%.

Myocardial infarction.

Scalp necrosis.

Limb ischemia.

Aortic rupture.

Differential diagnosis

Raised ESR

Other arteritides (rare in patients aged >70 years).
Myeloma.
Other skull metastases.
Subacute meningitis.
Infection with venous sinus thrombosis.

Normal ESR

Migraine.
Tension headache.
"Occipital neuralgia."
Cervical spine disease.
Paget's disease of the skull.
Vertebral or carotid dissection.
Temporomandibular joint disease.
Meningioma.

Etiology

• Cranial arteritis is presumed to be an autoimmune disorder, but the antigen is not known (perhaps component of internal elastic lamina).

• Immunoglobulin and complement deposits have been shown at the internal elastic lamina; other histological features suggest that cell-mediated mechanisms are also involved.

Epidemiology [4]

• The incidence is 9.3 in 100 000 population overall and 15–30 in 100 000 aged >50 years.

• The prevalence is 130 in 100 000 aged >50 years.

• Cranial arteritis rarely occurs in people aged <50 years.

• The median age of onset is 75 years (range, 56–92 years in published series).

• The female : male ratio is 3.7 : 1.

Pathology

• Cranial arteritis is an occlusive disease, involving large and medium-sized arteries arising from the aortic arch and sometimes the femoral arteries and aorta itself.

• Biopsy shows arterial luminal stenosis due to intimal proliferation, with disruption of the internal elastic lamina, mononuclear cell infiltration, necrosis of the media, giant cells, and granuloma formation; secondary thrombosis may be present. Involvement is patchy and may be missed by too small a biopsy.

Treatment

Diet and lifestyle
• No special precautions are necessary.

Pharmacological treatment [5]

General principles
• Cranial arteritis requires prompt treatment by corticosteroids to prevent the rare but serious complications, particularly blindness.

• Presenting symptoms are often nonspecific and "atypical" (*e.g.*, pyrexia of unknown origin, weight loss, anemia), so suspicion must be high and treatment initiated as soon as the diagnosis is seriously considered.

• Arterial biopsy is often taken after steroid treatment is started, but it should not be delayed by more than 2–3 days; the yield of positive histology in clinically probable cases falls from 60%–80% with early biopsy to only 10% in patients undergoing biopsy 1 week after starting steroid treatment.

• Traditional high doses of prednisolone are justifiable in all patients with visual symptoms or signs and in those with features of cerebral or myocardial ischemia.

• In critical cases (*e.g.*, visual loss in one eye and early symptoms in the other), infusion of high-dose methylprednisolone probably reduces the risk of complete blindness.

• In patients without visual symptoms, prospective trials suggest that most respond to much lower doses (even less needed for polymyalgia without symptomatic arteritis).

• The rate of reduction depends on clinical severity at presentation, starting dose, symptom control, and ESR.

• A maintenance dose of 5–10 mg daily is usually needed for 2–3 years.

• An alternate-day regimen is sometimes possible, when the dose is very low.

• 30%–50% of patients can discontinue treatment after 2 years.

• Some need treatment for several years, and a few apparently need long-term maintenance doses of 2–5 mg daily.

Steroid regimen [6]
Initial dose: prednisolone, 40–80 mg daily;
methylprednisolone, 1 g i.v. daily for 2–5 days in critical cases.

Months 1–2: reduced slowly to 20–40 mg daily.

Months 2–4: reduced slowly to 10–20 mg daily.

Months 4–24: reduced to maintenance dose 5–10 mg daily.

Months 24–36: withdrawal possible in ~50% of patients.

Complications of treatment
Vertebral compression fractures in 26%.

Other symptoms of osteoporosis.

Steroid myopathy in 11%.

Cataracts.

Gastrointestinal symptoms.

Other steroid side effects.

Other drugs
• Azathioprine has a modest steroid-sparing effect but is not of proven efficacy used alone.

• Cyclophosphamide is a possible third option but rarely used.

Treatment aims
To relieve symptoms.
To prevent complications.
To prevent and control steroid side effects.

Prognosis
• Prognosis is excellent with early and adequate steroid treatment, which is usually needed for at least 2–3 years.
• Subsequent morbidity is determined as much by steroid side effects as by the disease itself.

Follow-up and management
• Patients need regular monitoring of clinical symptoms, ESR, and potential steroid effects for at least 2 years, preferably in a specialist clinic (neurology or rheumatology).

Key references
1. Caselli RJ, Hunder GG, Whisnant JP: Neurologic disease in biopsy-proven giant cell (temporal) arteritis. *Neurology* 1988, **38**:352–359.
2. Hunder GG: Giant cell arteritis and polymyalgia rheumatica. *Med Clin North Am* 1997, **81**:195–219.
3. Turnbull J: Temporal arteritis and polymyalgia rheumatica: nosographic and nosologic considerations. *Neurology* 1996, **46**:901–906.
4. Nordborg E, Bengtsson BA: Epidemiology of proven giant cell arteritis (GCA). *Intern Med* 1990, **227**:233–236.
5. Evans J, Hunder GG: The implications of recognizing large-vessel involvement in elderly patients with giant cell arteritis. *Curr Opin Rheumatol* 1997, **9**:37–40.
6. Kyle V, Hazleman BL: Treatment of polymyalgia rheumatica and giant cell arteritis. Steroid regimens in the first two months. *Ann Rheum Dis* 1989, **48**:658–661.

Diagnosis

Symptoms
Diarrhea: nonbloody most common.
Abdominal pain.
Malaise and anorexia with subsequent weight loss.
Recurrent perianal pain and inflammation.
Arthropathy, skin, eye complaints in 10%–20%.

Signs
• Patients with mild to moderate disease most typically have a relatively normal examination.
Abdominal tenderness with occasional right lower quadrant mass or fullness: patients may present with signs of obstruction or peritonitis, in which case surgical consultation should be sought early.
Perianal abscess, fistula, or fissures outside of the midline: 50% of patients.
Muscle wasting, evidence of weight loss: in advanced or long-standing disease.
Pallor of mucous membranes, indicating anemia.
Clinical evidence of malabsorption such as chelosis, glossitis in vitamin B deficiencies, easy bruising in vitamin K deficiencies.
Skin findings (infrequent): tender red nodules of erythema nodosum, ulcerated lesions of pyoderma gangrenosum.
Arthritis of sacroiliac or other large axial joints: in a minority of patients.

Investigations
• The diagnosis of Crohn's disease can only be rendered after interpreting diagnostic studies in the context of the patient's clinical presentation (*i.e.*, radiographs, fiber-optic studies, or biopsies alone rarely in and of themselves make the diagnosis of Crohn's disease).
Stool studies: ova and parasites $\times$ 3, culture, *Clostridium difficile* toxin.
Complete blood count: to check for normochromic anemia of chronic disease, microcytic anemia of iron deficiency, macrocytic anemia (B_{12} and folate deficiency); increased platelets, and/or leukocytes may occur secondary to inflammation or infection.
ESR or CRP measurement: inflammatory markers of disease activity.
Electrolytes, blood urea nitrogen, creatine: abnormal in patients with dehydration.
Serum albumin: decreased in patients with malnutrition.
Colonoscopy: allows assessment of colonic disease and usually visualization of the terminal ileum and appropriate biopsy; Crohn's disease is characterized by intermittent disease (*e.g.*, aphthous or serpiginous ulcers) separated by areas of normal mucosa. Although perianal involvement is common, the rectum is often normal; strictures may be evidence of prior inflammation.
Mucosal biopsy.
Upper gastrointestinal endoscopy: if relevant symptoms; lesions must undergo biopsy to confirm that they are due to Crohn's disease.
Barium contrast radiography: small-bowel follow-through (or enteroclysis) allows assessment of small-bowel mucosal disease, such as rose-thorn ulceration, string sign, skip lesions, cobblestone mucosa, stricture, fistulous tracts; useful in assessing stricture formation and defining anatomy for surgery; barium enema may complement colonoscopy, particularly in checking for fistulas.
Abdominal CT scan: useful when checking for extraintestinal inflammation (*e.g.*, abscesses).
Radioisotope-labeled leukocyte scans: may be of use in localizing inflammation not detected by studies above or in defining extent of disease prior to surgical management.

Complications
Intestinal obstruction or perforation with abscess formation; intra-abdominal sepsis.
Fistula formation: to bowel, bladder, vagina, or skin.
Malnutrition, vitamin (*e.g.*, B_{12} deficiency).
Gastrointestinal bleeding, anemia.
Uveitis, episcleritis.
Skin lesions: erythema nodosum, pyoderma gangrenosum.
Cholestatic liver disease: *e.g.*, sclerosing cholangitis and rarely cholangiocarcinoma.
Renal oxalate stones: uncommon.
Deep venous thrombosis.
Secondary amyloidosis: rare.

Differential diagnosis [1]
Bacterial infections (*Salmonella, Shigella, Campylobacter* spp., *Escherichia coli, Yersinia*, tuberculosis, *C. difficile*).
Viral gastroenteritis, cytomegalovirus.
NSAID enteropathy.
Amebic infection, *Giardia* spp.
Ulcerative colitis.
Ischemia.
Colonic carcinoma.
Lymphoma.

Etiology
Unknown; environmental triggers such as smoking and unidentified infections in genetically susceptible individuals is the most popular opinion at this time. No specific dietary triggers have been identified [2].
Overall risk in first-degree relatives 5%–15%; higher with onset of disease in proband at a young age.

Epidemiology
• The prevalence of Crohn's disease is 1 in 1000.
• Ethnic clustering has been found.
• Onset may be in childhood.
• The disease most commonly presents in the third decade.
• The male : female ratio is equal.

Histology
Macroscopic
Patchy areas of disease with intervening areas of normal mucosa.
Terminal ileum involvement most common but disease can be found anywhere along the gastrointestinal tract.
Transmural inflammation.

Microscopic
Crypt distortion with inflammation.
Noncaseating granulomas: classic, but often not seen.
Lymphocytic infiltration.

Treatment

Diet and lifestyle

• Nutritional supplementation is needed in patients with severe illness, including parenteral nutrition in advanced disease. Elemental diets may be effective but are poorly tolerated because of unpalatability; remission induced by elemental diets does not continue after diets have been stopped.

• Patients should be urged to quit smoking.

• Patients with extensive small-bowel disease tolerate lactose poorly.

Pharmacological treatment [3–5]

Corticosteroids

• Corticosteroids are the most efficacious medication in the treatment of patients with moderate to severe disease.

Standard dose	Prednisone, 1 mg/kg up to a daily maximum of 60 mg/day; consider i.v. administration in patients with poor motility and absorptive function; topical steroids for rectal or perianal disease.
Contraindications	Overt sepsis; caution in hypertension and diabetes.
Special points	Does not prevent disease flair in patients in remission. Hip pain should immediately raise concern about possible aseptic necrosis. Long-term use should be avoided if possible, and steroid tapers should be initiated once the disease is in remission.
Main drug interactions	Significant immunosuppression with azathioprine: risk of opportunistic infections increased, immunization against varicella should be considered in patients without a history of chickenpox and negative antibody titer.
Main side effects	Fluid retention and hypertension, induction of glucose intolerance, osteoporosis, cushingoid features, mood lability, aseptic necrosis, hyperphagia, increased energy.

5-aminosalicylic acid preparations (*e.g.*, sulfasalazine, mesalamine, olsalazine) [3–5]

• These are used as sole agents in patients with mild to moderate disease and as supplemental medications to regimens for patients with more severe disease.

Standard dosage	Sulfasalazine, 4 g daily; mesalamine, 2.4–4.8 g daily.
Contraindications	Salicylate hypersensitivity, sulfonamide sensitivity with sulfasalazine, renal impairment with mesalamine.
Special points	Sulfasalazine causes reversible oligospermia, may cause hemolysis; slow-release preparation of mesalamine of particular benefit in small-bowel Crohn's disease.
Main side effects	Nausea, rashes, or occasional diarrhea.

Antibiotics

• Antibiotics are effective in some situations, particularly in perianal disease; they are of some benefit in small-bowel disease but mainly of use in colonic diseases.

• Metronidazole is the best-studied antibiotic but ciprofloxacin with the addition of azithromycin may also be shown in the future to be of benefit.

Standard dosage	Metronidazole, 500 mg orally 3 times daily.
Contraindications	Previous hypersensitivity, peripheral neuropathy.
Special points	Patients should avoid using alcohol (Antabuse effect).
Main drug interactions	Enhances effects of warfarin; inhibits metabolism of phenytoin.
Main side effects	Nausea, metallic taste, risk of neuropathy (long-term use).

Other immunosuppressive drugs

• These are useful as steroid-sparing agents and for additional immunosuppression in resistant disease.

• Azathioprine is the best-studied drug, but cyclosporine and methotrexate are also used in more refractory cases.

Special points	Risk of myelotoxicity maximal on starting treatment; whole blood count must be monitored closely, particularly in first few weeks, monthly thereafter.
Main drug interactions	Additive immunosuppressive effect with steroids.
Main side effects	Rashes, nausea, myelosuppression, increased risk of opportunistic infection, pancreatitis.

Key references

1. Kirsner JB, Shortr RG (eds.): *Inflammatory Bowel Disease*, edn 4. Baltimore: Williams & Wilkins; 1995.

2. Hanauer SB: Inflammatory bowel disease. *N Engl J Med* 1996, **334**:841–848.

3. Elton E, Hanauer SB: The medical management of Crohn's disease [review article]. *Aliment Pharmacol Ther* 1996, **10**:1–22.

4. Geier DL, *et al.*: New therapeutic agents in the treatment of inflammatory bowel disease. *Am J Med* 1992, **93**:1991–2008.

5. Reynolds PD, *et al.*: Pharmacotherapy of inflammatory bowel disease. *Dig Dis* 1993, **11**:334–342.

Diagnosis

Symptoms

Central weight gain: trunk more than arms and legs.

Hirsutism, thin skin, easy bruising, stretch marks, acne on back and chest.

Muscle weakness and aching, back and joint pain.

Menstrual disturbance, impotence, loss of libido.

Depression, anxiety, psychiatric and sleep disturbance.

Signs

Centripetal obesity.

"Moon face," hirsutism, facial plethora.

Thin skin relative to age, easy bruising, acne, red or purple wide abdominal striae: not just stretch marks, which are common in obese patients and after pregnancy.

Proximal myopathy: *e.g.*, difficulty rising from squat without assistance.

Hypertension: incidental finding or with symptoms of cardiovascular complications.

Kyphosis, loss of height.

Pedal edema.

Male-pattern balding in women: comparison with previous photographs can be extraordinarily helpful.

Investigations [1–5]

• The diagnosis of Cushing's syndrome is made biochemically, not radiologically. Imaging procedures should be used to confirm and extend the results of biochemical testing.

Screening tests for Cushing's syndrome

24-hour urinary-free cortisol (UFC): usually increased 2–3-fold in Cushing's syndrome. Smaller increases may be due to depression, alcoholism, or obesity (pseudo-Cushing's).

Overnight dexamethasone suppression test: dexamethasone, 1 mg, is given orally at 23.00 hours. Serum cortisol obtained at 08.00 hours the following day will normally be <5 mg/dL. Patients with Cushing's will fail to suppress. Higher false-positive rate than 24-hour UFC.

Differential diagnosis of Cushing's syndrome

Plasma corticotropin (ACTH) measurement: undetectable concentration confirms an adrenal source (adrenal adenoma or carcinoma). Values >400 ng/L suggest, but do not prove, ectopic ACTH secretion secondary to tumor.

Liddle test (6-day dexamethasone suppression test) [2]: 24-hour UFCs and 17-OH corticosteroids (17-OHS) are measured on 6 consecutive days. Days 1 and 2 are baseline. On days 3 and 4, patients receive dexamethasone, 0.5 mg orally every 6 hours (low dose). On days 5 and 6, they receive 2 mg every 6 hours (high dose). Suppression of UFCs and 17-OHS from the average of the baseline days to day 6 is calculated. Suppression of UFCs by >90% and 17-OHS by >64% is highly suggestive of Cushing's disease (84% sensitivity with 100% specificity).

8-mg overnight dexamethasone suppression test [3] and corticotropin-releasing hormone (CRH) simulation test [4]: newer tests that are emerging as efficient and effective in separating pituitary from nonpituitary causes of Cushing's syndrome.

Petrosal sinus sampling catheterization [5]: confirms pituitary ACTH secretion with high degree of confidence. Simultaneous use of CRH increases accuracy of test. Can also be used to lateralize the pituitary tumor. Requires a well-trained invasive radiologist.

CT or MRI of pituitary gland: if pituitary disease is suspected.

CT or MRI of adrenal glands: if primary adrenal disease is suspected.

CT or MRI of chest snd/or abdomen: if ectopic ACTH syndrome is suspected and source of ACTH is unknown.

Complications

Diabetes, infections, osteoporosis, thromboembolism, ischemic heart disease, cerebrovascular disease, peripheral vascular disease.

Differential diagnosis

Simple obesity.

Polycystic ovarian syndrome.

• Few patients with obesity, hirsutism, bruising, stretch marks, hypertension, or diabetes have Cushing's syndrome.

Etiology [1]

ACTH-dependent Cushing's syndrome

• Pituitary Cushing's disease (70% of patients) is usually due to a (basophil) corticotroph microadenoma, but can be due to macroadenoma or very rarely to corticotroph hyperplasia.

• Ectopic ACTH secretion (10%) is usually due to tumors of neuroendocrine origin (carcinoid, metastatic gastrointestinal endocrine tumors).

•Ectopic corticotropin-releasing hormone secretion is rare.

Adrenal Cushing's syndrome

• Causes include adrenal adenoma (10%), adrenal carcinoma (10%), and macronodular or micronodular adrenal hyperplasia (rare).

Iatrogenic Cushing's syndrome

• The most common cause of the clinical syndrome, this is due to steroid or ACTH treatment.

Epidemiology

• Endogenous Cushing's syndrome is rare.

• Cushing's syndrome and adrenal adenomas occur more often in women.

Ectopic ACTH syndrome

Occult ectopic ACTH syndrome

• This is usually seen when a neuroendocrine tumor (mostly carcinoid, of bronchial or thymic origin) secretes large amounts of ACTH and mimics a pituitary adenoma.

• The tumor may be only a few millimeters in diameter and only discovered after intensive imaging over extended periods of time; diagnosis may prove difficult with conventional tests.

Overt ectopic ACTH secretion

• Many malignant tumors secrete ACTH, most often bronchial small-cell carcinoma; usually the tumor is clinically obvious.

• Patients are rarely cushingoid; they may have no endocrine symptoms or may exhibit pigmentation, myopathy, weight loss, and debility, associated with high cortisol and ACTH concentrations and profound hypokalemic alkalosis.

Treatment

Diet and lifestyle

• Diet and lifestyle changes must be combined with medical or surgical treatment.

• Patients who maintain regular low-impact exercise and weight control probably have an improved postoperative recovery.

Pharmacological treatment

• Medical treatment for Cushing's syndrome is effective in improving the clinical syndrome but is a short-term measure to prepare the patient for surgery, while awaiting the long-term benefit of other treatment, or in patients with inoperable tumors.

• Drugs include metyrapone, ketoconazole, aminoglutethimide, and mitotane; all have significant problems and should be used only under specialist supervision.

Nonpharmacological treatment

For Cushing's disease

• Selective adenomectomy is the treatment of choice. Transsphenoidal surgery must be performed by a surgeon experienced in locating and removing ACTH-secreting microadenomas. Successful surgery results in temporary adrenal insufficiency due to the suppression of normal hypothalamic–pituitary function.

• Pituitary irradiation is combined with mitotane for patients with inoperable tumors or surgical failures. Bilateral adrenalectomy is reserved for patients who fail transsphenoidal surgery and external radiation therapy.

For ectopic ACTH syndrome

• Surgical excision is the treatment of choice if the hormone-secreting tumor can be localized and is resectable. Chemotherapy should be used when appropriate (*e.g.*, small cell cancers), with radiotherapy reserved for inoperable tumors (rarely effective).

• Long-term medical therapy (2–3 years) can be used with periodic (every 6 months) scanning to localize difficult-to-find tumors. Patients who begin to decompensate during this time due to excessive cortisol secretion should undergo bilateral adrenalectomy. Attempts to identify and resect the tumor should continue even after adrenalectomy.

For adrenal tumors

Excision of adrenal adenomas: usually complete, with cure of clinical syndrome and temporary adrenal insufficiency due to suppression of normal axis.

Excision of adrenal carcinomas: sometimes complete, although these carcinomas are often inoperable and usually recur (in which case, medical treatment is essential).

Micronodular or macronodular adrenal disease: bilateral adrenalectomy cures clinical syndrome and results in permanent adrenal insufficiency requiring hormone replacement (hydrocortisone and, in many cases, Florinef).

Treatment aims

To restore a normally functioning hypothalamo–pituitary axis, without damage to other endocrine axes.

Prognosis

• Young patients with mild Cushing's disease cured by transsphenoidal surgery without recurrence have no long-term sequelae.

• Patients with adrenal carcinoma usually suffer recurrence and death within months–years.

• Before effective treatment was available, 50% of patients with Cushing's syndrome died within 5 years of diagnosis.

• The overall "cure" rate for transsphenoidal surgery is usually 75%–80% but can be as low as 50% (depending on the criteria used to define cure).

• Bilateral adrenalectomy is 100% effective, but patients suffer from life-long hypoadrenalism and are at a small risk of Nelson's syndrome (pituitary hyperplasia).

• For adrenal adenomas, surgical excision cures most patients.

Follow-up and management

• Follow-up must be life-long because of the risk of recurrence and morbidity.

• Management depends on the individual patient and should be done by specialists.

Key references

1. Tsigos C, Chrousos GP: Differential diagnosis and management of Cushing's syndrome. *Ann Rev Med* 1996, **47**:443–461.

2. Flack MR, Oldfield EH, Cutler GB Jr, *et al.*: Urine free cortisol in the high-dose dexamethasone suppression test for the differential diagnosis of the Cushing syndrome. *Ann Intern Med* 1992, **116**:211–217.

3. Dichek HL, Nieman LK, Oldfield EH, *et al.*: A comparison of the standard high dose dexamethasone suppression test and the overnight 8-mg dexamethasone suppression test for the differential diagnosis of adrenocorticotropin-dependent Cushing's syndrome. *J Clin Endocrinol Metab* 1994, **78**:418–422.

4. Nieman LK, Oldfield EH, Wesley R, *et al.*: A simplified morning ovine corticotropin-releasing hormone stimulation test for the differential diagnosis of adreno-corticotropin-dependent Cushing's syndrome. *J Clin Endocrinol Metab* 1994, **77**:1308–1312.

5. Oldfield EH, Doppman JL, Nieman LK, *et al.*: Petrosal sinus sampling with and without corticotropin-releasing hormone for the differential diagnosis of Cushing's syndrome. *N Engl J Med* 1991, **325**:897–905.

Diagnosis

Symptoms

Cough that produces viscous and purulent sputum, shortness of breath, hemoptysis, wheezing.

Sinusitis, nasal polyposis.

Sterility in males, decreased fertility in females: due to absent or defective vas deferens in males and increased viscosity of vaginal secretions in females.

Signs of congestive heart failure and cor pulmonale in late disease.

Gastrointestinal symptoms: including meconium ileus or distal intestinal obstruction syndrome, malabsorption with weight loss, steatorrhea, failure to thrive in infancy and childhood, rectal prolapse, intussusception, volvulus, recurrent pancreatitis, cirrhosis.

Diabetes mellitus.

Salt depletion, heat stroke.

Signs

Inspiratory and expiratory rhonchi, rales, wheezes; barrel-shaped chest, reduced breath sounds, signs of hyperinflation; cyanosis, presence of *Pseudomonas* spp. in respiratory secretions, clubbing (hypertrophic osteoarthropathy).

Thin, anorexic appearance: however, normal size and weight does not rule out a diagnosis of cystic fibrosis.

Right ventricular heave, pedal edema: with cor pulmonale.

Pneumothorax.

Respiratory failure.

Investigations

• There is an increase in sweat chloride in patients with cystic fibrosis. Sweat chloride by quantitative pilocarpine iontophoresis is the standard for diagnosing cystic fibrosis. A level >60 mEq/L supports the diagnosis. Genetic testing is available commercially. It identifies the most frequent mutations that cause cystic fibrosis. Genetic testing identifies ~90% of the defective cystic fibrosis genes.

Pulmonary function testing: should be done to document severity of the obstructive respiratory defect. Pulmonary function studies may show airway hyperreactivity. Level of oxygenation by pulse oximetry or arterial blood gases should be done. PO_2 levels may be normal in mild disease, but eventually dip below 55 mm Hg on room air, signaling the need for oxygen supplementation. In end-stage disease, elevations of arterial PCO_2 occur.

• The most frequent organisms on sputum culture are *Staphylococcus aureus*, *Pseudomonas aeruginosa*, or *Burkholderia (Pseudomonas) cepacia*. These organisms are virtually never eradicated.

Pancreatic function studies: may be done to demonstrate steatorrhea, although clinical description suffices in most cases.

Chest radiography: shows hyperinflation increased linear streaking and nodular–cystic pattern, which involve all lung areas, most particularly the right upper lobe.

Complications

Infective exacerbations: common.

Malnutrition with weight loss.

Pulmonary hypertension.

Gastrointestinal obstruction.

Diabetes mellitus.

Atelectasis.

Massive hemoptysis.

Cor pulmonale.

Respiratory failure.

Death.

Differential diagnosis

Asthma.

Chronic bronchitis.

Emphysema.

Bronchiectasis from any other causes.

Chronic pancreatitis.

Hypogammaglobulinemia.

Alpha$_1$-antitrypsin deficiency.

Malabsorption from any other cause.

Cirrhosis from any other cause.

Etiology

• Cystic fibrosis is an inherited disease that follows an autosomal recessive pattern of transmission. An abnormality resulting in the loss of phenylalanine residue at position 508 on the long arm of chromosome 7 accounts for ~70% of all cystic fibrosis mutations. >600 other abnormalities at this site have been identified with the disease.

Epidemiology

• Cystic fibrosis is the most common life-limiting genetic disease in the United States; its frequency varies with ethnicity.

• The incidence is ~1:3 300 white newborns, ~1:15 300 in African-Americans, and 1:32 100 in Asian-Americans.

Treatment

Diet and lifestyle

• Many patients with cystic fibrosis have higher caloric needs both from the malabsorption and the increase workload of breathing. Replacement of pancreatic enzymes with normal diets and even increased caloric intake will help to maintain normal or near-normal weight.

• Fat-soluble vitamins (vitamins A, D, E, and K) are recommended as a supplement.

Pharmacological treatment

Antibiotic therapy

• Oral antibiotics are indicated for minor exacerbations of sensitive organisms. Agents selected should reflect the sputum culture and the susceptibilities. Because *P. aeruginosa* is a frequent pathogen, anti-pseudomonal oral agents are often used.

• Ciprofloxacin, 750 mg twice daily, or ofloxacin, 400 mg twice daily for 2- to 3-week course, would be common agents used against *Pseudomonas* spp. Patients with staphylococcus infection are often treated with dicloxacillin, 500 mg every 6 hours, or cephalexin, 500 mg every 6 hours.

• Patients with cystic fibrosis will have recurrent exacerbations. For major exacerbation, i.v. antibiotics are indicated; i.v. antibiotics should be chosen reflecting the culture and sensitivity of the sputum. In general two agents are used, especially to obtain synergy against *Pseudomonas* spp. Popular combinations include ceftazidime/tobramycin or tobramycin/piperacillin. Dosage of aminoglycoside should be determined by monitoring plasma levels.

• Nebulized anti-pseudomonal antibiotic (usually gentamycin or tobramycin) can be added as a prophylactic measure to minimize the infective exacerbations. Treatment for mild, moderate, and severe exacerbations usually are for 14–21 days, but sometimes are even longer. Patients should demonstrate return to baseline function in terms of pulmonary signs and symptoms for 3–4 days prior to discontinuation of the treatment.

• Home i.v. antibiotics are becoming increasingly common and guidelines have been established to select candidates for this therapy.

Bronchodilators

• These include inhaled beta-agonists, inhaled anticholinergics (which have been shown to be efficacious in a subset of patients with cystic fibrosis), and theophyllines (occasionally used in patients with cystic fibrosis, especially in the presence of reactive airway disease).

Standard dosage	Inhaled beta-2 agonists (*e.g.*, albuterol, metaproterenol, terbutaline), are used two puffs up to four times daily as needed. Ipratropium bromide inhaler (or another anticholinergic), two puffs 4 times daily. Theophylline, 300–600 mg daily.
Special points	*Theophyllines:* plasma concentrations must be monitored; they should be maintained between 10–15 µg/L.
Main drug interactions	*Inhaled beta-2 agonists*: none. *Inhaled anticholinergics*: none. *Theophyllines*: cimetidine, erythromycin, ciprofloxacin.
Main side effects	*Inhaled beta-2 agonists*: tremor. *Inhaled anticholinergics*: dry mouth in rare cases. *Theophyllines*: tachycardia and arrhythmias.

Mucolytic therapy

Standard dosage	DNase, aerosolized, 2.5 mg once daily.
Main drug interactions	None.
Special points	An approved nebulizer must be used to ensure adequate delivery.
Main side effects	Dysphagia or hoarseness, seen uncommonly.

Pancreatic enzymes

• Most patients with cystic fibrosis have exocrine pancreatic deficiency. Pancreatic enzymes are useful to minimize malabsorption. Dosing is emperic. The most common brands available in the United States are Pancrease, Ultrase, and Creon. Doses >6000 lipase U/kg/meal have been associated with colonic strictures in children. Fat-soluble vitamins (vitamins A, D, E, and K) are recommended (*e.g.*, ADEKs or Vitamax).

General references

Clinical Practice Guidelines for Cystic Fibrosis. Bethesda: The Cystic Fibrosis Foundation; 1977.

Davis PB, Drumm M, Konstan MW: Cystic fibrosis. *Am J Respir Crit Care Med* 1996, **154**:1229–1256.

Ramsey BW: Management of pulmonary disease in patients with cystic fibrosis. *N Engl J Med* 1996, 335:179–188.

Stern RC: The diagnosis of cystic fibrosis. *N Engl J Med* 1997, **336**:487–491.

Diagnosis

Symptoms

Loss of vision, floaters, decrease in visual acuity, unexplained fever: indicating retinitis (asymptomatic at early stage).

Fever, anorexia, odynophagia, weight loss, diarrhea, pain, cramps: indicating gastrointestinal tract infection (esophagitis, gastritis, colitis, or biliary involvement).

Fever, lower extremity weakness, headaches, seizures, somnolence: indicating polyradiculopathy or encephalopathy.

Fever, cough, dyspnea: indicating pneumonitis.

Signs

Fever: in 60%–80% of patients with cytomegalovirus disseminated infection.

Decreased visual acuity: indicating retinitis.

Weight loss, abdominal tenderness, hemorrhages: indicating gastrointestinal tract infections.

Neurological deficit, lethargy, coma: indicating CNS complications.

Increase of respiratory rate, minimal findings at auscultation: indicating pneumonitis.

Investigations

• The disease is caused by recrudescence of a latent infection, so serological tests are of limited value.

Fundoscopy: in retinitis, shows hemorrhagic exudates and necrotic areas.

Endoscopy: in gastrointestinal tract infection, shows submucosal hemorrhages, ulceration; each level of tract may be involved, *e.g.*, esophagus, stomach, duodenum, small intestine, or colon.

Ultrasonography: in cholangitis, shows dilatation of biliary tract.

Biopsy: in cholangitis, shows cytomegalovirus inclusions.

Fundoscopic appearance of cytomegalovirus retinitis. (*See* Color Plate.)

CSF culture: in encephalitis or myelitis, shows increased cells (nonspecific), presence of cytomegalovirus (unusual) in culture or polymerase chain reaction.

CT or MRI: in encephalitis or myelitis, shows ventriculitis or ependymitis, using contrast enhancement.

Transbronchial biopsy: in pneumonitis, shows cytomegalovirus inclusions.

Complications

Loss of vision, retinal detachment, acute retinal necrosis.

Gastrointestinal tract perforation, hemorrhages.

Respiratory failure.

Coma or death.

Differential diagnosis

Retinitis

Cotton-wool spot.

Toxoplasmosis.

Herpes simplex or varicella–zoster virus.

Acute retinal necrosis.

Syphilis.

Pneumocystis carinii choroiditis.

Gastrointestinal tract

Cryptosporidiosis or microsporidiosis.

Giardia, *Entamoeba*, *Shigella*, *Salmonella*, *Mycobacterium avium*, or *Campylobacter* spp. infection.

Lymphoma.

Kaposi's sarcoma.

Herpes simplex virus.

Encephalitis or myelitis

HIV encephalopathy or myelopathy.

Progressive multifocal leukoencephalopathy.

Aseptic meningitis.

Herpes virus encephalitis.

Spinal cord lymphoma.

Pneumonitis

P. carinii infection.

Mycobacteria infection.

Etiology

• Reactivation of latent cytomegalovirus infection due to underlying immune deficiency may be a cause.

• Cytomegalovirus infection is a potential cofactor of HIV disease.

Epidemiology

• >90% of homosexual or bisexual men have latent cytomegalovirus infection.

• Cytomegalovirus disease is found in 20%–40% of AIDS patients.

• End-stage opportunistic infection occurs in 90% of patients with CD4 counts of $<50 \times 10^6$/L (median, 25×10^6/L).

Treatment

Diet and lifestyle

• No special precautions are necessary.

Pharmacological treatment

Choice of treatment

• Systemic treatment is indicated in acute visceral localization. Ganciclovir and foscarnet have similar efficacy: 90% in retinitis, 80%–95% in gastrointestinal tract disorder, 60%–80% in pneumonitis. Cidovofir is effective for treatment of retinitis.

• Maintenance treatment is indicated for retinitis and gastrointestinal tract involvement (nonsystematically). Ganciclovir and foscarnet have similar efficacy: 50% relapse within 4 months.

Ganciclovir

• Intravenous ganciclovir is less toxic than foscarnet; intravitreal implants are available.

• Oral ganciclovir may be considered for maintenance therapy.

• It is active against cytomegalovirus and herpesvirus.

• Disadvantages include hemotoxicity and resistance in some strains of cytomegalovirus.

Standard dosage	*Acute:* ganciclovir, 5 mg/kg i.v. twice daily, 20 minutes infusion for 2–3 weeks. *Maintenance:* ganciclovir, 5 mg/kg i.v. once daily long term.
Contraindications	Neutropenia, anemia, resistant strains.
Main drug interactions	Zidovudine and other hemotoxic drugs.
Main side effects	Neutropenia, thrombocytopenia (frequent); rash-convulsion (unusual).

• Oral ganciclovir, 3 g daily, reduces progression of cytomegalovirus retinitis after i.v. induction. It may be considered for maintenance therapy following i.v. treatment for central retinitis and in additon to retinal implants.

Foscarnet

• Foscarnet may be considered in individuals who progress on ganciclovir.

• Advantages include absence of hemotoxicity and anti-HIV effect; disadvantages include the long infusion time.

Standard dosage	*Acute:* foscarnet, 90 mg/kg in 0.75–1.0 L saline isotonic solution i.v. twice daily, 90-minute infusion for 2–3 weeks. *Maintenance:* foscarnet, 90 mg/kg 0.75–1.0 L saline isotonic solution i.v. once daily, 90–120-minute infusion.
Contraindications	Renal impairment, concomitant nephrotoxic drugs.
Main drug interactions	Amphotericin B, i.v. pentamidine.
Main side effects	Nephrotoxicity, hypocalcemia, hypophosphatemia, nausea, genital ulcer.

Cidovofir

• Cidovofir may be considered in individuals who progress on ganciclovir.

Standard dosage	Cidovofir, 5 mg/kg/wk induction × 2–3 weeks; then every other week.
Contraindications	Renal impairment.
Main drug interactions	Amphotericin, pentamidine.
Main side effects	Nephrotoxicity.

Prognosis

• The incidence of visceral manifestations of cytomegalovirus is approximately 30%.

• Median survival is 12–18 months.

• With maintenance treatment, retinitis relapse has a high rate (>70%) and occurs approximately 2 months after therapy.

Follow-up and management

• Patients having acute treatment should be followed up every week.

• Patients having maintenance treatment must be followed up every 2–3 weeks.

General references

d'Arminio Monforte A, Mainini F, Testa L, *et al.*: Predictors of cytomegalovirus disease, natural history, and autopsy findings in a cohort of patients with AIDS. *AIDS* 1997, **11**:517–524.

Jabs D, SOCA group: Mortality in patients with acquired immunodeficiency syndrome treated with either foscarnet or ganciclovir for cytomegalovirus retinitis. *N Engl J Med* 1992, **326**:213–220.

Rodriguez-Barradas MC, Stool E, Musher DM, *et al.*: Diagnosing and treating cytomegalovirus pneumonia in patients with AIDS. *Clin Infect Dis* 1996, **23**:76–81.

Spector SA, McKinley GF, Lalczari JP, *et al.*: Oral ganciclovir for the prevention of cytomegalovirus disease in persons with AIDS. *N Engl J Med* 1996, **334**:1491–1497.

Diagnosis

Symptoms

Asymptomatic

Typical of isolated calf thrombi.

Common in high risk groups, *e.g.*, patients with acute cerebrovascular accident, spinal cord injuries, or malignancy, those undergoing general surgical or orthopedic surgical procedures, and hospitalized medical patients (*see* Prophylactic treatment).

Lower extremity pain

Dull ache or tightness in the calf or entire leg.

• Pain is generally worse when walking or standing.

Signs

Erythema, tenderness, and edema of the involved calf.

Slight fever and tachycardia.

Distention of superficial venous collateral vessels.

Palpable venous cord.

Homans' sign: limitation of dorsiflexion of the foot secondary to pain (insensitive and unreliable finding).

Phlegmasia cerulia dolens: pale, cool extremity resulting from severe venous obstruction and reflex arterial spasm.

Investigations

Venography: remains the gold standard of diagnosis: can define the location, extent, and degree of attachment of the thrombus; is the only reliable way to detect calf-vein or intra-abdominal thrombosis; limitations include the potential to induce thrombi at the injection site, the risk of contrast reaction, and decreased sensitivity for defining recurrent thrombosis.

Doppler ultrasound: diagnostic finding is noncompressibility of a venous segment; the addition of Doppler technology to standard two-dimensional ultrasound allows for detection of sonic differences in flow rates that occur with inspiration. Sensitivity for symptomatic patients is 93% by meta-analysis and it has been shown to be safe to withhold anticoagulation in patients with serial negative studies (*e.g.*, days 1, 2, and 6)[1]. Specificity is high; positive results are diagnostic and do not require confirmatory studies. Clinical models have been developed to identify low-risk patients with clinically suspected lower extremity deep-vein thrombosis (DVT) [2]. If validated, clinicians will be able to identify persons in whom a single negative Doppler ultrasound essentially rules out DVT.

Impedance plethysmography: with a proximal venous obstruction there is a delay in the characteristic increase in calf impedance when a thigh cuff is deflated. Sensitivity and specificity are comparable to Doppler ultrasound in the detection of symptomatic DVT. Unacceptably low sensitivity for asymptomatic clots.

Complications

Pulmonary embolism.

Postphlebitic syndrome.

Recurrent DVT.

Differential diagnosis

Cellulitis.

Venous stasis or lymphedema.

Popliteal inflammatory cysts (Baker's cysts).

Pathophysiology

Most thrombi originate as a platelet nidus within the valvular sinuses of the calf veins.

Platelets and fibrin aggregate to form a red fibrin clot that either dissolves or becomes organized and adherent to the vessel wall.

At any time during the process the clot may propagate or detach.

Risk factors: Virchow's triad

Trauma: direct lower extremity trauma, surgery (particularly orthopedic surgery), prior DVT, or varicose veins.

Hypercoagulable states: antithrombin III deficiency, protein C deficiency, protein S deficiency, resistance to activated protein C (factor V Leiden), antiphospholipid syndrome, malignancy, hyperhomocysteinemia, estrogen-containing medications, polycythemia.

Stasis: anesthesia, cerebrovascular accident, paraplegia, hospitalized medical patients.

Epidemiology

(Extrapolation to account for clinically unsuspected cases.)

Five million episodes of DVT annually in the United States.

500 000 pulmonary emboli annually.

50 000 attributable deaths annually.

Treatment

Lifestyle management

• Bedrest is recommended with the legs elevated and the knees slightly bent until the local tenderness and swelling have subsided.

• Support stockings should be worn at all times after a symptomatic DVT.

Pharmacological treatment

Initial therapy

• Therapy should begin with heparin for an immediate effect (80 U/kg bolus followed by 18 U/kg/h continuous infusion).

• A partial thromboplastin time (PTT) range of 1.5 – 2.5 times control should be targeted.

• Begin warfarin loading once target PTT is attained on heparin to a target international normalized ratio (INR) of 2.0–3.0.

• Five days of heparin infusion have been shown to be as effective as 10 days in terms of preventing recurrences.

• Thrombolytic agents are more effective at achieving early patency rates but are associated with an unacceptably higher incidence of serious bleeding.

Low molecular weight (LMW) heparin

• Treatment with LMW heparin at home during warfarin loading has been shown to be safe and effective.

• The fixed subcutaneous dosage is higher than dosages used for prophylaxis and it varies for different preparations.

• Monitoring of PTT is unnecessary.

Duration of treatment

• Oral anticoagulants should be continued for 3–6 months after an initial episode of DVT.

• Consider indefinite anticoagulation for recurrences and for events in the setting of permanent risk factors if there are no contraindications to anticoagulation.

Prophylactic treatment

Orthopedic surgery

• The rates for DVT are similar for LMW heparin vs. adjusted-dose warfarin to INR 2.0–3.0.

• Both warfarin and LMW heparin have shown limited efficacy in preventing DVT in patients undergoing knee replacement, although recent studies suggest a significant difference favoring LMW heparin (36.9% vs. 51.7% event rate) [3].

• Significantly fewer recurrences occur when prophylaxis with LMW heparin is continued for 1 month postoperatively rather than only during the hospitalization.

General surgery

Early ambulation only for low-risk patients (age <40 years, cases <60 minutes).

Heparin 5000 U twice daily, compression stockings, or intermittent pneumatic compression devices (IPC) for moderate-risk patients (age >40 years, major surgery).

Heparin 5000 U three times daily or LMW heparin for high-risk patients (age >40 years, major surgery, and other risk factors).

LMW heparin or adjusted-dose warfarin with IPC for very high-risk cases (multiple risk factors).

Hospitalized medical patients

• High-risk patients shown to benefit from heparin prophylaxis include intensive care unit patients, those with underlying malignancy, patients with spinal cord injuries or cerebro-vascular accident, patients with indwelling catheters, and hospitalized patients aged >65 years.

Treatment aims

To prevent pulmonary embolism.

To prevent recurrent DVT.

To prevent the postphlebitic state.

Other treatment options

Thrombectomy: can achieve high early patency rates; the majority will eventually reocclude; indicated only for phlegmasia cerulea dolens.

Vena caval interruption: Greenfield filter has an extremely low rate of recurrent pulmonary embolism (4%) over 20 years; indicated for recurrent events (DVT or pulmonary embolism while adequately anticoagulated or when there is a contraindication to systemic anticoagulation.

Prognosis

Postphlebitic syndrome: nearly 30% of patients with DVT may develop characteristic changes of pain, swelling, and discoloration after 8 years of follow-up.

Recurrent DVT: rates are estimated to be 20% at 2 years and 30% at 8 years; independent risk factors for increased rates of recurrence include an underlying diagnosis of malignancy, younger age at first presentation, and a history of thrombophilia [4].

Key references

1. Heijboer H, *et al*.: A comparison of real-time compression ultrasonography with impedance plethysmography for the diagnosis of deep-vein thrombosis in symptomatic outpatients. *N Engl J Med* 1993, **329**:1365–1369.

2. Wells PS, Hirsh J, Anderson DR, *et al*.: Accuracy of clinical assessment of deep-vein thrombosis. *Lancet* 1995, **345**:1326–1330.

3. Leclerc JR, Geerts WH, Desjardins L, *et al*.: Prevention of venous thromboembolism after knee arthroplasty: a randomized, double-blind trial comparing enoxaparin with warfarin. *Ann Intern Med* 1996, **124**:619–626.

4. Pradoni P, *et al*.: The long-term clinical course of acute deep venous thrombosis. *Ann Intern Med* 1996, **125**:1–7.

Diagnosis

Definition

• Dementia is the syndrome of impairment in multiple domains of cognition, which must include memory, with intact consciousness.

• Symptoms, signs, and investigations are used to differentiate potentially treatable causes of dementias from the degenerative dementias.

Symptoms

• Patients may be unaware of deficits and deny symptoms (anosognosia); a history from a caregiver is therefore essential.

Memory loss: the most common presenting symptom.

Psychiatric disturbances: including depression, hallucinations, or behavioral changes.

Dysphasia, dyspraxia, visuospatial dysfunction, behavioral change: usually progressive and may occur in any order.

• Additional symptoms depend on the cause, *e.g.*, the following:

Headache: due to space-occupying lesions or temporal arteritis.

Fatigue: due to systemic disease (*e.g.*, HIV, hypothyroidism).

Weight loss: due to neoplasia.

Peripheral neuropathy: due to vitamin B_{12} deficiency, alcohol.

Seizures: may occur in patients with Alzheimer's disease or may have a focal cause.

Gait disturbances: can be seen in normal pressure hydrocephalus.

Focal neurological symptoms: including hemiparesis can be seen in multi-infarct dementia.

Signs

• The primary degenerative dementias (*e.g.*, Alzheimer's disease) have few signs other than those relating to higher cortical function.

Primitive reflexes (grasp, rooting, sucking), spasticity: late in dementia.

More widespread dysfunction: in dementia plus syndromes, *e.g.*, Huntington's disease (dementia plus chorea), multi-infarct dementia (dementia plus focal motor signs).

Papilledema or focal signs: suggesting a potentially treatable intracranial cause.

Investigations [1]

• Few specific tests are available, and none for the most common cause, Alzheimer's disease.

• Investigations are aimed at excluding secondary causes, *e.g.*, cerebral neoplasms, metabolic disturbances.

Psychometry: to assess pattern and severity of cognitive impairment and influence of the affective components.

Complete blood count, ESR measurement, routine biochemistry, serum vitamin B_{12}, thyroid function tests, treponemal serology, and HIV antibody serology: in some patients.

EEG: to exclude Creutzfeldt–Jakob disease or concomitant epilepsy.

CT or MRI: to exclude mass lesions, assess vascular changes, and determine regional atrophy.

PET: if available, to assess regional metabolism.

Lumbar puncture: in selected patients with rapidly progressing symptoms to exclude inflammatory changes.

Cerebral biopsy: rarely used; can provide definitive histological diagnosis.

• Many markers are available (ApoE, and so on); no clear indication for these at present.

Complications

Bronchopneumonia: due to aspiration.

Parkinsonism or seizures: can be late complications of several degenerative dementias.

Incontinence.

Differential diagnosis

Acute confusional states or delirium with fluctuating impairment of arousal.

Korsakoff's and Wernicke's syndromes secondary to alcohol abuse.

Focal neuropsychological deficits, *e.g.*, dysphasia.

"Pseudodementia" resulting from impairment of cognitive function by anxiety or depression.

Etiology

• Any disease disrupting the function of corticocortical or subcorticocortical connections can cause dementia, *e.g.*, the following:

Causes of degenerative dementia [2]

Alzheimer's disease, frontal-lobe degeneration, Pick's disease, cortical Lewy body disease, Huntington's disease, prion disease.

• Some hereditary dementias are associated with specific genetic markers, *e.g.*, rare families with Alzheimer's disease and amyloid precursor protein gene mutations, later-onset disease with the apolipoprotein E4 genotype.

• Neuropathologically, dementia of Alzheimer's disease is associated with senile plaques and neurofibrillary tangles in the cerebral cortex.

• ~15% of Alzheimer's disease is familial.

Vascular causes

Multiple cortical or subcortical infarcts, small-vessel disease (Binswanger's disease).

Potentially treatable causes

Neoplasms, normal-pressure hydrocephalus, trauma, subdural and extradural hematomas, drugs or toxins.

Vitamin B_{12} deficiency, hypothyroidism, renal and hepatic dysfunction, inherited metabolic disease.

Multiple sclerosis, temporal arteritis, cerebral vasculitis, sarcoid.

HIV, neurosyphilis, chronic viral encephalitides, chronic meningitides, cerebral Whipple's disease.

Epidemiology

• Dementia is common in elderly patients, occurring in 2%–5% aged >65 years; 20%–40% aged >80 years.

• Alzheimer's disease is the most common cause, accounting for 50% of dementia patients and a further 15%–20% in association with vascular disease.

Treatment

Diet and lifestyle

- Patients must avoid fatigue, alcohol, and centrally active medications unless clearly indicated.

- Patients should use cognitive aids, *e.g.*, clear labeling, diary, calendars.

- Medicalert bracelets should be worn.

- Safety issues including driving, using potentially dangerous equipment, and wandering need to be addressed.

Pharmacological treatment [3]

- The treatment of dementia is first the treatment of the underlying cause when possible, *e.g.*, removal of meningioma, vitamin B_{12} replacement.

- The degeneration in Alzheimer's disease particularly affects the glutamatergic cortico-cortical association pyramidal neurons and the subcortico-cortical cholinergic projection neurons; cholinergic enhancement can improve memory in cholinergic-deficit states.

- Tacrine may be helpful to slow progression in some early cases [4].

Standard dosage	Tetrahydroaminoacridine (tacrine), 40–160 mg daily in divided doses.
Contraindications	Pregnancy, hepatic disease.
Main drug interactions	None.
Main side effects	Cholinergic effects, hepatotoxicity.

- Donepezil, another cholinesterase inhibitor, may slow progression of mild to moderate (MMSE 10-26) Alzheimer's dementia [5].

Standard dosage	Donepezil, 5 mg at bedtime.
Contraindications	Pregnancy.
Main drug interactions	None.
Main side effects	Nausea, diarrhea, dizziness.

- Other medications are under investigation.

- Many medications can be useful to manage psychiatric and behavioral problems, including antidepressants, anxiolytics, and antipsychotics.

Treatment aims

To treat the underlying cause, when possible.
To slow progression of disease.
To maintain patient safety and caregiver support.

Prognosis

- Prognosis depends on the causative disease.

Follow-up and management

- Management involves many disciplines: neurologists, psychiatrists, and geriatricians.
- Early involvement of social work and community psychiatric services is important.

Social support

Alzheimer's Association, 919 N. Michigan Ave., Suite 1000, Chicago, IL 60611-1676; phone (312) 335-870 or (800) 272-3900.

Legal issues

- Patients and families need to consider early living wills or medical, legal, and financial designation of power of attorney.

Key references

1. Cummings JL, Benson DF: *Dementia: a Clinical Approach*, edn 2. Oxford: Butterworth Heinemann; 1992.

2. Geldmacher DS, Whitehouse PJ Jr: Differential diagnosis of Alzheimer's disease. *Neurology* 1997, **48(suppl)**:S2–S9.

3. Rossor MN: Management of neurological disorders: dementia. *J Neurol Neurosurg Psychiatry* 1994, **57**:1451–1456.

4. Knapp MJ, *et al.*: A thirty week randomized controlled trial of high dose tacrine in patients with Alzheimer's disease. *JAMA* 1994, **271**:985–991.

5. Rogers SL, Friedhoff LT: Efficacy and safety of Donepezil in patients with Alzheimer's disease. *Dementia* 1996, **7**:293–303.

Diagnosis

Symptoms and signs

Risk factors for major depressive illness

Prior episodes of depression
  (especially if age of onset <40 years).
Family history of depressive disorder.
Lack of social support, stressful life events.
Current alcohol or substance abuse.

Stroke.
Disabling chronic diseases.
Prior suicide attempts.
Postpartum period.
Age >75 years.

Unexplained or ill-defined symptoms: *e.g.*, chronic pain, sleep complaints, somatic symptoms without organic cause after appropriate investigation.

Major depression [1]

Distinct periods (at least 2 weeks) of depressed mood (sometimes irritability in children or adolescents) or loss of interest of pleasure in usual activities, with at least four of the following:

Change in appetite or weight.
Difficulty in concentrating or making decisions.
Sleep disturbance (insomnia or hypersomnia).
Psychomotor agitation or retardation.

Anergia.
Suicidal thoughts or attempts.
Hopelessness, worthlessness,
  or guilt.

Dysthymia

Chronic disturbance with depressed mood, lasting 2 years—similar symptoms to a major depressive episode but less severe.

Depression in the elderly

Can manifest as decline in functional or cognitive status, or somatic complaints, often without depressed mood.

Other forms of depression

• Seasonal (winter) major depressive episodes suggest seasonal affective disorder.

• Symptoms of depression insufficient in number, severity, or duration to meet criteria for major depression or dysthymic disorder are termed "subsyndromal depression."

Investigations

Screening for depression [2]

• Screening instruments (*e.g.*, Centers for Epidemiological Studies–Depression instrument, Beck Depression Inventory) may help identify depression among patients at low to moderate risk.

• These are best used to rule out depression (negative result) and to identify patients for further investigation (positive result).

Laboratory investigations

• None are routinely indicated. In middle-aged and elderly patients, especially, investigations to rule out secondary depression (*e.g.*, associated with occult neoplasm or endocrine disturbance) may be warranted if the patient's symptoms suggest physical illness.

Assessment for complicated depression: identify and consider for immediate referral if suicidal thoughts or actions, frank delusions or hallucinations, prominent vegetative symptoms (*e.g.*, profound weight loss), or severe social role dysfunction is present.

Assessment for bipolar illness: symptoms of mania (periods of elevated or irritable mood, accompanied by hyperactivity, pressured speech, flight of ideas, euphoria, reduced sleep, distractability, or recklessness) should prompt consideration of lithium therapy and/or referral.

Screen for comorbidities: high prevalence of substance abuse (*e.g.*, alcohol), anxiety disorder, obsessive–compulsive disorder, personality disorder, somatization syndromes.

Complications

High suicide rate: 15%; highest risk groups are adolescents, middle-aged white males, and the elderly.

Distress to others in the patient's social network: *e.g.*, spouse, children.

Impairment in occupational function: *e.g.*, reduced productivity, absenteeism, unemployment.

Death due to dehydration and malnutrion: in elderly patients.

Differential diagnosis

Major depression

Medications: *e.g.*, steroids, antihypertensive agents, sedatives, alcohol, anticonvulsants.

Dementia: in elderly patients.

Schizophrenia, schizoaffective disorder.

Chronic anxiety state.

Uncomplicated bereavement.

Dysthymia

Major depression.

Personality disorder: *e.g.*, dependent, borderline, histrionic.

Normal fluctuation of mood.

Etiology

Biological factors: major depressive and bipolar disorders are familial; activity of biogenic amines (*i.e*, 5-hydroxytryptamine, noradrenaline) is altered in depressive and bipolar conditions.

Psychosocial factors: psychodynamic and cognitive factors and adverse life events have been associated with depressive illness.

Epidemiology

Prevalence of major depressive illness: in community-based populations, 2%–3% among men, 5%–10% among women.

Primary care outpatient settings: 4%–9%.

Patients with one or more general medical conditions: 12%–36%.

Poststroke: 10%–27%.

Subsyndromal depressive disorders: prevalence less well documented; estimated at 8%–10% of primary care patients.

Treatment

Diet and lifestyle

- No special precautions are necessary.

Pharmacological treatment [1,3]

- Depression is a recurrent disorder; optimal management is evaluated in terms of the following:

Response to initial therapy: reduction of symptoms with treatment.

Remission: resolution of symptoms for a continuous period in an episode.

Recovery: a stable remission lasting at least 4-6 months.

Relapse: symptoms recur during remission.

Recurrence: a new episode after recovery.

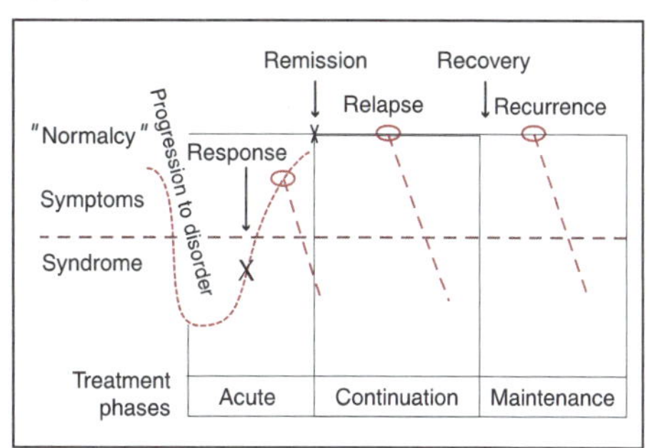

Stages of evaluation for major depression.

Standard dosage	Selective serotonin reuptake inhibitors (SSRIs), *e.g.*, fluvoxamine, 50-300 mg; paroxetine, 20-50 mg. Secondary amine tricyclic antidepressants (TCAs): nortriptyline, 25-250 mg; desipramine, 25-300 mg. Other agents: buproprion, 100-450 mg; nefazodone, 200-600 mg; venlafaxine, 75-375 mg.
Contraindications	*SSRIs*: relate mainly to potential drug interactions (*see* below); pregnancy rating C (fluvoxamine) or B (paroxetine). *TCAs*: relatively contraindicated in recent myocardial infarction, ischemic heart disease, heart block; pregnancy rating C (desipirmine) or D (nortryptiline).
Special points	*SSRIs*: generally have fewer side effects than older agents and may be considered first-line agents, especially for patients on few or no other medications; tricyclics and other new agents should be considered if drug interactions are likely with SSRI, or if no response to adequate doses of SSRIs.
Main drug interactions	*All agents*: potentially fatal interaction with monoamine oxidase inhibitors (MAOIs). *Tricyclics, SSRIs*: potentially fatal interaction with antiarrythmic agents. Most newer agents (fluvoxamine, nafazodone, paroxetine): hepatic cytochrome P_{450} isoenzyme inhibition, yielding a large number of potential drug interactions [3]. Serotonergic crisis (hypertension, hyperpyrexia, seizures) possible in patients on other serotonergic medications (*e.g.*, MAOIs, lithium, carbamazepine).
Main side effects	*SSRIs:* gastrointestinal upset, anorexia, vomiting, diarrhea, agitation, insomnia, sexual dysfunction. *TCAs:* cardiac dysrhythmias (high levels or underlying cardiac disease), anticholinergic effects (dry mouth, orthostasis, constipation, urinary retention), lower seizure threshold. *Venlafaxine:* supine hypertension, sexual dysfunction.

Key references

1. *Depression in Primary Care.* Rockville: US Department of Health and Human Services, Public Health Agency, Agency for Health Care Policy and Research (AHCPR), 1993. [AHCPR Publication no 93-055].

2. Mulrow CD, *et al.*: Case-finding instruments for depression in primary care. *Ann Intern Med* 1995, **122**:913–921.

3. Bhatia SC, Bhatia BK: Major depression: selecting safe and effective treatment. *Am Fam Physician* 1997, **55**:1683–1694.

Diagnosis

Symptoms

• Children may not admit to any symptoms until very late.

Thirst: including unusual forms, *e.g.*, drinking bath water.

Polyuria: bed wetting.

Weight loss.

Decreased appetite.

Vomiting: possibly with abdominal pain.

Confusion: without coma.

Signs

Uncomplicated
Irritability.

Dehydration.

Complicated
Semi-coma.

Deep but rapid respiration: Kussmaul's respiration.

Hypotension.

Infection: in ear, throat, lung, urinary tract.

Investigations (at presentation or with acute illness)

• The urine must always be tested for glucose in a sick child with some of the above symptoms or signs, even if atypical.

Blood glucose and plasma sodium, potassium, bicarbonate, and urea measurement: glucose >400 mg/dL; sodium usually within normal range (but is dependent on level of hypoglycemia and dehydration); potassium low, normal, or high (value governs i.v. replacement); bicarbonate low.

Urinalysis: for glucose and ketones.

Blood pH, oxygen, carbon dioxide, acid–base status analysis: if indicated, based on clinical findings and results of blood tests.

Blood, urine, and/or sputum cultures: as clinically indicated.

Chest radiography: to identify consolidation due to pneumonia.

Complications

Hypovolemia, circulatory failure, cardiac arrest.

Disequilibrium, with cerebral edema: caused by over-rapid correction of hyperglycemia or electrolyte imbalance.

Hypokalemia or hyperkalemia: due to inappropriate i.v. potassium replacement and insulin treatment.

Hypophosphatemia.

Hypoglycemia: due to insulin treatment.

Long-term complications of diabetes (*e.g.*, retinopathy, neuropathy, nephropathy, and macrovascular disease): unusual in childhood.

Differential diagnosis

Newly diagnosed child
Any condition manifest by nausea and vomiting.
Any condition manifest by polyuria.
Any condition manifest by coma.

Previously diagnosed child
Uncontrolled diabetes mellitus due to intercurrent infection.
Coma due to hypoglycemia.

Etiology

Failure of insulin production and secretion due to lymphocytic infiltration and destruction of beta cells of the islets of Langerhans of the pancreas.
Particular HLA phenotypes (HLA DQ8 and DQ2) and circulating compliment-fixing antibodies to islet tissue and antibodies to insulin itself.

Epidemiology

• ~3 in 1000 US children have insulin-dependent diabetes mellitus.

Treatment

Diet and lifestyle

• Parents should work closely with a dietitian to develop a realistic meal plan for their child.

• Meals should be regular, with snacks between main meals and at bedtime.

• No restrictions should be placed on children, but bouts of physical exercise may require additional carbohydrate intake. Hypoglycemia must be avoided during activities in which children are exposed to cold because their thermal regulation fails and hypothermia may occur.

• Glucose in the form of tablets or gel must be carried by a child or an accompanying adult. Parents should be taught to give glucagon, used when a hypoglycemic child cannot take oral glucose.

Pharmacological treatment [1]

• Oral agents have no place in the management of childhood-onset insulin-dependent diabetes mellitus.

• Long- and short-acting insulins are typically injected before meals, at a frequency and combination meant to achieve maximum glycemic control.

• Humalog insulin, with its rapid onset of action, can be administered at the end of a meal. This can be particularly useful for young children with irregular eating habits.

• In small children, insulin therapy may present a problem because of their sleep patterns. The evening injection can be divided so that short-acting insulin is given before the evening meal and intermediate-acting insulin later in the evening; this can be given while the child is asleep.

• Insulin-containing pens are available containing both short- and intermediate-acting insulin.

• Regimens can be altered so that insulin is injected before each meal and intermediate-acting insulin at bedtime, the latter to provide sufficient insulin during the resting period.

Standard dosage	Insulin, 0.5–1 U/kg daily, adjusted according to blood glucose concentration.
Contraindications	Very rare hypersensitivity (usually due to preservatives in insulin preparation).
Special points	Home blood glucose monitoring essential if hyper- and hypoglycemia are to be avoided.
Main drug interactions	High-dose beta-agonists cause severe insulin resistance.
Main side effects	Hyper- or hypoglycemia due to inappropriate dosing.

• Insulin can also be given by continuous infusions using pumps.

Treatment aims

To return child to health and normal lifestyle.
To achieve glycemic control.

Prognosis

• Childhood-onset diabetes mellitus can be associated with significant complications.

• In the past, life expectancy was reduced by one-third, although this is rapidly improving.

Follow-up and management

• Regular attendance at a combined pediatric and diabetic clinic is vital to monitor growth, provide advice on diet as child gets older, monitor long-term glycemic control, and check for complications [2].

• Management at presentation requires the following:

With hyperglycemia and ketonuria but no vomiting, outpatient management (i.v. fluids not needed).

Frequent visits to specialist diabetic unit or frequent visits of staff of the center to the child's home.

Adjustment of dose of insulin on the basis of blood glucose values.

Two or more s.c. insulin injections daily along with change in diet.

With vomiting, hospital admission for i.v. rehydration, insulin treatment, and identification of immediate cause of diabetic ketoacidosis.

Depending on age, education of child about the diabetic process and basic physiology of glucose homeostasis by a skilled member of the diabetic team, usually a specialist nurse.

Education of parents about their child's disease and its control (treatment of hyperglycemia, hypoglycemia, alteration of diet for physical activities, holidays, and sick days).

Counseling to enable parents to come to terms with their child's life-long disability.

Key references

1. Kostraba JN, *et al.*: Increasing trend of outpatient management of children with newly diagnosed IDDM. *Diabetes Care* 1992, **15**:95–100.

2. Diabetes Control and Complication Trial Group: The effect of intensive treatment of diabetes on the development and progression of longterm complications in insulin dependent diabetes. *N Engl J Med* 1993, **329**:977–986.

Diagnosis

Symptoms

• Symptoms are usually of short duration (days to weeks), often longer in older patients.

Polyuria.

Polydipsia.

Weight loss.

Lethargy.

Diabetic ketoacidosis or coma: if disease undetected or ignored; progression of above symptoms, with vomiting, abdominal pain, increased respiratory rate; may progress to altered mental status, including coma.

Signs

• Initially, few signs may be present.

Mild dehydration, weight loss: early signs.

Shock, severe dehydration, Kussmaul's respiration, ketones on breath (fruity), reduced level of consciousness: later signs.

Investigations

Laboratory blood glucose measurement: essential for diagnosis; in the absence of diabetic ketoacidosis, two fasting glucose levels >126 mg/dL are required for the diagnosis of diabetes [1].

Urinalysis: may show glycosuria; ketonuria may also be present.

Arterial blood gas measurement: shows metabolic acidosis.

Electrolyte analysis: wide variation in cases of diabetic ketoacidosis; typical findings include hyponatremia, hyperkalemia, hypophosphatemia, acidosis, and evidence of dehydration.

Anti-islet cell receptor antibody tests: usually unnecessary; can be used to confirm the diagnosis of type I diabetes.

Complications [2]

• Complications are rare before 5–10 years' duration of type I diabetes. Microvascular complications (retinopathy, nephropathy, and neuropathy) can be prevented or slowed with improved glucose control [3].

Diabetic retinopathy: background changes in >75% by age 30 years, only affects vision if near macula; proliferative affects fewer patients but threatens vision by vitreous hemorrhage/fibrosis; treated by laser; most common cause of new adult blindness in patients <65 years of age.

Diabetic nephropathy: affects up to 40% after age 30 years, but rate probably now falling; proteinuria is hallmark, with progressive renal impairment; can be slowed by early diagnosis (yearly screening for microalbuminuria) and vigorous antihypertensive treatment; angiotensin-converting enzyme inhibitors have been shown to slow the progression of diabetic nephropathy.

Diabetic neuropathy: many forms, most common being symmetrical sensory polyneuropathy leading to loss of temperature, vibration, and pain sense, hence easy progression to foot ulceration; also several painful forms.

Large-vessel disease (coronary, cerebrovascular, peripheral): also much more common, especially when nephropathy is present; possibly more diffuse than nondiabetic large-vessel disease, but otherwise generally similar.

• Other problems include skin disorders, especially necrobiosis, joint disorders, mononeuropathies, and cataracts.

Differential diagnosis

• In patients with altered mental status, the diagnosis of diabetic ketoacidosis is usually straightforward. However, a variety of illnesses can precipitate, exacerbate, or mimic diabetic ketoacidosis. Always consider infection, surgical abdomen, stroke, myocardial infarction, and alcohol and other drugs.

• Deciding whether the patient is insulin-dependent can be difficult if the diagnosis is made early; in case of doubt, short-term insulin treatment should be given.

Etiology

• Insulin-dependent diabetes mellitus is associated with HLA DR3 and DR4.

• The process occurs via an autoimmune mechanism with antibodies against pancreatic islet-cells, which show insulitis and are progressively destroyed.

• The triggering environmental agent is not known.

Epidemiology

• Insulin-dependent diabetes mellitus can occur at any age, but onset is frequently in children and young adults (hence the alternative term "juvenile-onset diabetes mellitus").

• It occurs most often in people of white race, especially in those furthest from the equator (Scandinavia, southern New Zealand); other races differ in genetic susceptibility.

• It affects ~3 in 1000 of the US population and represents ~10% of all patients with diabetes.

Treatment

Diet and lifestyle

• Annual dietary consultation is strongly recommended; the diet should be high in unrefined carbohydrate, low in simple sugars, with high fiber and low fat, spread throughout the day, including three meals and a bedtime snack.

• Normal activity is advised, except for a few career and driving limitations.

Pharmacological treatment [2]

• After insulin dependency has been established, exogenous insulin is required.

Types of insulin

• Mainly human biosynthetic insulins are used; pork and beef insulins are still available in some preparations.

Ultra-short acting: Humalog.

Short acting: regular or R.

Intermediate-acting (isophane): NPH or N.

Intermediate-acting (zinc): lente or L.

Long-acting: ultralente or U.

Premixed (NPH/R): 70%/50%, 60%/40%, 50%/50%.

Types of regimen (a sampling)

Once-daily: suited only for elderly, frail patients and those unable to self-inject.

Twice-daily: minimum for all other patients, including variable dose self-mixing.

Added bedtime dose: mixture in morning, short-acting before supper, intermediate-acting before bedtime; flexible regimen, especially for patients troubled by overnight hypoglycemia.

Multiple daily injections: long-acting overnight, short-acting boluses before meals.

Insulin pump: continuous s.c. infusion of regular insulin with premeal boluses.

Practical issues

Sites of injection: abdomen, leg or buttock, arm (s.c.).

Timing: usually 30 minutes before meal (at mealtime with Humalog).

Exercise: requires either extra food or reduced insulin dose.

Insulin infusion (variable rate): best method for ketoacidosis, for unstable diabetes, and during surgery.

Hypoglycemia

• This is the major unwanted effect of insulin treatment and the predominant concern of many patients.

• It is more common with long duration of diabetes and "tight control." Frequent episodes of hypoglycemia can result in subsequent hypoglycemic unawareness.

• Symptoms include sweating, shaking, hunger, palpitation, lack of concentration, confusion, and restlessness. In severe cases, seizure or coma may occur.

• Hypoglycemia should be treated by oral glucose or food (*e.g.*, skim milk or orange juice), i.v. glucose, or i.m. glucagon.

See Hypoglycemia *for details.*

Treatment aims

To restore normal sense of well-being.
To achieve optimal glycemic control without significant hypoglycemia.
To provide patient education and self-care.
To prevent complications.

Prognosis

• The prognosis is excellent and improving in the short and medium terms. Ketoacidosis and hypoglycemia are now rare causes of death.

• Longer-term prognosis largely depends on long-term glycemic control and compliance with screening and treatment [3].

• Major causes of death are end-stage renal failure and coronary artery disease.

• Major causes of morbidity include proliferative retinopathy leading to blindness, coronary artery disease and peripheral vascular disease, and neuropathy leading to foot ulceration, claudication, or gangrene.

Follow-up and management

• Long-term follow-up is essential for continued education, checks on long-term control (hemoglobin A_{1c}), home capillary blood glucose levels preprandially, and screening for complications (especially eye and foot examination, proteinuria).

• Potentially fertile women should have pre-conception counseling and optimal control before conception.

• Patient and family education by specialist nurses and dietitians is essential.

• Most patients should test their own blood glucose and learn to adjust insulin.

Patient support

American Diabetes Association, 1660 Duke Street, Alexandria, VA 22314; tel 1-800-ADA-DISC.

Key references

1. The Expert Committee on the Diagnosis and Classification of Diabetes Mellitus: Report of the Expert Committee on the Diagnosis and Classification of Diabetes Mellitus. *Diabetes Care* 1997, **20**:1183–1197.

2. American Diabetes Association: *Medical Management of Insulin-Dependent (Type I) Diabetes*, edn 2. Alexandria, VA: American Diabetes Association; 1994.

3. Diabetes Control and Complications Trial Research Group: The effect of intensive treatment of diabetes on the development and progression of long-term complications in insulin dependent diabetes. *N Engl J Med* 1993, **329**:977–986.

Diagnosis

Symptoms

• ~50% of patients are symptomatic; 50% found on routine or accidental screening.

• Common symptoms, often manifest over many months or years, include the following:

Polyuria, polydipsia.

Candidal vaginitis or balanitis.

Weight loss, fatigue, blurred vision.

Hyperglycemia nonketotic coma, with severe dehydration and hyperosmolality: rare manifestation.

Signs

• Generally, no signs are manifest.

• Patients may present with the following:

Obesity.

Foot ulceration or infection.

Diabetic retinopathy or peripheral neuropathy.

Signs of secondary causes of diabetes: *e.g.*, steroid use, acromegaly, Cushing's syndrome, thyrotoxicosis.

Investigations

Blood glucose measurement: two fasting levels >126 mg/dL is diagnostic; the National Institutes of Health recommends screening fasting glucose levels every 3 years in patients who are ≥45 years of age or at increased risk [1].

Glucose tolerance test: needed when diagnosis in doubt.

Measurement of hemoglobin A_{1c}: elevated concentration is strong evidence for diabetes [2].

Measurement of iron and total iron-binding capacity: to rule out hemochromatosis.

Measurement of thyroxine and thyroid-stimulating hormone: to rule out thyrotoxicosis.

• Glycosuria alone and self-monitoring of blood glucoses should not be considered diagnostic.

Complications

• Complications are often present at the time of diagnosis because patients may have had several years of asymptomatic hyperglycemia.

Diabetic retinopathy: may be present at diagnosis, only affects vision if near macula; macular edema frequent with major reduction of visual acuity; proliferative affects fewer but threatens vision by vitreous hemorrhage/fibrosis; both treated by laser.

Diabetic nephropathy: less common than in insulin-dependent diabetes mellitus, except in nonwhite races; proteinuria is marker for high cardiovascular risk, but not necessarily progressive renal impairment; can be slowed by vigorous antihypertensive treatment (*e.g.*, angiotensin-converting enzyme inhibitors).

Diabetic neuropathy: many forms, most common being symmetrical sensory polyneuropathy leading to loss of temperature, vibration, and pain sense, hence easy progression to foot ulceration.

Large-vessel disease (coronary, cerebrovascular, peripheral): much more common especially when patient has nephropathy; possibly more diffuse than nondiabetic large-vessel disease, but otherwise generally similar; these, especially coronary artery disease, are major causes of premature death.

Insulin

• Insulin is indicated for symptomatic or uncontrolled diabetes mellitus despite maximal oral agents, in addition to diet.

• Usually, it is needed only once or twice daily; a longer-acting formulation may be used to control basal hyperglycemia.

• *See* Diabetes mellitus, insulin-dependent *for details*.

Treatment

Diet and lifestyle

• Weight loss and exercise are critical components of any treatment plan.

• The diet should be high in unrefined carbohydrate, low in simple sugars, with high fiber and low fat, spread throughout the day.

• There are minimal limitations for those patients on insulin, including not driving commercial vehicles.

Pharmacological treatment [3]

• Diet and exercise should be used initially unless the patient is markedly symptomatic or has a significant elevation in hemoglobin A_{1c}.

• Each of the following oral therapies reduces hemoglobin A_{1c} levels by 0.5%–1.5%. Additive effects for some combinations have been reported.

Sulfonylureas
• These medications act as insulin secretagogues.

Standard dosage	Glyburide, 2.5–20 mg orally daily, given once or twice daily.
	Glipizide, 2.5–20 mg orally daily, given once or twice daily.
	Glibenclamide, 1–8 mg daily.
Contraindications	Breast-feeding, porphyria, pregnancy; caution in elderly patients and those with renal or hepatic dysfunction.
Main drug interactions	*See manufacturer's current prescribing information.*
Main side effects	Hypoglycemia is common; otherwise occasional rashes, jaundice, headache.

Biguanides
• Metformin reduces hepatic gluconeogenesis and may decrease carbohydrate absorption.

Standard dosage	Metformin, 1–2.5 g daily in divided doses.
Contraindications	Hepatic or renal impairment (creatinine >1.4 mg/dL in men or 1.3 in women), heart failure, pregnancy.
Special points	Does not cause hypoglycemia; may rarely cause lactic acidosis. Should be discontinued 2 days before and 2 days after any radiological study using i.v. contrast.
Main side effects	Flatulence, anorexia, diarrhea, sometimes transient.

Alpha-glucosidase inhibitors
• Acarbose decreases the rate of glucose absorption, which reduces postprandial rises in glucose.

Standard dosage	Acarbose, 25 mg with meals to start; titrate up to 50 mg with each meal.
Contraindications	*See manufacturer's current prescribing information.*
Special points	Does not cause hypoglycemia; can be used with other oral medications and insulin.
Side effects	Flatulence, diarrhea (usually, but not always, transient).

Insulin sensitizers
• Troglitazone increases insulin sensitivity in multiple tissues, most notably muscle.

Standard dosage	Troglitazone, 200–600 mg daily with food.
Contraindications	*See manufacturer's current prescribing information.*
Special points	Does not cause hypoglycemia; most expensive oral agent.
Drug interactions	Lowers serum levels of administered estrogens by 30%, which may reduce the efficacy of some oral contraceptives.
Side effects	Very well tolerated; however, there is a 2% incidence of elevated liver function tests.

Key references

1. The Expert Committee on the Diagnosis and Classification of Diabetes Mellitus: Report of the Expert Committee on the Diagnosis and Classification of Diabetes Mellitus. *Diabetes Care* 1997, **20**:1183–1197.

2. Peters AL, Davidson MB, Schriger DL, Hasselblad V, for the Meta-Analysis Research Group on the Diagnosis of Diabetes Using Glycated Hemoglobin Levels: A clinical approach of the diagnosis of diabetes mellitus. *JAMA* 1996, **276**:1246–1252.

3. American Diabetes Association: *Medical Management of Non-Insulin-Dependent (Type II) Diabetes*, edn 3. Alexandria, VA: American Diabetes Association; 1994.

Diagnosis

Symptoms and signs

• Diabetes may be a pre-existing condition (pregestational diabetes) or may develop during pregnancy (gestational diabetes). Also, some women with asymptomatic pregestational diabetes are first diagnosed during pregnancy. If this situation is suspected, the patient should be treated as a pregestational diabetic during the pregnancy.

• For women with pregestational diabetes, pre-conception counseling and optimal glucose control are of critical importance. A good rule of thumb is to inquire about contraception and prepregnancy planning at each visit.

• Gestational diabetes is usually asymptomatic; however, some patients may complain of an increase in their baseline polyuria. Because these patients have no history of diabetes, it is not necessary to screen for complications.

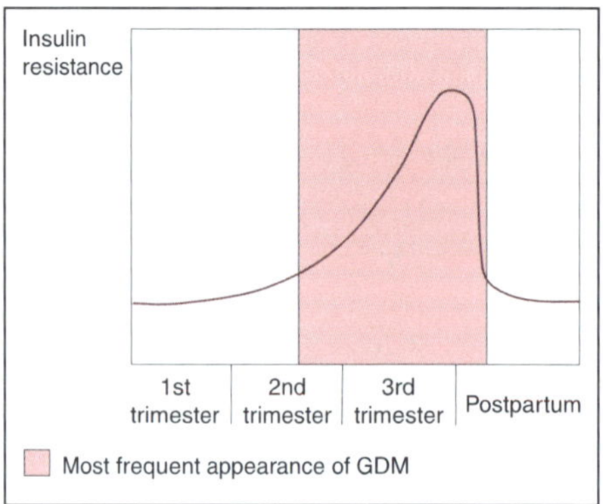

Increase of insulin resistance and the appearance of gestational diabetes mellitus (GDM).

Investigations [1,2]

• All women with risk factors for gestational diabetes mellitus should be screened at 12 weeks.

• All pregnant women should be screened at 24–28 weeks.

• If fasting blood glucose is >90 mg/dL, random blood glucose is >125 mg/dL, or if failed 1-hour screening test, a glucose tolerance test should be considered.

Screening test: give 50 g oral glucose solution and measure plasma glucose at 1 hour. All women with plasma glucose >140 mg/dL at 1 hour should have a 3-hour oral glucose tolerance test (GTT).

3-hour GTT: in pregnancy, 100 g glucose solution with blood glucose measured at fasting and at 1, 2, and 3 hours. Gestational diabetes is diagnosed if two or more values > these parameters: fasting >105 mg/dL; 1 hour >190 mg/dL; 2 hours >165 mg/dL; 3 hours >145 mg/dL.

Evaluation of pregnant women with pregestational diabetes

Hemoglobin A_{1c}: should be checked monthly and kept in the normal range throughout pregnancy; discrepancies between hemoglobin A_{1c} values and self-monitoring of glucoses need to be investigated; usually these can be explained by problems with home monitoring.

Dilated retinal examination (by a qualified examiner): during the first trimester, with follow-up as needed.

Electrolytes, blood urea nitrogen, creatinine, and complete blood count.

24-hour urine for protein and creatinine clearance: if both are normal in the first trimester, there is probably little need to repeat these studies unless specific problems arise.

Ultrasound for fetal abnormalities (including cardiac): performed at ~18 weeks.

Evaluation of all pregnant women with diabetes

Hemoglobin A_{1c}: *see above.*

Self-monitoring of glucoses: at least four times daily; targets vary from center to center, but are generally 65–95 mg/dL before meals, <110 mg/dL before bed, and <120 mg/dL 2 hours after meals.

Third-trimester monitoring of fetal weight and viability: *e.g.*, nonstress tests and biophysical profiles.

Complications

Maternal	Fetal
Worsening retinopathy, nephropathy.	Respiratory distress, jaundice, macrosomia.
Worsening macrovascular disease.	Hypoglycemia.
Increased pre-eclamptic toxemia.	Hypocalcemia.
Hydramnios.	Polycythemia.
Ketosis, hyperglycemia.	Microcephaly, sacral agenesis.
Death.	Congenital malformations.
	Congenital heart disease.
	Fetal demise.

Etiology

Causes of gestational diabetes (increased insulin resistance)

Increased concentrations of progesterone, cortisol, prolactin, and human placental lactogen, which also influence postinsulin receptor metabolism.

Poorly understood processes, which increase insulin need 2–3-fold during pregnancy.

Risk factors for gestational diabetes mellitus

Previous gestational diabetes.
First-degree relative with diabetes.
Fasting glycosuria.
Previous unexplained fetal death.
Previous "large for dates" baby.
Previous malformed baby.
Maternal obesity.
Hydramnios, macrosomia.

Epidemiology

• Prevalence of gestational diabetes mellitus in the United States is 2%–13%, depending on the diagnostic criteria and population studied.

Pregnancy counseling [2]

• Diabetic women must be advised of the following:

• The risk of maternal death is slightly higher than in nondiabetic women.

• Complications, *e.g.*, retinopathy, nephropathy, and heart disease, may worsen in pregnancy.

• Cesarean section is more probable.

• Numerous antenatal visits and close supervision will be needed.

• Home blood glucose monitoring will be needed several times daily.

• Multiple insulin injections will be needed daily.

• Diet must be adhered to, and smoking and drinking must be stopped.

• The baby may be at increased risk of malformations and serious neonatal complications. However, these risks can be reduced by close supervision and cooperation, and maintenance of euglycemia.

Treatment

Diet and lifestyle

• Known diabetic patients should already have consulted a dietitian; those with gestational diabetes must be referred.

• Patients must ensure that 50% of energy intake is carbohydrate and that their diet contains adequate calcium and vitamins.

• Iron and folate supplements are needed.

• Patients should aim to achieve the normal weight gain in pregnancy by appropriate food intake.

Pharmacological treatment [2]

During pregnancy

• All patients on oral agents [3] should be transferred to insulin, usually given 2–4 times daily; a mixture of short- and intermediate-acting insulin can be used depending on patient needs, or a late dose of intermediate-acting insulin before bed and short-acting insulin before meals.

• Two-thirds of patients with gestational diabetes mellitus may be treated by dietary advice; the remaining one-third need insulin, which can be given as a mixture of short- and intermediate-acting insulin twice daily, with possible supplement of short-acting insulin before lunch.

• Insulin needs increase during pregnancy; >100 U daily may be required.

• A decline in insulin requirements in the second or third trimester may be an indication of fetal problems and should be evaluated promptly.

During labor and delivery

• 1–4 U of insulin i.v. are needed hourly; insulin is adjusted based on hourly capillary and/or plasma glucose determination. Insulin requirements fall during and after labor.

• Blood glucose must be maintained at near-normal concentrations.

• In prolonged labor or in high-risk patients, an independent energy source, *e.g.*, 10% dextrose, 100 mL i.v. hourly, is needed.

• Insulin should be delivered by an infusion pump (regular insulin, 50 U in 50 mL normal saline solution).

• Beta-agonists used for premature labor may cause insulin resistance.

• General anesthesia and cesarean section increase insulin needs.

• After delivery, insulin needs fall dramatically.

• Patients with gestational diabetes mellitus often do not need further insulin treatment but may need medical review.

Other concerns

• Angiotensin-converting enzyme inhibitors are contraindicated in pregnancy and lactation.

• Oral agents are contraindicated in pregnancy and lactation.

• Glucocorticoids (for fetal lung maturation) may precipitate diabetic ketoacidosis in women with pregestational type I diabetes.

• Patients with gestational diabetes mellitus should have a standard 2-hour glucose tolerance test 6 weeks postpartum.

Treatment aims

To maintain preprandial blood glucose at 65–90 mg/dL, 2-hour postprandial blood glucose 120 mg/dL, and hemoglobin A_{1c} in normal range.
To achieve a mature fetus, with no neonatal or maternal complications.

Prognosis

• Retinopathy, nephropathy, and macrovascular disease can worsen during pregnancy, but this can be minimized by good metabolic control and supervision.

• Perinatal mortality is increased in diabetic pregnancies; half of the increase is associated with poor control.

• Maternal mortality is slightly higher than in nondiabetic patients.

Follow-up and management

Initial assessment

• Patients may benefit from a joint clinic with a diabetologist and an obstetrician.

• Patients should be screened for diabetic complications.

• Blood pressure should be monitored at each visit.

Subsequent assessment

• Follow-up should be every 1–2 weeks, depending on the patient's need.

• In gestational diabetes: risk of non–insulin-dependent diabetes mellitus at 5 years is 30%–50%.

Key references

1. The Expert Committee on the Diagnosis and Classification of Diabetes Mellitus: Report of the Expert Committee on the Diagnosis and Classification of Diabetes Mellitus. *Diabetes Care* 1997, **20**:1183–1197.

2. American Diabetes Association: *Medical Management of Pregnancy Complicated by Diabetes*. Alexandria, VA: American Diabetes Association; 1995.

3. Hellmuth E, Damm P, Molsted-Pedersen L: Congenital malformations in offspring of diabetic women treated with oral hypo-glycaemic agents during pregnancy. *Diabetic Med* 1994, **11**:471–474.

Diagnosis

Symptoms

• Well-controlled diabetic patients having an operation have no symptoms.

Thirst and polyuria: indicating poor control in patients with any type of diabetes.

Nausea and abdominal pain: indicating very poor control in insulin-dependent patients.

Signs

Tachycardia, ketosis, dehydration, hypotension: signs of poor diabetic control in insulin-dependent patients; these will most probably develop after the operation if preoperative control of diabetes was poor.

Investigations [1,2]

For elective surgery

Blood glucose profile: 2 days before patient has a major operation; hemoglobin A_{1c} should be within 10% of normal range.

• Other investigations are the same as for nondiabetic patients.

For emergency surgery

Blood glucose measurement: to assess hyperglycemia.

Electrolytes, blood urea nitrogen analysis: to assess renal function and electrolyte balance.

Blood gas analysis: to assess acid–base balance.

Complications

Cardiovascular problems: particularly myocardial infarction; the main perioperative causes of death in diabetic patients.

Infection and poor wound healing: in poorly controlled diabetic patients [3].

Differential diagnosis

• Acute surgical abdominal disorders can be confused with severely decompensated diabetes in insulin-dependent patients: a medical opinion is essential.

Etiology

• The stress response to surgery and anesthesia is characterized by hyperglycemia, suppression of insulin release, and insulin resistance.

• This is due to increases in cortisol, catecholamines, and other counterregulatory hormones.

• The stress response is greater with major surgery.

Epidemiology

• 50% of diabetic patients have operations at some point in their lives.

• Patients with macrovascular disease will probably have several operations.

Treatment

Diet and lifestyle

• Major operations are often followed by a period of relative or absolute starvation: adequate energy intake and insulin must be supplied to type I diabetic patients as insulin depletion leads to ketoacidosis.

• Breakfast and oral agents are omitted if the operation is in the morning.

• If the operation is minor, eating and oral agents can soon be restarted.

Pharmacological treatment [1,2]

• Patients with "brittle" diabetes may need a glucose insulin infusion for 24 hours before surgery.

• Regional anesthesia does not produce the same degree of stress response as general anesthesia.

• Infections should be treated aggressively by i.v. antibiotics.

For non–insulin-dependent diabetes: preoperative

• Metformin, which may cause lactic acidosis, and chlorpropamide, because its long action may lead to hypoglycemia, should be avoided for at least 48 hours prior to surgery.

• Patients should be given shorter-acting sulfonylureas instead, *e.g.*, glyburide, 2.5–20 mg daily, or glipizide, 2.5–20 mg daily.

• Blood glucose concentration must be monitored.

• The main side effect is hypoglycemia.

For non–insulin-dependent diabetes: perioperative

• Routine use of i.v. solutions containing glucose is not advised unless hypoglycemia is a risk.

• If the operation is major, treatment should be the same as for insulin-dependent diabetes until the stress response of surgery is finished [4].

For insulin-dependent diabetes: preoperative

• Preoperative admission for stabilization may be needed to achieve a blood glucose concentration of 100–180 mg/dL.

• If control is good, the insulin regimen need not be changed until the day of surgery; if control is poor before a meal, short-acting insulin achieves rapid metabolic control.

• Blood glucose concentration must be monitored.

For insulin-dependent diabetes: operative perioperative

Short-acting insulin, 50 U in 50 mL normal saline solution with an infusion pump; continuous insulin infusion is of critical importance to avoid ketoacidosis; if patients are hypoglycemic, dextrose infusion should be increased.

Dextrose solution with 10 mEq/L potassium chloride through a separate infusion pump; start with 5% dextrose at 125 mL/min or 10% dextrose at 60 mL/min.

• Blood glucose concentration must be maintained at 100–180 mg/dL; 1–4 U of insulin may be needed hourly via an infusion pump and can be titrated as needed [4].

• Premixed insulins are unsuitable as insulin need changes rapidly postoperatively.

• Glucoses should be monitored hourly.

• The insulin infusion must be continued until the patient's first meal, when s.c. insulin should be started 1–3 hours prior to cessation of insulin infusion; insulin needs will probably be higher than usual.

Treatment aims

To maintain blood glucose at 100–180 mg/dL during the operation.

Prognosis

• Mortality should be similar to that in nondiabetic patients.

Follow-up and management

• Blood glucose should be monitored 3–4 times daily before the operation.

• During and early after an operation, blood glucose should be monitored at least hourly.

• Creatinine and electrolytes should be measured daily, and any deficiencies replaced.

Timing of surgery

• Routine surgery should be postponed in newly diagnosed diabetic patients until good control is attained.

• Acute surgical conditions may lead to ketoacidosis; if possible, surgery should be delayed until metabolic control is achieved.

• Surgery should be done in the morning if possible.

Special situations

Cardiac surgery

• Hypothermic bypass surgery with pump priming and inotropic drugs leads to marked insulin resistance and much higher insulin needs.

• The rapidly changing insulin need makes a separate infusion line for insulin essential.

Pregnancy

• Control of diabetes during delivery is critical for mother and fetus.

Key references

1. Clark JDA, Currie J, Hartog M: Management of diabetes in surgery: a survey of current practice by anaesthetists. *Diabetic Med* 1992, **9**:271–274.

2. Gill GV: Surgery and diabetes mellitus. In *Textbook of Diabetes* vol 2. Edited by Pickup J, Williams G. Oxford: Blackwell Scientific Publications; 1991:820–825.

3. Sawyer RG, Pruett TL: Wound infections. *Surg Clin North Am* 1994, **74**:523–524.

4. Smith EA, Kilpatrick ES: Intra-operative blood glucose measurements. *Anaesthesia* 1994, **49**:129–132.

Diagnosis

Symptoms

Watery, large-volume diarrhea: >400 mL daily.

Abdominal pain, severe.

Vomiting.

Signs

Prominent weight loss and dehydration: possibly.

Investigations

Stool culture: for *Salmonella*, *Campylobacter*, and *Shigella* spp.

Stool staining and microscopy: possibly with concentration of stools; Ziehl–Neelsen stain for cryptosporidia, *Isospora* spp., and *Cyclospora* spp.; trichrome or fluorescent stain for microsporidia; microscopy of fresh stool for ameba and cysts of *Giardia* spp.

Small-intestinal biopsy: electron microscopy gold standard for diagnosis of microsporidia, although these are seen by stool staining or light microscopy.

Biopsy: for cytomegalovirus or *Mycobacterium avium* complex colitis, or involvement due to lymphoma or Kaposi's sarcoma.

Tests of malabsorption: protozoan infection associated with partial villus atrophy and malabsorption, particularly of vitamin B_{12} (Schilling test).

Complications

Toxic dilatation: unusual.

Right upper quadrant pain, cholangiographic appearances of "AIDS-related sclerosing cholangitis."

Gross wasting, inanition, death.

Differential diagnosis

Viral diarrhea: cytomegalovirus infection may be bloody and associated with abdominal pain.

Bacterial diarrhea: *Shigella*, *Salmonella*, and *Campylobacter* spp. cause acute diarrhea with systemic symptoms; opportunistic bacterial infection by *M. avium-intracellulare* causes watery diarrhea in patients with severely reduced CD4 counts (<100×10^6/L).

"Pathogen-negative diarrhea": after complete investigation, large-volume diarrhea with no cause is rare; low-volume irritable-bowel diarrhea is more common in patients with CD4 counts >200×10^6/L.

Etiology

Infectious

M. avium.

Cryptosporidia.

Microsporidia (at least two species: *Septata intestinalis* and *Enterocytozoon bieneusi*).

Cyclospora spp.

Isospora spp.

Entamoeba spp.

Giardia spp.

Cytomegalovirus.

Noninfectious

Lymphoma.

Kaposi's sarcoma.

Epidemiology

• Cryptosporidiosis occurs in animal handlers and is associated with sexual transmission; water-borne outbreaks are known.

• Microsporidiosis only occurs in severely immunosuppressed patients (CD4 lymphocyte count <100×10^6/L).

• *Isospora* infection is common in South Americans and Africans; it occasionally occurs in travelers to these continents.

• Infection by *Entamoeba* spp. is common in homosexual men, although these strains are usually not pathogenic.

• *Giardia* infection is common in homosexual men (possible sexual transmission); it is more common in HIV-seropositive men.

Treatment

Diet and lifestyle
- Safe sexual practices reduce sexual transmission.
- Immunosuppressed patients with a CD4 count $<200 \times 10^6$/L should boil drinking water.
- Care must be taken when gardening or handling pets or domestic animals.

Pharmacological treatment

General treatment
- Patients should be rehydrated, usually with oral rehydration fluids.
- Reduction with antimotility agents (*e.g.*, codeine phosphate, 30–80 mg daily) or stronger opiates may cause toxic megacolon.
- Specific vitamin supplementation should be given for malabsorption.
- Transient stool volume can be reduced during treatment by somatostatin analogues (*e.g.*, octreotide, 50–200 µg 2–3 times daily).

For cryptosporidiosis
- No standard treatment is of proven value.

Standard dosage	Paromomycin, 500 mg 4 times daily (not successful). Azithromycin, up to 1.5 g daily, may be used.
Contraindications	None.
Special points	*Paromomycin:* stool volumes reduced by 50%, but cryptosporidia not eradicated.
Main drug interactions	None known.
Main side effects	None known.

For microsporidiosis
- No standard treatment is of proven value.

Standard dosage	Albendazole, 400 mg twice daily, or metronidazole, 400 mg 3 times daily.
Contraindications	None.
Special points	*Albendazole:* eradicates *Septata intestinalis*, less effect on *E. bienusi.* *Metronidazole:* may produce symptomatic benefit.
Main drug interactions	*Metronidazole:* alcohol.
Main side effects	*Metronidazole:* nausea.

For *Entamoeba histolytica* infection
- Metronidazole, 400 mg 3 times daily for 1 week; iodoquinol for 3 weeks.

For giardiasis
- Patients can be given metronidazole, 1.2–2 g daily for 3 days; tinidazole, 2 g initially, repeated if necessary; or mepacrine, 100 mg 3 times daily for 5–7 days, repeated after 2 weeks if necessary.

For isosporiasis and cyclosporiasis
- Trimethoprim-sulfamethoxazole double-strength tablet by mouth twice daily $\times$ 2 weeks, then maintenance therapy.

Treatment aims

To resolve diarrhea.

To eradicate organism.

To promote weight gain or prevent weight loss.

Prognosis

Cryptosporidiosis
- In patients with CD4 counts $>200 \times 10^6$/L, the diarrhea resolves eventually.
- In patients with CD4 counts $<200 \times 10^6$/L, the diarrhea may be chronic.
- Diarrhea usually continues despite treatment.
- In patients with CD4 counts $>200 \times 10^6$/L, the prognosis depends on the CD4 count, rather than on the diarrhea.
- In patients with CD4 counts $<200 \times 10^6$/L, median survival is 1 year.

Microsporidiosis
- Diarrhea usually continues despite treatment.
- Median survival is <1 year.

Other infections
- Diarrhea usually resolves with treatment, but patients may relapse after treatment has stopped.
- The prognosis depends on the underlying CD4 count, rather than on the diarrhea.

Follow-up and management
- Eradication of organism must be checked.
- Continuing diarrhea leads to wasting due to severe anorexia; therefore, the need for supplements, elemental diets, or nasogastric or gastrostomy feeding must be reviewed.

General references

Babameto G, Kotler DP: Malnutrition in HIV infection. *Gastroenterol Clin North Am* 1997, **26**:393–415.

Clayton F, Clayton CH: Gastrointestinal pathology in HIV-infected patients. *Gastroenterol Clin North Am* 1997, **26**:191–240.

Framm SR, Soave R: Agents of diarrhea. *Med Clin North Am* 1997, **81**:427–447.

Diagnosis

Symptoms

• Disseminated intravascular coagulation occurs in a spectrum of guises from a chronic syndrome, diagnosed on laboratory tests, with no symptoms or signs (compensated), to an acute florid clinical bleeding state (uncompensated).

• It is always associated with an underlying disorder.

• The major symptoms are those of the underlying disorder.

Generalized bruising: especially over dependent areas.

Bleeding at surgical sites and incisions, around venipuncture sites, indwelling lines, and drainage tubes.

Hematemesis, melena, hemoptysis, hematuria, and vaginal bleeding.

Gangrene of fingers and toes, purpura fulminans, hemorrhagic bullae: microthrombotic lesions in 5%–10% of patients.

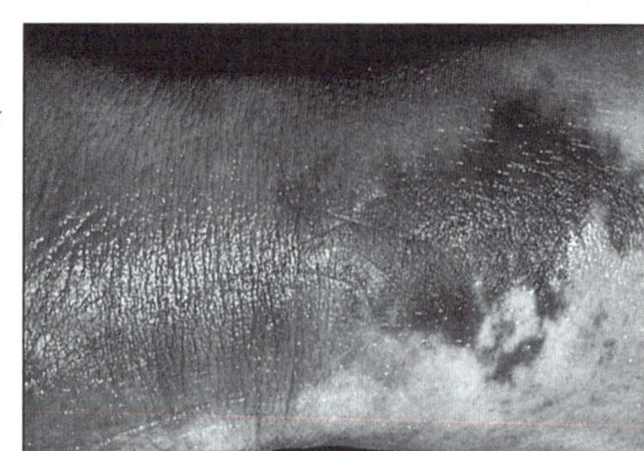

Purpura fulminans, with surrounding extensive subcutaneous hemorrhage. (*See* Color Plate.)

Signs

Evidence of bleeding: as detailed under symptoms, when present.

Investigations [1]

• Simple screening tests show reduced levels of clotting factors and platelets.

• Disseminated intravascular coagulation cannot be ruled out by a single set of normal results; serial values may be needed to show consumption.

Measurement of prothrombin time, activated partial thromboplastin time, thrombin time: all times prolonged; prolongation of thrombin time best guide to clinical significance of raised fibrinogen degradation products and low fibrinogen; thrombin time twice normal control value indicates impending overt clinical bleeding.

Fibrinogen measurement: concentration low.

Fibrinogen degradation products and D-dimers measurement: concentrations raised; fibrinogen degradation products sensitive but not specific for disseminated intravascular coagulation; D-dimer specific but not as sensitive.

Platelet count: low.

Blood film: many patients have associated microangiographic hemolytic anemia; erythrocytes fragmented by passing through deposited fibrin strands.

Complications

Uncontrollable hemorrhage.

Microvascular blockage and tissue necrosis of heart, liver, kidney, and brain.

Adult respiratory distress.

Treatment

Diet and lifestyle

• No special precautions are necessary.

Pharmacological treatment

Anticoagulants

• Although controversial, anticoagulants may have a role in acute promyelocytic leukemia (M3), acute intravascular hemolysis (incompatible blood transfusion), and purpura fulminans.

Standard dosage	Heparin, 5–10 U/kg/h continuous i.v. infusion.
Contraindications	Florid bleeding
Special points	Requires antithrombin III for its action, which is often low in patients with disseminated intravascular coagulation; fresh frozen plasma may also be needed to supply antithrombin III to maintain effective heparinization. Partial thromboplastin time should be kept at 1.5–2 times control. May increase bleeding tendency; close monitoring and specialist advice needed.
Main drug interactions	Other anticoagulants.
Main side effects	Bleeding (with overdose).

Fibrinolytic inhibitors

• Because of increased deposition, fibrinolysis is protective against microvascular organ damage in disseminated intravascular coagulation; inhibitors of fibrinolysis are therefore generally contraindicated. In special circumstances of predominant fibrinolysis, however, they may be useful.

• Specialist advice must be sought before use.

Nonpharmacological treatment

See Transfusion medicine *for further details.*

Fresh frozen plasma

• Fresh frozen plasma supplies all clotting factors and naturally occurring inhibitors of coagulation.

• Initially, 10–15 mL/kg should be given.

• It may cause fluid overload.

Cryoprecipitate

• Cryoprecipitate supplies fibrinogen and factor VIII.

• It is used, at a rate of 1 U/5 kg, when substantial fibrinogen replacement is needed.

Platelet concentrates

• Platelet concentrates are needed when consumptive thrombocytopenia is present.

• They are given, at a rate of 4 U/m² body surface area, if the platelet count falls below 50×10^9/L and overt bleeding occurs.

Packed erythrocytes

• Packed erythrocytes are needed to treat associated hemolysis or anemia at a rate sufficient to maintain hematocrit >0.3.

• Virus transmission is a risk with any blood product.

• Fluid overload may also be a problem.

Key references

1. Bick R: Disseminated intravascular coagulation: objective clinical and laboratory diagnosis, treatment, and assessment of therapeutic response. *Semin Thromb Hemost* 1996, **22**:69–88.

2. Levi M, *et al.*: Pathogenesis of disseminated intravascular coagulation in sepsis. *JAMA* 1993, **270**:975–979.

Diagnosis

Symptoms

• Diverticulosis is found in the majority of older adults but causes symptoms or signs of disease in only a minority [1].

Symptomatic diverticular disease

• Symptomatic diverticular disease may present with the following:

Fever, left lower quadrant pain (diverticulitis).

Maroon stools: from acute lower gastrointestinal bleeding from a diverticula.

Bowel obstruction: from a left-sided stricture caused by recurrent diverticulitis.

Signs

Symptomatic diverticular disease

Fever, tenderness, guarding, palpable inflammatory mass: indicating inflammation (*i.e.,* diverticulosis) and possible abscess formation, most typically in the left lower quadrant [2].

Shock, acute abdomen, paralytic ileus: indicating inflammation due to perforation.

Anemia, shock, fresh blood *per rectum*: indicating hemorrhage (*i.e.,* diverticular bleeding). Diverticular bleeding is commonly associated with hemorrhage of one or more units of blood. Occult gastrointestinal bleeding should suggest an alternative diagnosis.

Abdominal distension, obstruction: indicating stricture.

Investigations

• Laboratory tests are usually normal in asymptomatic diverticular disease but can help to exclude other diagnoses.

• Diverticula are easier to identify on barium enema than on colonoscopy.

• Symptomatic diverticular disease is a clinical diagnosis that relies more on presenting symptoms and signs as opposed to investigative studies of the colon. Investigative studies of the colon are used to exclude other competing diagnoses.

Complete blood count: to identify anemia due to bleeding or elevated leukocytes from inflammation.

Liver chemistry tests: to exclude biliary disease, which can occasionally mimic symptomatic diverticular disease.

Sigmoidoscopy: to exclude colitis or malignancy, which may mimic symptomatic diverticular disease.

Plain abdominal radiography: may show features of ileus or perforation.

Contrast enema: may show obstruction or stricture [3].

Ultrasonography or CT of abdomen and pelvis: may show abscess cavity.

Colonoscopy: may be needed for biopsy of stricture to exclude malignancy.

Tagged red blood cell nuclear scan: to investigate sites of ongoing bleeding.

Urinalysis: to exclude active renal inflammation.

Complications

Life-threatening gastrointestinal bleeding.

Abscess formation or perforation: leading to subphrenic or pericolic collections.

Intestinal obstruction.

Stricture formation.

Fistula: connection to bladder or vagina.

Differential diagnosis

General
Carcinoma of colon.
Inflammatory bowel disease.
Pseudomembranous colitis.

Abscess or perforation
Pelvic inflammatory disease.
Pyelonephritis.
Perforated peptic ulcer.
Ischemic colitis.
Appendicitis.
Crohn's disease.

Hemorrhage
Polyp in colon.
Angiodysplasia.
Upper gastrointestinal tract bleeding.

Stricture
Radiation damage.
Ischemic colitis.
Endometriosis.

Etiology

• Factors believed to be implicated in the development of diverticula include the following:

Low stool weight, leading to excessive intracolonic pressure.

Dietary fiber deficiency, reducing stool weight and colonic transit time.

Exaggerated colonic pressure due to abnormal colon muscular motility.

Weakness and poor elasticity of colon wall.

Epidemiology

• Colonic diverticula occur in 33% of people >40 years and 50% of people >70 years.

• Diverticulosis appears to be more common in developed countries.

• Diverticulitis and diverticular bleeding are completely different processes that rarely occur concomitantly in patients.

Treatment

Diet and lifestyle

• Increased dietary fiber intake may help some patients, especially those with marked constipation.

• Excessive dietary fiber is contraindicated in patients with excessive narrowing or stricture formation from previous inflammation.

• Regular exercise improves bowel function.

Pharmacological treatment

Diverticulitis

• Antibiotics are administered to patients with acute inflammation, abscess formation, or evidence of systemic toxicity for at least a 2-week course.

• Intravenous antibiotic regimens are indicated for patients with systemic manifestations of inflammation and include cefotetan, 2 g every 12 hours, or ciprofloxacin, 400 mg every 12 hours, and metronidazole, 500 mg every 6 hours and should be continued at least 48 hours after signs and symptoms have resolved.

• Oral antibiotic regimens include metronidazole, 500 mg every 8 hours, plus ciprofloxacin, 500 mg every 12 hours; trimethoprim, 160 mg/sulfamethoxazole, 800 mg every 12 hours; or an oral cephalosporin.

Diverticular bleeding

• Therapy is supportive, with volume expansion and blood products as necessary.

• Antibiotics have no role in the management of patients with diverticular bleeding.

Nonpharmacological treatment

For perforated diverticular disease of the colon: emergency decompression of the colon by colostomy, followed by elective resection of the diseased segment [4]. Abscess formation, sepsis, or failure to respond to medical therapy should prompt surgical consultation.

For life-threatening hemorrhage from diverticular disease: possible surgical control or embolization therapy at the time of selective mesenteric arteriography.

Treatment aims

To relieve acute symptoms.

To improve bowel function.

To reduce incidence of further symptom attacks.

Prognosis

• 70%–80% of patients with diverticular bleeding have spontaneous cessation, with recurrence in <50%.

• Most patients with diverticulitis respond to antibiotic management alone; a small subset will require drainage of an abscess or surgical management of stricutres.

Follow-up and management

• Recurrent symptoms are common, but new or different symptoms need further investigations.

• If symptoms are relieved by fiber supplementation, long-term treatment must be continued.

Key references

1. Cheskin LJ, Bohlman M, Schusler MM: Diverticular disease in the elderly. *Gastroenterol Clin North Am* 1990, **19**:391–403.

2. Jones DJ: Diverticular disease. *BMJ* 1992, **304**:1435–1437.

3. McKee RF, Deignan RW, Krukowski ZH: Radiological investigation in acute diverticulitis. *Br J Surg* 1993, **80**:560–565.

4. Kronberg O: Treatment of perforated sigmoid diverticulitis: a prospective randomized trial. *Br J Surg* 1993, **80**:505–507.

Diagnosis

Symptoms

Epigastric pain: often described as dull or burning; often occurring on an empty stomach and relieved with eating or antacids; pain may awaken patient from sleep during the early morning hours; pain may radiate to the back.

Hematemesis or melena: patients may present with gastrointestinal bleeding as their first symptom of peptic ulcer disease.

Anorexia and occasional vomiting in patients with outflow obstruction.

Weight loss.

Signs

• Most patients with duodenal ulcer disease have a normal examination. Epigastric tenderness is not a reliable parameter for the presence or absence of duodenal ulcer disease.

• Abnormalities when present may include the following:

Melena.

Hemetemesis.

Pallor and clinical evidence of anemia.

Peritonitis: patients who present with perforation (<5% of patients).

"Succussion splash" of gastric outflow obstruction: <5% of patients.

Investigations [1,2]

• *Helicobacter pylori* is very common in the healthy population and noninvasive testing alone does not distinguish patients with ulcer disease from patients with nonulcer dyspepsia who likely will not benefit from treatment for *H. pylori*.

• An imaging study of the gastroduodenal lumen is required to render a diagnosis of duodenal ulcer disease.

Contrast radiography: a barium upper gastrointestinal series is relatively inexpensive and safe; however, small lesions may be missed and tissue biopsies are not feasible.

Fiberoptic endoscopy: esophagogastro-duodenoscopy typically is performed under i.v. sedation and allows direct visual-ization of ulcers with biopsy and local treatment for bleeding when present. *H. pylori*, the greatest risk factor for duodenal ulcer disease, may be diagnosed from tissue samples immediately at the time of endoscopy (*e.g.*, CLO test) or histologically on formalin-fixed biopsies.

Testing for *H. pylori* in patients who have ulcer but no tissue studies for *H. pylori*: urea breath test, serology for *H. pylori*.

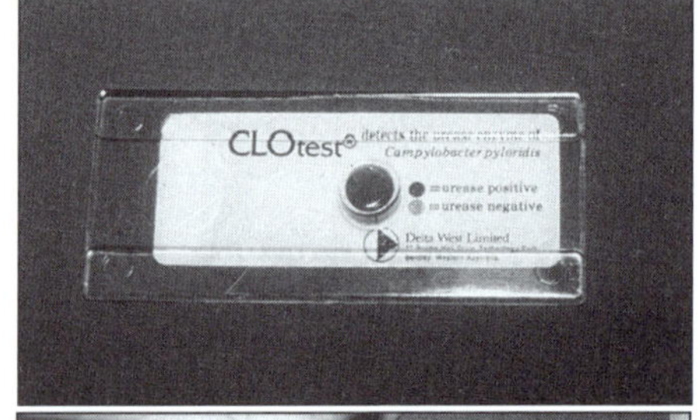

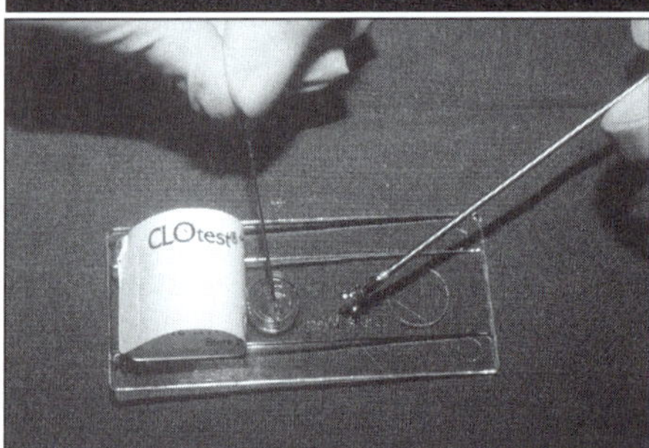

CLO test detects urease activity in gastric biopsy. (*See* Color Plates.)

Complete blood count: to evaluate for anemia or systemic evidence of inflammation.

Serum gastrin levels: in patients with unexplained recurrent disease or severe disease without evidence of nonsteroidal drug ingestion or *H. pylori*.

Complications

Acute hemorrhage: in 10% of patients.

Perforation: in 1% (often asymptomatic in elderly or immunosuppressed patients).

Penetration: pancreatitis.

Outlet obstruction from scarring of the duodenum.

Treatment

Diet and lifestyle

• Patients should restrict alcohol consumption, eat balanced meals daily with no bedtime snacks, avoid aspirin and other NSAIDs, and stop cigarette smoking.

• Bland or milk diets have not been shown to decrease acidity, promote healing, or relieve symptoms.

Pharmacological treatment

H. pylori–positive patients [3,4]

• Empiric treatment of symptomatic patients with positive *H. pylori* noninvasive testing in the absence of diagnostic imaging studies for peptic ulcer disease is controversial.

• A large number of regimens have been shown to eradicate *H. pylori*; the best regimens have eradication rates of ≥90% with low toxicity and little recurrence. All of these regimens require at least 7 days of therapy with a preference of 2 weeks of therapy using 3–4 medications. Three particularly popular regimens are given below.

Standard dosage	Omeprazole, 20 mg (or lansoprazole, 30 mg twice daily), plus amoxicillin, 1 g twice daily (or metronidazole, 500 mg twice daily), plus clarithromycin, 500 mg twice daily, all for 10-14 days with careful instructions to patients concerning compliance.
	Omeprazole, 20 mg (or lansoprazole, 30 mg twice daily), plus bismuth subsalicylate, 2 tablets 4 times daily, plus metronidazole, 250 mg 4 times daily, plus tetracycline, 500 mg 4 times daily (or amoxicillin, 500 mg 4 times daily), all for 14 days with emphasis on patient compliance.
	Omeprazole, 40 mg daily, or ranitidine/bismuth citrate, 400 mg twice daily, plus clarithromycin, 500 mg 3 times daily, all for 14 days.
Contraindications	Pregnancy, drug sensitivity.
Main drug interactions	Coumadin.
Special points	Avoid ethanol when taking metronidazole; bismuth may temporarily darken oral mucosa and result in black-appearing stools.

H. pylori–negative patients

Antacids

• Antacids are effective for duodenal ulcer treatment and should be taken 1 and 3 hours after meals; some patients may find complying with this regimen difficult.

• Sucralfate, 1 g 4 times daily, is another alternative regimen to promote healing.

H$_2$-receptor antagonists

• These produce symptomatic relief in days and ulcer healing in 80% of patients at 4 weeks and 95% at 8 weeks; they are also used as maintenance treatment to prevent recurrence at half the usual dose [5].

Standard dosage	Ranitidine, 300 mg; cimetidine, 800 mg; famotidine, 40 mg; or nizatidine, 300 mg in the evening.
Contraindications	Rare hypersensitivity; avoid in pregnancy and lactation.
Main drug interactions	*Cimetidine:* oral anticoagulants, theophylline, phenytoin, warfarin.
Main side effects	Altered bowel habits, headache (both rare). *Cimetidine:* gynecomastia, confusion in elderly.

Proton-pump inhibitors

• Proton-pump inhibitors are associated with faster healing (*e.g.*, 93% healing after 4 weeks of treatment), but they are not approved for long-term management.

Standard dosage	Omeprazole, 20 mg daily [6], lansoprazole, 30 mg daily.
Contraindications	Pregnancy and lactation.
Main drug interactions	Diazepam, phenytoin, warfarin.
Main side effects	Diarrhea, headache, rash (all rare); increased risk of enteric infection.

Key references

1. Peterson WL: *Helicobacter pylori* and peptic ulcer disease. *N Engl J Med* 1991, **324**:1043–1048.

2. Vander Hulst RWM: *Helicobacter pylori* and peptic ulcer disease. *Scand J Gastroenterol* 1996, **31(suppl 220)**:10–18.

3. Graham DY, *et al.*: *Helicobacter pylori*: current status. *Gastroenterology* 1993, **105**:279–282.

4. Yamada T, *et al.*: *Helicobacter pylori* in peptic ulcer disease. *JAMA* 1994, **272**:65–69.

5. Feldman M, Burton ME: Histamine 2-receptor antagonists: standard therapy for acid-peptic diseases. *N Engl J Med* 1991, **323**:1672–1678; 1749–1755.

6. Maton PN: Omeprazole. *N Engl J Med* 1991, **324**:965–975.

Diagnosis

Symptoms

Myocardial infarction, angina, claudication, transient ischemic attacks, cerebrovascular accident: indicating accelerated atheroma.

Pancreatitis, confusional states: rare, caused by chylomicronemia.

• Adverse lipid profiles without symptoms are often revealed by well-person screening or through other risk associations, *e.g.*, bad family history.

Signs

• Ectopic lipid deposits should be sought because they suggest the duration of lipidemia (and thus the degree of risk) and alert to asymptomatic lipidemia.

Corneal arcus: traces in 50% of adults by age 50 years; heavy or early presence can reveal hypercholesterolemia; differential arcus can reveal carotid stenosis.

Xanthomas of tendons: heels, knees, knuckles; indicating long-standing severe hypercholesterolemia, almost always familial.

Xanthomas of soft tissues: elbows, eyelids, palmar creases, rarely elsewhere; typical of mixed lipidemia and triglyceride excess.

Lipidemia retinalis and eruptive xanthomas: indicating chylomicronemia.

Corneal clouding: rare major disorder of high-density lipoprotein.

Carotid bruit, poor or absent peripheral pulses: vascular abnormalities.

Investigations

• The aim of investigations is to clarify the pattern of lipid abnormality and its cause.

• Lipid profiles can be disturbed and difficult to interpret for up to 3 months after myocardial infarction.

Lipid profile: for concentrations of cholesterol, triglycerides, and high-density lipoprotein cholesterol after overnight fasting; random sample adequate for cholesterol.

Secondary lipidemia tests: for thyroid-stimulating hormone concentration, glucose tolerance, alcohol markers; other tests suggested by history or examination.

Second-level tests: apolipoprotein E typing for moderate mixed excess or palmar xanthomas; fibrinogen level, platelet function, lipoprotein (a) concentration also of interest.

Special procedures: for major hypertriglyceridemia, measurement of apolipoprotein CII and lipoprotein lipase; for major high-density lipoprotein deficiency, measurement of lecithin cholesterol acyltransferase activity and apolipoprotein AI and DNA studies.

Family screening: to review suspected genetic problem, notably polygenic or familial hypercholesterolemia.

• Other problems, notably blood pressure, cardiac status, cigarette smoking, and fibrinogen concentration, should be considered in the overall assessment of clinical risk and options for benefit.

Complications

Progressive atheromatous disease.

Graft or angioplasty restenosis.

Attacks of abdominal pain and pancreatitis.

Treatment

Diet and lifestyle

• Reduction in total fat intake (with a greater proportion taken as unsaturates), weight loss, and more steady physical activity should be encouraged.

• Much ingenuity and interpersonal skill is needed to maintain compliance, and committed support by skilled dietitians is invaluable.

• Diet change can also sharpen responses to any subsequent lipid drug treatment.

Pharmacological treatment

• The cause of the abnormal lipid profile must be identified and treated.

• No single drug is universally appropriate; combinations are useful.

Priorities for lipid-lowering treatment in diet-resistant patients

1. Existing coronary heart disease or previous coronary artery bypass grafting, angioplasty, or cardiac transplantation. For such pateints, effective therapy of moderate to severe hypercholesterolemia improves overall survival and freedom from myocardial infarction, revascularization, and cardiac death [3].
2. Asymptomatic dyslipoproteinemia in men or in postmenopausal women, particularly with several risk factors or major genetic lipid disorder (*e.g.*, familial hypercholesterolemia). This condition should lead to statin therapy if the LDL cholesterol remains severely elevated on dietary therapy [4].

Statins

• Statins are powerful cholesterol-lowering agents, alone or with resins.

Standard dosage	Statins, 10–40 mg single daily dose, depending on product (*e.g.*, lovastatin, fluvastatin, pravastatin, simvastatin).
Contraindications	Liver disease, pregnancy, breast-feeding.
Special points	Not licensed for children.
Main drug interactions	Occasional severe myositis or rhabdomyolysis when used with cyclosporine or fibrates.
Main side effects	Rheumatic complaints, severe myositis alone or in combination treatment; reaction time may be delayed.

Resins

• Resins divert bile acids, lower cholesterol, and raise triglycerides; they are first-line treatment in children with familial hypercholesterolemia.

Standard dosage	Resins, 1–2 sachets twice daily (up to 4 sachets daily).
Contraindications	Biliary obstruction.
Special points	Compliance is better with newer formulations.
Main drug interactions	May reduce absorption of other medication (should be given before or well after).
Main side effects	Gastric irritation, constipation, gas.

Fibrates

• Fibrates are used in patients with mixed lipidemia or low high-density lipoprotein levels; they promote turnover of triglyceride lipoproteins and can generate high-density lipoproteins; some lower fibrinogens, and the level may affect choice.

Standard dosage	Depends on product.
Contraindications	Severe renal or liver disease, pregnancy.
Special points	Some fibrates are licensed for children but rarely so used.
Main drug interactions	If used with statins, can affect prothrombin time on oral anti-coagulants.
Main side effects	Changed bowel habit, rashes, myositis (rare).

Second-line drugs

• Probucol can cause xanthoma regression, but high-density lipoprotein concentrations are reduced.

• Fish oils or polyunsaturates (vegetable or marine) may be antithrombotic.

• Nicotinates can raise high-density lipoproteins and lower lipoprotein (a), but compliance is difficult.

Treatment aims

To improve overall lipid profile in patients with or at risk of coronary heart disease.
To reduce coronary progression [5] and improve outcomes, including death [3].

Prognosis

• Increase in high-density lipoprotein levels is associated with plaque regression.

Follow-up and management

• Dietary support must be reinforced, enthusiastic, and family-based.

• For failing lipid response, compliance and the prospect of a second lipid-related disorder (*e.g.*, hypothyroidism, alcoholism) must be checked.

• Diet or medication changes must be given time to act (*e.g.*, review after 4 months).

Key references

1. Barth JD, Arntzenius HC: Progression and regression of atherosclerosis, what roles for LDL cholesterol and HDL cholesterol. *Eur Heart J* 1991, **12**:952–957.

2. Betteridge DJ, *et al.*: Management of hyperlipidaemia: guidelines of the British Hyperlipidaemia Association. *Postgrad Med J* 1993, **69**:359–369.

3. Scandinavian Simvastatin Survival Study Group: Randomized trial of cholesterol lowering in 4444 patients with coronary heart disease (4S). *Lancet* 1994, **344**:383–389.

4. Shepard J, *et al.*: Prevention of coronary heart disease with pravastatin in men with hypercholesterolemia. *N Engl J Med* 1995, **333**:1301–1307.

5. Brown BG, *et al.*: Lipid-lowering and plaque regression: new insights into prevention of plaque disruption and clinical events in coronary disease. *Circulation* 1993, **87**:1781–1791.

Diagnosis

Symptoms

Itching.

Dryness, discoloration, thickening of involved areas; blistering and oozing of skin.

Signs

Xerosis.

Keratosis pilaris.

Dennie-Morgan lines (infraorbital fold of skin).

"Allergic shiners" (infraorbital darkening).

Excoriations.

Lichenification of skin: with predilection for flexural creases.

Follicular prominence: especially in patients with dark skin.

Associated pityriasis alba.

Increased fine line markings of the skin of the palms of bilateral hands.

Secondary impetiginization of excoriated skin.

Investigations

• Atopic eczema is a clinical diagnosis, although family history is helpful.

• Patients often have all or part of the atopic triad (*i.e.*, asthma, allergic rhinitis, atopic eczema).

Skin scrapings: to rule out scabies or dermatophyte infections.

Cultures: to rule out staphylococcal superinfections.

Skin biopsy: rarely performed by experienced clinicians.

Complications

Secondary infection: usually with *Staphylococcus aureus*; Kaposi's varicelliform eruption (eczema herpeticum) occurs when atopic patients get herpes simplex infections that become disseminated over the involved cutaneous surface (may be very severe and life-threatening in young children); molluscum contagiosum not uncommon [1].

Erythroderma (exfoliative erythroderma): possible in severe cases; requires hospital admission with close monitoring to fluid and electrolyte status as well as treatment of any secondary infection that could have triggered the flare.

Differential diagnosis

Scabies.

Tinea.

Psoriasis.

Ichthyosis.

Dermatitis herpetiformis.

Premycosis fungoides (T-cell lymphoma).

Netherton's syndrome (atopic dermatitis is one of the hallmark features).

Wiskott-Aldrich syndrome.

Acrodermatitis enteropathica.

Neurodermatitis.

Contact dermatitis.

HIV infection (especially in children).

Phenylketonuria patients often have atopic eczema during the first year of life.

Etiology

• Although a host of immunological abnormalities have been identified, there is no real consensus as to the cause of atopic dermatitis; it is probable that many factors play a role.

Immunological abnormalities have included the following:

Elevated serum IgE levels.

Reduced cell-mediated immunity.

Slowed chemotaxis of neutrophils and monocytes.

Relative increase in the number of CD4-positive T-cells that secrete interleukin (IL)-4.

Decrease in CD4-positive T-cells that secrete IL-2 [2].

Epidemiology

• Prevalence of atopic dermatitis (atopic eczema) is 7–24 per 1000.

• The highest prevalence is in children.

• Onset of disease is in the first year of life in ~50% of patients and before the age of 5 years in 85% of patients.

Treatment [3]

Diet and lifestyle

• Rare patients have a definite cutaneous response to certain foods, which obviously should be avoided.

• Children as well as adults should be educated regarding the disease and taught how to apply emollients when they "itch" instead of scratching.

• Patients specifically need to know everything that can aggravate their skin condition, *i.e.*, dry ambient environment (especially in households with woodburning stoves), hot baths, harsh soap, wool, fabric softener, dusty environments, stress, scratching, and so forth.

Pharmacological treatment

Topical

• Emollients are the mainstay to prevent dryness.

• Steroids may be used at mild, intermediate, or most potent strength, as follows:

Mild potency: topical steroids, over-the-counter or prescription, 1%–2.5% hydrocortisone; class VI and VII steroids.

Intermediate potency: triamcinolone, flurandrenolide, fluocinolone; class III–V steroids.

Most potent: desoximetasone, clobetasol, betamethasone; class I and II steroids.

Standard dosage	All topical steroids should be applied once or twice a day; intermediate and potent topical steroids should not be used for more than a few days on the face, axillary region, or groin.
Contraindications	None.
Special points	Potent topical steroids should be tapered off as soon as possible to avoid side effects.
Main drug interactions	Atrophy of the skin, steroid folliculitis, systemic absorption (especially in children).
Main side effects	Atrophy of the skin, steroid folliculitis, systemic absorption (especially in children).

Systemic therapy

• Systemic treatment is used only in the following situations:

Acyclovir: for secondary infection with herpes.

Antibiotics: for secondary bacterial infection.

Systemic steroids: used only in exceptional cases.

Antihistamines: to relieve pruritis.

Ultravoilet radiation [4]

May be a useful adjunct in the treatment of chronic recalcitrant dermatitis.

Standard dosage	Artificial UVB or PUVA (oral or topical psoralens followed by UVA) requires 3–4 treatments per week under professional supervision; can be localized to hands and/or feet.
Contraindications	*Relative*: fair-skinned patients. *Absolute*: any photoexacerbated dermatosis such as lupus erythematosus, polymorphic light eruption, photoallergic dermatosis, or photoexacerbated atopic dermatitis.
Special points	Patients who do not possess any contraindications to UV therapy should expose themselves to moderate amounts of natural sunlight. However, they should be warned not to sunburn and to avoid hot or humid conditions, which may actually induce more pruritus. Home sunlamp treatment is generally not recommended because of the dangers of overexposure.
Main drug interactions	Photosensitivity-causing agents such as tetracycline, fluoroquinolone antibiotics, phenothiazines, or sulfonamides.
Main side effects	*Acute*: phototoxicity. *Chronic*: increased risk or skin cancer.

Treatment aims

To decrease pruritis.

To prevent secondary infection.

To educate patients so that they can control the disease themselves.

• The main objective is to control, not cure, the disease, as it is a chronic skin disease.

Prognosis

Resolves in approximately 40% of patients by adulthood.

• The remainder of patients have a chronic course characterized by intermittent flares and remissions.

Follow-up and management

• Most patients are treated with topical agents and are followed up until their disease clears.

• Some physicians continue to follow-up at 3- to 6-month intervals to educate their patients appropriately.

Key references

1. Bork K, Brauninger W: Increasing incidence of eczema herpeticum: analysis of seventy-five cases. *J Am Acad Dermatol* 1988, **19**:1024–1029.

2. Van der Heijden FL, *et al.*: High frequency of IL-4-producing CD4 positive allergen-specific T-lymphocytes in atopic dermatitis lesional skin. *Invest Dermatol* 1991, **97**:389–394.

3. Hanafin JM: Atopic dermatitis: new therapeutic considerations. *J Am Acad Dermatol* 1991, **24**:1097–1101.

4. Sams WM Jr, Lynch PJ: *Principles and Practice of Dermatology*. New York: Churchill Livingstone; 1990:377.

Diagnosis

Definition

Eisenmenger's complex
• Originally described by Eisenmenger, this is defined as pulmonary hypertension at systemic levels due to raised pulmonary vascular resistance, with reversed shunting (*i.e.*, right to left) through a large ventricular septal defect [1].

Eisenmenger's syndrome
• This extension of the term by Wood includes all defects associated with pulmonary hypertension at systemic levels and pulmonary vascular disease; this includes all shunts whether they are atrial, ventricular, or even at the aortopulmonary level [2].

Symptoms

Dyspnea: related to degree of hypoxia; breathlessness least marked in an Eisenmenger patent ductus arteriosus because blue blood is shunted to lower body.

Angina of effort.

Exertional syncope: low cardiac output.

Hemoptysis: pulmonary infarction or capillary rupture.

Ankle swelling: right ventricular failure.

Palpitation: sinus tachycardia, atrial arrhythmias.

Signs

Central cyanosis.

Clubbing: with patent ductus arteriosus, toes clubbed and more cyanosed than hands.

Low-volume pulse, arrhythmias.

Raised venous pressure: with a dominant "a" wave.

Prominent right ventricular impulse with palpable pulmonary second sound.

Right atrial fourth heart sound, pulmonary ejection click, loud pulmonary second sound.

Murmurs: not from defects; low flow across large defects, thus murmurs from effects of pulmonary hypertension; early diastolic murmur due to pulmonary regurgitation, pansystolic murmur of tricuspid regurgitation.

Second sound fixed and split with atrial septal defect, single with ventricular septal defect, normally split with patent ductus.

Ankle edema: with right ventricular failure.

Investigations

ECG: shows P pulmonale (right atrial hypertrophy), right axis deviation, with tall R waves and inverted T waves in right precordial leads (right ventricular hypertrophy).

Chest radiography: shows large main pulmonary artery with narrowed "pruned" peripheral vessels.

Two-dimensional echocardiography: shows anatomy of defect and effects of right ventricular disease (enlarged right ventricle compressing small left ventricle).

Cardiac catheterization: pulmonary pressures at systemic levels, with evidence of shunting on saturation samples.

Complications

Right ventricular failure.

Sudden death.

Polycythemia.

Cerebral abscess.

Hemorrhage.

Paradoxical embolus.

Infective endocarditis.

Hemoptysis.

Hyperuricemia.

Differential diagnosis

Tetralogy of Fallot.

Transposition with pulmonary stenosis.

Primary pulmonary hypertension.

Secondary pulmonary hypertension: *e.g.*, pulmonary vasculitis or pulmonary thrombo-embolic disease.

• Any of these may coexist with a patent foramen ovale and may confuse the significance of the defect.

Etiology

• Associated defects include the following:

Ventricular septal defect.

Atrial septal defect.

Patent ductus arteriosus.

Aortopulmonary defect.

Double outlet right ventricle.

Truncus arteriosus.

Transposition of great vessels.

Epidemiology

• The incidence of congenital heart disease is ~10 in 1000 live births; only a few of these progress to Eisenmenger's syndrome.

Treatment

Diet and lifestyle

- Pregnancy carries significant mortality and should be avoided.

- Travel to high altitude is extremely poorly tolerated.

- Strenuous exertion and competitive sports must be avoided.

- Oxygen should be given during flights and dehydration avoided.

Pharmacological treatment

Diuretics

- Standard diuretic treatment is appropriate for right ventricular failure, but care must be taken to avoid dehydration.

Digoxin

- Digoxin remains the mainstay for rate control of atrial fibrillation. Role of primary antiarrhythmic agents such as amiodarone has been little studied.

Standard dosage	Digoxin, 0.0625–0.25 mg daily.
Contraindications	Renal failure.
Special points	Hypokalemia must be avoided.
Main drug interactions	None.
Main side effects	Anorexia, nausea, vomiting, arrhythmias.

Antibiotics

- Antibiotics are indicated for invasive procedures and to treat infective endocarditis (*see* Endocarditis *for specific details*).

Anticoagulants

- Anticoagulants are indicated when thromboembolism is clinically evident (*e.g.*, transient ischemic attacks) and for patients with atrial fibrillation and are frequently prescribed for severe pulmonary hypertension to prevent in situ thrombosis.

Standard dosage	Warfarin guided by INR.
Contraindications	Pregnancy, peptic ulcer, severe hypertension.
Main drug interactions	*See manufacturer's current prescribing information.*
Main side effects	Hemorrhage.

Other options

- Nonpharmacological methods of contraception are preferred, but the progesterone-only pill may be used.

- No effective pulmonary vasodilators can be recommended routinely; controlled trials on an individual patient basis may be appropriate. Early experience with continuous infusion of prostacycline is encouraging.

- Hemoptysis should be treated as a medical emergency; specialist treatment at a cardiac center is recommended.

Treatment aims

To improve symptoms and prolong survival.

Other treatments

- Surgical correction of the anatomical defect is not possible when pulmonary vascular resistance is raised.

- Heart–lung transplantation offers the best chance of survival in severely disabled patients, but they must be free from other disease, *e.g.*, renal failure.

- Phlebotomy should be done, with simultaneous fluid replacement, to avoid symptoms of polycythemia.

Prognosis

- Death occurs most often in the fourth decade, with sudden death being the most common mechanism [3].

- Long-term survival after heart–lung transplantation is possible, but studies are in progress at present,

Follow-up and management

- Patients need careful follow-up.

- Attention must be paid to hematocrit and phlebotomy in polycythemic patients.

- Cardiological input to all aspects of the patient's medical care is essential (*e.g.*, contraception and pregnancy, noncardiac surgery, infections).

Key references

1. Graham TP Jr: The Eisenmenger syndrome. In *Adult Congenital Heart Disease*. Edited by Roberts WC. Philadelphia: FA Davis; 1987:567–582.

2. Wood P: The Eisenmenger syndrome, or pulmonary hypertension with reversed central shunt. *BMJ* 1958, **ii**:755–762.

3. Liberthson RR: *Congenital Heart Disease: Diagnosis and Management in Children and Adults*. Boston: Little Brown; 1989:87–94.

Diagnosis

Symptoms

Headache, behavioral abnormality, fever, photophobia, drowsiness; may progress to confusion, coma, convulsions.

Speech disturbance, limb weakness, incoordination, involuntary movements: indicating focal cerebral involvement.

Seizures.

Signs

Drowsiness, confusion, irritability, coma.

Neck stiffness: due to associated meningeal inflammation (may be absent).

Associated focal cerebral hemisphere signs: *e.g.*, hemiparesis and dysphasia (consider herpes simplex encephalitis).

Ataxia, nystagmus, myoclonus, involuntary movements, extensor plantar responses.

Investigations

CT and MRI of brain: help to exclude other causes and may show brain edema; focal inferior temporal and orbital frontal damage with herpes simplex can take several days to become apparent on plain CT but may be seen earlier on contrast-enhanced CT.

Lumbar puncture and CSF analysis: CSF may be under increased pressure and usually shows lymphocytic pleocytosis, modestly elevated protein, and normal glucose concentration; showing a fourfold rise in specific viral antibody titers is only helpful in retrospect; enzyme-linked immunoassays for viral antigens and gene amplification with polymerase chain reaction are increasingly available to aid early specific diagnosis [1,2].

EEG: shows widespread slow activity with diffuse brain disorder and may show periodic complexes or focal slowing over temporal region in herpes simplex encephalitis.

Complications

Seizures and status epilepticus: often occur and need vigorous treatment.

Cerebral edema: may cause herniation and calls for measures to reduce intracranial pressure.

Differential diagnosis

Meningitis: bacterial, tuberculous, fungal, or viral.

Acute disseminated encephalomyelitis.

Toxic encephalopathy with systemic infection.

Metabolic encephalopathy: usually no fever, headache, or CSF abnormality.

Cerebral abscess, empyema, subdural hematoma, and other mass lesions.

Meningeal carcinomatosis.

Etiology

• Viral invasion of brain parenchyma causes an inflammatory reaction of varying intensity, associated with perivascular cuffing with lymphocytes and other mononuclear cells and with destruction of nerve cells and glia; hemorrhagic necrosis may occur.

Epidemiology [3,4]

• Herpes simplex virus is the most common cause of sporadic encephalitis.

• Other herpes viruses, especially herpes zoster, cytomegalovirus, and Epstein-Barr virus, are common causes, particularly when immunity is impaired, as in transplant or AIDS patients.

• Arboviral encephalitis occurs in epidemics in which mosquitoes bite humans.

• Mumps encephalitis and subacute sclerosing encephalitis have declined in incidence with vaccination; the latter is a progressive late complication of measles infection.

• Progressive multifocal leukoencephalopathy, common in AIDS patients, is due to a human polyoma virus (JC) complicating immunodeficiency.

• HIV may cause meningoencephalitis at seroconversion and, later, a slowly progressive dementia.

Treatment

Diet and lifestyle

Not relevant.

Pharmacological treatment

• No effective treatment is available against many of the viruses causing encephalitis; often, the specific causative virus is not identified.

• Seizures need prompt anticonvulsant administration to reduce the deleterious effects of further seizures.

• Full supportive measures are necessary during what is often a self-limiting illness with good recovery.

• Ventilation, mannitol, and dexamethasone can be used acutely to manage edema.

• Intravenous acyclovir started early reduces the morbidity and mortality of herpes simplex encephalitis; treatment should not await the outcome of brain biopsy, which is seldom appropriate [2].

Standard dosage	Acyclovir, 10 mg/kg i.v. infusion every 8 hours for 10 days (adults), 500 mg/m² every 8 hours (children aged 3 months–12 years).
Contraindications	Hypersensitivity.
Special points	Renal impairment necessitates dose reduction.
Main drug interactions	Possible interaction with zidovudine.

• Ganciclovir may be of benefit when cytomegalovirus is the probable cause.

• Improvement of HIV encephalopathy has been reported with zidovudine.

Treatment aims

To treat herpes simplex encephalitis.

To prevent recurrent seizures.

To control raised intracranial pressure.

To provide optimal rehabilitation when necessary.

Prognosis

• The outcome varies with different causative viruses, the age of the patient, and associated underlying disease.

• Death and serious residual disability are frequent with herpes simplex when the diagnosis and treatment are delayed.

Follow-up and management

• Specialized neurological rehabilitation may be important for patients with residual disability in the wake of the illness.

Key references

1. Aurelius E, *et al.*: Rapid diagnosis of herpes simplex encephalitis by nested polymerase chain reaction assay of cerebrospinal fluid. *Lancet* 1991, **337**:189–192.

2. Whitley RJ: Viral encephalitis. *N Engl J Med* 1990, **323**:242–250.

3. Skoldenberg B: Herpes simplex encephalitis. *Scand J Infect Dis* 1996, **100**:8–13.

4. Armbas JR, Storch GA, Clifford DB, Tselis AC: Cytomegalovirus encephalitis. *Ann Intern Med* 1996, **125**:577–587.

Diagnosis

Definition

• Endocarditis is an infection (usually bacterial) of the lining of the heart (usually the valves); the hallmark is endocardial vegetations consisting of platelet or fibrin thrombi with bacteria and mononuclear cells.

Subacute endocarditis: low-virulence organisms on previously abnormal valves.

Acute endocarditis: high-virulence organisms on previously normal valves.

Culture-negative endocarditis: negative blood cultures may be due to previous partial treatment, infection by an unusual organism (*e.g.*, chlamydiae, rickettsiae, *Brucella* spp., fungi), or noninfective endocarditis.

Noninfective endocarditis: Libman–Sacks endocarditis in SLE; noninfected vegetations occur (mitral more than aortic) with valvular stenosis or regurgitation.

Marasmic endocarditis in terminal illnesses: sterile vegetations, rarely embolizing, often chance postmortem finding.

Symptoms

Fever, malaise, anorexia, weight loss, rigors: nonspecific symptoms of inflammation.

Progressive heart failure: due to valve destruction (can be dramatic).

Stroke, pulseless limb, renal infarct, pulmonary infarct: due to embolization of vegetations.

Arthralgia, loin pain: due to immune-complex deposition.

Signs

Fever: unless patient is moribund or immunosuppressed.

Murmurs: except in right-sided endocarditis.

Pallor, purpura, petechiae, vasculitis, splinter hemorrhages, erythematous nodules in finger pulps, flat red spots on palms and soles, hemorrhagic retinal infarcts.

Rashes.

Heart failure.

Clubbing, café-au-lait pigmentation, splenomegaly: if disease is chronic.

Investigations

• Diagnosis depends on a high index of suspicion; no single test is "diagnostic."

Blood culture: at least three cultures needed to attempt to identify organism.

Complete blood count: shows anemia, raised leukocyte count, hemolysis with para-prosthetic leaks.

Urinalysis: shows microscopic hematuria, proteinuria.

Urea and creatinine analysis: concentrations raised with glomerulonephritis.

CRP, ESR, plasma viscosity analysis: raised as markers of inflammation.

ECG: may reveal conduction disturbances indicative of septal abscess formation (*e.g.*, onset of left bundle branch block may presage heart block or sudden death).

Two-dimensional echocardiography: may reveal vegetations to support diagnosis (absence does not exclude diagnosis); can be used to assess valvular regurgitation or heart chamber size; may detect complications early (*e.g.*, abscess formation).

Transesophageal echocardiography: more sensitive than two-dimensional; indicated if diagnosis in doubt and in patients with prosthetic valves.

Serological tests: *e.g.*, to diagnose infection with *Brucella* spp., chlamydiae, rickettsiae.

Complications

Valve destruction: acute regurgitation, pulmonary edema, heart failure.

Embolism: leading to infarction; in any vascular bed.

Local extension of infection: purulent pericarditis, aortic root abscess (may cause sinus of valsalva fistula), myocardial abscess (conduction disturbance).

Septic emboli to vasa vasorum: may lead to mycotic aneurysms anywhere on vascular tree; most worrying in cerebral vessels, resulting in cerebral hemorrhage.

Distal infection (metastatic): due to septic emboli, *e.g.*, brain abscess, cerebritis.

Candidal endocarditis: may be manifest by fungal endophthalmitis.

Glomerulonephritis.

Differential diagnosis

Pyrexia of unknown origin, tuberculosis, staphylococcal septicemia, paraneoplastic phenomenon (lymphoma, carcinoma).

Systemic vasculitis.

Chordal rupture, aortic dissection, left atrial myxoma.

Etiology

• Damaged valves carry small, short-lived, sterile platelet or fibrin thrombi on their surfaces; these thrombi become infected during transient bacteremia.

• Bacteremia can result from dental manipulations (*Streptococcus viridans*), genitourinary instrumentation or surgery (*Escherichia coli, Streptococcus faecalis*), mucosal damage due to carcinoma of the colon (*Streptococcus bovis*), or insertion of i.v. lines or injections (*Staphylococcus aureus* or *epidermidis*).

• Alpha hemolytic (*S. viridans* group) account for 50% of patients.

• Other bacteria include *Streptococcus pyogenes, Haemophilus parainfluenzae*, and *Neisseria, Pseudomonas*, and *Brucella* spp.

• Nonbacterial organisms include fungi (*e.g., Candida* spp., *Aspergillus* spp.), chlamydiae (*e.g., Chlamydia psittaci*), and rickettsiae (*e.g., Coxiella burnetii*).

• Groups at risk include the following: Patients with previously damaged endocardium (75% of cases: 25% rheumatic heart disease; 25% prosthetic heart valves; 15% bicuspid aortic valve, mitral valve prolapse; 10% congenital heart disease). Intravenous drug abusers. Patients with long-standing i.v. lines, *e.g.*, for feeding, chemotherapy, or hemodynamic monitoring: recurrent bacteremia, immunosuppression, and valve trauma caused by the line itself.

Epidemiology

• An average community hospital admits one patient with endocarditis each month.

• An average primary care physician sees one patient with endocarditis every 10 years.

Treatment

Diet and lifestyle

• No special precautions are necessary.

Pharmacological treatment

• The key is accurate, early diagnosis and close cooperation between cardiologist, microbiologist, and cardiac surgeon.

• Patients presenting with fever and suspected endocarditis do not need emergency antibiotic treatment (unless acutely unwell); a delay of 48–72 hours allows efforts to make an accurate diagnosis.

• Positive blood cultures allow the initiation of antibiotic treatment based on probable sensitivities, while laboratory confirmation is awaited.

• If the blood culture is negative, appropriate serology for culture-negative organisms should be sent, while "best-bet" antibiotics are given.

• Successful treatment should result in a fall in fever within 10 days and a fall in CRP within 2 weeks.

Standard dosage	*For S. viridans:* penicillin G, 8–24 MU i.v. daily as 6-hourly boluses or continuous infusion. *For S. aureus:* nafcillin or oxacillin, 2 gm i.v. every 4 hours. Each with aminoglycoside in synergistic doses (*e.g.*, 60 mg i.v. twice daily), depending on renal function and blood concentrations. *For S. faecalis:* ampicillin and gentamicin. *For S. epidermidis:* vancomycin. *For fungi:* amphotericin B.
Contraindications	Penicillin allergy: vancomycin.
Special points	Adequacy of dosing can be checked by using patient's serum to inhibit or kill organisms in vitro (back titrations should be >1:8).
Main drug interactions	Warfarin dose needs may be altered. Risk of ototoxicity and nephrotoxicity with combined vancomycin and gentamicin, especially if renal function impaired, also when given with high-dose furosemide.
Main side effects	Anaphylaxis, rashes, fever (allergic reactions to initial treatment), oropharyngeal candidiasis, and, rarely, neutropenia (penicillin G), cholestatic jaundice (floxacillin), hepatitis (floxacillin, rifampicin, amphotericin), ototoxicity (vancomycin, gentamicin).

Nonpharmacological treatment

• If the portal of entry was bad teeth, these should be removed.

• After the need for surgery has been identified, treatment must not be delayed.

• Surgery is indicated in the following situations [1]:

Failure of medical treatment to control infective process (possible abscess formation), indicated by continuing fever >10 days, rising CRP concentration, worsening nephritis.

Indications of abscess formation, *e.g.*, conduction abnormalities, cavity on echocardiography, or prosthetic valve dehiscence.

Hemodynamic deterioration, *e.g.*, pulmonary edema or increasing cardiomegaly.

Infection by organisms that are difficult to eradicate, *e.g.*, *S. aureus*, *Candida* spp., *Aspergillus* spp.

Infection on a prosthetic valve.

Recurrent embolization or enlarging, large-size vegetations while patient is on effective antimicrobial therapy.

Treatment aims

To eradicate infection and prevent valve damage.

Prognosis

• Despite advances in diagnosis and treatment, mortality remains high at >20%; avoiding delay before diagnosis, isolation of an organism, use of high-dose antibiotics, and appropriate use of cardiac surgery should reduce this figure.

• Some patients have recurrent infection (<10%), and all are at risk of re-infection.

Follow-up and management

• Blood culture, blood count, CRP concentration, and echocardiograph should be checked 3–4 weeks after apparently successful antibiotic treatment has been stopped.

• Removal of the predisposing factor (*e.g.*, ventricular septal defect, patent ductus arteriosus) should be considered.

Prevention

• Patients at risk should maintain good dental hygiene and receive antibiotic prophylaxis for potentially bacteremic maneuvers, *e.g.*, tooth extraction, genitourinary surgery, instrumentation [2].

• This will, however, probably prevent only 10% of cases.

Key references

1. Larbalestier RI, *et al.*: Acute bacterial endocarditis: optimizing surgical results. *Circulation* 1992, **86(suppl):**II68–II74.

2. Working Party of the British Society of Antimicrobial Chemotherapy: Antibiotic prophylaxis of infective endocarditis. *Lancet* 1990, **335:**88–89; 1992, **339:**1292–1293.

Diagnosis

Symptoms

Seizures: usually abrupt onset, transient, stereotyped.

Somatic, visual, auditory, olfactory, gustatory, or visceral sensations.

Déjà vu, jamais vu, macropsia, micropsia.

Abnormal posture, tone, movements.

Loss of or altered awareness.

Signs

• Usually no signs are manifest.

• Patients should be checked for the following:

Mental status and cognitive function.

Focal neurological deficit, head circumference, hemiatrophy.

Evidence of raised intracranial pressure.

Evidence of adverse effects from antiepileptic drugs.

Cutaneous lesions suggestive of tuberous sclerosis, neurofibromatosis, and so on.

Investigations [1]

EEG: routine, with hyperventilation and photic stimulation; if normal and diagnosis in doubt, sleep-deprived and sleep EEG, 24-hour ambulatory tape, video-EEG monitoring can be considered (if episodes frequent); yield increased with repeat EEG up to 4.

Neuroimaging: MRI superior to CT, necessary for intractable partial seizures or focal deficit, if CT normal or unclear, or if surgical treatment of epilepsy contemplated.

Antiepileptic drug concentration measurement: if prescribed treatment, to check compliance and to assess role of medication levels in symptoms and seizure control.

Blood chemistry: fasting glucose, liver, renal, and complete blood count profiles.

Lumbar puncture: for acute assessment where indicated.

Neuropsychology: if cognition or memory causes concern.

Chest radiography, ECG, HIV and syphilis serology: can also be considered.

Complications

Trauma.

Status epilepticus.

Sudden unexpected death, atrial arrythmias.

Psychosocial handicap.

Differential diagnosis

Altered or lost awareness
Syncope, vagal overactivity, breath holding (children), arrhythmia, cardiac outflow obstruction, drug abuse, hypoglycemia, toxic confusional state, narcolepsy or cataplexy, sleep attacks, transient global amnesia, psychologically mediated disorders.

Abnormal movements
Paroxysmal movement disorder, oculogyric crisis, tetany from hyperventilation, psychologically mediated disorders.

Neurological deficit
Transient ischemic attack, stroke, migraine, psychologically mediated disorders.

Nocturnal spells
Parasomnias, paroxysmal nocturnal dystonia.

Etiology

• Causes include the following:
Cryptogenic.
Idiopathic (often familial).
Hippocampal sclerosis.
Cortical dysplasia.
Tumor.
Trauma.
Infection: encephalitis, bacterial meningitis.
Vascular: infarct, hemorrhage.
Hypoxia.
Granuloma: tuberculosis, cystercercosis (in developing countries).

Epidemiology

• 1 person in 40 has a nonfebrile seizure at some time in his or her life.

• The prevalence of active epilepsy (seizure within past 2 years) is 1 in 200 of the general population and 1 in 150 people aged <15 years.

Classification

• Classification of epilepsy is important for investigation, treatment, and prognosis.

Partial epilepsy
Seizures arising from one or more discrete foci with mixture of simple partial, complex partial, and secondarily generalized seizures.

Generalized epilepsy
Primary: normal cerebral function with normal background EEG, high incidence of familial and young onset, absence, myoclonic tonic–clonic seizures.
Secondary: abnormal cerebral function, slowed EEG, mixed tonic, atypical absence, myoclonic, or tonic–clonic seizures.

Treatment

Diet and lifestyle

- Patients must avoid sleep deprivation.
- Alcohol lowers seizure threshold and may affect antiepileptic levels.
- Patients are not allowed to drive, swim, go to heights alone, or operate dangerous tools.

Pharmacological treatment [2]

- Drug interactions are complex.
- The following doses are for adults.

First line

Phenytoin: for all seizure types; may give 20 mg/kg loading dose; i.v. phosphenytoin now available with less toxicity (maintenance 300–500 mg/day).

Carbamazepine: for simple, complex, or secondarily generalized partial seizures and for tonic or clonic generalized seizures; 100 mg initially, average maintenance dose 600–2400 mg daily in 3–4 doses. Available in long-acting equivalent twice-daily dose.

Clonazepam: for myoclonic seizures (second-line treatment for absences, atonic seizures); 0.5 mg initially, average maintenance dose 0.5–3.0 mg daily in 1–2 doses.

Ethosuximide: for absences only; 250 mg initially, average maintenance dose 500–1500 mg daily in 1–2 doses.

Valproate: primarily for generalized or myoclonic seizures; also useful for some partial epilepsies; 750 mg initially, average maintenance dose 1500–3000 mg daily in 3 divided doses.

Second line

Gabapentin: for partial seizures; 300 mg initially, average maintenance dose 1800–3600 mg daily in 3 doses.

Lamotrigine: for partial seizures, tonic, clonic, tonic–clonic, or atonic seizures, and absence or atypical absence; 25 mg initially, average maintenance dose 300–500 mg daily in 2 doses; if combined with valproate, initial dosage should be 25 mg increasing on alternate weeks.

Phenobarbitol: for partial seizures, tonic, clonic, tonic–clonic, atonic, and atypical absences; 60 mg initially, average maintenance dose 60–180 mg daily as single dose.

Topiramate: for partial seizures, 50 mg increasing gradually up to 400 mg daily.

General adverse effects

Acute, dose-related: sedation, dizziness, nausea, headaches, sometimes tremor.

Idiosyncratic: skin rash, severe bone-marrow suppression, diplopia, liver failure, behavioral disorder, weight gain, tremor, gingival hyperplasia, soft-tissue changes, peripheral neuropathy.

Treatment aims

To control seizures without drug side effects.

Other treatments

- In patients with refractory mesial temporal lobe epilepsy, anterior temporal lobectomy produces an 80% chance of remission, in well-chosen patients.
- Lesional and extratemporal partial epilepsy remission rate is 30%–50% after surgery.

Prognosis

- Remission occurs in 70%–80% of patients in 2–5 years; patients have a 30% chance of remission if epilepsy is active for 5 years.
- After the patient is in remission, the overall risk of relapse is 20% in 2 years if the patient remains on medication, and 40% if medication is tapered.
- Risk factors for relapse include early onset, frequent generalized seizures, generalized spike-wave on EEG, structural brain damage, and difficulty obtaining seizure control.

Follow-up and management

Staged treatment strategy

- This can be followed as far as necessary.
1. Minimizing of epileptogenic stimuli: fever (in children), alcohol, excessive fatigue, epileptogenic drugs, photosensitivity.
2. Initial small dose of first-line drug.
3. Dosage increase if needed, up to maximum tolerated dose.
4. Review of diagnosis, cause, and compliance if no response after treatment.
5. Trial of other drugs alone or combined (80% of patients best treated by monotherapy, 10%–15% by two drugs).
6. Gradual withdrawal of unhelpful drugs or drugs causing adverse effects.
7. Referral for investigational drugs.
8. Referral for possible neurosurgical treatment of partial epilepsies.
9. Gradual drug withdrawal considered in patients free of seizures for 2–3 years.

Essential counseling

- Patients should be advised of the need to take medication regularly, driving regulations, contraception and pregnancy, safe bathing, and safe cooking with a microwave.

Key references

1. Wylie E: *The Treatment of Epilepsy*. Philadelphia: Lea and Febiger; 1993.
2. MacDonald RL, Greenfield LJ Jr: Mechanisms of action of new antiepileptic drugs. *Curr Opin Neurol* 1997, **10**:121–128.

Diagnosis

Symptoms

• These conditions form a spectrum from the relatively mild erythema multiforme minor to the severe and potentially life-threatening Stevens–Johnson syndrome.

Nonspecific upper respiratory tract infection: prodromal syndrome.

Intensely itchy skin rash.

Painful, bullous lesions: involving two or more mucous membranes in Stevens–Johnson syndrome; shallow ulcers result if the bulla ruptures.

Fever, malaise, cough, sore throat, chest pain, vomiting, diarrhea, myalgia, arthralgia: severe systemic reaction in Stevens–Johnson syndrome.

Signs

Erythema multiforme

Classic "target" lesions: develop abruptly and symmetrically, heaviest peripherally; often involve palms and soles.

Urticarial plaques: may develop but do not evolve rapidly as with a true urticaria.

Vesicles and bullae: may develop in pre-existing lesions, usually heralding a more severe form of disease; severe disease with mucosal involvement and constitutional upset indicates Stevens–Johnson syndrome.

Stevens–Johnson syndrome

Bullous lesions on mucous membranes: abrupt appearance 1–14 days after other symptoms; often on oral mucosa, lips, and conjunctivae, often with variable involvement of other mucous surfaces; urethral, vulvo-vaginal, and balanitic involvement may lead to urinary retention.

Pain from oral lesions: possibly severe enough to compromise fluid intake and breathing.

Patchy pulmonary disease, pneumonia, renal failure, diarrhea, paronychia, nail loss, polyarthritis, otitis media, and coma.

Investigations

History of drug ingestion: very important.

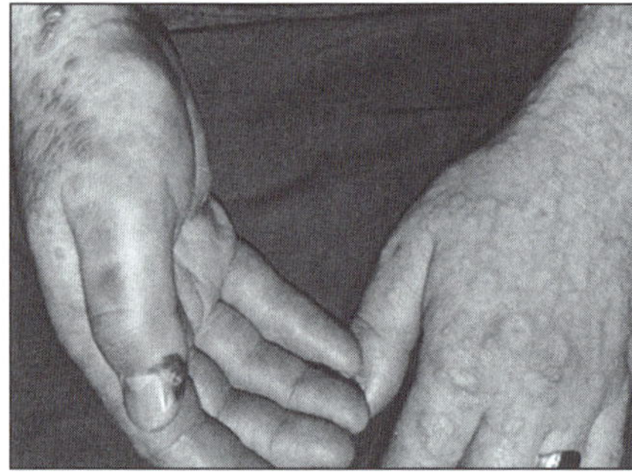

Typical "target" lesions on hands. (*See* Color Plate.)

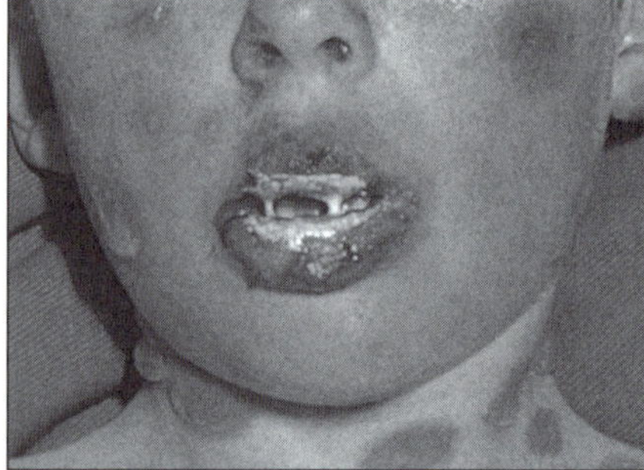

Buccal mucous membrane involvement. (*See* Color Plate.)

Throat swab: to detect coxsackieviruses, herpes simplex virus, adenoviruses.

Serology: for *Mycoplasma pneumoniae*, coxsackie, herpes simplex virus, adenovirus.

Autoimmune serology: to detect collagen diseases.

Complete blood count and ESR measurement: total leukocyte count often raised and may show excess of eosinophils; ESR and CRP usually raised.

Urea and albumin measurement: urea raised because of catabolic state and fluid loss if skin lesions extensive; exudation from lesions may cause hypoalbuminemia.

Skin biopsy: shows characteristic range of changes from mild dermal inflammation to full epidermal necrosis.

Complications

Blindness: caused by corneal involvement.

Recurrence: especially of disease caused by herpes simplex virus or drugs.

Differential diagnosis

• Classic cases with target lesions should prove no problem; atypical cases may resemble any of the following:

Chronic urticaria.

Toxic erythema (drugs or infection).

Collagen diseases.

Secondary syphilis.

Acute HIV seroconversion.

Hemorrhagic fevers.

Kawasaki syndrome.

Toxic epidermal necrolysis.

Chronic meningococcemia.

Etiology

• The condition is produced by a hypersensitivity reaction mediated by immune complexes in dermal blood vessels.

• In ~50% of patients, no cause is identified.

• Common antigenic triggers involve the following:

Infection by virus (especially herpes simplex, enteroviruses), *M. pneumoniae*, chlamydiae, histoplasmosis.

Drugs: antibiotics (*e.g.*, penicillins, sulfonamides), anticonvulsants (especially phenytoin), aspirin, corticosteroids, cimetadine.

Allopurinol, oral contraceptives.

Neoplasia: leukemia, lymphoma, multiple myeloma, internal (cryptic) malignancy.

Collagen diseases: lupus erythematosis, polyarteritis, rheumatoid arthritis.

Others: sarcoidosis, foods (*e.g.*, emulsifiers in margarine).

Epidemiology

• Erythema multiforme and Stevens–Johnson syndrome account for up to 1% of dermatology outpatient consultations.

• Children <3 years and adults >50 years are rarely affected.

• The incidence peaks in the second and third decades, with 50% of patients aged <20 years.

• The male : female ratio is 1.5 : 1.

• The illness is most severe in young adults and children, especially boys.

• Seasonal epidemics occur, related to the common provoking agents, *e.g.*, *Mycoplasma* spp., herpesvirus, and adenoviral infections.

Treatment

Diet and lifestyle

- In rare cases of a dietary "trigger," *e.g.*, emulsifiers in margarine, this must be avoided.

- If the oral contraceptive is implicated, obvious lifestyle changes must follow.

Pharmacological treatment

For the underlying "trigger" condition

- Possible drug precipitants should be withdrawn.

- Acyclovir is indicated for herpes simplex virus, and the appropriate antibiotic for *Mycoplasma* infection (macrolide or tetracycline).

Standard dosage	Acyclovir applied directly every 4 hours (ointment) or 200 mg 5 times daily. Acyclovir or valacyclovir, 500 mg twice daily. Erythromycin, 500 mg 4 times daily.
Contraindications	*Acyclovir*: renal impairment, severe dehydration. *Erythromycin*: hypersensitivity.
Main drug interactions	*Acyclovir*: other antivirals, *e.g.*, zidovudine (produces lethargy). *Erythromycin*: increase in theophylline concentrations.
Main side effects	*Acyclovir*: rashes, gastrointestinal disturbances. *Erythromycin*: gastrointestinal disturbances, nausea, vomiting, pain, diarrhea.

For skin lesions

- Antihistamines are indicated for pruritus, salicylates or NSAIDs for symptomatic relief (salicylates have been implicated as causative agents). For bullous skin lesions, Domeboro compresses applied twice daily for 20 minutes followed by applications of silver sulfadiazine cream twice daily.

Standard dosage	Chlorpheniramine, 4 mg orally every 6–8 hours. Naproxen, 250 mg every 6–8 hours.
Contraindications	*Naproxen*: active peptic ulceration; to be avoided in children (acetaminophen analgesia instead).
Special points	*Chlorpheniramine*: patients must not drive if drowsiness ensues.
Main drug interactions	*Chlorpheniramine*: alcohol or sedatives. *Naproxen*: oral anticoagulants.
Main side effects	*Chlorpheniramine*: drowsiness, headache, gastrointestinal disturbances. *Naproxen*: gastrointestinal disturbances.

For severe cases (Stevens–Johnson syndrome)

- Withdrawal of any drug precipitant and treatment of infective causes is vital.

- No data from well-controlled trials are available, but the dermatological manifestations respond to a short course of high-dose steroids.

- Because of mouth involvement, enteric or parenteral feeding may be needed and should be considered during the first week.

- Intravenous fluid replacement should be instituted early.

Standard dosage	Prednisolone, 80–100 mg daily.
Contraindications	Active peptic ulceration.
Special points	Possible adrenal suppression on withdrawal.
Main drug interactions	NSAIDs, oral anticoagulants.
Main side effects	Cushing's syndrome, growth retardation in children.

General references

Hurwitz S: Erythema multiforme: a review of its characteristics, diagnostic criteria, and management. *Pediatr Rev* 1990, **11**:217–222.

Renfro L, *et al.*: Controversy: are systemic steroids indicated in the treatment of erythema multiforme? *Pediatr Dermatol* 1989, **6**:43–50.

Diagnosis

Symptoms

Painful red nodules: on lower legs and occasionally on thighs and forearms; pain worse on weight-bearing; gradual appearance; can become almost confluent; gradual healing (3–6 weeks), with bruising but no scarring.

"Crops" of lesions: occurring at different times, so that lesions manifest at different stages of evolution.

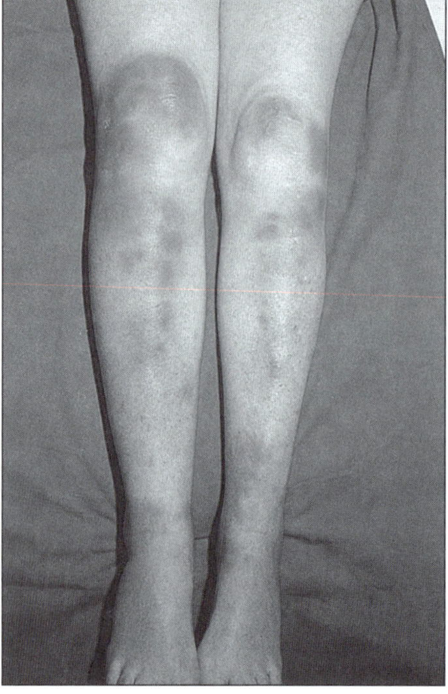

Classic lesions over pretibial region. (*See* Color Plate.)

Signs

Tender erythematous nodules: 1–5 cm diameter; usually bilateral over pretibial areas; no ulceration or blistering; involution over 3–6 weeks, with yellow–purple bruising.

Fever and systemic reaction: variable but may precede lesions by 1–7 days.

Investigations

• Discovering the cause is important because treatment of this prevents recurrences.

History: for drugs (*e.g.*, oral contraceptive), pregnancy, contact with tuberculosis, inflammatory bowel disease, yersiniosis, histoplasmosis, streptococcal infection.

Complete blood count, ESR analysis: acute-phase reactants always raised.

Chest radiography: to detect features of sarcoidosis, tuberculosis, disseminated fungal infection.

Bacteriology: sputum or early morning urine for acid/alcohol-fast bacilli; throat swab or antistreptolysin O titer for evidence of streptococcal infection; stool culture.

Mantoux test: strongly positive in tuberculosis, negative in sarcoidosis.

Complications

• The skin lesions have no complications.

• Any complications relate to the underlying condition; if this is not controlled, the skin lesion may continue to be manifest (lasting up to 4–5 months).

Differential diagnosis

Erythema nodosum leprosum: in multibacillary leprosy, unrelated acute reactional state to the release of mycobacterial protein during treatment.

Erythematous skin lesions of pretibial area: *e.g.*, pretibial myxedema.

Rheumatoid nodules (usually on elbows, wrists, or palms).

Battered child syndrome.

Henoch-Schönlein purpura (also associated with abdominal and joint pain.

Infectious cellulitis (especially in the immunodeficient patient).

Subcutaneous granuloma annulare (more chronic history, usually asymptomatic).

Etiology

• Erythema nodosum is a septal panniculitis in subcutaneous fat due to a hypersensitivity reaction to antigenic or other stimulus.

• Causes include the following:

Drugs: *e.g.*, penicillin, sulfonamides, oral contraceptive pill in 25% of patients.

Infections: *e.g.*, tuberculosis, streptococci, *Yersinia, Salmonella, Campylobacter* spp., deep fungal infection, leprosy.

Inflammatory conditions: *e.g.*, sarcoidosis, inflammatory bowel disease, Behçet's syndrome, pregnancy, thyroid disease.

• 20%–40% of cases are idiopathic.

Epidemiology

• Erythema nodosum is the most frequent cause of acute panniculitis.

• The most common cause in children is infection with streptococci (usually of the pharynx).

• The peak age is 20–30 years, but erythema nodosum can occur at any age.

• The female : male ratio is 3 : 1.

• Patients with tuberculosis-related disease are usually <20 years of age.

• Patients with disease caused by pregnancy or inflammatory bowel disorders are usually 15–40 years of age.

• Patients with disease caused by Behçet's syndrome or sarcoidosis are usually 20–40 years of age.

• Fever and systemic reactions occur more often and for longer in older patients.

Treatment

Diet and lifestyle

• During the acute phase of the inflammation, prolonged weight-bearing should be avoided.

Pharmacological treatment

• Treatment of skin lesions is primarily symptomatic.

• Management of the underlying condition prevents further erythema nodosum.

For pain relief

• NSAIDs should be sufficient.

Standard dosage	Naproxen, 250 mg every 6–8 hours.
Contraindications	Hypersensitivity, active peptic ulceration; caution with concomitant anticoagulation and asthma.
Main drug interactions	Warfarin.
Main side effects	Gastrointestinal disturbances, discomfort, nausea, ulceration.

Systemic steroids

• Steroids are effective, but extreme caution must be observed; they should be used only if the underlying conditions, *e.g.*, tuberculosis, have been adequately treated.

Standard dosage	Prednisolone, 20–40 mg initially, reduced rapidly over 10 days to nil.
Contraindications	Active peptic ulceration.
Special points	Possible adrenal suppression on sudden withdrawal.
Main drug interactions	NSAIDs, oral anticoagulants.
Main side effects	Cushing's syndrome, growth retardation in children, glucose intolerance, osteoporosis.

Treatment aims

To provide symptomatic relief of lesion-related pain or discomfort.

To remove or treat underlying cause.

Other treatments

Potassium iodide.

Wet dressings to the lesions for symptomatic relief.

Prognosis

• Lesions usually clear in 3–6 weeks.

• Spontaneous resolution is usual.

Follow-up and management

• The most important aspect of erythema nodosum management is diagnosis of any underlying precipitant.

General references

Fox MD, Schwartz RA: Erythema nodosum. *Am Fam Physician* 1992, **46**:818–822.

Hannuksela M: Erythema nodosum. *Clin Dermatol* 1986, **4**:88–95.

Diagnosis

Symptoms

Dysphagia: solids > liquids is the classic presentation.

Weight loss, fatigue.

Unexplained cessation of reflux symptoms: in patients with untreated pyrosis.

• Gastrointestinal bleeding occasionally is the chief presenting symptom.

Signs

• Most typically, patients have a normal physical examination on presentation. When present, abnormalities may include the following items:

Clinical evidence of weight loss (*e.g.,* muscle wasting).

Pallor when anemia is present.

Supraclavicular or cervical lymphadenopathy.

Hepatomegaly secondary to metastasis.

Respiratory findings (*i.e.,* rales or rhonchi) from aspiration.

Investigations

• Primary investigation should be directed at the integrity of the esophageal lumen.

Barium swallow (esophagram): least-expensive imaging modality but does not allow tissue identification of the lesion or therapeutic dilation if necessary; malignant findings must be confirmed with biopsy.

Upper endoscopy: offers direct examination of the lesion and allows sampling of abnormalities for histological confirmation.

Endoscopic ultrasonography: allows staging of the tumor in patients who are potential candidates for surgical resection.

Thoracic-abdominal CT scanning: best initial study to determine the extensiveness of disease once malignancy has been identified.

Complete blood count: may reveal iron-deficiency anemia.

Liver chemistry tests: may reveal metastatic disease to the liver with elevated alkaline phosphatase or transaminases.

Complications

Esophageal obstruction.

Malnutrition.

Bleeding.

Fistula to bronchial tree: cough with swallowing.

Invasion of mediastinum.

Aspiration: recurrent pneumonia.

Differential diagnosis

Benign esophageal stricture.
Motility disorders, particularly achalasia.
Extrinsic compression of esophagus: *e.g.,* carcinoma of bronchus.
Schatzki's ring.

Risk factors

Squamous carcinoma: most common in African-American males; associated with alcohol and tobacco use.

Adenocarcinoma: most common in whites with a slight predominance in males; reflux predisposes to Barrett's esophagus (premalignant tissue of specialized columnar epithelium in the distal esophagus that may progress to adenocarcinoma of the esophagus) [1,2].

• Achalasia and previous caustic ingestion injuries predispose to later development of esophageal malignancies.

Epidemiology [3]

• Esophageal carcinoma is one of the most common cancers in the world, but wide geographical variations are found.

• Environmental factors are poorly characterized (*e.g.*, high-risk regions in Iran, China, and Russia identified).

• It is relatively less frequent in western Europe and North America (incidence, 5 in 100 000).

Histological types

• Worldwide, squamous carcinoma predominates, accounting for 90% of esophageal malignancies.

• Adenocarcinoma of the stomach cardia and distal esophagus is increasing in frequency, probably because of the association with gastroesophageal reflux and Barrett's esophagus (a preneoplastic lesion).

Treatment

Diet and lifestyle

• Adequate nutrition should be ensured, preferably orally (soft foods and high-calorie nutritional supplements should be emphasized).

• The need for a fine-bore enteral feeding tube or percutaneous endoscopic gastrostomy tube should be anticipated, and the tube should be placed prior to high-grade obstruction of the esophagus.

Pharmacological treatment [4,5]

• Simple analgesics are used for pain control in the early stages, but opiates are needed later.

• Avoid prokinetic agents such as metoclopramide or cisapride, which may potentiate dysphagia.

Standard dosage	Morphine, 5–10 mg every 4 hours, titrate as needed.
Contraindications	Raised intracranial pressure.
Special points	Concerns about side effects should not deter use.
Main drug interactions	Synergistic effect with other CNS depressants.
Main drug effects	Constipation, nausea, drowsiness.

• Chemotherapy is reserved for patients who are not surgical candidates and involves 5-fluorouracil– and cisplatin-based protocols that are ideally used concomitantly with radiation therapy.

Nonpharmacological treatment [5,6]

• Curative surgery is attempted whenever possible, but most patients have evidence of extensive disease on presentation and are suitable for only palliative treatment [3–5].

Surgical resection: suitable in only about one-third of patients; esophagectomy with primary esophagogastrostomy most frequently chosen. Investigational protocols involving perioperative radiation and/or chemotherapy show some promise but are often quite cumbersome for the patient.

Endoscopic palliation: simple dilatation (by bougie or balloon), endoscopic intubations (prosthetic stents available), laser therapy, thermal devices (*e.g.*, bipolar coagulation) may be used to facilitate patency of the esophageal lumen allowing maintenance of hydration and nutrition.

Palliative radiotherapy: intracavitary irradiation with cobalt or iridium or external beam irradiation; can be beneficial for pain from mediastinal extension.

Esophageal carcinoma

Treatment aims

To delay physical deterioration by improving and maintaining swallowing and nutrition.
To diminish pain.
To avoid respiratory complications.

Prognosis

• The 5-year survival for patients with esophageal cancer is <10% and most patients die within 4–12 months of diagnosis. Radiation and/or chemotherapy can offer only modest improvements in this prognosis.

• Patients who are candidates for surgical resection have a 5-year survival of ~20%. This may be further enhanced with perioperative chemotherapy/radiation investigational protocols. Perioperative mortality in general is <15% and attributed to cardiopulmonary complications, sepsis, and anastamotic leaks with malnutrition as an additional potentiating influence.

Follow-up and management

• Patients who have had curative treatment should be monitored for features of relapse with CT scans and imaging studies of the esophageal lumen.

• A fistula communicating with the bronchial tree should be considered in patients with progressive disease who develop a cough; stent placement may be beneficial in these patients.

Key references

1. Cameron AJ: Barrett's esophagus and adenocarcinoma. *Gastroenterology* 1993, **102**:1421–1424.

2. Kruse P, *et al.*: Barrett's oesophagus and oesophageal adenocarcinoma. *Scand J Gastroenterol* 1993, **28**:193–196.

3. Blot WJ: Esophageal cancer trends and risk factors. *Semin Oncol* 1994, **21**:403–410.

4. Griffin SM, Robertson CS: Nonsurgical treatment of cancer of the oesophagus. *Br J Surg* 1993, **80**:412–413.

5. Haller DG: Treatments for esophageal cancer. *N Engl J Med* 1992, **326**:1629–1630.

6. Walsh TN, *et al.*: A comparison of multimodal therapy and surgery for esophageal adenocarcinoma. *N Engl J Med* 1996, **335**:462–467.

Diagnosis

Symptoms

• Symptoms do not predict the severity of mucosal inflammation.

Heartburn: retrosternal or epigastric burning is the most common symptom; dull ache may resemble angina.

Regurgitation of food, acid, or bitter juice: may be confused with "vomiting" (but without nausea).

Respiratory symptoms: *e.g.*, nocturnal cough or dyspnea, asthma.

Hoarseness.

Dysphagia: stricture or motility disorder.

Odynophagia (painful swallowing): suggests infectious etiology or pill-induced ulcer.

Signs

• Signs are frequently absent.

Pulmonary consolidation or bronchospasm: rarely, if aspiration has occurred as a result of regurgitation.

Melena or hematochezia.

Evidence of immunocompromise.

Investigations

• Uncomplicated reflux esophagitis often requires no diagnostic testing prior to initiation of therapy.

• For patients with dysphagia, weight loss, bleeding, or refractory symptoms, diagnostic imaging must be performed.

Radiography: not reliable for showing esophagitis (particularly mild forms) or reflux; may be of some use in assessing esophageal motility.

Endoscopy: preferred to radiography because it offers visualization of mucosa and option of obtaining cytology and histology; allows determination of severity of esophagitis. Indicated for patients with dysphagia, complicated recurrent or refractory symptoms.

pH monitoring: for diagnosis of acid reflux without esophagitis; for quantifying reflux to assess effectiveness of treatment or before antireflux surgery.

Manometry: useful to exclude associated motility disorders before antireflux surgery.

Cardiac tests: to exclude cardiac disease as a source of symptoms.

Complete blood count: in complicated cases to evaluate for anemia or systemic manifestations of inflammation.

Complications

Stricture [1].

Barrett's esophagus.

Aspiration, leading to night cough, bronchospasm, pneumonia, asthma.

Bleeding: may be life-threatening.

Differential diagnosis

Peptic ulcer disease.

Esophageal malignancy.

Esophageal motility disorder.

Gallstone disease.

Ischemic heart disease.

Etiology

• Esophagitis is mucosal damage most commonly caused by gastroesophageal reflux, which occurs when the lower esophageal sphincter is incompetent or esophageal clearance is impaired.

• Reflux esophagitis is caused by prolonged exposure of esophageal mucosa to gastric contents and is more intense if the mucosa is compromised or if gastric emptying is delayed.

• Reflux symptoms are often erroneously attributed to hiatal hernia, a common condition that is most often asymptomatic.

• Infectious esophagitis due to *Candida* spp., herpesvirus, or cytomegalovirus may occur in immunocompromised patients.

Epidemiology

• Two-thirds of the population may suffer from reflux at some time, but only a small proportion seek medical advice.

• Mechanical and hormonal factors make reflux common during pregnancy.

• Infectious esophagitis is a common component of HIV infections.

• Pill-induced ulcers of the esophagus are most common in bedridden patients with medications such as NSAIDs, tetracyclines, quinidine.

Savary-Miller endoscopic classification

Grade I: nonconfluent mucosal lesions.

Grade II: confluent mucosal lesions.

Grade III: circumferential mucosal lesions.

Grade IV: deep ulcer, stricture, or Barrett's esophagus.

Treatment

Diet and lifestyle

• Reducing weight, stopping smoking, eating small meals, avoiding certain foods (*e.g.*, chocolate, coffee, mints, alcohol), and sleeping with the head of the bed raised are crucial measures that decrease reflux [2,3].

• Patients should be advised to remain upright for 2–4 hours after a meal.

• NSAIDs, slow-release potassium chloride, theophylline, nitrates, and calcium blockers (*e.g.*, nifedipine) may also aggravate symptoms.

Pharmacological treatment [4]

Acid antisecretory agents (first-line agents)

• These diminish gastric acid production, thus decreasing exposure of the esophageal mucosa. Healing requires 6–8-week courses with further maintenance therapy as required.

• Proton-pump inhibitors (*e.g.*, omeprazole, lansoprazole) are more powerful than H_2 antagonists (*e.g.*, ranitidine) and are favored in severe cases.

Standard dosage	Ranitidine, 150–300 mg twice daily. Omeprazole, 20–40 mg daily. Lansoprazole, 30 mg daily. Dose can be titrated against symptoms.
Contraindications	Known hypersensitivity.
Main drug interactions	*Omeprazole, lansoprazole:* warfarin, phenytoin, diazepam.
Main side effects	*Ranitidine:* the following side effects are rare and usually not clinically significant: headache, blood disorders, increased liver enzyme levels. *Omeprazole:* skin reactions, diarrhea, headache, enteric infections are rarely observed.

Motility-enhancing agents

• These are not widely used, with the exception of cisapride, which is as effective as some H_2 antagonists.

Standard dosage	Cisapride, 10–20 mg 3–4 times daily, 30 minutes before meals.
Contraindications	Gastrointestinal hemorrhage or perforation, mechanical bowel obstruction.
Main drug interactions	Anticoagulants: effect possibly enhanced; erythromycin.
Main side effects	Diarrhea, abdominal discomfort.

Mucosal-protecting agents

• Only sucralfate has proved reasonably effective.

Standard dosage	Sucralfate, 1 g 4 times daily.
Contraindications	Caution in renal impairment (aluminum toxicity).
Main drug interactions	Decreased bioavailability of tetracycline, phenytoin, cimetidine (avoided by separating administration from sucralfate by 2 hours).
Main side effects	Constipation.

Antacids

• Antacids may provide reasonable but short-lasting relief; they have little effect on mucosal inflammation.

Standard dosage	30–60 mL 3–4 times daily.
Contraindications	Renal failure (magnesium based).
Main drug interactions	Iron, phenytoin, penicillamine, tetracycline.
Main side effects	Constipation (aluminum based), diarrhea (magnesium based).

Treatment aims

To control symptoms.
To prevent complications, especially for stricture formation [5].

Other treatments

Antireflux surgery

• Nissen fundoplication and its modifications using a laparoscopic approach are the most popular techniques.

• Surgery is indicated for the following: refractory, debilitating symptoms that are complicated by bleeding, asthma, or severe strictures or that are refractory to aggressive medical management.

Prognosis

• This is a chronic and relapsing condition, but up to 40% of patients remain in remission.

Follow-up and management

• Permanent reflux-reducing measures (particularly weight reduction) must be implemented in order to avoid relapse. Some form of treatment may be necessary to maintain remission.

• Long-term treatment is indicated in patients who have had frequent relapse.

• Identification of Barrett's esophagus is an indication for more careful monitoring for esophageal malignancy. Esophago-gastroduodenoscopy with biopsies are routinely performed every 1–3 years.

Key references

1. Marks AD, Richter JE: Peptic strictures of the esophagus. *Am J Gastroenterol* 1993, **88**:1160–1173.

2. Pope CE: Acid-reflux disorders. *N Engl J Med* 1994, **331**:656–660.

3. Richter JE: Esophageal chest pain: current controversies in pathogenesis, diagnosis, and therapy. *Ann Intern Med* 1989, **110**:66–78.

4. Vignieri S, *et al.*: A comparison of five maintenance therapies for reflux esophagitis. *N Engl J Med* 1995, **333**:1106–1110.

5. Sontag SJ: Gastro-oesophageal reflux disease. *Aliment Pharmacol Ther* 1993, **7**:293–312.

Diagnosis

Symptoms [1,2]

Total body aches.

Total body exhaustion.

Fatigue.

Intractable chronic pain.

Myalgias, arthralgias.

Low-grade fever.

Exercise limitation.

Sleep disturbance.

Signs

Absence of objective inflammation.

Trigger points.

Normal range of motion.

Investigations

Normal complete blood count.

Normal serologies: Westegren erythrocyte sedimentation rate, rheumatoid factor, antinuclear antibodies.

Electromyography.

Radiography.

Complications

Impaired quality of life.

Deconditioning.

Work limitation.

Analgesic dependency.

Depression.

• Chronic deformity and/or crippling does not occur with fibromyalgia.

Differential diagnosis

Chronic fatigue syndrome.
Depression.
Osteoarthritis.
Rheumatoid arthritis.
SLE.

Terminology issues

The term "fibrositis" is best avoided because inflammation is not present in this condition; "myofascial pain syndrome" is an acceptable alternative.

Etiology [1,2]

Unknown.
• Hypotheses include the following:
A disorder of central pain perception.
Abnormal muscle metabolism.
Abnormality of nonrestorative deep sleep.

Epidemiology

Prevalence: 5% of patients in general medicine practice, 2%–4% of the general population.
More common in women.
Age of onset 20–45 years of age.
Overrepresented in highly educated, high-achieving, perfectionistic individuals.

Treatment

Diet and lifestyle

• A gentle, continuous exercise program may be the most helpful intervention overall. Rigorous exercise programs are uniformly poorly tolerated (and abandoned early).

Pharmacological treatment [2,3]

• Low-dose antidepressants, *e.g.*, amitriptyline, 10–25 mg daily, may be helpful in 20%–30% of patients. It may work via effects on central pain, biochemical pathways, and sleep disturbance. Main side effects include dry mouth, fatigue, and somnolence. The low dosages help to minimize these side effects.

Nonpharmacological treatment

Reassurance: nondestructive, not deforming.

Chronic pain management: referral may be very helpful, including techniques such as visual imagery, relaxation, meditation, etc.

Physical therapy: gentle, long-term exercise program with special emphasis on evidence of injury and exhaustion.

Treatment aims

To control pain.

To improve sense of well being.

To improve exercise tolerance.

To improve work tolerance.

Prognosis

• The prognosis is highly variable.

• It is controversial whether life expectancy is normal or slightly diminished.

Follow-up and management

• The primary care provider can follow the patient at mutually agreeable intervals.

• Narcotic analgesia should be avoided (and frequently does not significantly reduce pain).

Key references

1. Krsnich-Shriwise S: Fibromyalgia syndrome: an overview. *Phys Ther* 1997, **77**:68–75.

2. Simms RW: Fibromyalgia syndrome: current concepts in pathophysiology, clinical features, and management. *Arthritis Care Res* 1996, **9**:315–328.

3. Goldenberg D, Mayskiy M, Mossey C, *et al.*: A randomized double-blind crossover trial of fluoxetine and amitriptyline in the treatment of fibromyalgia. *Arthritis Rheum* 1996, **39**:1852–1859.

Diagnosis

Symptoms and signs

Candida infections

White plaques in mouth or tongue, angular cheilitis.
Vulvovaginal discharge, pruritus.
Cutaneous candidiasis, intertrigo, folliculitis, balanitis, perianal or interdigital infection, diaper rash.
Paronychia or onychomycosis.
Cystitis, urethritis.
Disseminated candidiasis involving several organs; endophthalmitis, endocarditis, cerebral or hepatic microabscesses.
Pneumonia, allergic wheeze, breathlessness.
Peritonitis, esophagitis.

Aspergillus infections

Wheeze, breathlessness: indicating allergic bronchopulmonary aspergillosis.
Fever, cough, hypoxia, chest discomfort or pleuritic pain, hemoptysis, pneumonia: indicating invasive aspergillosis.
Blocked nose, facial pain, nasal discharge, chronic headache: indicating allergic or saprophytic sinus infection.
Chronic otitis media or externa, meningitis or cerebral microabscesses, endocarditis, endophthalmitis, osteoarticular disorders.

Cryptococcal infections

• Onset is insidious.

Fever, headache, nausea, vomiting, neck stiffness, photophobia: indicating meningitis.
Dyspnea, cough: indicating pneumonia.

Histoplasmosis, coccidiomycosis, blastomycosis

Breathlessness, lung infiltrates: indicating pulmonary histoplasmosis.
Pancytopenia, pneumonia, lymphadenopathy, hepatosplenomegaly, oral or gastrointestinal ulcers, adrenal masses: indicating disseminated histoplasmosis.
Enlarged lymph glands: indicating lymphadenopathy.

Agents of mucormycosis (zygomycosis)

Headache, facial pain, orbital cellulitis, lower cranial nerve palsies: indicating rhinocerebral infection.
Pneumonia, disseminated disease.

Investigations

Biopsy of tissue and bone marrow with culture and histology (histoplasmosis only), culture of blood, sputum, fluid (including CSF), and sinuses.
Antigen tests: for cryptococcal infections.
CT for *Aspergillus* infections: of thorax for aspergilloma and invasive infections; of sinuses for allergy, saprophytic, acute invasion; of brain for brain abscess.
Endoscopy, colonoscopy, barium meal, swallow, follow-through: for esophagitis, gastritis, small and large bowel plaques, and ulceration.
Radiography of chest, thorax, and sinuses.
Bronchoscopy: lavage, biopsy, for pulmonary disease and diagnosis.
Serology: fungal immunodiffusion testing and serum cryptococcal antigen.

Complications

Candida infections

Esophageal candidiasis, azole-resistant thrush, endometritis, ascending renal infection in intensive care or surgical patients, prostatitis, multiple organ involvement, hepatosplenic candidiasis in leukemic patients.

Other infections

Pulmonary fibrosis: after 5–10 years; complication of allergic bronchopulmonary aspergillosis.
Hemoptysis: in *Aspergillus* infections and zygomycosis.
Hydrocephalus, impaired mental function, blindness: complications of cryptococcal infections; hydrocephalus usually communicating.

Differential diagnosis

Other infections.
Lymphoma.
Tuberculosis.

Etiology

• Predisposing causes include the following:

Superficial *Candida* infections
Antibiotics, steroids, diabetes mellitus, AIDS, pregnancy, oral contraceptives, macerated skin, occupation, abnormal T-cell response to *Candida* antigens.

Systemic *Candida* infections
Urinary catheterization, immunosuppression, surgery, burns, premature birth, endocarditis, valvular heart disease, prosthetic valves, peritoneal dialysis, abdominal surgery, bowel perforation, hematological malignancies, CSF shunts.

Aspergillus infections
Asthma, cystic fibrosis, neutropenia, organ transplantation, AIDS, steroids, chronic granulomatous disease, previous pulmonary tuberculosis, sarcoidosis, bronchiectasis, chronic lung disease, diabetes mellitus, alcoholism, previous ear disease, i.v. drug abuse, valve replacement.

Cryptococcal infections
AIDS, lymphoma, steroids, sarcoidosis.

Histoplasmosis, coccidiomycosis, blastomycosis
History of exposure, *e.g.*, endemic area, bat caves (acute), emphysema (chronic), AIDS.

Mucormycosis
Acidosis, diabetes mellitus, neutropenia, bone-marrow transplantation, i.v. drug abuse, deferoxamine treatment.

Epidemiology

Environmental saprophytes.
• Vaginal candidiasis affects 70% of all women, and 5% have frequent recurrences.
• Oral thrush affects 90% of AIDS patients and 15%–30% of leukemia patients.
• Invasive aspergillosis affects 5%–40% of immunocompromised patients.
• Cryptococcal meningitis affects 4%–35% of AIDS patients, depending on country.

Treatment

Diet and lifestyle

• No special precautions are necessary.

Pharmacological treatment

Amphotericin B

• Amphotericin B is indicated for the following:

Candida infections (oropharyngeal, urogenital tract, candidemia, endocarditis, pneumonia, visceral, CNS).
Aspergillus infections (invasive or chronic necrotizing aspergillosis, acute invasive sinus, or paranasal granuloma).
Cryptococcal infections (meningitis).
Histoplasmosis (chronic pulmonary, disseminated).
Agents of mucormycosis (rhinocerebral).

Standard dosage	Amphotericin B, 0.5–1.5 mg/kg i.v.
Contraindications	Hypersensitivity.
Special points	Resistant strains include *Candida krusei*, *Fusarium* spp., *Pseudallescheria boydii*, *Trichosporon beigelii*, Mucorales (limited activity).
Main drug interactions	Increased nephrotoxicity with aminoglycosides or cyclosporine.
Main side effects	Infusion-related fever or rigors, nausea, phlebitis, renal toxicity, anemia, electrolyte disturbances.

Azoles

• Fluconazole is indicated for *Candida* infections (oropharyngeal, vulvovaginal, nail infections, chronic mucocutaneous candidiasis, urogenital tract, visceral candidiasis) and for cryptococcal infections (meningitis in AIDS).

• Itraconazole is indicated for *Aspergillus* infections (pulmonary, acute invasive sinus, paranasal granuloma) and for histoplasmosis (severe acute, chronic pulmonary, less seriously ill, disseminated; maintenance in AIDS and coccidiomycosis).

Standard dosage	Fluconazole, 50–400 mg orally or i.v. daily. Itraconazole, 100–200 mg orally daily; 200 mg loading doses 3 times daily initially in severe or life-threatening disease. Ketoconazole, 200–400 mg orally daily.
Contraindications	Azole hypersensitivity.
Special points	*Fluconazole*: resistant strains include *Histoplasma capsulatum*, Mucorales, *Candida krusei* and *glabrata*, *Aspergillus* and *Fusarium* spp. *Itraconazole*: resistant strains include *C. glabrata*, *Fusarium* spp., Mucorales. *Ketoconazole*: resistant strains include *C. glabrata*, *Cryptococcus neoformans*, *Aspergillus* and *Fusarium* spp.
Main drug interactions	Altered azole or drug concentrations with phenytoin, cyclosporine, rifampin, phenobarbital, carbamazepine, warfarin, astemizole, digoxin.
Main side effects	*Fluconazole:* nausea, rash, liver dysfunction (rare). *Itraconazole:* gynecomastia, peripheral edema, hypokalemia, liver dysfunction (rare). *Ketoconazole:* liver dysfunction, nausea, reduced libido, menstrual irregularities, gynecomastia.

Other drugs

Flucytosine, 150 mg/kg orally daily in 4 divided doses only in combination with amphotericin B: for *Candida* infections (candidemia, endocarditis, CNS infections), *Aspergillus* infections (invasive aspergillosis), and cryptococcal infections (meningitis).

Topical nystatin: for mucosal *Candida* infection.

Topical antifungals: for cutaneous *Candida* and dermatophyte infections.

Inhaled steroids, bronchodilators: for allergic pneumonitis.

Oral steroids: for exacerbations of allergic bronchopulmonary aspergillosis.

General references

British Society for Antimicrobial Chemotherapy Working Party: Antifungal chemotherapy in patients with acquired immunodeficiency syndrome. *Lancet* 1992, **340**:648–651.

Denning DW, Stevens DA: Antifungal and surgical treatment of invasive aspergillosis: review of 2121 published cases. *Rev Infect Dis* 1990, **12**:1147–1201.

Minamoto GY, Rosenberg AS: Fungal infections in patients with aquired immunodeficiency syndrome. *Med Clin North Am* 1997, **81**:381–409.

Diagnosis

Symptoms

Cosmetic embarrassment.

Mechanical problems: onychodystrophic nails get snagged on clothing; pressure and irritation from footwear.

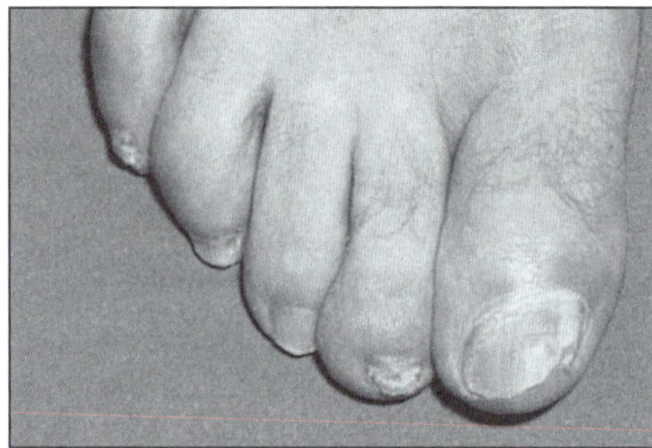

Distal and lateral subungual onychomycosis secondary to dermatophyte infection. (*See* Color Plate.)

Signs

•Signs can be divided into three varieties of clinical manifestations based on the type of nail infection: distal variety, proximal infection, or superficial infection.

Distal infection

Onycholysis: distal or distal-lateral nail separation from nail bed with hyperkeratotic subungual debris and crumbling friable nails; over time extends proximally.

Proximal infection

Discoloration: white to yellow, affecting the proximal ventral nail plate; extends distally and toward the dorsal surface of the nail plate but rarely involves the whole nail (least common type).

Superficial infection

Discoloration: patchy chalk-white, mainly of toenails, known as "superficial white onychomycosis."

Investigations

Microscopic examination: potassium hydroxide preparation of subungual debris (as proximal as possible) will be positive only in 50% of cases.

Culture: positive in only 50% of cases in which microscopy is positive.

Complications

Spread of infection: to other nails or adjacent skin.

Secondary pseudomonas infection (green nail syndrome).

Complete onycholysis: disruption and separation of the entire nail plate from the nail bed.

Treatment

Diet and lifestyle

• Prophylaxis using antifungal foot powder and prevention of overhydration of feet in occlusive, nonbreathing footwear undoubtedly has merit.

Pharmacological treatment

Topical treatment

• Topical treatment is prophylactic only to control tinea pedis.

• Superficial white onychomycosis can be treated by simply scraping off the superficial fungi from the nail.

Systemic treatment

• Allylamines (terbinafine) and triazoles (itraconazole and fluconazole) are much more effective over a much shorter treatment period than is griseofulvin, which is more effective in fingernail infection than in toenail infection, requires a course of 12–18 months in toenail infections, and has a cure rate of only 10%–50% [1–3].

Standard dosage	Terbinafine, 250 mg orally once daily for at least 3 months. Itraconazole (pulse therapy), 200 mg orally twice daily for the first 7 days of months 1, 2, 3, and 4. Itraconazole, 400 mg orally daily for 1 week, then repeated at monthly intervals for 4 months. Fluconazole, 150 mg orally every week for up to 9 months.
Contraindications	Pregnancy.
Main drug interactions	*Terbinafine*: rifampin or phenobarbital will result in decreased serum levels of terbinafine. Cimetidine will increase terbinafine levels. *Itraconazole*: minimal risk of drug interactions because of the lack of significant inhibitory or inducing effect on hepatic microsomal enzymes; otherwise, same as terbinafine. *Fluconazole*: primary route of excretion is renal not hepatic; high specificity for fungal cytochrome P-450, otherwise similar to itraconazole and terbinafine.
Main side effects	*Terbinafine*: gastrointestinal upset, skin reactions (drug rash). *Itraconazole*: nausea, gastrointestinal upset, elevated liver function tests (0.3%–5% of patients). *Fluconazole*: gastrointestinal upset, elevated liver function tests, Stevens–Johnson syndrome (especially patients who are HIV-positive).

Treatment aims

To eradicate the infection.
To prevent recurrence.

Other treatments

• Amorolfine 5% nail lacquer may be an alternative to systemic therapy, especially when the nail matrix is not involved [4]. Nail avulsion combined with systemic therapy.

Prognosis

Better for fingernail involvement (~50% cure rate).
High relapse rate.

Follow-up and management

• It is very important to monitor liver function tests because of the possibility of hepatotoxicity (as with ketoconazole).

• The systemic drugs are relatively new agents that should be used cautiously and monitored carefully.

Key references

1. Roberts DT: Oral therapeutic agents in fungal nail disease. *J Am Acad Dermatol* 1994, **31**:578–581.

2. Raza A: Ecology and epidemiology of dermatophyte infections. *J Am Acad Dermatol* 1994, **31**:521–525.

3. Cohen PR, Scher RK: Geriatric nail disorders: diagnosis and treatment. *J Am Acad Dermatol* 1992, **26**:521–531.

4. Gupta A, Sauder D, Shear N: Antifungal agents: an overview. Part II. *J Am Acad Dermatol* 1994, **30**:911–933.

Diagnosis

Symptoms
• Up to 70% of patients are asymptomatic or have nonspecific dyspeptic symptoms.

Uncomplicated
Biliary colic: sudden-onset severe epigastric or upper right quadrant abdominal pain, lasting for several hours, usually radiating to back, sometimes associated with nausea and vomiting.

Complicated
Fever, persistent abdominal pain, nausea and vomiting: indicating acute cholecystitis.

Fever, pain, jaundice: indicating acute cholangitis.

Abdominal pain radiating to the back, vomiting: indicating acute pancreatitis.

Signs

Uncomplicated
• Few signs are manifest.

Tenderness in right upper quadrant: usually during or after episodes of biliary colic.

Complicated
Jaundice: indicating stone impaction in common bile duct.

Murphy's sign (a halt in deep inspiration when deep palpation in the right upper quadrant results in pain): indicating acute cholecystitis.

Hypotension: indicating acute pancreatitis or sepsis from cholangitis.

Investigations

Ultrasonography: first choice test to identify stones; may also detect small stones and biliary sludge; detects dilated bile ducts and can occasionally identify disease in the liver, pancreas, or kidneys.

• Gallstones are frequently found incidentally by ultrasonography or abdominal radiography (if calcified).

• Laboratory tests are not diagnostic but are useful for identifying complications and excluding other abnormalities.

Serum alkaline phosphatase and bilirubin measurement: elevation suggests biliary tract disease.

Leukocyte count: frequently elevated with inflammation of the biliary tract.

Serum amylase measurement: >100 IU/dL suggests acute pancreatitis.

Antimitochondrial antibody tests: in atypical cases (*e.g.*, pruritis, painless jaundice) to exclude primary biliary cirrhosis.

Plain abdominal radiography: identifies stones that are calcified (~20%).

Oral cholecystography: identifies radiolucent stones, good for determining gallbladder contraction and cystic duct patency and for identifying anatomical abnormalities in gallbladder; not sensitive for detecting small stones and invalid in case of nonopacifying gallbladder.

CT: less sensitive than ultrasonography for detecting gallbladder stones or bile duct dilatation.

Cholescintigraphy: using [99mTc]-HIDA (hepatic iminodiacetic acid) helpful in suspected acute cholecystitis (*i.e.*, gallbladder does not fill); parenchymal liver disease or significant cholestasis may lead to false-positive results.

Complications
Acute cholecystitis.
Acute cholangitis.
Acute pancreatitis.
Hydrops, empyema of gallbladder.
Malignancy of gallbladder.
Perforation.
Internal and external biliary fistulas.
Gallstone ileus.
Hemobilia.
Choledocholithiasis.

Differential diagnosis

Obstructive jaundice
Pancreatic neoplasm.
Bile-duct stricture.
Cholestatic hepatitis

Biliary colic
Pancreatitis.
Esophagitis.
Peptic ulcer.
Irritable bowel syndrome.

Etiology

• No unifying cause has been found, but the following may have a role:

Pathogenesis
Cholesterol supersaturation of bile.
Impaired gallbladder emptying.
Rapid cholesterol nucleation.

Predisposing factors
Obesity.
High-fat diet.
Disease: cirrhosis of liver, ileal dysfunction.
Drugs: *e.g.*, octreotide, oral contraceptives.

Epidemiology

• 10%–15% of the adult population have cholesterol gallstones.

• The incidence is 0.6% of the population.

• Gallstones occur more often in women, and their occurrence increases with age.

Treatment

Diet and lifestyle

• No evidence suggests that diet high in fiber and low in cholesterol dissolves stones or prevents their recurrence.

• Patients at risk of gallstones should avoid obesity.

• Rapid weight reduction should be avoided.

• Diets high in polyunsaturated fat should be avoided.

Pharmacological treatment

• Drugs are indicated for patients with other major medical problems that are contraindications for nonpharmacological treatment and in those with infrequent or mild symptoms, radiolucent stones, and functioning gallbladder [1,2].

• Bile-acid treatment is used for patients with small stones (<15 mm diameter); bile acids dissolve cholesterol gallstones by micellar solubilization or liquid crystal formation; they also reduce cholesterol absorption by intestine or secretion by liver.

Standard dosage	Ursodeoxycholic acid (UDCA), 10 mg/kg daily. Chenodeoxycholic acid (CDCA), 15 mg/kg daily. UDCA and CDCA, 5 mg/kg each daily. All as single bedtime dose for up to 2 years.
Contraindications	Pregnancy and lactation. *CDCA:* chronic liver disease or diarrhea. *UDCA:* active peptic ulcers.
Special points	Dissolution of stones requires 12 months or more of treatment, and recurrence is common when the medication is discontinued; UDCA or combination better than CDCA alone.
Main drug interactions	Sex hormones, oral contraceptives, blood cholesterol-lowering agents.
Main side effects	*CDCA:* diarrhea, hypertransaminasemia (reversible and dose-dependent). *UDCA:* gallstone calcification resulting in treatment failure.

Nonpharmacological treatment

Surgery

• Surgery is the preferred management for almost all patients with symptomatic gallstones.

• Open cholecystectomy is the traditional treatment.

• Laparoscopic cholecystectomy is rapidly becoming the procedure of choice.

Endoscopic retrograde cholangiography with sphincterotomy and stone extraction

• This treatment is for patients with choledocholithiasis.

• It is often performed in conjunction with laparoscopic cholecystectomy [3].

Extracorporeal shock-wave lithotripsy

• Lithotripsy is possible for 1–3 stones <30 mm in diameter; however, surgical management or dissolution therapy is the preferred approach.

• Expensive equipment is needed.

• The incidence of biliary colic and hematuria hematobilia is higher than with other approaches.

• It is contraindicated in hemolytic disorders.

Treatment aims

To dissolve stones, with consequent relief of symptoms and prevention of complications [4,5].

Prognosis

• Gallstones recur after dissolution therapy in 50% of patients within 5 years.

• If recurrent stones are detected early and treated, >80% of patients remain gallstone-free in the long term.

Follow-up and management

• Regular ultrasonography is needed every 6–12 months after dissolution to detect early recurrence.

• Bile acid treatment (full dose) is needed for recurrent stones.

Causes of pharmacological treatment failure

Patients' noncompliance with treatment.

Presence of radiolucent pigment stones or subradiographic calcification of stones.

Development of nonfunctioning gallbladder.

Inadequate dose (especially in obese patients).

Key references

1. Jonston DE, Kaplan MM: Pathogenesis and treatment of gallstones. *N Engl J Med* 1993, **328**:412–421.

2. Jazrawi RP, *et al.*: Optimum bile acid therapy for rapid gallstone dissolution. *Gut* 1992, **33**:381–386.

3. Cuschieri A, *et al.*: The European experience with laparoscopic cholecystectomy. *Am J Surg* 1991, **161**:385–387.

4. Sauerbruch T, Paumgartner G: Gallbladder stones: management. *Lancet* 1991, **338**:1121–1124.

5. Ransohoft DF, *et al.*: Treatment of gallstones. *Ann Intern Med* 1993, **119**:606–619.

Diagnosis

Symptoms

Epigastric pain: often aggravated by eating.

Early satiety, fullness.

Dysphagia: with adeocarcinoma of the cardia or distal esopohagus.

Vomiting.

Hematemesis or melena.

Weight loss.

Signs

• Often no signs are manifest.

Pallor: due to anemia.

Abdominal epigastric mass: palpable gastric tumor.

Nodular, enlarged liver: with metastatic disease.

Succussion splash: suggests gastric outlet obstruction.

Hard fixed supraclavicular node: sentinel node of Virchow; in left supraclavicular fossa.

Rectal mass: rectal shelf of Blumer; on digital examination (uncommon).

Infiltration of the umbilicus: "Sister Joseph's" nodule (uncommon).

Investigations

• Laboratory tests are not diagnostic but may suggest bleeding or liver metastases.

Complete blood count: to identify anemia.

Liver chemistry tests: raised alkaline phosphatase common with metastatic disease.

Fiberoptic endoscopy: allows direct visualization of cancer and assessment of obstruction to cardia or pylorus; allows biopsy (a minimum of eight tissue samples should be obtained, especially from the edge) and cytology; infiltrating cancer (linitis plastica) and lymphoma may need deep or large biopsies at repeat endoscopy to establish the diagnosis; superficial cancers may be difficult to recognize [1].

Double-contrast barium meal: blunting, fusion, clubbing, or tapering of mucosal folds suggests cancer; less accurate than endoscopy.

CT: to assess extent of disease, metastases.

Ultrasonography: conventional abdominal ultrasonography helpful when assessing for liver metastases; endoscopic ultrasonography is very useful for determining resectability if other imaging studies are negative for metastatic disease.

Complications

Obstruction.

Hemorrhage.

Tumor spread: lymphatic, hematogenous (liver, lungs, bone, adrenals), local dissemination into esophagus, invasion of adjacent organs (pancreas, mesocolon, liver).

Differential diagnosis

Ulcer or nonulcer dyspepsia.

Reflux esophagitis.

Ischemic gastropathy.

Hepatic or pancreatic cancer.

Anemia of other causes.

Depression.

Etiology

• Risk factors include the following:
Helicobacter pylori infection.

Smoked foods, salt fish, pickled foods.

Inverse association with refrigeration, vitamin C, fresh fruit and vegetable intake.

Genetic factors: including blood group A, family history, and Lynch syndrome II.

Epidemiology

• In the United States, the annual incidence is 10 cases per 100 000 population; more common in patients from Japan and other regions of east Asia.

• The male:female ratio is 1.5:1.

• There has been a considerable decline in the incidence of gastric cancer over the past 30 years.

• Patients with early gastric cancer are, on average, 8 years younger than those with advanced disease [2].

Pathology

Malignant neoplasm of stomach
90% adenocarcinoma; 5% lymphoma; 5% others (carcinoid, leiomyosarcoma, adeno-acanthoma, squamous, hepatoid, liposarcoma).

• Advanced cancer may be polypoidal or fungating, ulcerating with a raised border, or diffusely infiltrating (linitis plastica).

Early gastric cancer
Confined to gastric mucosa or submucosa, irrespective of lymph-node invasion.
Three types: protruded (type I), superficial (type II, most common), excavated (type III).

Premalignant conditions

Chronic atrophic gastritis/achlorhydria.

Pernicious anemia: 8% may develop gastric tumors (cancers and carcinoids).

Dysplasia.

Adenomatous polyps.

Previous gastrectomy (especially 10–20 years after Billroth II with gastrojejunostomy).

Hypertrophic gastropathy (Menetrier's disease): 10% may develop gastric cancer.

Treatment

Diet and lifestyle

• Patients with dysphagia should have a semi-liquid diet, with enteral feeding supplements.

• After gastrectomy, patients are at risk for dumping syndrome. Liquids should be taken prior to a meal but not during or immediately after ingestion of solid food. Patients should be advised to ingest frequent, small meals. Lying down immediately after a meal may be helpful.

Pharmacological treatment

• Chemotherapy has not been shown in trials to produce increased survival; it can produce effective reduction in tumor size and has been used for palliation.

• Symptoms may respond to treatment, as follows:

Ulcer-type pain: H_2 blockers (*e.g.*, ranitidine, cimetidine, nizatidine, or famotidine) or proton pump inhibitors (*e.g.*, omeprazole or lansoprazole).

Thrush or odynophagia pain: nystatin or ketoconazole if candidal infection is present.

Infiltrative pain: narcotic analgesics.

Constipation: laxatives.

Vomiting (infiltrative: incompetence of gastroesophageal sphincter): metoclopramide or cisapride (rarely responds and may aggravate obstructive symptoms).

Nonpharmacological treatment

• Curative resection: for the 30%–50% of patients without evidence of distant metastases [3,4].

Total gastrectomy: if tumor is extensive or close to cardioesophageal junction; higher mortality and morbidity than partial gastrectomy; side effects include small reservoir or bilious vomiting, diarrhea, and malabsorption.

Partial gastrectomy: for early gastric cancer or infiltrative advanced cancer with 5 cm distance clear of cancer from the cardia; side effects include weight loss and altered eating ability.

Dissection of lymph glands draining stomach: important even in early gastric cancer.

Palliation of symptoms, as follows:
Gastric bypass surgery: for obstructive pain or obstructive vomiting due to pyloric stenosis.
For dysphagia: laser treatment or repeat dilation.
For bleeding: surgery, endoscopic laser or electrocautery treatment.
For depression, anxiety, or anger: careful discussion, enlistment of family, and palliative care team support with appropriate use of antidepressants, anxiolytics, and analgesics.

• Palliative surgery for locally advanced disease involving adjacent organs may benefit patients with bleeding or pyloric obstruction even with metastatic spread.

• Complications after surgery include anastomotic leakage and small gastric reserve.

Treatment aims

To provide curative resection when still possible.

To provide effective symptomatic palliation when cure not possible [5].

Prognosis

• In patients with unresectable disease, mean survival is 4–12 months, with almost no 5-year survivors.

• In patients having apparent curative resection, mean survival is 28 months, and the 5-year survival rate is 40%.

• The prognosis of early gastric cancer is much better, with a 5-year survival rate of 80%, compared with 20% for advanced gastric cancer after resection (types I and II better prognosis than type III) [6,7].

Follow-up and management

• Gastrectomy patients may need iron and vitamin B_{12} or D supplements.

• Some total gastrectomy patients need careful nutritional support.

• Endoscopy, ultrasonography, or CT may be needed during follow-up to diagnose local or distant recurrence.

Key references

1. Takemoto T, *et al.*: Impact of staging on treatment of gastric carcinoma. *Endoscopy* 1993, **25**:46–50.
2. Lechago J, Correa P: Prolonged achlorhydria and gastric neoplasia: is there a causal relationship? *Gastroenterology* 1993, **104**:1554–1557.
3. Cushieri A: Gastrectomy for gastric cancer: definitions and objectives. *Br J Surg* 1986, **73**:513–514.
4. Gouzi JL, *et al.*: Total versus subtotal gastrectomy for adenocarcinoma of the gastric antrum. *Ann Surg* 1989, **2**:162–166.
5. Valen B, *et al.*: Treatment of stomach cancer: a national experience. *Br J Surg* 1988, **75**:708–710.
6. Thompson GB, van Heerden JA, Sarr MG: Adenocarcinoma of the stomach: are we making progress? *Lancet* 1993, **342**:713–718.
7. Green PHR, *et al.*: Increasing incidence and excellent survival of patients with early gastric cancer. *Am J Med* 1988, **85**:658–661.

Diagnosis

Symptoms

Often clinically indistinguishable from duodenal ulcer.

Epigastric pain: described as dull, burning discomfort; variably affected by food; relieved by antacids; nocturnal pain common.

Nausea, early satiety, or vomiting: with gastric outflow obstruction.

Hematemesis or melena.

Weight loss: suggesting malignant gastric ulceration.

Signs

• Most commonly, the physical examination is normal; epigastric tenderness on physical examination is an unreliable parameter of disease activity.

Signs of hemodynamic compromise: tachycardia, orthostatic hypotension in acute hemorrhage.

Local or generalized peritonitis: if ulcer has perforated.

Upper abdominal distension, succussion splash: with gastric outflow obstruction.

Hematemesis or melena with gastrointestinal bleeding.

Investigations

• A diagnosis of gastric ulcer can only be made after imaging the gastric lumen.

Fiberoptic endoscopy: esophagogastroduodenoscopy (EGD) is the investigation of choice (biopsy and cytology essential to exclude malignancy); allows direct visualization of ulcer; may help to diagnose small lesions or mucosal abnormalities; allows histological confirmation of diagnosis; allows assessment of *Helicobacter pylori* status.

Contrast radiography: barium upper gastrointestinal studies compare favorably with EGD at a lower cost, although small lesions may be missed and biopsies are not possible.

Complete blood count: to detect anemia or systemic evidence of inflammation.

Serum gastrin measurement: to evaluate for Zollinger-Ellison syndrome in recurrent or multiple ulceration not due to NSAID gastropathy or *H. pylori* [1].

• Patients with gastric ulcers should be tested for *H. pylori* (*see* Duodenal ulcer).

Complications

Perforation.

Hemorrhage.

Gastric outflow obstruction.

Differential diagnosis [2]

Duodenal ulceration.

Nonulcer dyspepsia.

Pancreatic carcinoma.

Gastroesophageal reflux disease.

Chronic gastritis.

Irritable bowel syndrome.

Biliary disease.

Pancreatitis.

Gastric carcinoma.

Ischemic gastropathy.

Lymphoma.

Etiology

Basal and peak acid secretion usually within normal range; mucosal defenses impaired, with subsequent back-diffusion of acid into mucosa.

• Causes include the following:

NSAIDs inhibiting protective prostaglandin synthesis.

H. pylori infection in 70% of patients.

Epidemiology

• The incidence of gastric ulceration increases with age.

• The male : female ratio is equal.

• Gastric ulceration is more prevalent in low socioeconomic groups.

• The ratio of duodenal to gastric ulcers is 9:1.

Treatment

Diet and lifestyle

• Bland diets, spicy foods, acid-containing fruits do not affect the healing process.

• Caffeine, ethanol, and smoking should be avoided.

• Patients must be explicitly asked about NSAID use and instructed to refrain from all such medications except acetaminophen.

Pharmacological treatment

• If *H. pylori* is present in patients with gastric ulcers, eradication should be attempted [3] (*see* Duodenal ulcer *for further details*).

Antacids

• These may give temporary symptomatic relief if taken 1 and 3 hours after meals and at bedtime.

• Healing may be achieved in patients motivated to comply with this regimen.

H$_2$-receptor antagonists

• The mainstay of treatment, these produce symptomatic relief within days and have ulcer healing rates of 80% at 4 weeks and 90% at 8 weeks [4].

Standard dosage	Ranitidine, 300 mg; cimetidine, 800 mg; famotidine, 40 mg; all given as single dose at night.
Contraindications	Known hypersensitivity (rare), pregnancy and lactation.
Main drug interactions	*Cimetidine:* oral anticoagulants, theophylline, phenytoin.
Main side effects	*Cimetidine:* headache, constipation or diarrhea, gynecomastia (all unusual).

Proton-pump inhibitors

Standard dosage	Omeprazole, 20 mg, or lansoprazole, 30 mg daily for 8 weeks [5].
Contraindications	Known hypersensitivity.
Special points	Faster healing has been noted when compared with other agents.
Main drug interactions	Diazepam, phenytoin, warfarin.
Main side effects	Headache, diarrhea, nausea, skin rashes (all unusual).

Prostaglandins

• Prostaglandins are probably most useful as prophylatic agents in patients with peptic ulcer disease who require ongoing NSAID treatment. Healing rates are inferior to those of H$_2$ antagonists [6].

Standard dosage	Misoprostol, 400 µg daily in 4 divided doses.
Contraindications	Pregnancy or planned pregnancy.
Special points	Small doses of synthetic prostaglandins have been shown to exhibit a cytoprotective effect and to inhibit gastric acid secretion.
Main drug interactions	None known.
Main side effects	Diarrhea, abdominal pain, flushing, menorrhagia.

Treatment aims

To relieve symptoms.

To heal ulcer.

To exclude malignancy.

Other treatments

• Surgery is indicated for uncontrolled ulcer-related hemorrhage (early operation important in elderly patients), perforation, malignant ulceration, delayed healing, or gastric outlet obstruction due to structure.

Prognosis

• After completion of a healing course of H$_2$ antagonists, the chance of recurrence in 1 year is 50% unless predisposing factors (NSAIDs, *H. pylori*) are removed.

Follow-up and management

• Endoscopic confirmation of mucosal healing at 8–12 weeks is essential, with repeated biopsy and further endoscopy if ulcer healing has not occurred.

• After ulcer healing, treatment is usually discontinued unless an obvious and continuing predisposing factor is present.

• Recurrence of symptoms must be reassessed with further endoscopy.

• Significant gastrointestinal bleeding is managed by maintenance treatment with half-dose H$_2$ blockade and the therapeutic treatment regiment is completed.

Key references

1. Soll H: Pathogenesis of peptic ulcer and implications for therapy. *N Engl J Med* 1990, **322**:909–916.

2. Bernersen B, *et al.*: Non-ulcer dyspepsia and peptic ulcer. *Gut* 1996, **38**:822–825.

3. Peterson WL: *Helicobacter pylori* and peptic ulcer disease. *N Engl J Med* 1991, **324**:1043–1048.

4. Feldman M, Burton ME: Histamine 2-receptor antagonists: standard therapy for acid peptic disease. *N Engl J Med* 1991, **323**:1672; 1749–1755.

5. Maton PN: Omeprazole. *N Engl J Med* 1991, **324**:965–975.

6. Walt RP: Misoprostol for the treatment of peptic ulcer and antiinflammatory-drug-induced gastroduodenal ulceration. *N Engl J Med* 1992, **327**:1575–1580.

Diagnosis

Definition

• Glomerulonephritis is an immunologically mediated glomerular inflammation, often with associated tubulointerstitial lesions, which may be chronic or acute.

• The following classification is based in part on that of the World Health Organization:

Nonproliferative

Minimal-change glomerulonephritis: normal on light microscopy.

Membranous glomerulonephritis: thick-basement membranes, subepithelial immune complexes.

Focal segmental glomerulosclerosis: mesangial and capillary loop scarring.

Fibrillary or immunotactoid glomerulonephritis: extracellular, nonbranching microfibrils.

Proliferative: endocapillary

Diffuse proliferative glomerulonephritis: overcellular glomeruli.

Focal segmental proliferative glomerulonephritis: overcellular glomeruli.

Mesangial IgA disease: large deposits of IgA in mesangium.

Mesangiocapillary glomerulonephritis: thick capillary loops with expanded over-cellular mesangium; also called "membranoproliferative glomerulonephritis."

Focal necrotizing glomerulonephritis: segment of necrosis in peripheral capillary loop.

Proliferative: extracapillary

Crescentic glomerulonephritis: sheaves of macrophages and other cells filling all or part of Bowman's space with variable underlying glomerular lesions.

Symptoms and signs

Proteinuria: asymptomatic (usually <2 g/24 h); nephrotic (>3 g/24 h).

Hematuria: microscopic (detected by stick test); macroscopic (smoky urine).

Hypertension.

Acute nephritic illness.

Acute renal failure.

Chronic renal failure.

Investigations

Urine microscopy: dysmorphic erythrocytes and casts imply glomerular inflammation.

24-hour urinalysis: for creatinine clearance and urine protein.

Blood urea nitrogen and creatinine measurement.

Renal biopsy (light, electron, and immunofluorescent microscopy all needed): necessary to diagnose and manage almost all types of glomerulonephritis.

Albumin and lipid measurement.

Tests for lupus and vasculitis: *e.g.*, anti-double-stranded DNA antibody, anti-neutrophil cytoplasmic antibody (ANCA).

Antiglomerular basement membrane antibody measurement.

Investigation for appropriate associated infections.

Complement studies: CH50, C3, C4.

Plain abdominal radiography and ultrasonography or intravenous pyelography.

Complications

Hypertension: can be severe.

Acute or chronic renal failure.

Nephrotic syndrome: venous and arterial thromboses, pleural effusions, ascites, intravascular volume depletion, infection, accelerated atherosclerosis.

Differential diagnosis

Nephritic syndrome

Severe hypertension.

Scleroderma renal crisis.

Thrombotic microangiopathies (*e.g.*, hemolytic uremic syndrome).

Acute interstitial nephritis.

Nephrotic syndrome

Pre-eclampsia.

Amyloidosis.

Diabetes mellitus.

Congestive cardiac failure.

Cirrhosis with edema and ascites.

NSAID use.

Other

Orthostatic proteinuria.

Other causes of hypertension or acute or chronic renal failure.

Etiology

Immunopathogenesis

Immune complex: in situ formation (built up within glomerulus) or, less commonly, deposition of preformed immune complexes from circulation.

Direct antibody-mediated injury: antiglomerular basement membrane antibody (Goodpasture's syndrome); this is rare.

Unknown, but possibly cell-mediated; probably important in many forms of glomerulonephritis.

Associated diseases

Primary: no known association (idiopathic).

Secondary: postinfectious, *e.g.*, viruses, (hepatitis B, HIV), bacterial (poststrepto-coccal), protozoal (malarial); drug-induced, *e.g.*, gold or penicillamine; vasculitis; neoplasia.

Epidemiology

• Glomerulonephritis is one of the most common causes of chronic renal failure.

• Minimal-change glomerulonephritis is the most common cause of nephrotic syndrome in children.

• Mesangial IgA disease is the most common cause of recurrent episodes of macroscopic hematuria in young adults.

Treatment

Diet and lifestyle

- Patients must not have added salt if they have edema or hypertension.
- Nephrotic patients should have a normal protein intake.
- Renal failure patients should have a low protein intake (0.5 g/kg daily).
- Oral intake of fluids should be restricted if the patient is edematous.
- Pregnant patients are at increased risk of pre-eclampsia (high risk if creatinine raised).
- Occasionally, pregnant patients experience deterioration of renal function.

Pharmacological treatment

Immunosuppression

- Patients are chosen on the basis of clinical syndrome and histology.
- Aggressive treatment is indicated for heavy proteinuria or falling glomerular filtration rate.
- Histology is most helpful for choosing treatment.

For minimal-change glomerulonephritis:
remission induction: high-dose steroids, cyclosporine;
maintenance: low-dose steroids or cyclosporine;
prevention of relapse: cyclophosphamide.

For membranous glomerulonephritis: trial of steroids, possibly with chlorambucil or cyclophosphamide in selected patients.

For focal segmental glomerulosclerosis: high-dose steroids or cyclosporine, or both (prolonged treatment needed).

For mesangial IgA disease: fish oil (eicosapentaenoic acid).

For postinfectious diffuse proliferative glomerulonephritis: treat infection.

For mesangiocapillary glomerulonephritis: no treatment effective; trial of immunosuppression in selected patients.

For focal necrotizing or crescentic glomerulonephritis: steroids with cyclophosphamide (pulse i.v. methylprednisolone for 3 days may help); additional plasma exchange in selected patients (immediate plasma exchange mandatory in Goodpasture's syndrome).

Supportive

Control of fluid balance: diuretics (combinations may be needed).

Control of blood pressure: angiotensin-converting enzyme inhibitors if possible; calcium channel blockers may worsen edema.

Aggressive treatment of intercurrent infections (cellulitis, pneumonia, spontaneous bacterial peritonitis).

Anticoagulation: should be considered for nephrotic patients, especially if they are immobile.

Treatment aims

To suppress glomerular inflammation.
To prevent progressive glomerular scarring and progression to chronic renal failure.
To minimize proteinuria.
To control hypertension and fluid balance.
To avoid overimmunosuppression.

Prognosis

- A poor prognosis is associated with severe hypertension, heavy persistent proteinuria, and raised creatinine.
- Prognosis is closely related to histology, *e.g.*:
Minimal-change glomerulonephritis: excellent, resolves despite relapses.
Membranous glomerulonephritis: 30% resolve, 30% remain static, 30% progress to CRF.
Mesangial IgA disease: 25% progress to CRF.
Postinfectious diffuse proliferative glomerulonephritis: >90% resolve.
Mesangiocapillary glomerulonephritis: >75% progress to CRF.

Follow-up and management

- Follow-up should be for life in most patients.
- Strict control of blood pressure is needed, use angiotensin-converting enzyme inhibitors whenever possible
- Immunosuppressive drugs must be titrated to disease activity.
- Lipids must be controlled.

General references

D'Amico G, Sinico RA, Ferrario F: Renal vasculitis. *Nephrol Dial Transplant* 1996, **11(suppl 9)**:69–74.

Ferrario F, Rastaldi MP, D'Amico G: The crucial role of renal biopsy in the management of ANCA-associated renal vasculitis. *Nephrol Dial Transplant* 1996, **11**:726–728.

Gaskin G: Management of rapidly progressive glomerulonephritis. *J R Coll Physicians Lond* 1997, **31**:15–18.

Glassock R, Cohen AH: The primary glomerulopathies. *Dis Mon* 1996, **42**:329–383.

Klahr S: Role of dietary protein and blood pressure in the progression of renal disease. *Kidney Int* 1996, **49**:1783–1786.

Reisman L, *et al.*: Renal biospy: why and when. *Mt Sinai J Med* 1996, **63**:178–190.

Diagnosis

Symptoms

Acute pain in a single joint: usually base of great toe; often starting at night; self-limiting but tendency to recur.

Mild systemic disturbance, with irritability and low-grade fever.

Polyarticular attacks: in 5%–10% of patients (50% of elderly patients).

Chronic asymmetrical polyarthritis: after repeated acute attacks.

Signs

Exquisite tenderness.

Swollen, shiny, red, tender joints.

Desquamation: as attack subsides.

Tophi in helix of ear, elbow, and over small joints of hands and feet: in severe cases.

Olecranon bursitis: "imbiber's elbow"; common.

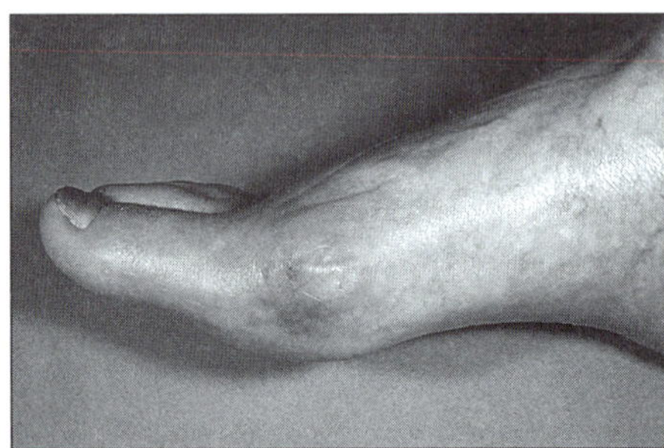

Acute gout in big toe. (*See* Color Plate.)

Investigations

Polarized light microscopy: needle-shaped, negatively birefringent crystals in synovial fluid from the affected joint are diagnostic.

Serum uric acid measurement: concentration usually raised but may fall to normal during acute attack.

Complete blood count: to exclude secondary cause, *e.g.*, lymphoproliferative disorder.

ESR measurement: may be raised during acute attack.

Creatinine measurement: renal failure may result from or be caused by hyperuricemia.

Fasting lipids measurement: hyperlipidemia common.

Urinary urate excretion measurement: differentiates overproducers from under-excretors (while on low-purine diet).

Radiography: may show characteristic juxta-articular punched-out erosions without accompanying osteoporosis around joints ("overhanging edges") in patients with chronic arthritic gout.

Complications

Prolongation of acute attack: by incorrect use of allopurinol.

Gastrointestinal bleeding: due to high-dose NSAIDs.

Renal impairment: due to drug interference with renal cortical blood flow.

Differential diagnosis

Acute gout
Septic arthritis.
Cellulitis.
Pyrophosphate arthritis ("pseudogout").

Chronic tophaceous gout
Rheumatoid arthritis.
Septic arthritis.
Hyperlipidemia with xanthomata.

Nongout
Painful bunion with asymptomatic hyper-uricemia.

Etiology

• Gout is often precipitated by alcohol over-indulgence, surgery, or intercurrent illness.

• Primary gout may be caused by a genetic predisposition to overproduction or under-excretion of urate or failure to inhibit crystallization in tissues.

• Secondary gout may be caused by diuretics (particularly in older women), renal impairment, diet (high purine intake coupled with obesity), high cell turnover (malignant disease), alcohol excess, or heavy-metal poisoning, especially lead (saturnine gout).

Epidemiology

• Gout is particularly prevalent in middle-aged men, postmenopausal women, and patients with renal failure.

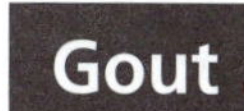

Treatment

Diet and lifestyle

• Patients with associated obesity may benefit from caloric restriction.

• Alcohol intake should be moderated because alcohol inhibits urate excretion by the kidney and is often associated with acute attacks [1].

• Consumption of high-purine foods (*e.g.*, shellfish) should be restricted because they may provoke acute attacks; a purine-free diet is impractical.

Pharmacological treatment

For acute attack

Standard dosage	Rapidly acting NSAID, *e.g.*, indomethacin, 25–50 mg initially, followed by 25–50 mg 3 times daily until attack starts to subside, then reduced dose [1,2]. Colchicine, 0.5 mg hourly to a maximum of 6 mg in first 24 hours; do not repeat dose for 7 days.
Contraindications	*Indomethacin:* peptic ulcer, anticoagulants, renal impairment. *Colchicine:* hypersensitivity.
Special points	*Colchicine:* can be used to prevent recurrence at 0.5 g once or twice daily. Alternatives for resistant or difficult cases include intra-articular or oral steroids.
Main drug interactions	*Indomethacin:* warfarin.
Main side effects	*Indomethacin, diclofenac:* indigestion, gastric bleeding, headache, nausea, dizziness (worse with indomethacin). *Colchicine:* nausea, diarrhea.

For hyperuricemia

• Treatment can be considered between attacks if the serum urate concentration remains raised [1,2].

• Allopurinol is indicated for recurrent attacks of gout, chronic tophaceous gout, renal impairment due to hyperuricemia, induction of chemotherapy, and asymptomatic hyperuricemia (>12 mg/dL) or for any gouty patient with a history of renal stones.

Standard dosage	Allopurinol, 300 mg initially; reduce dosage for renal insufficiency.
Contraindications	Acute gout, hypersensitivity.
Special points	Lower dose in renal failure to prevent build up of metabolites; additional prophylactic NSAID or colchicine for first 3 months to prevent multiple attacks of gout.
Main drug interactions	Azathioprine.
Main side effects	Rash.

Key references

1. Star VL, Hockberg MC: Prevention and management of gout. *Drugs* 1993, **45**:212–222.

2. Tan N, Lertratanakul W, Barr WG: Acute gouty arthritis: modern approaches to an ancient disease. *Postgrad Med* 1993, **94**:73–75; 78; 83–84.

Diagnosis

Symptoms

Sweats, chills, or rigors.

Cough, possibly with sputum, pleuritic chest pain, breathlessness.

Dysuria, urinary frequency.

Abdominal pain, nausea, vomiting, diarrhea.

Headache, neck stiffness, confusion.

Signs

• Focal clinical signs, if present, may help to localize the site of infection.

Tachycardia: >90 beats/min.

Tachypnea: >20 breaths/min.

Temperature >38°C or <35.6°C: hypothermia associated with worse prognosis.

Hypotension: systolic blood pressure <90 mm Hg or fall of 40 mm Hg from baseline.

Oliguria: <20 mL/h.

Petechial or purpuric skin rash: suggesting meningococcal septicemia; ecthyma gangrenosum associated with *Pseudomonas* infection in neutropenic patients.

Investigations

• Investigations are directed toward ascertaining the microbiology, site of infection, severity, and complications of gram-negative sepsis.

• Ideally, culture specimens should be taken before antimicrobial treatment, but treatment should not be unduly delayed in seriously ill patients.

Blood cultures: at least two, preferably three.

Urine and sputum microscopy and culture.

Gram-stain and culture of available pus or body fluids: may provide rapid diagnosis.

Chest radiography, further radiography directed by clinical picture.

Hemoglobin count: to detect severe anemia (may need to be corrected).

Leukocyte count: to detect neutrophil leukocytosis or toxic granulation; leukopenia associated with poor prognosis.

Platelet count and coagulation studies: for evidence of disseminated intravascular coagulation.

Arterial blood gas analysis: shows respiratory alkalosis early and metabolic acidosis later; possibly hypoxia.

Liver function tests: abnormal results in 40%-60% of patients.

Complications

Renal failure: acute tubular necrosis, usually reversible.

Disseminated intravascular coagulation.

Adult respiratory distress syndrome: in 15%–40% of patients.

Hepatic failure.

Differential diagnosis

• More than one factor may contribute to shock in an individual patient.

Other causes of shock: cardiogenic, hypovolemic, redistribution of fluid (*e.g.*, burns, pancreatitis, anaphylaxis), toxins.

Other infections: *e.g.*, gram-positive bacteria, fungi, malaria, or viral infections, staphylococcal or streptococcal toxic shock syndrome.

Etiology

• Gram-negative septicemia is usually associated with *Escherichia coli*, *Klebsiella*, *Enterobacter*, *Serratia*, *Proteus*, *Pseudomonas* spp., and *Neisseria meningitidis*; enteric gram-negative bacteria account for most cases.

• The most common sources are intra-abdominal or urinary tract infections and pneumonia.

• Host risk factors include the following:

Surgery (especially gastrointestinal, genitourinary, hepatobiliary).

Abnormalities of genitourinary tract.

Intravenous lines.

Hospitalization.

Cancer.

Neutropenia.

Immunosuppression.

Epidemiology

• Gram-negative septicemia and shock have been increasing over the past 30 years.

• Bacteremia is found in ~7 in 1000 hospital admissions.

• Septic shock complicates 20% of bacteremias.

Pathogenesis of gram-negative shock

• Bacterial endotoxin (lipopolysaccharide) and other bacterial products initiate the release of inflammatory mediators from monocyte/macrophages, endothelial cells, and polymorphonuclear leukocytes.

• The interaction of these mediators leads to an "inflammatory cascade" of reactions, leading to widespread endothelial damage, hypotension, refractory shock, multiorgan failure, and death.

Treatment

Diet and lifestyle

• No special precautions are necessary.

Pharmacological treatment

Indications

• Antibiotic treatment depends on the site of the infection and host and environmental factors.

Urinary tract (community-acquired): quinolone.

Urinary tract or pneumonia (hospital-acquired): ceftazidime, or piperacillin with gentamicin.

Intra-abdominal: cefotaxime with metronidazole, or piperacillin with gentamicin.

Biliary tract: piperacillin with gentamicin.

Cefotaxime or ceftazidime

Standard dosage	Ceftriaxone, 1–2 g daily, or ceftazidime, 1–2 g 8-hourly.
Contraindications	Previous cephalosporin hypersensitivity.
Special points	Dose adjusted in moderate to severe renal failure.
Main drug interactions	None.
Main side effects	Rashes, diarrhea, hemolysis, or raised transaminases (rare).

Gentamicin

Standard dosage	Gentamicin, 4 mg/kg daily (normal renal function).
Contraindications	Myasthenia gravis, pre-existing renal failure.
Special points	Concentrations must be monitored before and after dose.
Main drug interactions	Loop diuretics, curare-type anesthetic agents.
Main side effects	Nephrotoxicity, ototoxicity.

Quinolones

Standard dosage	Ciprofloxacin, 500 mg twice daily.
Contraindications	Pregnancy, childhood.
Special points	Dose adjusted in severe renal failure.
Main drug interactions	None.
Main side effects	Diarrhea, renal failure.

Piperacillin

Standard dosage	Piperacillin, 2 g 6-hourly.
Contraindications	Penicillin hypersensitivity.
Special points	Dose adjusted in moderate to severe renal failure.
Main drug interactions	Inactivates aminoglycosides if mixed in solution.
Main side effects	Hypersensitivity, hepatotoxicity in 3% of patients, platelet dysfunction.

Treatment aims

To control infection.
To maintain organ perfusion and tissue oxygen delivery.
To minimize complications

Other treatments

Drainage of infected collections of pus. Surgical debridement of dead or infected material.

Prognosis

• Mortality is 10%–20% in patients with bacteremia, 40%–60% in those with shock, and >90% in those with multiorgan failure.

Follow-up and management

• Patients need careful management in the convalescent stage, which may be prolonged after acute septic shock; they may relapse if the predisposing condition remains.

Management of gram-negative bacterial shock

• Monitoring of the following is needed: Systolic blood pressure (must be kept >90 mm Hg or high enough to maintain renal perfusion).
Central venous pressure or postcapillary wedge pressure (to exclude hypovolemia).
Cardiac output.
Systemic vascular resistance (normal, >1000; in septic shock, generally <1000).
Catheterization (for urine measurement).
Oxygen saturation (arterial pressure falls, venous pressure rises because of failure in tissue oxygenation).
• Treatment includes the following:
Colloid to restore intravascular volume (blood for severe anemia).
Pressor or inotropic agents, if necessary.
Renal dopamine 2–4 µg/min to maintain renal perfusion.
Inspired oxygen at minimum to maintain arterial oxygenation.
Nutritional support.

General references

Edwards JD: Management of septic shock. *BMJ* 1993, **306**:1661–1664.

Parillo JE: Pathogenetic mechanisms of septic shock. *N Engl J Med* 1993, **328**:1471–1477.

Pollack M, Ohl CA: Endotoxin-based molecular strategies for the prevention and treatment of gram-negative sepsis and septic shock. *Curr Top Microbiol Immunol* 1996, **216**:275–297.

Diagnosis

Symptoms

• Symptoms are often nonspecific, with a wide variety of manifestations.

Initial or indolent phase

Cough, dyspnea.

Nasal and ocular symptoms: in Wegener's granulomatosis.

Wheezing or asthma, abdominal pain: in Churg-Strauss syndrome.

Active or aggressive phase

Fever, malaise, anorexia, weight loss.

Cough, dyspnea, hemoptysis, chest pain.

Skin rash, arthralgia.

Signs

• Manifestations are widely varied.

Chest signs: often little, compared with extent of radiographic changes.

Wheezing: feature of Churg-Strauss syndrome and bronchocentric granulomatosis.

Nasal inflammation and granulation: in Wegener's and lymphomatoid granulomatoses.

Ocular inflammation or proptosis: in Wegener's granulomatosis.

Vasculitic or nonspecific skin rash.

Peripheral or cranial neuropathy.

Investigations [1]

Complete blood count: anemia common; eosinophilia >1.5 × 10^9/L in Churg-Strauss syndrome.

ESR: usually raised.

Renal function test: abnormalities frequent in Wegener's granulomatosis.

Chest radiography: varied appearances; can show mass lesion, consolidation, or diffuse shadowing; cavitating nodules typical of Wegener's granulomatosis.

Antineutrophil cytoplasmic antibodies (ANCA): cANCA present in 90% of patients with active Wegener's granulomatosis, pANCA present in some Churg-Strauss, lymphomatoid, or Wegener's sufferers; other serology usually negative.

Biopsy: ideally open lung biopsy; bronchoscopic or renal biopsy may give specific histology; nasal and skin biopsy usually nonspecific.

Complications

General

Pulmonary hemorrhage: uncommon.

Infection: common.

Peripheral or cranial neuropathy, mononeuritis multiplex.

Wegener's granulomatosis [2]

Renal impairment: in 75% of patients.

Deafness: in 30%.

Artharlgios, myalgias: in 70%-90%.

Churg–Strauss syndrome [3]

Cardiac involvement: in 50% (most common cause of death).

Treatment

Diet and lifestyle

• Stopping smoking should be encouraged in view of the risk of chest infection from disease and treatment.

Pharmacological treatment [2,6,7]

Prednisone

• Prednisone is important in all initial treatment and in maintenance for Churg–Strauss syndrome, necrotizing sarcoid granulomatosis, and bronchocentric granulomatosis.

Standard dosage	Prednisone, 60–80 mg orally daily initially. Optional initial pulse methylprednisolone 1 g i.v. on 3 successive days. Steady dose reduction and alternate-day use after 1 month. Wegener's patients should be weaned off drug entirely after remission.
Contraindications	Caution in diabetes mellitus, hypertension, or peptic ulceration.
Special points	Patients must be given a steroid-warning card; blood glucose and blood pressure must be checked.
Main drug interactions	Rifampin, carbamazepine, phenytoin, phenobarbital.
Main side effects	Fluid retention, hypertension, proximal myopathy, mental disturbance, osteoporosis, skin fragility, increased risk of infection.

Cyclophosphamide

• Cyclophosphamide is essential in Wegener's granulomatosis, advised in lymphomatoid granulomatosis, and sometimes needed in Churg–Strauss syndrome.

Standard dosage	Cyclophosphamide, 1–2 mg/kg orally daily, with prednisone. Optional initial pulse cyclophosphamide, 0.5 g i.v., followed by 0.5–1 g i.v. monthly, according to leukocyte count.
Contraindications	Porphyria, pregnancy.
Special points	Dose reduced in patients with renal impairment; should be adjusted according to regular leukocyte counts and side effects; usually continued for 1 year after remission has been induced.
Main drug interactions	Allopurinol, succinylcholine.
Main side effects	Bone-marrow suppression, nausea and vomiting, hair loss, cystitis, sterility, bladder cancer, lymphoma.

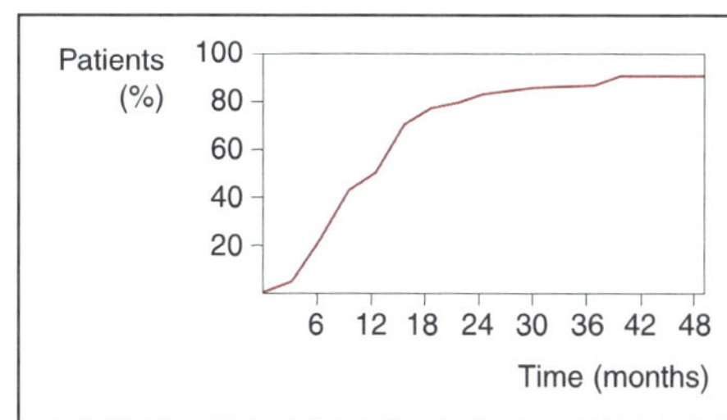

Cumulative remission rate on standard treatment for Wegener's granulomatosis (in the 75% of patients who achieve complete remission).

Prognosis

Wegener's granulomatosis

• Long-term survival is >80%, but relapse is common, and >80% of patients suffer permanent morbidity.

Churg–Strauss syndrome

• Long-term survival is high, but cardiac complications are the main cause of death.

Lymphomatoid granulomatosis

• The 5-year survival rate is 50%, less if lymphoma is present.

Bronchocentric granulomatosis

• The prognosis and response to steroids are good.

Follow-up and management

• Long-term monitoring is required; ESR and chest radiography are guides of disease activity.

• ANCA titers are helpful guides in Wegener's granulomatosis; they do not rise in infective episodes but may rise some time before relapse occurs.

• Renal function in Wegener's granulomatosis should be monitored.

Key references

1. Rao JK, Weinberger M, Oddone EZ, *et al.*: The role of antineutrophil cytoplasmic antibody (c-ANCA) testing in the diagnosis of Wegener granulomatosis: a literature review and meta-analysis. 1995, **123**:925–932.

2. Duna GF, Galperin C, Hoffman GS: Wegener's granulomatosis. *Rheum Dis Clin North Am* 1995, **21**:949–986.

3. Lanham JG: Churg–Strauss syndrome. *Br J Hosp Med* 1992, **47**:667–673.

4. Hoffman GS, *et al.*: Wegener's granulomatosis: an analysis of 158 patients. *Ann Intern Med* 1992, **116**:488–498.

5. Pisani RJ, DeRemee RA: Clinical implications of the histopathologic diagnosis of pulmonary lymphomatoid granulomatosis. *Mayo Clin Proc* 1990, **65**:151–163.

6. Fauci A, *et al.*: Wegener's granulomatosis: prospective clinical and therapeutic experience in 85 patients for 21 years. *Ann Intern Med* 1983, **98**:76–85.

7. Hammar SP: Granulomatous vasculitis. *Semin Respir Infect* 1995, **10**:107–120.

Diagnosis

Symptoms

Height less than the third height centile or short for family.

Delayed puberty: in some patients.

Signs

- Signs are not always manifest.
- Features of hypothyroidism with goiter may be seen.

Disproportionate growth: *e.g.*, short legs.

Dysmorphic features: *e.g.*, in Turner's syndrome, intrauterine growth retardation.

Investigations [1,2]

Anthropometry: height of child should be recorded on at least two occasions separated by at least 3 months to calculate growth velocity; assessments of nutrition (weight, skinfold thickness) helpful; Tanner stages of puberty must be elicited; heights of parents should be measured.

Radiography: bone age; skeletal survey (for disproportionate short stature); pituitary MRI (if hypothalamic or pituitary dysfunction is suspected).

Hematology: to identify anemia (vitamin B_{12}, folate, ferritin malabsorption).

ESR measurement: to exclude inflammatory disease.

Chemistries: standard chemistry panel including electrolytes, blood urea nitrogen, creatinine, calcium, and liver function tests; growth hormone and/or somatomedin C (insulin-like growth factor–1); thyroid function tests (thyrotropin, free thyroxine); luteinizing hormone, follicle-stimulating hormone, gonadal steroids, prolactin (if delayed puberty is suspected).

Karyotyping: XO in Turner's syndrome.

Complications

Premature fusion of epiphyses: through injudicious treatment with gonadal steroids.

Differential diagnosis

- The vast majority of short children have no abnormalities and will go on to achieve their normal adult heights. These children, and particularly their parents, should be reassured following an appropriate medical evaluation.

Etiology [1,2]

- All disease in childhood causes a decrease in growth velocity that ultimately becomes manifest as short stature.
- The following may play a role:

Nutritional disorders: in infants.

Diminished growth hormone secretion: in the absence of physical signs in children (hypoglycemia may sometimes be present).

Delayed or absent puberty.

Some hypothalamic–pituitary disorders associated with obesity and short stature (*e.g.*, Prader Willi).

Disease in any body system: in thin patients.

Epidemiology

- Boys with delayed puberty (and its consequent short stature) outnumber girls by 20:1.
- Most other conditions have a roughly equal gender distribution.

Treatment

Diet and lifestyle

• In infants, adequate nutrition must be promoted, including correction of malabsorption.

Pharmacological treatment [1,2]

• In childhood, growth hormone is appropriately prescribed to correct insufficiency; sex steroids are appropriate first-line treatment (*see* below).

• Long-term alleviation of short stature is achievable only when an abnormal growth velocity can be corrected; the height of a normal child cannot be increased.

Thyroxine: 100 µg/m^2 orally as single daily dose.

• The following should be prescribed by the appropriate specialist:

Growth hormone: 0.04 mg/kg daily.

Ethinyl estradiol: initially 2 µg daily, increased to 5, 10, 15, 20, and 30 µg daily at 6-monthly intervals; progestogen added when dose of 15 µg achieved or if breakthrough bleeding occurs earlier; use caution if family history of thrombotic disorder is present.

Testosterone: initially 50 mg testosterone esters at 4-weekly intervals, increased to 100 mg every 4 weeks after 6 months; increased to 3-weekly intervals over a further 6 months and then to 2-weekly intervals; causes accelerated fusion of epiphyses.

Treatment aims

To redress abnormal growth.

To reassure patients and parents.

Prognosis

• Medical therapy does not turn normal short children into tall children.

• Adult height is fixed once epiphyses have fused.

• Early diagnosis and treatment maximizes the chances of achieving maximal potential adult height.

• Best case scenario with treatment is achieving expected height based on parents' height.

Follow-up and management

• 6-monthly anthropometry is needed to record effects on growth and to readjust doses for increase in size.

Key references

1. Brook CGD: *A Guide to the Practice of Paediatric Endocrinology.* Cambridge: Cambridge University Press; 1993.

2. Brook CGD (ed.): *Clinical Paediatric Endocrinology,* edn 3. Oxford: Blackwell Scientific Publications; 1995.

Diagnosis

Symptoms

• Symptoms are usually minimal (other than being tall for one's age).

Signs

• Tall children usually look normal.

Signs of precocious puberty or thyrotoxicosis.

Signs of virilization: pubic hair, acne, cliteromegaly; adrenal androgen excess should be ruled out.

Joint hypermobility, arachnodactyly, iridonodesis, high arch palate: signs of Marfan syndrome.

Investigations [1]

• Height and weight should be monitored on standard growth charts. Patients whose height and weight percentiles remain constant over time are less likely to have a pathological cause of tall stature.

• Tall stature associated with true precocious puberty must be fully investigated.

Anthropometry: height of child and both parents should be measured; Tanner stages of puberty should be recorded; measurement of sitting height to determine leg length more helpful than measurement of span.

Radiography: assessment of skeletal maturity (including bone age) enables height prediction; radiographical appearance of iliac apophyses helps to assess potential for spinal growth.

Special tests: measurement of thyroxine and thyroid-stimulating hormone may reveal thyrotoxicosis; gigantism is associated with elevated somatomedin-C levels and may also be accompanied by hypogonadism (resulting in nonclosure of epiphyses).

Complications

• There are no complications in normal tall individuals.

• Complications are related to underlying disease in patients with pathological tall stature.

• Patients with tall stature due to congenital adrenal hyperplasia may complete puberty early, resulting in a short final adult height.

Treatment

Diet and lifestyle

• No special precautions are necessary.

Pharmacological treatment [1]

• Precocious puberty and adrenal, thyroid, and pituitary conditions should be referred for appropriate treatment, including surgery.

• Patients with Klinefelter's syndrome and inadequate puberty need androgens to prevent gynecomastia and osteoporosis.

• Sex steroids can be used to accelerate epiphyseal closure in tall children with hypogonadism or delayed puberty.

Ethinyl estradiol: initially 2 µg daily, increased to 5, 10, 15, 20, and 30 µg daily at 6-monthly intervals; progestogen added when dose of 15 µg achieved or if breakthrough bleeding occurs earlier; contraindicated if family history of thrombotic disorder.

Testosterone: initially 50 mg testosterone esters at 4-weekly intervals, increased to 100 mg every 4 weeks after 6 months; increased to 3-weekly intervals over a further 6 months and then to 2-weekly intervals; causes accelerated fusion of epiphyses.

Treatment aims

To reduce adult stature.

Prognosis

• The prognosis depends on the diagnosis.

Follow-up and management

• Children with Marfan syndrome need ophthalmological and cardiac opinions.

Key reference

1. Brook CGD (ed.): *Clinical Paediatric Endocrinology*, edn. 3. Oxford: Blackwell Scientific Publications; 1995.

Diagnosis

Symptoms [1]

Ascending, symmetrical weakness in all limbs: legs usually affected first, with patient initially noticing difficulty climbing stairs, rising from sitting, and, eventually, walking and standing.

Paresthesias of extremities, with distal sensory loss: in 95% of patients.

Neck, shoulder, back, and sciatic pain: may be severe.

Diplopia, drooling, nasal regurgitation of food or drink, slurred speech, weak cough: indicating cranial nerve involvement.

Dyspnea: late symptom, reflecting intercostal and diaphragmatic weakness.

Fatigue: possibly profound and often persisting after return of muscle strength.

Hesitancy and urinary retention: usually when weakness more advanced (vs. acute myelopathy, in which sphincter symptoms appear early).

Signs

Weakness in limbs: flaccid, usually symmetrical, arms usually less severely affected.

Cranial nerve palsies: facial nerve most often affected, followed by bulbar muscles.

Hyporeflexia, areflexia: early.

Sensory deficit: may be absent or minor despite prominent symptoms.

Profound sensory loss: in some patients.

Ataxia, ophthalmoplegia, areflexia, with little or no weakness: Miller–Fisher syndrome; rare.

Investigations

Initial

Lumbar puncture: classically, raised protein concentration associated with normal cell count (albuminocytological dissociation); protein possibly normal within first week.

Serum potassium measurement: to exclude hypo- or hyperkalemic paralysis.

Antinuclear antibodies analysis: positive in rare cases associated with SLE.

Liver function tests: often abnormal.

Heavy metal screening: only if clinically indicated.

Porphyrin screening: positive in acute intermittent porphyria, which may manifest like Guillain–Barré syndrome.

Lyme titers.

Stool *Campylobacter* antibodies analysis: associated with axonal involvement.

Specialist

Nerve conduction studies: to identify multifocal conduction block and slowed conduction, confirming demyelinating neuropathy; studies early in disease may be only mildly abnormal, *e.g.*, delayed or absent F waves; axonal degeneration may also occur [2].

Electromyography: in patients without sensory involvement, to help to rule out neuromuscular conduction block or muscle disease and to document axonal degeneration.

Antiganglioside antibody analysis: anti-GM_1 antibodies present in 20%–30% of patients; anti-GQ1b antibodies associated with Miller–Fisher syndrome.

Complications

Death: if airway not adequately protected.

Atelectasis, pneumonia, deep-vein thrombosis, pulmonary embolism, joint contractures, pressure sores, anxiety and depression, pain.

Cardiac arrhythmias, including bradycardic and asystolic episodes, labile blood pressure: due to autonomic instability.

Differential diagnosis

Brain stem encephalitis or infarct.

Acute myelopathy.

Poliomyelitis.

Other neuropathies: porphyria, vasculitis, critical-illness neuropathy, drug-induced neuropathy, toxins (*e.g.*, heavy metals, organophosphates), Lyme disease, or HIV.

Neuromuscular conduction block: myasthenia gravis, botulism.

Muscle disease: hypokalemia (with or without periodic paralysis), polymyositis, acute rhabdomyolysis.

Functional disease: hysteria, malingering.

Etiology

• The cause of Guillain–Barré syndrome is unknown, but, in 60%–70% of patients, it is associated with antecedent infection.

• Inflammatory demyelination with variable axonal degeneration in the peripheral nervous system due to autoimmune mechanisms is triggered by many different agents, including the following:

Viruses: cytomegalovirus, Epstein–Barr virus, HIV (usually around seroconversion).

Bacteria: *Mycoplasma pneumoniae*, *Campylobacter jejuni*.

Vaccines against rabies or swine influenza.

Surgery.

Epidemiology

• Guillain–Barré syndrome has become the most frequent cause of acute generalized neuromuscular paralysis in developed countries since the virtual eradication of poliomyelitis.

• The incidence is 1–2 in 100 000 population.

• More men than women are affected.

• The disease occurs more often in young women and elderly patients.

• It is not contagious.

• No seasonal variation is evident.

Treatment

Diet and lifestyle
• No special precautions are necessary.

Pharmacological treatment

General measures
Frequent measurement of vital capacity and continuous ECG monitoring during progressive phase.

Admission to intensive care unit if vital capacity falling rapidly or patient unable to swallow saliva.

Regular turning, mouth and eye care, aspiration of secretions.

Heparin, 5000 units s.c. twice daily.

Nasogastric feeding if patient has bulbar palsy or is too weak to eat.

Plasma exchange
• Plasma, 50 mL/kg, exchanged five times over 5–10 days is indicated for any patient unable to walk unaided.

• Treatment should be initiated as soon as the diagnosis is made because it is more effective in early disease.

Immunoglobulin [3]

Standard dosage	Immunoglobulin, 0.4 g/kg i.v. daily for 5 days or 1 g/kg daily for 2 days.
Contraindications	IgA deficiency due to circulating anti-IgA antibodies.
Special points	May cause aseptic meningitis and acute or chronic renal failure and exacerbate underlying ischemic disease.
Main side effects	Fever, hypersensitivity reactions, fluid overload.

Treatment aims

To prevent respiratory failure.

To relieve pain.

To prevent complications of immobility.

To optimize functional recovery.

Other treatments

Early tracheostomy: to assist tracheal toilet and increase patient comfort.

Ventilatory assistance: if vital capacity 20 mL/kg or falling rapidly (oxygen saturation best monitored by pulse oximetry) or patient unable to protect airway.

Endocardial pacemaker: for episodes of bradycardia or sinus arrest.

Prognosis

• ~5% of patients relapse; 80% make a good recovery (median time to full independence, 9 months); 20% have permanent disability; 5% die.

• Poor prognostic indicators include age >40 years, rapid onset of weakness, ventilation, high titers of IgG anti-ganglioside GM_1 antibodies, and previous diarrheal illness.

Follow-up and management

• A high level of vigilance must be maintained until recovery has started and the tracheostomy has been closed.

• The patient should be reassured that recovery is probable and is nearly complete in most cases.

• Rehabilitation, *e.g.*, physical therapy, must be continued after discharge.

• Immunization injections must be avoided, especially tetanus toxoid, which has been associated with relapse.

Key references

1. Fulgram JR, Wijdicks EF: Guillain-Barré syndrome. *Crit Care Clin* 1997, **13**:1–15.

2. Albers JW: Acquired inflammatory demyelinating polyneuropathies: clinical and electrodiagnostic features. *Muscle Nerve* 1989, **12**:435–451.

3. van der Meché FGA, Schmitz PIM, the Dutch Guillain–Barré Study Group: A randomized trial comparing intravenous immune globulin and plasma exchange in Guillain–Barré syndrome. *N Engl J Med* 1992, **326**:1123–1129.

Diagnosis

Definition

• Heart block is a disturbance of conduction of the electrical impulse from atrium to ventricle.

• Failure of the sinus impulse to penetrate the atrium (sinoatrial block) and bundle branch block are not considered here.

First-degree atrioventricular block: delayed conduction of impulses from atrium to ventricle, with a prolonged PR interval, but all impulses are conducted.

Second-degree atrioventricular block: intermittent complete failure of conduction of atrial impulse to ventricle, with dropped (nonconducted) P waves on ECG.
Mobitz type I (Wenckebach): progressive lengthening of PR interval until conduction completely fails; atrioventricular conduction recovers after dropped beat, and sequence is repeated.
Mobitz type II: occasional or repetitive failure of conduction without previous lengthening of PR interval; may be every second (2:1) or third (3:1) beat or occasional random dropped P waves [1].

Third-degree (complete) atrioventricular block: complete failure of conduction of all atrial impulses to ventricles; escape rhythm is either narrow complex (if level of block is in atrioventricular node, escape pacemaker arises in bundle of His) or broad complex (if block is infranodal).

Symptoms

First-degree and Mobitz type I

• Patients are usually asymptomatic but may progress to higher-grade atrioventricular block.

Mobitz type II and complete heart block

Syncope (Adams–Stokes attack): loss of consciousness is abrupt, without warning, and the patient appears pale; rare in Mobitz type II.

Presyncope and dizzy spells, fatigue, dyspnea, sudden death.

Signs

First-degree

• No signs are manifest.

Mobitz type I
Irregular pulse with dropped beats.

Mobitz type II
Occasional dropped beats: irregular pulse.
2:1/3:1 block, etc.: bradycardia, edema, raised venous pressure.

Complete heart block
Bradycardia, large-volume pulse, raised venous pressure with occasional cannon waves, variable intensity of first heart sound, peripheral edema.

Investigations

Resting ECG: usually diagnostic.

24-hour Holter monitoring: if heart block is intermittent or continuous "event recorder" if symptoms are infrequent.

Complications

Injury: from syncope.

"Heart failure": underlying ventricular function may be normal, but low cardiac output due to bradycardia and loss of atrioventricular synchrony may mimic ventricular disease.

Ventricular tachycardia and fibrillation: leading to sudden death, may complicate complete heart block.

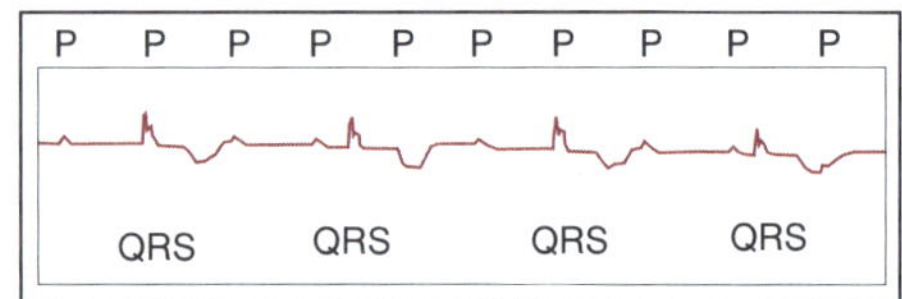

Rhythm strip of ECG for complete heart block demonstrating complete dissociation between P waves and QRS complexes and slow ventricular escape rhythm of 32 beats/min.

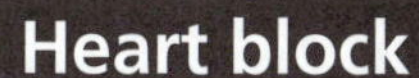

Treatment

Diet and lifestyle

• Patients should lead a normal life after heart block has been treated.

• Permanent pacemaker implantation places certain restrictions on patients, *e.g.*, avoidance of contact sports, which might damage the device or lead.

Pharmacological treatment

• Atropine (0.5–1 mg i.v. bolus) and isoproterenol (200 μg i.v. bolus or 0.5–10 μg/min infusion) may be used as temporary measures before temporary or permanent pacemaker implantation or when heart block needs treatment during resuscitation, although external temporary pacing should also be considered in such circumstances.

Nonpharmacological treatment

• Implantation of a permanent pacemaker in a patient with complete heart block is one of the most cost-effective interventions in modern medicine.

Indications for permanent pacemaker implantation

Second-degree Mobitz type II heart block.

Complete heart block.

Indications for temporary pacing

Symptomatic second-degree Mobitz type II and complete heart block, pending implantation of a permanent pacemaker.

Acute myocardial infarction: complete heart block, second-degree Mobitz type II, development of alternating bundle branch block, development of right bundle branch block with left axis deviation, especially when in combination with first- or second-degree heart block.

Treatment aims

To return patient to a full and active life.

Prognosis

• Implantation of a permanent pacemaker dramatically improves the prognosis of patients with complete heart block.

Follow-up and management

• Patients with first-degree or second-degree Mobitz type I heart block should be followed carefully to check for development of higher-grade atrioventricular block.

• Patients with a permanent pacemaker need regular follow-up in a pacemaker clinic to ensure continued normal function of the device.

• Permanent pacemakers must be changed every 7–10 years.

Key reference

1. Rowlands DJ: Conduction disturbances. In *Understanding the Electrocardiogram: Rhythm Abnormalities*. Macclesfield: ICI; 1987:483–507.

Diagnosis

Definition

• Hemolytic uremic syndrome (HUS) is a syndrome, not a disease; it is defined by the following:

Acute renal insufficiency.

Microangiopathic hemolytic anemia.

Thrombocytopenia.

• Thrombotic thrombocytopenic purpura (TTP) is closely related and often indistinguishable from HUS; the term should be reserved for the following:

A relapsing form of HUS.

Associated fever and fluctuating CNS signs.

• Both HUS and TTP are associated with normal clotting times. Thrombocytopenia and a microangiopathic hemolytic anemia with prolonged clotting times indicate septicemia and disseminated intravascular coagulation.

Symptoms

Malaise, nausea, tiredness: nonspecific symptoms of renal insufficiency.

Oliguria, discolored urine, difficulty concentrating, other subtle CNS changes.

Abdominal cramps; watery diarrhea, then bloody diarrhea; fever <38°C: indicating infection by *Escherichia coli*.

Signs

Pallor: from anemia.

Yellow tinge: occasionally, from the hemolysis.

Purpura, petechia, or prolonged bleeding: if thrombocytopenia is severe.

Investigations

Complete blood count: thrombocytopenia; schistocytes seen on film.

Clotting times: prothrombin time and partial thromboplastin time typically normal.

Biochemistry: raised urea, creatinine, and urate concentrations, hyponatremia, hypoalbuminemia in severely ill patients.

Renal biopsy: usually not needed in children; contraindicated during severe thrombocytopenia; may show glomerular and arteriolar thrombosis, acute tubular necrosis, intimal proliferation of preglomerular arterioles and small arteries, varying degrees of glomerular endothelial injury.

Stool culture for *E. coli* 0157:H7 and isolation of verotoxin: can confirm diagnosis in patients with associated diarrhea.

Serology: for neutralizing antibodies to *E. coli* 0157:H7.

Hemolysis studies: increased lactate dehydrogenase, increased free hemoglobin, decreased serum haptoglobin.

Complications

Bloody diarrhea, gut infarction, rectal prolapse: in patients with associated diarrhea.

Severe malignant hypertension, cardiomyopathy: in patients without diarrhea.

Irritability, restlessness, twitching, generalized or focal seizures, transient visual disturbance, drowsiness, cerebellar ataxia, reduced level of consciousness, decerebrate spasms, coma.

Differential diagnosis

Septicemia associated with disseminated intravascular coagulation
Gram-negative bacilli.
Infection by *Staphylococcus aureus*, *Pneumococcus* spp., or *Meningococcus* spp.
Psittacosis.
Mycoplasma.

Viral and other diseases: thrombocytopenia without hemolysis
Hantavirus.
Dengue hemorrhagic fever.
Malaria.
Leptospirosis.
Snake bite.

Associated with pregnancy (associated with disseminated intravascular coagulation)
Septic abortion.
Amniotic fluid embolus.
Prolonged intrauterine fetal death.
Antepartum hemorrhage.

Other medical conditions
Organ and bone-marrow transplantation.
Scleroderma crisis.
Delayed postpartum or contraceptive pill–associated HUS.
Mytomycin-C cancer chemotherapy.

Etiology

Infectious causes
E. coli associated with diarrhea (in most patients): infection acquired from contaminated beef or dairy products.
Shigella spp.
HIV.

Sporadic, noninfectious causes
Idiopathic or familial disorders, drugs (mitomycin, cyclosporine), tumors, pregnancy, SLE, transplantation, scleroderma, malignant or accelerated hypertension.

Epidemiology

• Patients with diarrhea-associated HUS are usually aged <5 or >65 years.

Treatment

Diet and lifestyle

• No special precautions are necessary.

Pharmacological treatment

Intravenous saline solution and furosemide: to correct circulating volume and reverse prerenal failure and to establish diuresis.

Antiplatelet drugs (*e.g.*, aspirin, dipyridamole): have a logic but no proven benefit.

Prostacyclin infusions: of theoretical value and useful to control hypertension.

Nonpharmacological treatment

Erythrocyte transfusion: for anemia.

Hemodialysis: when indicated, *i.e.*, for volume overload, hyperkalemia, "uremia," acidosis.

Infusions of fresh frozen plasma: may induce remission; amount necessary not known but probably 1–2 L daily; mechanism of benefit not known but may include neutralizing toxins, restoring antioxidant activity, and inducing prostacyclin synthesis; infusions should be continued until erythrocyte fragmentation ceases and platelet count rises $\sim100 \times 10^9$/L.

Plasma exchange: typically used to create intravascular space for repeated infusions of fresh frozen plasma, and may be of benefit by removing humoral factors. Treatment course is typically 6–12 exchanges, the total number depending on response to therapy, *i.e.*, increasing platelet count, decreasing LDH.

Treatment aims

To establish diuresis if possible.

To provide dialysis if necessary.

To control blood pressure.

To try to induce hematological remission.

To prevent seizures.

Prognosis

• The natural history of HUS, when preceded by a diarrheal illness and associated with glomerular thrombi, is one of spontaneous recovery, although patients may have some residual injury; most children are in this category.

• Idiopathic patients, particularly adults, often have major preglomerular vascular disease and irreversible renal failure.

• 3%–25% of patients die during the acute illness (usually from CNS involvement); 10%–20% remain dependent on dialysis; 10% have long-term neurological sequelae; 70% recover with no residual evidence of renal disease.

Follow-up and management

Recovery of renal function and disappearance of proteinuria.

Long-term follow-up if persistent renal insufficiency.

• Blood pressure should be controlled by angiotensin-converting enzyme inhibitors, if possible.

General references

Conlon PJ, Howell DN, Macik G, *et al.*: The renal manifestations and outcome of thrombotic thrombocytopenic purpura/hemolytic uremic syndrome in adults. *Nephrol Dial Transplant* 1995, **10**:1189–1193.

Melnyk AM, Solez K, Kjellstrand CM: Adult hemolytic-uremic syndrome: a review of 37 cases. *Arch Intern Med* 1995, **155**:2077–2084.

Remuzzi G, Ruggenenti P: The hemolytic uremic syndrome. *Kidney Int* 1995, **48**:2–19.

Ruggenenti P, Lutz J, Remuzzi G: Pathogenesis and treatment of thrombotic microangiopathy. *Kidney Int Suppl* 1997, **58**:S97–S101.

Siegler RL: The hemolytic uremic syndrome. *Pediatr Clin North Am* 1995, **42**:1505–1529.

Siegler RL, Pavia AT, Cook JB: Hemolytic-uremic syndrome in adolescents. *Arch Pediatr Adolesc Med* 1997, **151**:165–169.

Diagnosis

Symptoms

Hemophilia

Episodic spontaneous hemorrhage: into joints and muscles.

Deep-tissue hematoma: particularly after trauma or surgery.

Von Willebrand's disease

Bruising.

Epistaxis and melena.

Excessive bleeding after dental extraction or surgery.

Postpartum bleeding, rarely hemarthroses and muscle hematomas.

Signs

Hemophilia

Acute: Hot, swollen, painful joint; unexpected bleeding after surgery.

Chronic: Crippling joint deformity.

Investigations

Hemophilia

Activated partial thromboplastin time measurement: prolonged.

Hemophilia A, factor VIII; hemophilia B, factor IX; and hemophilia C, factor XI assays: all three show low values.

Coagulation factor activity measurement: correlated with disease severity in hemophilia A and B (normal range, 50–150 U/dL):
<2 U/dL indicates severe disease, manifest as frequent spontaneous bleeding episodes, joint deformity, and crippling;
2–5 U/dL indicates moderate disease, manifest as posttraumatic bleeding, occasional spontaneous episodes;
5–20 U/dL indicates mild disease, manifest as posttraumatic bleeding.

Von Willebrand's disease [1]

Bleeding time measurement: prolonged.

Factor VIII clotting activity, von Willebrand factor antigen and activity measurement: low values.

Platelet function tests: reduced aggregation of platelets with ristocetin.

• Von Willebrand's disease is classified on the basis of the type of protein abnormality; this is important for deciding treatment.

Complications

Transfusion-transmitted disease [2]

Hepatitis A: has been a problem with a solvent detergent sterilized product; all patients with bleeding disorders should be vaccinated.

Hepatitis B: although all blood donors are tested for this, sterilization processes for clotting factor concentrate cannot be regarded as 100% safe; vaccination mandatory in patients with bleeding disorders [3].

Hepatitis C: all patients treated by unsterilized clotting factor concentrates have been infected (sterilization introduced in 1985); some patients progress to chronic liver disease; treatment by interferon may normalize transaminases; HIV co-infection results in faster progression of hepatitis C liver disease [3].

HIV infection: occurred in patients receiving concentrates between 1979 and 1985 [4,5].

Inhibitors

Neutralizing antibodies: occurring after infusion of concentrates.

Chronic arthropathy

Chronic disabling arthritis: caused by recurrent hemarthroses.

Differential diagnosis

Other clotting factor deficiencies or platelet function disorders.

Etiology

Causes of hemophilia
Quantitative deficiency of clotting factors.
Factor VIII: hemophilia A (most common).
Factor IX: hemophilia B.
Factor XI: hemophilia C.

Causes of von Willebrand's disease
Quantitative or qualitative deficiency of von Willebrand factor, important in primary platelet hemostasis, acting as an adhesive protein and a carrier protein for factor VIII.

Genetics
Hemophilia A and B: X–linked (men affected, but some women carriers may need concentrate for surgery or trauma).
Von Willebrand's disease: autosomal-dominant.
Hemophilia C (severe disease): autosomal-recessive or compound heterozygote.

Epidemiology

• 1 in 5000 men is affected by hemophilia A or B; 1 in 6 patients with hemophilia has hemophilia B.

• Hemophilia C is common in Ashkenazi Jews; it may occur in any ethnic group.

• Von Willebrand's disease is the most common inherited bleeding disorder if all grades of severity are considered; clinically significant disease occurs in ~125 in one million population.

Carrier detection and antenatal diagnosis [6]

• Carrier status and presence of the disorders in fetuses can be detected by the following:
Restriction fragment length polymorphisms.
Variable-number repeat sequences.
Direct mutational analysis (research).
Chorionic villus sampling before 10 weeks (for carriers with a molecular marker).
Fetal sexing and choriocentesis (for carriers without a molecular marker).

Treatment

Diet and lifestyle

• Patients should avoid contact sports, but regular exercise, *e.g.*, swimming, should be encouraged.

Pharmacological treatment

• Intramuscular injections must be avoided in patients with bleeding disorders.

• Aspirin or NSAIDs that impair platelet function must also be avoided.

Indications

For hemophilia A: factor VIII concentrate or DDAVP (desmopressin).

For hemophilia B: factor IX concentrate.

For hemophilia C: factor XI concentrate or fresh frozen plasma [7].

For von Willebrand's disease: factor VIII concentrate rich in von Willebrand's factor or DDAVP.

Clotting factor preparations [8]

Recombinant: Recombinate (VIII), Kogenate (VIII), Benefix (IX).

Extracted by immunoaffinity chromatography: Hemofil M (VIII), Antihemophilic factor (American Red Cross) Monoclate P (VIII), Mononine (IX), Humate P (von Willebrand's factor).

Extracted by conventional separation: *very high purity (>100 U/mg):* Alphanine (IX) SD; *intermediate purity (<50 U/mg):* Humate P (von Willebrand's factor) (VIII).

• The units of clotting factor needed, x, can be calculated by the following equation:
x = [rise in clotting factor required (%) × weight (kg)] ÷ K
where K = 1.5 for factor VIII, 1 for factor IX, and 2 for factor XI.

• Approximate levels for hemostasis are as follows:

15–20 U clotting factor/dL plasma for minor spontaneous hemarthroses and hematomas.

20–40 U clotting factor/dL plasma for severe hemarthroses and muscle hematomas, minor surgery.

80–100 U clotting factor/dL plasma for major surgery or intracranial/intra-abdominal hemorrhage.

DDAVP

• DDAVP releases von Willebrand's factor from endothelial cells.

• It is used to raise endogenous factor VIII von Willebrand's levels during minor procedures in patients with mild hemophilia and von Willebrand's disease.

• It is not indicated for severe hemophilia or type III form of von Willebrand's disease.

Standard dosage	DDAVP, 0.3 µg/kg in 100 mL normal saline solution i.v. infusion over 20 minutes.
Contraindications	Vascular disease, type II B von Willebrand's disease [9].
Special points	Response should be monitored using factor assays.
Main drug interactions	None.
Main side effects	Hyponatremia and seizures (in children aged <2 years), coronary occlusion (in patients aged >60 years).

Tranexamic acid and aminocaproic acid

• Tranexamic acid, an inhibitor of fibrinolysis, reduces blood loss, particularly in mucosal bleeding, *e.g.*, oral surgery, epistaxis, and tonsillectomy.

Standard dosage	Tranexamic acid, 1 g orally or i.v. 3–4 times daily; in children, 25 mg/kg 3 times daily. Aminocaproic acid, 5–30 g in divided doses every 3–6 hours for 5–7 days.
Contraindications	*Tranexamic acid and aminocaproic acid:* hematuria, risk of "clot colic."
Special points	*Tranexamic acid and aminocaproic acid:* dose should be reduced in patients with renal impairment.
Main drug interactions	None.
Main side effects	*Tranexamic acid and aminocaproic acid:* nausea, dizziness.

Key references

1. Nichols WC, Ginsburg D: von Willebrand disease. *Medicine* 1997, **76**:1–20.

2. Vermylen J, Briet E: Factor VIII preparations: need for prospective pharmacovigilance. *Lancet* **342**:693–694.

3. Lee CA, Dusheiko G: Hepatitis and hemophilia. In *Viral Hepatitis.* Edited by Zuckerman AJ, Thomas HC, New York: Churchill Livingstone; 1993.

4. Goerdert JJ, *et al.*: A prospective study of human immunodeficiency virus type I infection and the development of AIDS in subjects with hemophilia. *N Engl J Med* 1989, **321**:1141–1148.

5. Lee CA, *et al.*: Progression of HIV disease in a hemophilic cohort followed for 11 years and the effect of treatment. *BMJ* 1991, **303**:1093–1094.

6. Peake I: Molecular genetics and counselling in haemophilia. *Thromb Haemost* 1995, **74**:40–44.

7. Bolton-Maggs PHB, *et al.*: Production and therapeutic use of a factor XI concentrate from plasma. *Thromb Haemost* 1992, **67**:314–319.

8. Mannucci PM: Modern treatment of hemophilia: from shadows towards light. *Thromb Haemost* 1993, **70**:17–23.

9. Holmberg L, Nilsson IM, Borge L, *et al.*: Platelet aggregation induced by 1-desamino-8-D-arginine vasopressin (DDAVP) in type IIB von Willebrand's disease. *N Eng J Med* 1983, **309**:816–821.

Diagnosis

Symptoms

Painless bleeding: blood typically on surface of stool or toilet paper from an otherwise normal bowel movement; occult blood loss should never be attributed to hemorrhoids without excluding more serious diseases (*see* Differential diagnosis).

Protruding tissue following defecation.

Perianal irritation, pruritis.

Acute, severe perianal pain: suggests acute thrombosis or strangulation.

Signs

Internal hemorrhoids: visible and occasionally palpable hemorrhoidal plexus above the dentate line (seen best with an anoscope).

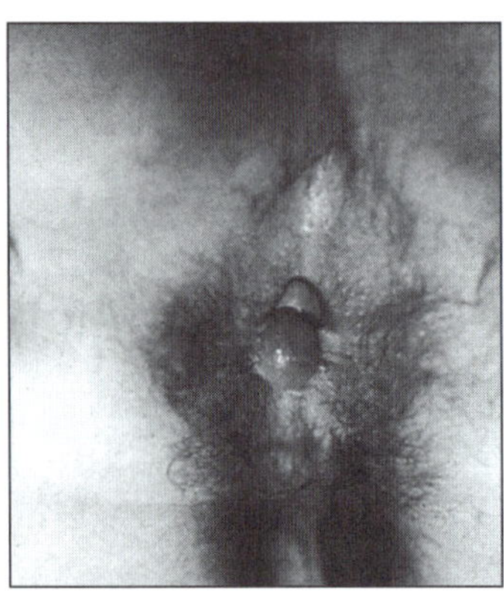

An acutely thrombosed external hemorrhoid. (*See* Color Plate.)

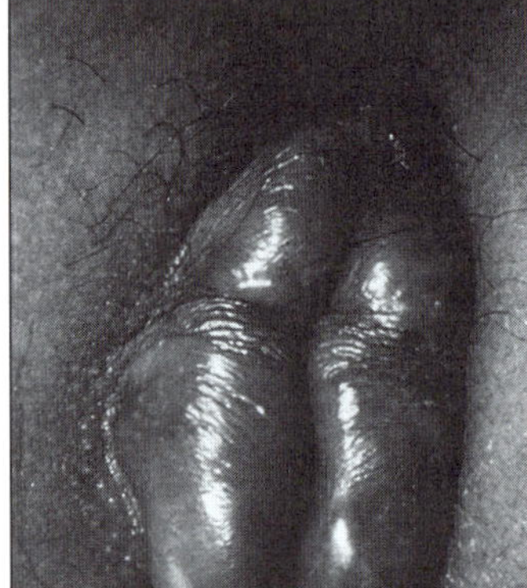

Acutely prolapsed large, bilateral external and internal (mixed) hemorrhoids. (*See* Color Plate.)

External hemorrhoids: palpable venous engorgement below the dentate line, covered by squamous epithelium; exquisitely tender when thrombosed, which eventually results in small, benign-appearing external skin tags.

Perianal inflammation: attributed to compromised hygiene because of redundant tissue.

Investigations

Anoscopy: should be performed to assess the nature and severity of hemorrhoids, although patients with acute thrombosis or strangulation will not be able to tolerate this procedure.

Sigmoidoscopy: required to exclude other competing diagnoses, *e.g.*, malignancy; visualization of the entire colon by colonoscopy or air-contrast barium enema should also be performed in patients >45 years of age, patients with a family history of colonic malignancy, and patients who do not respond to conservative therapy.

Complications

Thrombosis resulting in severe pain.

Strangulation of internal hemorrhoids with possible gangrene and life-threatening infection: rare.

Treatment

Diet and lifestyle

- Patients should be placed on a high-fiber diet.
- Patients should avoid excessive straining during defecation.
- Patients should take sitz baths.

Pharmacological treatment [1]

• Stool softening agents (*e.g.*, synthetic mucilloids or psyllium preparations) should be titrated at a dose that will minimize straining and achieve 1–2 soft bowel movements each day. A typical starting dose consists of one heaping tablespoon in 8 oz of water once or twice each day. The patient should be instructed to drink the preparation immediately after mixing. A few days of increased flatus or bloating is commonly experienced at the start of therapy.

• Topical emollients with local anesthetics (*e.g.*, benzocaine, witch hazel) may be used to provide symptom relief but do not contribute to a reduction in the hemorrhoids or control of bleeding. Preparations containing a topical steroid (*e.g.*, 1% hydrocortisone) or efficacious in reducing the symptoms of perianal inflammation. Patients should be instructed to apply these preparations locally twice daily as needed for symptom control.

Treatment aims

To reduce pain, bleeding, and perianal inflammation.

Other treatment options [2]

• Rubber band ligation is perhaps the most popular treatment for symptomatic internal hemorrhoids, although injection sclerotherapy, cryosurgery, electro-coagulation, or laser obliteration are alternatives; the innervation of the covering squamous epithelium prevents the use of these modalities in the management of external hemorrhoids.

• The acute pain of a thrombosed external hemorrhoid may be managed with injection of local anesthesia and a limited decompression if performed within the first 48 hours of symptoms. It is often difficult to evacuate the hematoma and achieve optimal control of bleeding after this time period. Surgical therapy of internal hemorrhoids is usually reserved for persistent symptoms despite the use of the conservative approaches noted previously or strangulation.

Prognosis

• Hemorrhoidal disease can be a nuisance but rarely has a significant effect on an individual's health.

• The presence of palpable or visual hemorrhoids alone is not an indication for treatment and is not predictive of future symptoms.

Follow-up and management

• Routine follow-up of hemorrhoidal disease is not typically required; the nature of the patient's symptoms rather than the presence of hemorrhoids should direct the management plan of the physician.

Key references

1. Johnson JF, Rimm A: Optimal nonsurgical treatment of hemorrhoids. *Am J Gastroenterol* 1992, **87**:1601–1605.

2. Barnett JL, Raper SE: Anorectal disease. In *Textbook of Gastroenterology*, edn 2. Edited by Yamada T. Philadelphia: JB Lippincott; 1995:2027–2032.

Diagnosis

Symptoms

• In most patients, symptoms occur 24–48 hours after infection (usually upper respiratory tract infection) or drug ingestion (antibiotics).

• ~50% of adults develop only the characteristic rash and malaise.

Florid palpable purpuric skin rash: predominantly on lower legs but also on buttocks and arms (cardinal symptom).

Cramping abdominal pains: in 60%–70% of patients

Joint pains: in 60%–70%.

Blood in urine or stool: in 20%–30%.

Symptoms of intestinal obstruction: due to intussusception, in young children.

Fever and toxicity: if severe.

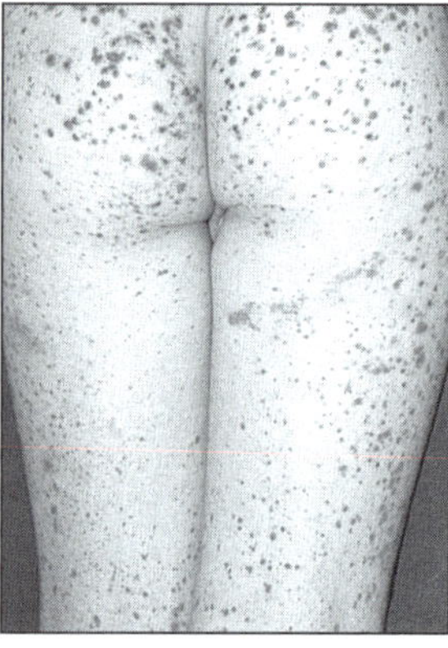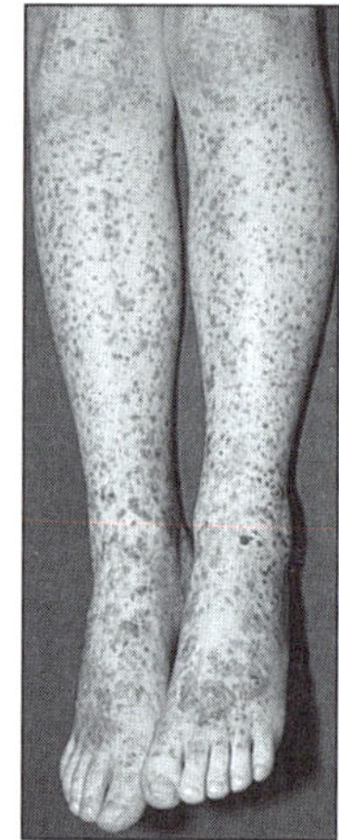

Typical purpuric lesions on buttocks (*left*) and pretibial areas and lower legs (*right*). (*See* Color Plates.)

Signs

Rash: "papular purpura" lesions that do not blanch on pressure, some forming a necrotic center that may vesiculate, usually on buttocks, gluteal cleft, and extremities; usually painless; in adults, may persist or recur for up to 2 months.

Joint involvement: mild to moderate symmetrical arthropathy in 60%–70%; some periarticular swelling; a few patients also have angioedema of hands and feet.

Gut involvement: cramping abdominal pain, and some rebound tenderness in 25%; frank blood in stool in 10%–20%; obstructive symptoms (intussusception) or perforation.

Renal involvement: ~30% of patients develop nephritis.

Investigations

Skin biopsy: may show cutaneous necrotizing venulitis but does not indicate cause.

History: may be positive for recent infective episodes or drug ingestion (antibiotic).

Complete blood count: may show mild polymorphonuclear leukocytosis.

Serology: for recent viral or streptococcal infection.

Stool and urine analysis: regularly during and after rash, with formal microscopy if positive; 30% of patients show evidence of erythrocytes, raised protein concentration, and casts on urinalysis.

Formal renal investigations, including biopsy: if findings indicate renal disease.

Complications

• In children, this condition is often thought of as "harmless."

Secondary infection of vasculitic lesions.

Glomerulonephritis, IgA nephropathy: in ~30% of patients; 15%–20% of these progress to renal failure in 6 months (adults).

Renal failure: in 5%–10% of all patients.

Gastrointestinal or surgical problems: *e.g.*, intussusception or perforation in young children; of the 60%–70% of patients with gastrointestinal complications, a few develop intramural hematomata, associated with intussusception, infarction, or gut perforation; protein-losing enteropathy.

Renal problems: *e.g.*, immunoglobulin nephropathy in older children and adults.

Differential diagnosis

Other forms of vasculitic or purpuric rash (*e.g.*, meningococcal septicemia).

Embolic phenomena from acute or subacute bacterial endocarditis.

Systemic gram-negative sepsis.

Collagen vascular disease, especially polyarteritis nodosa.

Etiology

• Henoch–Schönlein purpura is essentially idiopathic.

• Triggers include the following:

Nonspecific upper respiratory infection (in ~33% of patients).

Sulfonamide or penicillin treatment.

Streptococcal infection.

Streptokinase treatment for myocardial infarction.

Epidemiology

• Henoch–Schönlein purpura can occur at any age, but it predominantly affects children.

• It has a seasonal variation, occurring most often in winter months in temperate climates.

Treatment

Diet and lifestyle

• Other than bed rest during the acute phase, no special precautions are necessary.

Pharmacological treatment

• Treatment is symptomatic and does not alter the course or outcome of the condition or its complications.

• Local treatment of the rash, if needed, should be designed to prevent secondary infection, *e.g.*, potassium permanganate soaks.

• Steroids have no effect on renal abnormalities and are associated with a significant incidence of gastrointestinal side effects.

For pain relief

Standard dosage	NSAIDs, *e.g.*, naproxen, 250 mg every 6–8 hours (adults).
Contraindications	Active peptic ulceration.
Special points	Asthma may be exacerbated.
Main drug interactions	Oral anticoagulants.
Main side effects	Gastrointestinal disturbances, discomfort, nausea, or ulceration.

For joint abnormalities

Standard dosage	Corticosteroids, *e.g.*, prednisolone, 40–60 mg daily.
Contraindications	Active peptic ulceration.
Special points	Possible adrenal suppression on sudden withdrawal.
Main drug interactions	NSAIDs, oral anticoagulants.
Main side effects	Cushing's syndrome, growth retardation in children, osteoporosis.

Treatment aims

To prevent secondary infection in vasculitic skin lesions.

To relieve symptoms of joint or abdominal pain.

Other treatments

• Renal replacement therapy may be needed in the 5%–10% of patients who develop renal failure or nephrotic syndrome.

Prognosis

• The prognosis of the rash alone is good.

• Crops of lesions may recur within 4–8 weeks, especially in adults.

• Spontaneous remission is the norm.

• Relapses of the rash alone often occur in adults.

• 15%–20% of adults with IgA nephropathy progress to renal failure in 6 months.

• Generally, 5%–10% of patients develop renal failure; this is most probable in adults or adolescents.

Follow-up and management

• Renal function or urinary sediment must be monitored for evidence of renal involvement.

• If renal involvement is detected, full renal investigation, including biopsy is needed.

General references

Fogazzi GB, *et al.*: Long term outcome of Schönlein Henoch nephritis in the adult. *Clin Nephrol* 1989, **31**:60–66.

Ford EG, Jennings LM, Andrassay RJ: Management of Henoch–Schönlein purpura and polyarteritis nodosum. *Tex Med* 1987, **83**:54–58.

Schreiner DT: Purpura. *Dermatol Clin* 1989, **7**:481–490.

Szer IS: Henoch-Schönlein purpura: when and how to treat. *J Rheumatol* 1996, **23**:1661–1665.

Diagnosis

Definition

• Hepatic encephalopathy is a reversible neuropsychiatric syndrome that is a complication of fulminant or chronic liver disease [1].

• Hepatic encephalopathy may also be present in the rare cases of urea-cycle enzyme defects and portosystemic shunting in the absence of liver disease.

• Latent encephalopathy is a subclinical form occurring in chronic liver disease, only detected by psychometric testing.

Symptoms

• Wide differences are seen in presentation and evolution (*see* Classification).

Inversion of normal sleep pattern.

Deterioration of intellectual function.

Slurred speech.

Tremor: absent at rest.

Personality changes: features of frontal-lobe syndrome.

Coma.

Symptoms of precipitating causes: *e.g.*, infection or gastrointestinal bleeding.

Signs

• Patients with impaired consciousness have intact pupillary reflexes.

Asterixis.

Fetor hepaticus.

Constructional apraxia: Reitan trail test.

Brisk tendon reflexes: except in coma.

Increased muscle tone and rigidity.

Hyperventilation in deep coma.

Signs of precipitating causes: *e.g.*, spontaneous bacterial peritonitis.

Investigations

• No single parameter confirms the diagnosis.

• The underlying liver disease or its complications must be identified.

• A precipitant cause must always be sought.

• A careful evaluation for infection is warranted including paracentesis if ascites is present.

Psychometric testing: essential to detect subclinical encephalopathy; number connection test (Reitan trail) and drawing a clock face easiest to perform.

EEG: slowing of normal frequency to severe slowing; characteristic triphasic waves; changes appearing first in frontal regions.

CT of head: to exclude subdural hematomas and other intracranial diseases; some atrophy of brain usually manifest, particularly in chronic encephalopathy.

Blood ammonia measurement: concentration usually raised, but false-positive and false-negative results may occur.

Complications

Increase in intracranial pressure: in patients with fulminant liver failure; due to cerebral edema, which can lead to brain death.

Complications of coma: *e.g.*, aspiration in patients with encephalopathy.

Structural neuronal damage: with demyelination and a spastic paraplegia, in patients with chronic encephalopathy (rare); chronic cerebellar or basal ganglia signs may also be present with Parkinsonian features.

Focal seizures: rare, other causes must be sought.

Differential diagnosis

Alcoholic brain damage.

Alcohol withdrawal syndrome.

Wernicke's encephalopathy.

Chronic subdural hematoma or other space-occupying lesion.

Other causes of metabolic coma.

Postictal state.

Meningitis, encephalitis.

Etiology

• Precipitant causes include the following:

Constipation.

Gastrointestinal bleeding (occult or apparent).

Infection.

Overdiuresis.

Hypovolemia.

Sedative and opiate drugs.

Diarrhea and vomiting.

Dietary indiscretion.

Protein excess.

Acute worsening of chronic liver disease.

Urea and electrolyte abnormalities.

Uncontrolled diabetes.

Hypoglycemia.

Surgery.

Epidemiology

• Chronic liver disease is usually progressive, so that most patients develop hepatic encephalopathy at some time, particularly secondary to a precipitant cause.

• Intermittent encephalopathy is the most common pattern.

• Subclinical or latent encephalopathy is present in most patients, but its clinical significance is unclear.

• Fulminant liver failure is a rare disorder that warrants immediate referral to a liver transplant center.

Classification

	Mental status	Signs
Stage 1	Mild confusion	None
	Slowness in mentation	Mild apraxia
	Slurred speech	Impaired
	Euphoria	handwriting
Stage II	Increased confusion	Brisk reflexes
	Disoriented to time	Increased tone
	Lethargy	Asterixis
		Ataxia
Stage III	Somnolent but arousable	Asterixis
	Marked confusion	Babinski's sign
	Incoherent speech	Clonus
Stage IV	Coma	Absent reflexes
		Decerebrate

Treatment

Diet and lifestyle

• Careful attention must be paid to adequate nutrition, and this should take priority over protein restriction which is required (*e.g.*, <30 g/day), only in a subset of patients with encephalopathy that is difficult to control pharmacologically.

• The early warning signs of encephalopathy must be explained to patients and their families so that early medical attention can be obtained.

Pharmacological treatment

• Encephalopathy typically resolves when the precipitating cause is corrected [2].

For acute encephalopathy in chronic liver disease

Lactose or sorbitol administered by nasogastric tube or enema.

Correction of electrolyte abnormalities.

Intravenous thiamine in alcoholics.

Long-term treatment

Standard dosage	Lactulose or sorbitol, 30 mL 4 times daily initially and titrated to produce two soft bowel movements daily.
Contraindications	Known hypersensitivity.
Special points	Demyelination, electrolyte abnormalities should be watched for.
Main drug interactions	None known.
Main side effects	Abdominal bloating, flatulence.

Encephalopathy of fulminant liver failure

Correction of hypoglycemia: 20% dextrose i.v.

Correction of electrolyte abnormalities.

Bowel decontamination: oral antibacterial agents.

Early treatment of infection.

Other options

• Flumazenil, a benzodiazepine receptor antagonist, may temporarily reverse symptoms.

Treatment aims

To correct or remove precipitating cause.
To prevent recurrence.

Other treatments

Refashioning, embolization, or ligation of surgical shunt (if present).

• Oral, nonabsorbable antibiotics (*e.g.*, neomycin) may be considered for patients refractory to treatment with lactulose or sorbitol.

Liver transplantation: for recurrent acute or chronic encephalopathy, and fulminant liver failure with adverse prognostic factors.

Prognosis

• Prognosis is determined by the underlying liver disease and avoidance of precipitating factors.

Follow-up and management

• Follow-up depends on the severity of the underlying liver disease, but clinic visits every 1–3 months are common; patients usually should keep a 3-monthly diary and stool chart.

Key references

1. Fraser CL: Hepatic encephalopathy. *N Engl J Med* 1985, **313**:865–873.

2. Butterworth RF: Pathogenesis and treatment of portal-systemic encephalopathy. *Dig Dis Sci* 1992, **37**:321–327.

Diagnosis

Symptoms

• Acute hepatitis is often asymptomatic, and hepatitis C is typically asymptomatic.

• Symptoms, when present, may include malaise, headaches, myalgias, arthralgias, anorexia, nausea, right upper quadrant discomfort, fever, jaundice, pruritis, dark urine, acholic stools.

• Children <2 years of age rarely develop symptoms with hepatitis A virus (HAV) or hepatitis B virus (HBV) infection, but most adults who become infected develop symptoms [1].

Signs

• Signs are usually absent but may include the following:

Jaundice, right upper quadrant tenderness, hepatomegaly.

Hepatic encephalopathy, asterixis, fetor hepaticus: associated with acute hepatic failure.

Skin rash secondary to leukocytoclastic vasculitis: less common symptoms.

Investigations [2]

Biochemical assays: should confirm hepatitis, with elevated serum transaminases, mild increase in alkaline phosphatase, variable increase in bilirubin; as disease progresses, cholestatic picture may evolve before recovery.

Complete blood count or blood film: not usually helpful; features consistent with hypersplenism, however, suggest underlying chronic liver disease.

Prothrombin time: If elevated, fulminant hepatic failure should be watched for; underlying chronic liver disease should be considered.

Virology tests: should be ordered based on probable cause.
Hepatitis A: check for IgM antibody (indicates acute infection; IgG antibody present for life and suggests previous infection) [3].
Hepatitis B: check for IgM anticore antibody (develops early in illness) and surface antigen (present in most symptomatic patients but may be eliminated quickly) [4].
Hepatitis C: antibody may take several months to convert, although most patients become positive within 2 months (hepatitis C virus RNA using polymerase chain reaction is positive early in the infection) [5].
Hepatitis D: presence of anti-hepatitis D virus antibody indicates infection: as coinfection with acute hepatitis B infection or as a superinfection in a chronic carrier of HBV.
Hepatitis E: can be sought by enzyme-linked immunosorbent assay (very rare) [6].
Cytomegalovirus and Epstein-Barr virus: should be sought when viral cause suspected and other serological tests negative.
Hepatitis G: probably does not cause clinical disease and should not be tested for at this time.

Liver biopsy: may be indicated in rare circumstances when diagnostic confusion exists or when underlying liver damage is suspected.

Complications

Fulminant liver failure: in 1%–5% of cases.

Progression to chronic hepatitis: may occur with hepatitis B (~10%), hepatitis C (50%–70%); chronic infection never occurs in hepatitis A.

Anemia.

Aplastic anemia, vasculitis, cryoglobulinemia: rarely, in cases of hepatitis B or C.

Arthritis.

Renal disease.

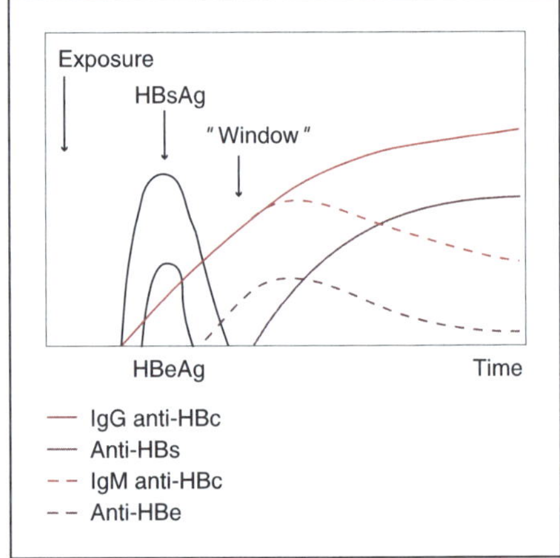

Serological diagnosis of acute hepatitis B (HB) infection. HBeAg, HBe antigen; HBsAg, HB surface antigen.

Treatment

Diet and lifestyle

• Abstinence from alcohol until recovery should be recommended.

• Excessive amounts of acetaminophen (>4 g/day) should be avoided.

• Rest is recommended; many patients are unable to return to work for weeks or months and, even after return, may need time before normal function fully returns.

• Patients must understand the routes by which the hepatitis infection has been acquired and may therefore be transmitted; this may place certain restrictions on professional or sexual activities in the short term.

Pharmacological treatment

• The onset of jaundice is often associated with loss or significant reduction of infectivity in patients with hepatitis A and B; no specific treatment is available for acute viral hepatitis.

• Symptomatic improvement may be obtained in patients with prolonged cholestasis using ursodeoxycholic acid, 600 mg at night.

• For HAV, an effective vaccine is available for protective immunization; immunoglobulin has a well defined role in short-term prophylaxis and for household contacts of patients with acute hepatitis.

• For HBV, an effective vaccine is available; vaccination soon after exposure may still be effective; hepatitis B immunoglobulin is given with vaccination to infants born of mothers who are hepatitis B surface antigen–positive and for postexposure prophylaxis.

• Acute hepatitis C infection is rarely diagnosed. Given the high rate of chronic hepatitis C infection and its uncertain prognosis, interferon, 3 MU 3 times a week, should be considered in acute infection.

Treatment aims

To palliate symptoms.
To observe for progression to fulminant hepatic failure.

Prognosis

• Acute hepatitis is often a debilitating illness, but recovery is usual, although patients may experience fatigue for several months before full recovery.

• Over 40% of patients infected by hepatitis C virus and ~10% infected by hepatitis B become carriers; for the latter, chronic infection is less common after a severe, acute illness.

• The immediate prognosis for patients with hepatitis C who become carriers is excellent; chronic liver disease often develops, however.

Follow-up and management

• Patients with acute hepatitis A, B, or E should be followed until the liver function tests have returned to normal.

• Patients with hepatitis B should also be followed until hepatitis B surface antigen is eliminated; persistence of hepatitis Be antigen beyond 6 weeks suggests that a carrier state may be evolving.

• For hepatitis D, the prognosis depends ultimately on the outcome of the hepatitis B infection; a patient who remains hepatitis B surface antigen–positive may develop chronic liver disease.

• In the present state of uncertainty about the prognosis of patients with hepatitis C, they should be followed every 6–12 months unless evidence for persistent hepatitis C is lacking, *i.e.*, disappearance of hepatitis C virus antibody or RNA.

Key references

1. Lieberman JM: Hepatitis A and B vaccines in children. *J Pediatr Infect Dis* 1996, **11**:333–363.

2. Sjogren MH: Serologic diagnosis of viral hepatitis. *Med Clin North Am* 1996, **80**:856–929.

3. Ross BL, *et al.*: Hepatitis A virus and hepatitis A infection. *Ad Virus Res* 1991, **39**:209–257.

4. Brown JL, *et al.*: The hepatitis B virus. *Baillières Clin Gastroenterol* 1990, **4**:721–747.

5. Sharara AI: Hepatitis C. *Ann Intern Med* 1996, **125**:658–668.

6. Krawczynski K: Hepatitis E. *Hepatology* 1993, **17**:932–941.

Diagnosis

Symptoms

• Most patients with chronic hepatitis are asymptomatic.

Fatigue, malaise: most common symptoms.

Gastrointestinal bleeding, altered mental status, abdominal pain or distention: in patients with long-standing chronic hepatitis who progress to end-stage liver disease.

Signs

• If signs are present they usually indicate advanced liver disease.

Muscle wasting, ascites, palmar erythema, Dupuytren's contracture: nonspecific findings.

Spider telangiectasis, splenomegaly, testicular atrophy, gynecomastia, encephalopathy, caput medusae.

Investigations

Liver chemistry tests: ALT and AST typically elevated to a greater degree than alkaline phosphatase; elevation in bilirubin variable.

Coagulation screening: impaired hepatic synthetic function causes prolonged prothrombin time in addition to low albumin.

Complete blood count: hypersplenism may result in leukopenia and thrombocytopenia.

Liver ultrasonography or CT: often normal but may show small liver with splenomegaly.

Liver biopsy for histology: shows the following:
Hepatitis B/D virus: inflammatory cells spreading into parenchyma from enlarged portal tracts; hepatitis B sAg on immunohistochemistry; hepatitis D infection increases severity and can be detected by immunohistochemistry.
Hepatitis C virus: usually mild chronic hepatitis with lobular component, prominent lymphoid follicles in portal tracts, acidophil body formation, focal hepatocellular necrosis; no immunohistochemical staining currently available.
Autoimmune disease: periportal inflammatory infiltrate and piecemeal necrosis; negative to hepatitis B/D staining on immunohistochemistry.

• Additional investigations are usually directed at identifying either infectious causes or treatable causes (*e.g.*, hemochromatosis, autoimmune liver disease, Wilson's disease, alcoholic liver disease, or drug-induced liver disease). These may include:

Serum ferritin: elevated in hemochromatosis. Iron saturation (*i.e.*, iron/transferrin) >60% should be evaluated with liver biopsy for quantitative iron.
Autoantibody analysis: antinuclear antibody, double-stranded DNA, and smooth-muscle antibody often positive in autoimmune disease.
Serum protein electrophoresis: loss of alpha spike in alpha-1 antitrypsin, immunoglobulins elevated in chronic liver disease but particularly prominent in autoimmune hepatitis (especially IgG).
Ceruloplasmin: decreased and 24-hour urine copper increased in Wilson's disease.
Hepatitis C serology: interpreted as follows:
Positive, active disease: ELISA+, RIBA+ (2–4 bands), ALT increased, RNA+.
False-positive: ELISA+, RIBA– or indeterminate (1 band), ALT normal, RNA–.
Hepatitis B serology: interpreted as follows:
Immune, postvaccination: sAb+, sAg–, cAb–, eAg–, eAb–, DNA–.
Immune, past exposure to hepatitis B virus: sAb+, sAg–, cAb+, eAg–, eAb+, DNA–.
Infected, carrier: sAb–, sAg+, cAb+, eAg–, eAb+, DNA–.
Infected, high risk of transmission: sAb–, sAg+, cAb+, eAg+, eAb–, DNA+.
Hepatitis D (delta) serology: hepatitis D can present as coinfection with hepatitis B virus (HBV) or as superinfection of a HBV carrier; anti–hepatitis D antibody positive indicates superinfection.

Complications

Cirrhosis: in 20%–50% of patients.
Variceal bleeding, encephalopathy, ascites: due to portal hypertension.
Hepatocellular carcinoma: increased incidence in patients with cirrhosis.

Differential diagnosis

Primary biliary cirrhosis.
Primary sclerosing cholangitis.
Granulomatous hepatitis: multiple granulomata (on liver biopsy), sarcoid, tuberculosis, histoplasmosis, Q fever, brucella, lymphoma.
Alcoholic liver disease.
Hemochromatosis.
Wilson's disease.

Definition

Hepatic dysfunction (*i.e.*, abnormal liver enzyme levels, often with progression to abnormal synthetic function) of at least 6 months' duration secondary to inflammation of the hepatic parenchyma [1].

Etiology

Hepatitis C virus, 34%.
Alcohol, 38%.
Unknown, 17%.
HBV, 9%.
Autoimmune, 1%.
• Remaining causes include drugs, Wilson's disease, hemochromatosis, alpha$_1$-antitrypsin deficiency, and steatohepatitis.

Abbreviations

ALT	alanine aminotransferase (SGPT)
AST	aspartate aminotransferase (SGOT)
cAb	Hepatitis B core antibody
eAb	Hepatitis B e antibody
eAg	Hepatitis B e antigen
ELISA	enzyme-linked immunosorbent assay
RIBA	recombinant immunoblot assay
sAb	Hepatitis B surface antibody
sAg	Hepatitis B surface antigen

Treatment

Diet and lifestyle

- Alcohol must be avoided.

- Patients infected by HBV should be advised on barrier methods of contraception unless the partner is vaccinated; sexual transmission of hepatitis C occurs, but at a much lower frequency.

- Avoid excessive amounts of acetaminophen (>4 g/day).

Pharmacological treatment

- Treatment should be given under specialist supervision.

For HBV infection

- Treatment is indicated for patients who have histological evidence of chronic hepatitis and are positive for hepatitis B e antigen or virus DNA [2].

- Meaningful remission can be achieved in 40%–50% of patients with HBV.

Standard dosage	Interferon-α, 10 MU s.c. 3 times a week for 4–6 months [3]. Alternative regimens also available.
Contraindications	Hypersensitivity, evidence of liver failure (*e.g.*, ascites, varicies, thrombocytopenia).
Main drug interactions	None.
Main side effects	*Induction:* low-grade fever, malaise, arthralgia, myalgia, headache, anorexia, nausea, vomiting, diarrhea. *Maintenance:* fatigue, anorexia, weight loss, alopecia, depression, neutropenia, thrombocytopenia, exacerbation of autoimmune disease, induction of thyroid disease, myalgia.

- Steroid pretreatment may cause rebound immune stimulation; available data do not indicate that combination is superior to interferon alone.

- Drug-resistant HBV mutants may occur.

For hepatitis C virus infection

- Treatment is indicated for patients with histological evidence of hepatitis who are positive for recombinant immunoblot assay (2–4 bands) or virus RNA by the polymerase chain reaction.

- Remission persists in only 20% of patients after treatment is stopped.

Standard dosage	Interferon-α, 3 MU s.c. 3 times weekly for 4–12 months [4].
Contraindications	Hypersensitivity, evidence of liver failure (*e.g.*, ascites, varices, thrombocytopenia).
Main drug interactions	None.
Main side effects	As above.

For hepatitis D virus infection

- Patients may respond to interferon-α, but remission does not usually persist after treatment is discontinued.

For autoimmune disease

- Treatment is indicated for patients with raised transaminase and IgG, histological evidence of chronic hepatitis, and serologic test results consistent with autoimmune hepatitis (*e.g.*, ANA, SMA, LKM antibodies) [5].

Standard dosage	Prednisone, 20–40 mg initially, reduced gradually (depending on clinical response); 5–10 mg daily maintenance dose may be needed. Azathioprine, 50–70 mg orally daily as adjunct.
Contraindications	Systemic infection; previous serious reaction to corticosteroids (*e.g.*, psychosis).
Main drug interactions	None.
Main side effects	*Steroids:* osteoporosis, proximal myopathy, skin thinning, cataracts, diabetes mellitus, weight gain, amenorrhea, depression, hypertension. *Azathioprine:* pancreatitis, bone-marrow suppression.

Surgical treatment

Orthotopic liver transplantation: liver transplantation is a treatment option for all patients with end-stage liver disease from chronic hepatitis; the 5-year survival rate is 50%–70% depending on the cause.
For HBV patients, recurrence of HBV accompanied by aggressive progression of liver disease is common [6].

Follow-up and management

- During interferon-α treatment, patients must be monitored closely for leukopenia and thrombocytopenia.

- Thyroid function must be checked because autoimmune disease can be exacerbated.

- Patients on long-term corticosteroid treatment should be monitored for steroid side effects and should have annual bone densitometry to check for osteoporosis.

- Patients who have progressed to cirrhosis are at risk of hepatocellular carcinoma; some investigators advocate surveillance with alpha fetoprotein and ultrasound evaluations every 6 months.

Key references

1. Scheuer PJ: Classification of chronic viral hepatitis: a need for reassessment. *J Hepatol* 1991, **13**:372–374.

2. Niederau C: Long term follow up of hepatitis e antigen positive patients treated with interferon alpha for chronic hepatitis B. *N Engl J Med* 1996, **334**:1422–1427.

3. Perillo RP: Interferon in the management of chronic hepatitis B. *Dig Dis Sci* 1993, **38**:577–593.

4. Poynard P: Meta-analysis of interferon randomized trials in the treatment of viral hepatitis C: effects of dose and duration. *Hepatology* 1996, **24**:778–789.

5. Johnson RL, *et al.*: The natural course and heterogeneity of autoimmune chronic active hepatitis. *Semin Liver Dis* 1991, **11**:187–196.

6. Lake JR, Wright TL: Liver transplantation for patients with hepatitis B: what have we learned from our results? *Hepatology* 1992, **13**:796–799.

Diagnosis

Symptoms

• Small hepatocellular carcinomas (<3 cm diameter) are usually asymptomatic; symptoms have insidious onset and usually consist of the following:

Upper abdominal pain: right hypochondrial or epigastric.

Weight loss, weakness, anorexia.

Abdominal swelling: may be due to ascites or enlarged liver.

Low-grade pyrexia.

Features of cirrhosis.

Metastatic symptoms: *e.g.*, bone pain.

Signs

• The liver is often enlarged and tender but may be normal when the tumor is relatively small.

Stigmata of chronic liver disease.

Arterial bruit: heard in 20% of patients.

Ascites.

Splenomegaly: in 20–30%.

Wasting: with more advanced disease.

Jaundice: in later stages of illness.

Investigations

Biochemistry: elevation of alkaline phosphatase without elevation in bilirubin common; aspartate aminotransferase and alanine aminotransferase elevations often mild.

Hematology: may show evidence of pancytopenia (hypersplenism) or erythrocytosis.

Alpha-fetoprotein: combined with ultrasonography for early detection; alpha fetoprotein possibly normal in small hepatocellular carcinoma; can be falsely elevated in patients with chronic hepatitis.

Chest radiography: may show raised right hemidiaphragm or metastases.

CT: useful to stage tumor; MRI scanning can be used to complement CT scanning and is of particular use in differentiating hemangiomas from other tumors.

Ultrasonography: may be useful for screening patients with cirrhosis for small hepatocellular carcinoma; 1-cm lesions can be detected, often as hypoechoic lesions.

Celiac axis angiography: tumors usually hypervascular; useful for staging disease that does not appear confined or in distinguishing benign nodules from malignant lesions.

Lipiodol CT: sensitive method for detecting small hepatocellular carcinoma; lipiodol, an oil contrast medium, cleared by hepatocytes but not by hepatocellular carcinoma; CT done 2 weeks after intra-arterial injection.

Liver biopsy: directed biopsy usually indicated; aspiration biopsy can be performed but is less diagnostic.

Complications

Acute intraperitoneal hemorrhage: often the terminal event.

Intravascular and intraductal growth.

Portal vein, inferior vena cava, and right atrial involvement.

Metastases: lung, bone, skin, brain, adrenal, and lymphogenous.

Hypoglycemia, hypercalcemia, polycythemia, hyperlipidemia.

Hepatic failure.

Variceal bleeding.

Differential diagnosis

Cystic lesions, hepatic metastatic carcinoma from other sites, abscess, adenoma, focal nodular hyperplasia.
Benign hemangioma.

Etiology

• Most cases of hepatocellular carcinoma develop in the setting of cirrhosis, including disease caused by the following [1]:
Chronic hepatitis B or C virus infection.
Alcoholic liver disease.
Autoimmune hepatitis or primary biliary cirrhosis.
Hemochromatosis.
Other inherited disorders of metabolism.
Tyrosinosis, alpha-1-antitrypsin deficiency.
Environmental carcinogens: aflatoxin is a potent chemical carcinogen, produced by *Aspergillus flavus*, which contaminates food in high-incidence areas; genetic changes have been documented.
Membranous inferior vena cava obstruction.
Androgenic anabolic steroids.
Contraceptives (controversial).

Epidemiology

• Areas of high, intermediate, and low incidence correspond crudely to prevalence of hepatitis B and C infection; low-incidence areas include northern Europe and North America.

• Hepatocellular carcinoma is more frequent in immigrants from high- and intermediate-prevalence countries (sub-Saharan Africa, China, southern and eastern Europe, Middle East).

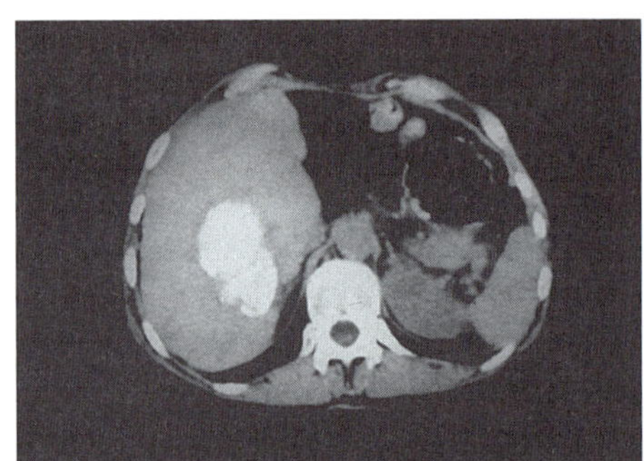

Retention of lipiodol within a hepatocellular carcinoma.

Treatment

Diet and lifestyle

• No special precautions are necessary.

Surgical treatment [2–5]

• Surgical resection is the treatment of choice for hepatocellular carcinoma when possible. Resection is recommended for solitary lesions without vascular evasion or extrahepatic metasasis: extensive resection is not recommended for patients with cirrhosis.

Orthotopic liver transplantation: for patients with underlying cirrhosis, orthotopic liver transplantation can be performed with solitary lesions <5 cm or with three tumor nodules each <3 cm.

Pharmacological treatment

Chemotherapy for palliation

• The response rate and survival in patients undergoing chemotherapy has been disappointing. Treatment should be given under special supervision.

Standard dosage	Doxorubicin, epirubicin, cisplatin, mitoxantrone every 3–4 weeks.
Contraindications	*All:* hypersensitivity. *Doxorubicin:* bone-marrow suppression, buccal ulcerations (after first dose). *Cisplatin:* pre-existing renal impairment, hearing disorders, bone-marrow suppression.
Special points	Other adjunctive agents, *e.g.*, tamoxifen, interferon, and interleukin-2, may be used. *Doxorubicin:* ECG, ejection fraction, and echocardiogram must be monitored. *Cisplatin:* hydration must be maintained; blood count, serum creatinine, and blood urea nitrogen must be monitored; audiometry needed.
Main drug interactions	*Cisplatin:* use with aminoglycoside or cephalosporins may cause increased ototoxicity or nephrotoxicity.
Main side effects	*Doxorubicin:* mucositis, bone-marrow suppression, alopecia, nausea, vomiting, diarrhea, cardiotoxicity. *Cisplatin:* nephrotoxicity, myelosuppression, neurotoxicity, ototoxicity, immunosuppression, nausea, vomiting. *Mitoxantrone:* leukopenia, thrombocytopenia, anemia, nausea, vomiting, alopecia, diarrhea, mucositis, cardiovascular effects (rare), blue-green discoloration of urine.

Percutaneous ethanol injection [6]

• Percutaneous ethanol injection is most effective in solitary tumors <3 cm (injection of tumor using alcohol or lipiodol, *e.g.*, alcohol, 10–20 mL intratumoral injection 3 times weekly for 12 treatments). This form of palliative treatment has become widely used in the past several years. Injection therapy is recommended for those patients with cirrhosis who are not good surgical candidates.

Treatment aims

To cure disease or prolong survival without recurrence.
To alleviate symptoms.

Other treatments

Transcatheter arterial embolization: for unresectable carcinoma, not for portal-vein thrombosis or Child's C cirrhosis; side effects include abdominal pain and fever; can be used with lipiodol-targeted chemotherapy.

Prognosis

• <25% of patients have partial responses to current chemotherapeutic regimens.

• 60% 5-year survival rates have been reported after intratumoral injection of alcohol for small tumors, but injection is without benefit in other series.

• 1-year survival rates as high as 78% after transcatheter arterial embolization have been reported.

• The 5-year survival rate after surgery is 25%; patients with encapsulated tumors, negative resection margins, no intracapsular or intravascular invasion of tumor cells, and Child's class A have better prognosis for surgical management [4].

Follow-up and management

• Serial imaging of the liver, lung, and bones is suggested to detect recurrence.

• Serial alpha-fetoprotein concentrations should be measured if initially high.

Key references

1. Simonetti RG, *et al.*: Hepatocellular carcinoma: a worldwide problem and the major risk factors. *Dig Dis Sci* 1991, **36**:962–972.

2. Dusheiko GM, *et al.*: Treatment of small hepatocellular carcinomas. *Lancet* 1992, **340**:285–288.

3. Di Bisceglie AM, *et al.*: Hepatocellular carcinoma. *Ann Intern Med* 1988, **108**:390–401.

4. Okuda K: Hepatocellular carcinoma: recent progress. *Hepatology* 1992, **15**:948–963.

5. Mazzafermo V: Liver transplantation for treatment of small hepatocellular carcinomas in patients with cirrhosis. *N Engl J Med* 1996, **334**:693–699.

6. Bruix J: Treatment of hepatocellular carcinoma. *Hepatology* 1997, **25**:259–262.

Diagnosis

Symptoms

Pain, burning, itching, tingling lasting 6–12 hours, vesicles (generally ulcerating or crusting within 48 hours): recurrent orolabial herpes (cold sores).
Fever, malaise, headache, altered personality, confusion, convulsions, paresis, paralysis, or coma: herpes encephalitis.
Fever, malaise, headache, nausea, vomiting, photophobia, neck stiffness: herpes meningitis.
Pain, photophobia, edema of the eyelid, lacrimation, blurring of vision: ocular herpes (spectrum ranges from superficial infections to stromal keratitis and iridocyclitis affecting inner eye).
Fever, sore mouth, swelling of gums, vesicles, ulceration in anterior half of mouth, tender anterior cervical lymph nodes: primary gingivostomatitis (frequently asymptomatic).
Pain, burning, itching, tingling, vesicles followed by ulcers and crusts in perineum, vaginal discharge, dysparunia: genital herpes; symptoms vary in severity, extent, and duration, depending on whether the infection is primary (usually most severe) or recurrent; may be asymptomatic.
Vesicles, ulcers, crusts, malaise, fever, lymphadenopathy: eczema herpeticum.
Pruritus, severe localized pain, vesicles, ulcers, crusts, fever, lymphadenopathy: other cutaneous herpes infections (herpes whitlow or gladiatorum, herpetic nipple).

Signs

Erythema progressing to vesicles, ulcers, and crusts: cutaneous lesions.
Altered personality, fluctuating levels of consciousness, focal or generalized convulsions, focal neurological findings, drowsiness, stupor, coma: herpes encephalitis.
Neck stiffness, positive Kernig's test: herpes meningitis.
Small blister or predendritic ulcers on cornea: ocular herpes; dendritic ulcers have serpentine branching appearance on fluoroscopy after fluorescein instillation.

Investigations

Cutaneous lesions

• Laboratory tests are usually not needed because symptoms and signs are diagnostic.

Tzanck test: may show multinucleated giant cells.
Immunofluorescence: can show viral antigens in cell smears.
Virus culture: from vesicle fluid or ulcers.

Herpes encephalitis

CT, MRI, EEG: show temporal lobe localization; EEG shows temporal spike and slow wave activity in 80% of patients.
CSF analysis: shows pleocytosis, usually 50–500 cells/mm^3, with lymphocyte predominance; erythrocytes often present, specimen may be xanthochromic; protein or red erythrocyte count may be raised, sugar usually normal; CSF can be examined for virus DNA (polymerase chain reaction) or viral antigens (immunology), but treatment should not await results.

Herpes meningitis

Lumbar puncture: to show CSF abnormalities of aseptic meningitis; herpes meningitis assumed when findings accompany mucocutaneous herpes, usually primary genital.
EEG: localized abnormalities in temporal lobe.

Ocular herpes

Ophthalmic examination and fluorescein: show presence of dendritic ulceration.
Abrasion of corneal cells: shows viral antigens; can be used for virus isolation.

Complications

Erythema multiforme, aseptic meningitis, urethritis, urinary retention, myelitis: due to mucocutaneous herpes.
Death, severe neurological sequelae: due to herpes encephalitis.
Visual loss, rupture of the globe (rare): due to recurrent ocular herpes.

Differential diagnosis

Mucocutaneous lesions
Causes of gingivitis and stomatitis.
Aphthous ulceration.
Coxsackievirus infection (hand, foot, and mouth).
Behçets syndrome.
Inflammatory bowel disease.
Varicella–zoster virus.
Sexually transmitted disease.

Herpes encephalitis
Other encephalitides.
Space-occupying lesions (*e.g.*, abscess, tumor, tuberculoma).

Herpes meningitis
Other causes of meningitis (*e.g.*, viruses, bacteria, fungi).

Ocular herpes
Ocular infections.

Etiology

Herpes simplex virus types 1 and 2: enveloped DNA viruses.

Exposure to strong sunlight, ultraviolet light, pneumonia, meningitis and malaria: cause reactivation (cold sores).

Fever, stressful events, depression, menstruation, sexual activity: causes of recurrences of genital herpes.

Immunosuppression: cause of mucocutaneous herpes.

Inoculation of virus into a finger or direct contact: cause of herpetic whitlow and herpes gladiatorum.

Bites and other traumatic forms of viral inoculation (*e.g.*, from needles, razors, contaminated finger nails): causes of herpetic nipple.

Epidemiology

• Seroepidemiological studies show that 30%–50% of patients in higher socio-economic groups and 100% of those in lower groups are infected with herpes simplex virus 1 by puberty.

• The prevalence of antibodies to herpes simplex virus 2 varies from 3% in nuns to ~70% in prostitutes.

• The prevalence of herpes encephalitis is 0.1–0.4 in 100 000 people.

Treatment

Diet and lifestyle

• Parents or grandparents with cold sores should not kiss young children.

• Laboratory tests have shown latex condoms to be effective mechanical barriers to herpes simplex virus.

Pharmacological treatment

• Acyclovir is of proven clinical value in some infections.

• It is not recommended for orolabial herpes or treatment of recurrent genital herpes.

• No other licensed compound has the combined safety and efficacy of acyclovir.

• Famcyclovir is now available and quite effective.

Standard dosage	*For initial genital herpes:* acyclovir, 200 mg 5 times daily for 10 days. *For recurrent genital herpes (prophylaxis):* acyclovir, 400–800 mg daily in 2–4 divided doses (continuous suppressive therapy). *For mucocutaneous herpes in immunocompromised patients:* acyclovir, i.v. or oral. *For herpes encephalitis:* acyclovir, 10 mg/kg i.v. 3 times daily for 10 days. *For ocular herpes simplex:* acyclovir, 400 mg 5 times daily, more effective than 3% ointment.
Contraindications	Hypersensitivity.
Special points	Limited experience in pregnancy and lactation so should be used only when potential benefits outweigh risks. Bioavailability of drug possibly reduced in patients being treated for malignancy so i.v. route advised.
Main drug interactions	Probenecid increases acyclovir half-life. No detrimental interactions recognized.
Main side effects	Raised urea and creatinine concentrations due to deposition of acyclovir crystals in tubules after rapid bolus doses, occasional nausea and vomiting, inflammation and ulceration at site of infusion if extravasation of drug occurs.

Treatment aims

To accelerate healing.

To reduce virus replication and dissemination.

To prevent recurrence, death and neurological complications, and blindness.

Prognosis

• Treatment of mucocutaneous herpes results in accelerated healing and reduced viral shedding.

• Treatment of herpes encephalitis results in reduced mortality and morbidity, especially in young patients with high Glasgow Coma Scale scores who are treated early.

• Treatment of ocular herpes has varying outcomes, depending on previous inflammation and scarring.

• Prophylactic treatment reduces the incidence and severity of recurrences in patients with recurrent genital herpes and viral shedding in immunocompromised patients.

Follow-up and management

• Pregnant women should inform their obstetrician of a past history of genital herpes.

General references

Conant MA, Berger TG, Coates TJ, *et al.*: Genital herpes: an integrated approach to management. *J Am Acad Dermatol* 1996, **35**:601–605.

Prober CG, *et al.*: The management of pregnancies complicated by genital infections with herpes simplex virus. *Clin Infect Dis* 1992, **15**:1031–1038.

Woo SB, Sonis ST: Recurrent aphthous ulcers: a review of diagnosis and treatment. *J Am Dent Assoc* 1996, **127**:1202–1213.

Diagnosis

Symptoms

Chickenpox (varicella)
Fever and malaise: in prodromal phase, variable.

Headache, myalgia.

Vesicular rash: frequently itchy.

Shingles (herpes zoster)
Pain in affected dermatome: may precede rash by a few days.

Mental confusion, depression: common in elderly patients.

• Symptoms often continue for weeks or months.

Signs

Chickenpox
Vesicular rash: maximal on face and trunk; rapidly evolving from macules and papules to vesicles and crusts; crops of new vesicles continuing to appear for 3–4 days; drying up in 7–10 days; possibly involving conjunctivae, oropharynx, vulva, vagina; larger lesions and slow evolution suggest underlying immune deficiency.

Shingles
Unilateral, segmental skin rash: lesions similar to chickenpox but often confluent; possibly ulcerating; often a few scattered lesions elsewhere; severe multiple dermatome or recurrent disease suggests underlying immune deficiency, including HIV infection.

Investigations

• Virological investigations are needed only when the clinical diagnosis is uncertain.

Tzanck smear: of material from vesicular skin lesions for rapid confirmation of herpes virus infection.

Tissue culture: to distinguish varicella–zoster virus from herpes simplex virus.

Complications

Chickenpox
Secondary bacterial infection of skin: usually *Staphylococcus aureus* or *Streptococcus pyogenes*.

Chickenpox pneumonia: particularly in adults and pregnant women.

Systemic spread: to liver, brain, lung of immunocompromised patients.

Hemorrhagic rash: in immunocompromised patients.

Encephalitis, polyneuritis, transverse myelitis: rare.

Reye's syndrome: in children, rare.

Hemolytic anemia, coagulopathy with hemorrhagic rash: rare.

Shingles
Uveitis, keratitis: in patients with ophthalmic herpes zoster.

Lower motor neuron paralysis.

Ramsey Hunt syndrome: herpes zoster of geniculate ganglion, with facial palsy, loss of taste, ipsilateal oral ulcers and skin lesions in pinna of ear.

Bowel and bladder dysfunction: in patients with sacral herpes zoster infection.

Encephalitis: rare.

Cerebral vasculopathy: trigeminal herpes zoster virus infection, with delayed cerebral infarction and hemiplegia; rare.

Differential diagnosis
Herpes simplex virus.
Other vesicular rashes, especially erythema multiforme.

Etiology
• Chickenpox is caused by direct contact or airborne transmission of varicella–zoster virus from either chickenpox or shingles.
• After primary infection, the virus probably incorporates its DNA into the satellite cells of dorsal-root or cranial-nerve ganglion cells.
• Later reactivation causes shingles.

Epidemiology
•2% of cases of chickenpox but 25% of deaths due to the disease occur in people aged >20 years.
• The prevalence of shingles rises steadily with age, 1 in 100 people >80 years being affected.
• Shingles in infants and young children probably is caused by a reactivation of intrauterine infection.
• Both chickenpox and shingles are cross-infection hazards in hospitals.

Infection in pregnancy
• Chickenpox in pregnant women may be severe and complicated by varicella pneumonia; patients should be monitored closely.
• Intrauterine infection may damage the fetus and cause limb scarring and hypoplasia, microcephaly or hydrocephalus, and eye abnormalities.
• This fetal varicella syndrome has an incidence of 1%–3% in the first trimester (much lower risk in subsequent trimesters).
• Termination of pregnancy on the grounds of maternal chickenpox is not indicated, because the risk to the fetus is small and unpredictable.
• Maternal herpes zoster infection is not a risk to the fetus.

Infectivity
Incubation period (chickenpox): 17 days.
Infectivity: from 2 days before onset of rash until lesions have dried.
Increased infectivity and susceptibility with immunodeficiency or immunosuppression.

Treatment

Diet and lifestyle

• Patients should avoid contact with susceptible individuals (*e.g.*, immunocompromised) until their skin lesions have dried.

Pharmacological treatment

Acyclovir

• Acyclovir is a highly selective antiviral agent that inhibits viral DNA polymerase and causes premature DNA chain termination.

Standard dosage	*For chickenpox and shingles in immunocompromised patients, chickenpox pneumonia:* acyclovir, 10 mg/kg i.v. 8-hourly.
	For cutaneous shingles: acyclovir, 800 mg orally 5 times daily for 7 days (started within 72 hours of rash onset).
	For ophthalmic shingles: acyclovir orally as above for 10 days.
	For severe maternal or neonatal chickenpox: acyclovir i.v.
Contraindications	Hypersensitivity.
Special points	High cost; no effect on latency or recurrence; not licensed for uncomplicated chickenpox.
Main drug interactions	Extreme lethargy has been reported on administration of zidovudine with i.v. acyclovir.
Main side effects	Rashes and gastrointestinal disturbances (occasionally), alterations in biochemical and hematological indices (more rarely), headaches and neurological reactions, particularly with i.v. administration, some risk of crystalluria and renal impairment at high dose (maximum oral dose in renal failure, 800 mg 3 times daily).

Varicella–zoster immune globulin

• This is distributed by the Public Health Laboratory Service (in short supply).

• It is used for highly susceptible contacts of chickenpox or shingles, including the following:

Bone-marrow transplant recipients (despite history of previous chickenpox).
Patients with debilitating disease (despite history of previous chickenpox).
HIV-positive patients with symptoms but no known varicella–zoster virus antibody.
Pregnant women without antibody (patients without a definite history of previous chickenpox must be screened for antibody).
Immunosuppressed patients who have been treated by high-dose steroids within the 3 months before contact (screened first).
Neonates up to 4 weeks of age whose mothers develop chickenpox between 1 week before and 1 month after delivery or those in contact with chickenpox or shingles whose mothers have no history of previous varicella–zoster infection or no antibody.
Premature babies <30 weeks gestation or weighing <1 kg at birth in contact with chickenpox.

Standard dosage	Varicella–zoster immune globulin, depending on age: *0-5 years,* 250 mg; *6-10 years,* 500 mg; *11-14 years,* 750 mg; *≥15 years,* 1000 mg.
Contraindications	Hypersensitivity to human immunoglobulin.
Special points	Must be given as soon as possible and not more than 10 days after exposure.
Main drug interactions	None.
Main side effects	Hypersensitivity reactions (rare).

• Live attenuated varicella vaccine is available, on a named-patient basis, for immunocompromised patients, especially children with leukemia.

Treatment aims

Chickenpox
To relieve symptoms in previously healthy patients.
To contain infection and reduce morbidity and mortality in immunocompromised patients or those with chickenpox pneumonia or maternal or neonatal infection.

Shingles
To accelerate healing and curtail pain.
To prevent complications in patients with ophthalmic herpes zoster.
To prevent progressive disease in immunocompromised patients.

Prognosis

• Mortality from chickenpox is increased in patients aged >20 years.

• Morbidity and mortality are reduced by acyclovir treatment in immunocompromised patients.

Follow-up and management

• Patients must be monitored for the development of complications.

• Pain continuing at the site of herpes zoster infection 30 days or more after an acute attack indicates postherpetic neuralgia, which should be treated by amitriptyline or sodium valproate. *See* Neuralgia, postherpetic *for details.*

General references

Anonymous: Acyclovir in general practice. *Drug Ther Bull* 1992, **30**:101–104.

Arvin AM: Varicella-zoster virus: overview and clinical manifestations. *Semin Dermatol* 1996, **15(suppl)**:4–7.

Bowsher D: Neurogenic pain syndromes and their management. *Br Med Bull* 1991, **47**:644–666.

Flamholc L: Neurological complications in herpes zoster. *Scand J Infect Dis* 1996, **100(suppl)**: 35–40.

Gilbert GL: Chickenpox during pregnancy. *BMJ* 1993, **306**:1079–1080.

Wallace MR, *et al.*: Treatment of adult varicella with oral acyclovir. A randomized, placebo-controlled trial. *Ann Intern Med* 1992, **117**:358–363.

Diagnosis

Symptoms

- The usual presentation is a lymph-node mass noticed by the patient.
- Fluctuation in size is not unusual.
- ~25% of patients have other symptoms.

"B" symptoms: unexplained fever >38ºC, loss of >10% body weight in 6 months, night sweats.

Pruritus: may lead to extensive excoriation from scratching.

Alcohol-induced nodal pain: rare and nonspecific.

Anorexia, lethargy.

Signs

Palpable lymphadenopathy: usually; careful examination of all node-bearing areas essential.

Extranodal involvement: *e.g.*, bone-marrow, liver, CNS; in 10%–20% of patients.

Investigations

- Initially, a good biopsy specimen must be carefully examined to make the diagnosis. Reed–Sternberg cells are the hallmark of Hodgkin's disease and the putative malignant cell.
- Investigation is then systematic to "stage" the disease.

Full blood count: possible neutrophilia, eosinophilia, lymphopenia, leukoerythroblastic picture if bone-marrow is involved.

ESR measurement: rate sometimes raised; can be useful disease marker and prognostic feature.

Liver function tests: abnormalities raise possibility of liver involvement.

Lactate dehydrogenase measurement: useful disease marker and prognostic feature.

Chest radiography: to look for nodal and pulmonary disease.

CT of chest and abdomen: to detect nodes; poor at detecting hepatic and splenic disease.

Lymphangiography: in centers with expertise, better than CT for assessing retroperitoneal nodes.

Bone-marrow examination: with trephine; rarely reveals unsuspected bone-marrow involvement.

Staging laparotomy: controversial now; in theory, might detect unsuspected splenic disease and change treatment plan.

Complications

Infection related to underlying defect in cell-mediated immunity: herpes zoster seen in 20%, and tuberculosis not unusual.

Differential diagnosis

Non-Hodgkin's lymphoma.

Infections, *e.g.*, Epstein-Barr virus, toxoplasma, cytomegalovirus.

Angioimmunoblastic lymphadenopathy.

Etiology [1]

- The origin of the Reed–Sternberg cell, the putative malignant cell, is still debated; cell surface marker CD15 is usually expressed; T- or B-lymphocyte markers are also sometimes expressed.
- Recent evidence implicates Epstein–Barr virus (EBV) in the cause of some cases of Hodgkin's disease; the EBV genome has been found incorporated into DNA in Reed–Sternberg cells, and serological evidence links EBV with Hodgkin's disease.

Epidemiology [1]

- Hodgkin's disease has a bimodal distribution, with a first peak at 15–40 years, then increasing incidence with increasing age.
- Male patients are more frequently affected than female patients.
- The incidence is higher in whites.

Classification

Based on the Rye system:

1. Nodular sclerosing (>80% of patients): dense bands of collagen with nodules of tumor.
2. Lymphocyte predominant: infiltrate of small lymphocytes.
3. Mixed cellularity: pleomorphic infiltrate.
4. Lymphocyte depleted: few Reed–Sternberg cells seen.

Staging

- Hodgkin's disease appears to start unifocally and to spread to adjacent lymph nodes in an orderly fashion. Staging (based on the Ann Arbor Scheme) is important for rational planning of treatment.

Stage I: involvement of single lymph-node region.

Stage II: two or more lymph-node regions on same side of diaphragm.

Stage III: lymph-node involvement on both sides of diaphragm, including spleen.

Stage IV: diffuse involvement of extranodal sites.

Suffix A: no systemic symptoms.

Suffix B: "B" symptoms as described earlier.

Treatment

Diet and lifestyle

• Some patients continue a normal lifestyle during chemotherapy; others feel quite unwell.

Pharmacological treatment

• Hodgkin's disease is a chemo- and radiosensitive disease.

• Treatment decision depends on accurate staging and should also take into account current clinical trials.

Radiotherapy [2]

• Patients with stage I and IIA disease and no other adverse prognostic features can be cured by radiotherapy alone.

• This is usually given to an extended field beyond the area of overt nodal disease over 1 month.

• Initial treatment with combined chemo- and radiotherapy provides no survival advantage in early-stage disease and may lead to increased toxicity.

Chemotherapy [3]

• For more advanced disease, several standard four-drug combinations are used, *e.g.*, MOPP (mechlorethamine, vincristine, procarbazine, prednisone), LOPP (chlorambucil, vincristine, procarbazine, prednisone), ABVD (doxorubicin, bleomycin, vinblastine, dacarbazine), or EVAP (etoposide, vincristine, doxorubicin, prednisone).

• Precise details of treatment should always be decided by an experienced hematologist or oncologist.

• Good i.v. access is needed because some drugs, particularly vinca alkaloids and anthracyclines, are vesicant.

• Admission to the hospital is not usually required for treatment, although treatment should commence as soon as practical after initial diagnosis and staging.

Treatment after relapse

• Relapse after initial treatment may still be compatible with long-term survival.

• Patients who relapse after radiotherapy can be "salvaged" with chemotherapy with similar overall survival to those who were initially treated with both modalities; the converse is rarely true.

• The longer the duration of first remission, the greater is the chance of obtaining a second remission on standard treatment.

• Increasing dose intensity of treatment is of benefit in Hodgkin's disease; ~50% of patients resistant to standard treatment can still achieve long-term survival with high-dose chemotherapy regimens such as BEAM (BCNU [carmustine], etoposide, cytarabine, melphalan) and autologous hematopoietic stem cell support [4,5].

Complications of treatment

Skin reactions and pneumonitis after radiotherapy.

Myelosuppression, emesis, hair loss, and neurotoxicity after chemotherapy.

Second malignancy: lung cancer; acute myeloid leukemia (~ 1%), peak incidence 4–11 years after initial treatment.

Impaired fertility after chemotherapy.

Pulmonary fibrosis.

Treatment aims

To cure the disease with minimal toxicity from the treatment.

Prognosis

• The overall survival at 10 years is ~60%.

• Poor prognostic features include the following:

Older age.

Presence of B symptoms.

Mixed cellularity/lymphocyte-depleted histology.

Stage III or IV disease at presentation.

ESR >40 mm/h.

Lactic dehydrogenase >normal.

Mass >10 cm.

Failure to obtain complete remission after adequate first-line treatment.

Follow-up and management

• Regular review during treatment is essential to detect complications and assess response.

• Full blood count is mandatory before administration of each cycle of treatment.

• After treatment is finished, full restaging is needed.

• Follow-up interval may gradually lengthen but should be continued indefinitely to detect late complications of treatment or relapse.

Key references

1. Collins RH Jr: The pathogenesis of Hodgkin's disease. *Blood Rev* 1990, **4**:61–68.

2. DeVita VT Jr, Hubbard SM: Drug treatment: Hodgkin's disease. *N Engl J Med* 1993, **328**:560–565.

3. Linch DC, *et al.*: Dose intensification with autologous bone marrow transplantation in relapsed and resistant Hodgkin's disease: results of a BNLI randomised trial. *Lancet* 1993, **341**:1051–1054.

4. Diehl V, Engert A (eds.): Proceedings of the Third International Symposium on Hodgkin's Lymphoma. *Ann Oncol* 1996, **7(suppl 4)**:1–143.

5. Horning SJ, Chao NJ, Negrin RS, *et al.*: High-dose therapy and autologous hematopoietic progenitor cell transplantation for recurrent or refractory Hodgkin's disease: analysis of the Stanford University results and prognostic indices. *Blood* 1997, **89**:801–813.

Diagnosis

Symptoms

• Hypercalcemia causes either no symptoms or nonspecific symptoms, *e.g.*, the following:

Tiredness and lethargy.

Nausea and vomiting.

Constipation.

Polydipsia and polyuria.

Muscle weakness.

Impaired mental function and occasional loss of consciousness: in severe cases.

Signs

• Specific signs of hypercalcemia are rare.

Signs of dehydration: caused by moderate to severe hypercalcemia.

Nephrolithiasis: may be seen in hyperparathyroidism.

Corneal and soft-tissue calcification.

Investigations

Serum calcium measurement: total serum calcium influenced by serum protein concentration, especially albumin.

Parathyroid hormone measurement: high concentration indicates probable hyperparathyroidism; measurement of intact parathyroid hormone molecule is preferred.

Tests for anemia, liver function tests, alkaline phosphatase and serum protein electrophoresis: malignancy more probable if concentrations are abnormal or raised.

Chest and skeletal radiography: indicated if malignancy probable.

• Specific investigations of other causes of hypercalcemia are indicated when the more common causes have been excluded.

Complications [1]

Dehydration: common and, unless corrected, causes worsening of hypercalcemia.

Bone pain: common in malignancy, rare in hyperparathyroidism.

Pancreatitis: rare complication of chronic hypercalcemia.

Differential diagnosis

Not applicable.

Etiology

• 97% of cases of hypercalcemia in general medical practice are due either to primary hyperparathyroidism or to malignancy, which is usually disseminated.

• Other causes include the following:

Severe thyrotoxicosis.

Vitamin D excess.

Vitamin A excess.

Calcium treatment to bind phosphate in chronic renal failure.

Sarcoidosis.

Familial benign or hypocalciuric hypercalcemia.

Diuretic phase of acute renal failure.

Milk-alkali syndrome.

Addison's disease.

Epidemiology

• Primary hyperparathyroidism increases markedly after middle age and is three times more common in women than in men.

• Hyperparathyroidism is typically present in multiple endocrine neoplasia type I (90%–95%), but is less common in type II (20%–30%).

• Many malignancies can be complicated by hypercalcemia.

Treatment

Diet and lifestyle

• A low-calcium diet is of little value in treating hypercalcemia, although high calcium intake exacerbates the disorder.

• Patients with hyperparathyroidism treated conservatively should be advised to maintain an adequate fluid intake, especially when they are unwell.

Pharmacological treatment [2]

For hyperparathyroidism [3]

• The only definitive treatment of hypercalcemia due to primary hyperparathyroidism is surgical.

• Estrogen therapy helps to maintain bone mass in women with hyperparathyroidism.

For malignancy [3]

• Intravenous rehydration *followed* by diuresis is of primary importance.

• The bisphosphonate drugs are frequently first-line pharmacological therapy for significant hypercalcemia.

Standard dosage	Pamidronate, 60–90 mg i.v. by continuous infusion.
	Etidronate, 5–10 mg daily, can also be used.
Contraindications	Caution in renal failure.
Special points	Serum calcium falls to or toward normal within 3–5 days. Oral bisphosphonates must be taken on an empty stomach; they are much less effective than i.v. preparations.
Main drug interactions	Absorption of oral drug reduced by antacids, iron, and calcium.
Main side effects	Gastrointestinal upset.

For sarcoidosis

• Hypercalcemia responds rapidly to steroids.

Standard dosage	Prednisone, 20 mg daily, reduced to lowest dose that controls hypercalcemia.
Contraindications	Systemic infections; caution in peptic ulceration or diabetes.
Main drug interactions	None.
Main side effects	Cushingoid appearance (with maintained high doses), dyspepsia.

Adjunctive therapy

• Calcitonin may be used early as an adjunct to treat hypercalcemia.

Standard dosage	Calcitonin, 4 IU/kg s.c. or i.m. every 12 hours; dose may be increased to 8 IU/kg every 12 or every 6 hours if necessary.
Contraindications	Allergy to synthetic salmon calcitonin.
Main drug interactions	Effective within 12 hours but effectiveness greatly diminished by 72–96 hours.
Main side effects	Hypocalcemia.

Nonpharmacological treatment

For hyperparathyroidism

• Surgery should be seriously considered for all younger patients and those with complications of the disease (*e.g.*, renal stones).

• Elderly asymptomatic patients can be followed conservatively [4].

• Surgery *must* be done by an experienced parathyroid surgeon.

• After successful surgery, serum calcium is usually normal or low within 24 hours.

• Transient hypocalcemia may occur; rarely, permanent hypoparathyroidism may follow.

For malignancy

• Surgical cure is rare because of early metastases.

Key references

1. Larsson K, *et al.*: The risk of hip fractures in patients with primary hyperparathyroidism: a population based cohort study with a follow-up of 19 years. *J Int Med* 1993, **234**:585–593.

2. Bilezikian JP: Management of hypercalcaemia. *J Clin Endocrinol Metab* 1993, **77**:1445–1449.

3. Heath DA: The treatment of hypercalcaemia of malignancy. *Clin Endocrinol* 1991, **34**:155–157.

4. Proceedings of the NIH Consensus Development Conference on diagnosis and management of asymptomatic primary hyperparathyroidism. Bethesda, Maryland, October 29–31, 1990. *J Bone Miner Res* 1991, **6(suppl 2)**:81–166.

Diagnosis

Symptoms

Hyperglycemia
Polyuria, thirst, polydipsia.

Weight loss.

Lassitude, general malaise.

Decreasing level of consciousness.

Ketoacidosis
Nausea, vomiting, abdominal pain.

Dyspnea.

Precipitating cause
Symptoms of infection, myocardial infarction, or other illness.

Signs

General
Dehydration: particularly marked in hyperosmolar coma.

Hypotension.

Variable level of consciousness.

Signs of precipitating cause, especially fever: however, infection may be present in absence of fever in patients with ketoacidosis.

Ketoacidosis
Kussmaul's respiration, ketones on breath.

Peripheral vasodilatation, warm skin, tachycardia, generalized abdominal tenderness.

Investigations [1,2]

To rapidly establish diagnosis
Capillary blood glucose analysis.

Urinalysis: for glucose, ketones.

To confirm diagnosis
Laboratory blood glucose analysis.

Serum sodium, potassium, bicarbonate, phosphate, blood urea nitrogen, and creatinine measurement.

Arterial blood gas: if indicated.

To identify precipitating cause
Complete blood count: to look for anemia or leukocytosis.

Blood, urine, and throat cultures.

ECG: may show acute myocardial infarction or signs of electrolyte disturbance.

Chest radiography: may show infection or pulmonary edema.

Abdominal ultrasonography or paracentesis: to exclude acute abdominal disease if abdominal signs do not resolve quickly.

Complications

Cardiac arrest.

Thromboembolism: particularly if patient is hyperosmolar.

Aspiration pneumonia.

Renal failure.

Rhabdomyolysis: rare; may result from hypophosphatemia.

Differential diagnosis

Ketotic
Hyperventilation, chest infection, lactic acidosis, sepsis.
Acute abdominal disease.

Nonketotic
Hypercalcemia.
Cerebrovascular disease.
Thyrotoxicosis.

Etiology [2]

• Causes include the following (in both type I and II diabetes):
Initial presentation of diabetes.
Physical stressors, precipitating rise in counter-regulatory hormones and relative deficiency of insulin (*e.g.*, infection, myocardial infarction, stroke).
Omission of insulin.

Epidemiology

• The incidence is not declining, despite advances in diabetes education.

• 3–8 episodes occur in 1000 diabetic patients each year.

Treatment

Diet and lifestyle

• Patients should be told not to stop insulin treatment if they become acutely ill. Instead, they should call their physician for "sick-day" management.

Pharmacological treatment [3]

• Rehydration and correction of electrolyte imbalance must begin immediately.

• A central venous pressure measurement may be a useful guide to fluid replacement in elderly patients or those with cardiac or renal disease.

• If the patient is comatose, a nasogastric tube should be passed.

• Urinary catheterization may be needed to allow accurate monitoring of urinary output.

Rehydration

0.9% saline solution, 1 L in first hour to restore circulating volume, raise blood pressure, and open renal circulation; then infusion rates should be adjusted as clinically indicated.

• 0.45% saline solution should be used if serum sodium is >155 mEq/L.

• Colloid solution can be given if the patient remains hypotensive.

Insulin

By continuous i.v. infusion (preferred): *if ketotic*: 6 U/h by pump; *if nonketotic*: 3–4 U/h.

• Adjustments in these insulin doses may be required in some patients.

• Treatment is continued until blood glucose is 250 mg/dL; then the dose of insulin should be halved, and i.v. infusion of 10% dextrose commenced at 80 mL/h.

Continue i.v. insulin therapy until serum bicarbonate has returned to near normal levels.

Potassium

• The total body deficit of potassium is ~1000 mEq.

• Infusion should be started when serum potassium is <5.0 mEq/L and urine output has been demonstrated.

• Potassium chloride, 20–80 mEq/h, well diluted in rehydration fluid, should be given.

• Treatment should be monitored by serum potassium measurement (and ECG, if hyperkalemic).

Sodium bicarbonate

• This is rarely of benefit. It may be given if pH is <7.1.

• Sodium bicarbonate, 100 mL 8.4% in 30 minutes, with 20 mEq potassium chloride, should be given.

Other options

Anticoagulation: low-dose s.c. heparin, if no contraindications; consider full-dose i.v. heparin if serum osmolality >360 mOsmol/kg.

Antibiotics: broad spectrum if there is any suspicion of infection.

• Replacement of other electrolytes (magnesium, phosphate) is rarely required.

Complications of treatment

• Most complications are avoidable with meticulous care and attention to detail.

Hypo- or hyperkalemia.

Hypoglycemia.

Fluid overload, especially in elderly patients.

Cerebral edema.

Adult respiratory distress syndrome.

Treatment aims

To save the patient's life.
To rehydrate the patient.
To restore acid-base and electrolyte balance to normal.
To achieve euglycemia in 24–48 hours.

Prognosis

• Mortality remains at 5%–15% in diabetic ketoacidosis and 30%–50% in hyperosmolar coma, even in experienced units.
• In elderly patients, the cause of death is often the underlying precipitating disorder rather than the metabolic upset.

Follow-up and management

Response to treatment

• Response should be monitored at the bedside (pulse, blood pressure, respiratory rate every 30–60 minutes, capillary glucose hourly) and in the laboratory (glucose, sodium, potassium, bicarbonate, creatinine, pH on admission and at 2-hour intervals until clinically stable).

Later management

• Patients should be given fluids or a light diet when able to eat, but i.v. insulin should be continued.
• When patients can tolerate oral intake, they should be transferred to s.c. insulin regimen that includes long-acting insulin.
• A 1–3-hour overlap must be allowed before i.v. insulin is discontinued, to allow time for s.c. absorption.

Follow-up

• The events leading to admission should be reviewed in an effort to educate the patient and prevent further admissions; all patients should be taught "sick-day" rules, including advice on seeking professional help early.
• Patients presenting in hyperosmolar coma may not need long-term insulin, but continuing it for a few weeks is probably safer, before stopping under close supervision.

Key references

1. Siperstein MD: Diabetic ketoacidosis and hyperosmolar coma. *Endocrinol Metab Clin North Am* 1992, **21**:415–432.

2. Marshall SM: Hyperglycaemic emergencies. *Care Crit Ill*, 1993, **9**:220–223.

3. Berger W, Keller U: Treatment of diabetic ketoacidosis and non-ketotic hyperosmolar coma. *Clin Endocrinol Metab* 1991, **6**:1–22.

Diagnosis

Symptoms

• Often no symptoms are manifest.

Hyperkalemia
Skeletal muscle weakness.

Diarrhea.

Hypokalemia
Muscle weakness and fatigue.

Polyuria and polydipsia.

Palpitations.

Signs

Hyperkalemia
Skeletal muscle weakness.

Irregular pulse.

Ileus.

Bradycardia, heart block, cardiac arrest (asystolic).

Hypokalemia
Postural hypotension.

Ileus.

Skeletal muscle weakness: rarely, respiratory distress.

Cardiac arrhythmias: atrial and ventricular premature beats, atrial or ventricular tachycardia.

Investigations

• Markedly abnormal potassium levels should be repeated immediately with optimal venipuncture technique and rapid transfer to laboratory.

Renal function tests: blood urea nitrogen, creatinine.

ECG.

Acid–base analysis.

Magnesium, phosphate, and glucose measurements.

Urinary potassium and pH measurement.

Creatine kinase measurement.

Complications

Hyperkalemia
Sudden death: asystole.

Hypokalemia
Rhabdomyolysis on vigorous exertion (acute).

Growth retardation in children.

Nephrogenic diabetes insipidus.

Negative nitrogen balance.

Interstitial nephritis: renal impairment.

Glucose intolerance.

Myocardial fibrosis.

Differential diagnosis

Artifact of sampling technique (hyperkalemia).

Etiology

Hyperkalemia

• The most common cause is a combination of renal impairment (may be minimal or transient) with the following:

Excessive potassium intake: due to diet, salt substitutes, potassium penicillins, transfusion of stored blood.

Redistribution: due to acidosis, exercise, hyperkalemic familial periodic paralysis, hormonal deficiencies (insulin, aldosterone, cortisol), drugs (beta-blockers, alpha-antagonists), release from damaged tissues, hyperosmolality.

Impaired renal excretion: due to acute or chronic renal failure, potassium-conserving diuretics, inadequate mineralocorticosteroid hormones, angiotensin-converting enzyme inhibitors, NSAIDs, cyclosporine, pentamidine, type IV renal tubular acidosis.

Impaired gut excretion: due to colectomy in patients with pre-existing renal failure.

Hypokalemia

Inadequate intake: due to diet.

Redistribution: due to anabolic states, correction of severe anemia, transfusion of washed or frozen erythrocytes, metabolic alkalosis, some myeloproliferative disorders, beta-agonists, correction of hyperglycemia, hypokalemic periodic paralysis.

Gut losses: due to vomiting or nasogastric aspiration, diarrhea, purgative abuse.

Urinary losses: due to diuretics, hyperaldosteronism, Bartter's syndrome, Cushing's syndrome, licorice abuse, excess adrenocorticotropic hormone, renal tubular acidosis, tubular toxins (*e.g.*, cisplatin, amphotericin, aminoglycosides), urinary diversion into gut, magnesium depletion.

Epidemiology

• Hyperkalemia rarely occurs without renal impairment.

• Hypokalemia is more common, being associated with the use of common drugs (diuretics and purgatives) and as a common complication of diarrheal states.

Treatment

Diet and lifestyle

• Hyperkalemic patients with underlying chronic renal failure need dietary advice to restrict the daily potassium intake to 40–60 mEq/day; high-potassium foods include fruits, chocolate, nuts, and instant coffee.

• Hypokalemia can rarely be corrected by dietary means.

Pharmacological treatment

For hyperkalemia: moderate

• For moderate hyperkalemia with an acute rise in potassium to <6.5 mEq/L and a normal ECG, the following measures should be taken:

Intake of potassium decreased.

Offending drug removed.

Good urinary output ensured.

Plasma potassium concentration measured every 6 hours to ensure falling values.

For hyperkalemia: severe

• An acute rise in potassium to >6.5 mEq/L and abnormal ECG or chronically raised potassium >8 mEq/L is a medical emergency.

• ECG monitoring is needed.

• Rapid correction is vital.

• Emergency dialysis is needed if the patient is oliguric and volume overloaded.

Standard dosage	*Acute therapies:* 10% calcium gluconate solution, 10 mL i.v. slowly. 50% glucose solution 50 mL, containing insulin, 10 U, i.v. *Longer-term therapies:* 8.4% sodium bicarbonate solution, 50 mL i.v. only if acidotic. Sodium polystyrene sulfonate, 15 g, and lactulose, 10 mL orally 6-hourly *or* sodium polystyrene sulfonate by rectal retention enema if no ileus present. Furosemide or bumetanide i.v. every 4–6 hours to achieve urine flow rate >50 mL/h, *e.g.*, bumetanide 1 mg initially, increased to 5 mg.
Contraindications	None.
Special points	Patient must be checked for hypoglycemia after i.v. glucose and insulin. *Calcium gluconate:* a cardioprotective agent, does *not* lower plasma potassium concentration.
Main drug interactions	None.
Main side effects	None.

For hypokalemia

Standard dosage	Effervescent potassium chloride, 80–200 mEq orally daily. Potassium chloride, 60–120 mEq i.v. over 24 hours.
Contraindications	None.
Special points	Oral supplements should be used whenever possible. Intravenous repletion is potentially dangerous: 10 mEq/h is usually safe; higher rates may be used, but ECG monitoring is essential. Potassium as chloride should be used in patients with alkalosis to minimize continued urinary losses of potassium.
Main drug interactions	Hypokalemia exacerbates digoxin toxicity.
Main side effects	Late hyperkalemia due to delayed gastrointestinal absorption after oral potassium supplements.

Treatment aims

To restore acid–base balance and plasma potassium slowly over 24–72 hours.

Prognosis

• Prognosis depends on the underlying condition.

Follow-up and management

• If deviations are gross, frequent and repeated measurements of plasma potassium are essential for several days.

General references

Androgue HJ, Wesson DE: Potassium. In *Blackwell's Basics of Medicine*. Oxford: Blackwell Scientific Publications; 1994.

Jacobsen HR, Rector FC (eds.): Renal regulation of extracellular fluid composition. *Kidney Int* 1990, **38**:569–743.

Schrier RW (ed.): *Renal and Electrolyte Disorders*, edn 4. Boston: Little Brown & Co; 1992.

Tannen RL: Potassium metabolism. In *Current Nephrology*, vol 15. Edited by Gonick HC. St Louis: Mosby Year Book; 1992:109–148.

Diagnosis

Symptoms

• Symptoms depend on both absolute sodium level and rate of change.

Hypernatremia
Restlessness.

Irritability.

Lethargy, somnolence.

Hyponatremia
Lethargy.

Confusion and disorientation.

Anorexia.

Nausea.

Muscle cramps.

Signs

Hypernatremia
Increased reflexes.

Increased muscle tone.

Depressed consciousness.

Convulsions.

Altered consciousness, coma.

Hyponatremia
Decreased reflexes.

Hypothermia.

Pseudobulbar palsy.

Convulsions.

Cheyne–Stokes respiration.

Altered consciousness, coma.

Investigations

• Most sodium is extracellular, so changes in sodium balance are reflected in changes in extracellular fluid volume (ECFV).

• Changes in serum sodium concentration reflect alterations in the sodium : water ratio in the extracellular fluid and can occur with increased, normal, or decreased ECFV (increased, normal, or reduced total body sodium).

Detection of edema, estimation of jugular venous pressure, tissue turgor, erect and supine pulse and blood pressure, peripheral perfusion, auscultation of lung bases, and patient weighing: vital for accurate documentation of state of ECFV; edema always indicates raised total body sodium.

Renal function tests, chest radiography, ECG, liver function tests, albumin and glucose measurement, urine and plasma osmolality, endocrine tests (thyroid and adrenal); echocardiography if cardiac disease suspected.

Complications

Hypernatremia
Seizures

Shrinkage of brain cells.

Rupture of cerebral veins.

Cerebral venous (sinus) thrombosis.

Intracranial hemorrhage.

Hyponatremia
Seizures

Cerebral edema.

Raised intracranial pressure.

Herniation of brain stem.

Central pontine myelinolysis: attributed to over-rapid correction; causes permanent residual neurological deficits; rare.

Differential diagnosis

Hyperlipidemia or hyperproteinemia: may cause pseudohyponatremia; serum osmolarity in these patients will be normal.

Hyperglycemia: also causes pseudohyponatremia. To estimate the decrease in serum sodium, divide serum glucose by 62.

Etiology

Causes of hypernatremia

Normal or slightly reduced ECFV: diabetes insipidus, dry ventilation, hypodipsia, sweating.

Increased ECFV (edema): excessive sodium intake, excessive adrenocortical hormones.

Decreased ECFV (without free access to water): excessive loss of sodium in urine, excessive loss of gastrointestinal secretions, burns, sweating.

Causes of hyponatremia

Normal or slightly expanded ECFV: excessive water intake, syndrome of inappropriate antidiuretic hormone secretion (drug-induced).

Increased ECFV (edema): acute or chronic renal failure, cardiac failure, cirrhosis with ascites, nephrotic syndrome, pregnancy.

Decreased ECFV (with free access to water): excessive loss of sodium in urine, excessive loss of gastrointestinal secretions, burns, sweating.

Epidemiology

• Hypernatremia is common in the elderly, and in immobile or unconscious patients, all of whom may lack access to water.

• Hyponatremia is common in hospitals because of inappropriate fluid replacement, usually with dextrose saline solution or over-diuresis of patients with cardiac failure.

Treatment

Diet and lifestyle

• Hypernatremia and hyponatremia usually develop in hospitals; thus the primary underlying disease dominates the clinical picture.

• Alterations in sodium intake are needed for patients with changes in their extracellular fluid volume, *e.g.*, sodium restriction for those with edema.

• Compulsive water drinkers and drug abusers may need psychiatric counseling.

Pharmacological treatment

Hypernatremia

• Extracellular fluid volume must first be defined and corrected; a decrease should be corrected by normal saline solution, an increase by diuretics or dialysis.

• Then the hypernatremia can be corrected *slowly* by 0.5% dextrose, dextrose with saline, or 0.9% saline solution, giving about half of the calculated volume replacement over the first 24 hours.

• Central venous pressure monitoring and urethral catheterization for monitoring urine output may be needed.

Hyponatremia

• For mild to moderate chronic dilutional hyponatremia, restriction of water intake alone may be sufficient.

• For edematous states, diuretics should be given.

• Patients with true sodium depletion should be given 0.9% saline (often with diuretics) or 3% hypertonic saline (without diuretics) solution infused slowly, to correct serum sodium concentrations—over-rapid correction may cause brain damage (hyponatremia should be corrected by 1.5–2 mEq/h if acute onset or ≤1 mEq/h if chronic). Serum sodium should be frequently monitored, and saline infusion discontinued when serum sodium reaches 120–125 mEq/L.

• Administration of sodium to edematous patients may precipitate cardiac failure; diuretics may be needed to normalize intravascular volume.

• In severe cases, central venous pressure monitoring and urethral catheterization to monitor urine output are needed.

Treatment aims

To correct extracellular fluid volume.

To correct serum sodium concentration.

To avoid morbidity secondary to rapid changes in serum sodium or ECFV.

Prognosis

• Prognosis depends on the underlying condition.

• Acute changes in onset or correction are more dangerous than slow changes.

• Very old or very young patients are most vulnerable.

• Permanent neurological deficits are common, especially if correction is over-rapid.

Follow-up and management

• Follow-up depends on the underlying condition.

General references

Richardson RMA: Water metabolism. In *Current Nephrology*, vol 15. Edited by Gonick HC. St Louis: Mosby Year Book; 1992:149–206.

Schrier RW: Body fluid volume regulation in health and disease: a unifying hypothesis. *Ann Intern Med* 1990, **113**:155–159.

Sterns RH: Central nervous system complications of hyponatremia. In *International Year Book of Nephrology*. Edited by Andreucci VE, Fine LG. Berlin: Springer-Verlag; 1992:55–74.

Diagnosis

Symptoms

• Symptoms can be subdivided into those directly related to hyperprolactinemia and those due to the mass effect of a pituitary macroadenoma (if present).

Hyperprolactinemia

Galactorrhea.

Amenorrhea, oligomenorrhea: in women.

Impotence: in men.

Infertility.

Reduced libido.

Macroadenoma

Headache.

Visual field defect: typically bitemporal hemianopia or diplopia.

Convulsions: temporal-lobe epilepsy due to local extension of tumor (rare).

Cerebrovascular accident: rare.

Signs

Macroadenoma

Hypopituitarism.

Optic atrophy: if tumor compressing optic nerve.

Loss of secondary sexual characteristics, postural hypotension, hypothyroidism, delayed or arrested puberty: signs of hypopituitarism.

Investigations [1,2]

Detailed drug history.

Serum prolactin measurement: thyroid-releasing hormone and other dynamic stimulation tests are of no value.

Thyroid function tests: hypothyroidism is a cause of raised serum prolactin.

Gonadotropin and gonadal steroids measurement: to determine if hypogonadism is present.

Pituitary MRI or CT: to identify tumor.

If macroadenoma is present

Visual field study.

Corticotropic hormone and cortisol measurement.

Dynamic pituitary function testing.

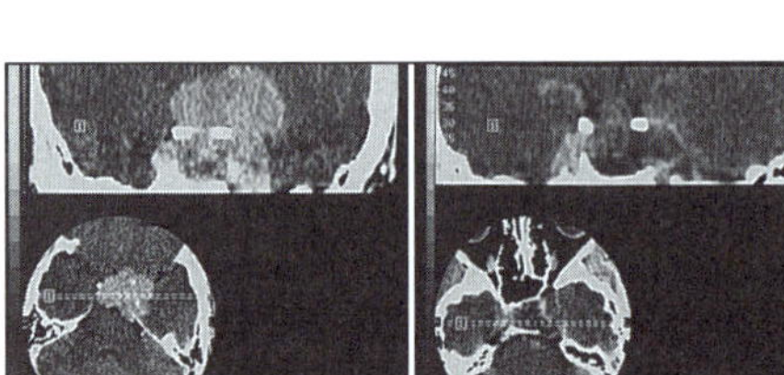

Axial and coronal view of large prolactinoma (*left*). Repeat scan (*right*) showing virtual disappearance of tumor on treatment by bromocriptine.

Complications

Hyperprolactinemia

Infertility, impotence.

Osteoporosis: due to hypogonadism.

Macroadenoma

Hydrocephalus.

Blindness.

Hypopituitarism.

Cranial nerve palsy.

Treatment

Diet and lifestyle

• Prolactinoma therapy will restore fertility to many women. Therefore, counseling regarding contraception is very important.

Pharmacological treatment [1–4]

Standard dosage	Bromocriptine, 1.25 mg initially, in the middle of a snack last thing at night; dose titrated against serum prolactin. Cabergoline (Dostinex), 0.25 mg twice weekly, slowly increased to 1.0 mg twice weekly [5]. Recently approved for treatment of prolactinomas; major advantage is twice-weekly dosing.
Contraindications	Toxemia of pregnancy, sensitivity to ergot alkaloid, history of psychosis.
Special points	An alternative dopamine agonist in cases of bromocriptine or cabergoline intolerance or resistance is pergolide. However, pergolide is not specifically approved for the treatment of hyperprolactinemia.
Main drug interactions	None.
Main side effects	Gastrointestinal disturbance, particularly nausea; postural hypotension; first-dose hypotension (effect negated by drugs that raise prolactin concentration).

Special considerations

Oral contraceptive use

• Estrogens can stimulate prolactinoma growth. If oral contraceptives are used, prolactin levels should be monitored. If they rise, or patients develop symptoms of pituitary enlargement, then a pituitary MRI, visual fields, or both, should be obtained. Low-dose oral contraceptives (ethinyl estradiol, ≤30 μg daily) are preferred, and physicians should have a low threshold for discontinuing oral contraceptives if complications develop.

Pregnancy

• Neither prolactinoma nor bromocriptine therapy is an absolute contraindication to pregnancy. Prolactin rises normally during pregnancy, and may therefore be misleading in pregnant patients with pre-existing hyperprolactinemia. Instead, patients with prolactinomas should be followed closely for evidence of pituitary enlargement (*e.g.*, visual field abnormalities). Bromocriptine is not approved for use during pregnancy and should be discontinued if possible.

Treatment aims

To normalize serum prolactin concentration. To retain normal pituitary function.

Other treatments [1,2]

Transsphenoidal surgery: typically reserved for patients who either fail therapy with dopamine agonists or have symptoms secondary to tumor mass. Resection of a microadenoma can be curative, and some authors believe this a viable alternative to long-term bromocriptine agonist therapy. Pituitary radiotherapy: adjunct to surgery and medical therapy; associated with significant risk of long-term panhypopituitarism.

Prognosis

• 15%–20% of microprolactinomas resolve during long-term dopamine agonist treatment.

• 40% of patients with macroadenomas have normal serum prolactinomas after transsphenoidal hypophysectomy.

Follow-up and management

• Patients should be maintained on the minimum dose of bromocriptine necessary to normalize serum prolactin concentrations.

• Bromocriptine should be stopped every 2 years and serum prolactin concentration checked.

• Long-term follow-up is necessary.

Key references

1. Aron DC, Tyrrell JB, Wilson CB: Pituitary tumors: current concepts in diagnosis and management. *West J Med* 1995, **162**:340–352.

2. Cunnah D, Besser GM: Management of prolactinomas. *Clin Endocrinol* 1991, **34**:231–235.

3. Jones TH: The management of hyperprolactinemia. *Br J Hosp Med* 1995, **53**:374–378.

4. Faglia G: Should dopamine agonist treatment for prolactinomas be life-long? *Clin Endocrinol* 1991, **34**:173–174.

5. Webster J, *et al.*: A comparison of cabergoline and bromocriptine in the treatment of hyperprolactinemic amenorrhea. Cabergoline Comparative Study Group. *N Engl J Med* 1994, **331**:904–909.

Diagnosis

Symptoms

• Patients are usually symptomless; hypertension is discovered at opportunistic or organized screening visits or detected after a hypertensive complication has intervened (myocardial infarction, cardiovascular accident, peripheral vascular disease, heart failure).

• Patients should be asked about symptoms of underlying causes of hypertension, *e.g.*, flushing and palpitations with pheochromocytoma, also other endocrine causes.

Headaches: occasionally.

Poor vision, shortness of breath, angina: rare.

Signs

Uncomplicated mild hypertension
• No signs other than raised blood pressure are manifest.

Moderate to severe hypertension
Displaced forceful apex beat, fourth heart sound, left atrial lift: signs of cardiac hypertrophy.

Silver wire arterioles, arteriovenous nipping, hemorrhages, exudates, papilledema.

Hypertensive complications
Signs of heart failure, renal failure, peripheral vascular disease, strokes.

Underlying causes (much less common than essential hypertension)
Signs of Cushing's syndrome, renal artery stenosis, aortic coarctation, pheochromocytoma, acromegaly, Conn's syndrome.

Investigations

Blood pressure measurement: to confirm diagnosis; repeated over several visits or by ambulatory monitoring.

Chest radiography: for coarctation, *e.g.*, rib-notching and double aortic shadow.

Renal function and electrolyte analysis: to check for renal failure, low potassium in Conn's syndrome.

Urine microscopy: for hematuria, casts, proteinuria in nephritis.

24-hour urinary catecholamines, metanephrines, vanillylmandelic acid analysis: for pheochromocytoma.

Ultrasonography of kidneys: show small scarred kidneys of pyelonephritis or end-stage renovascular disease; obstructive nephropathy.

Nuclear renography or renal angiography: for renal artery stenosis.

Endocrine tests: for Cushing's syndrome, acromegaly, thyroid disease.

ECG or echocardiography: for left ventricular hypertrophy in patients with moderate to severe hypertension.

Microalbuminuria measurement: for kidney damage in patients with moderate to severe hypertension.

Complications

Atrial fibrillation, ischemic heart disease, heart failure.

Peripheral vascular disease.

Nephrosclerosis, renovascular disease, renal failure.

Transient ischemic attacks, cardiovascular accidents, encephalopathy.

Hemorrhage, infarction, papilledema, blindness.

Etiology

• In most patients, no cause is found (essential hypertension).

• Underlying causes include the following:
Renal artery stenosis, nephritis, obstructive uropathy.

Coarctation.

Pheochromocytoma, Cushing's syndrome, Conn's syndrome, acromegaly, thyroid disease.

Cyclosporine, steroids, NSAIDs.

Pre-eclampsia, occasional autonomic neuropathy.

Epidemiology

• The frequency of hypertension depends on diagnostic cut-off levels of blood pressure: 10%–15% of the adult population have hypertension, increasing with age.

• Incidence and associations differ in nonwhite populations: *e.g.*, with insulin resistance in Asians, low-renin hypertension in Afro-Caribbeans.

Treatment

Diet and lifestyle

• Patients should be encouraged to lose weight, increase physical exercise, reduce salt intake, moderate alcohol intake, stop smoking, and consider other risk factors, *e.g.*, hyperlipidemia.

Pharmacological treatment

Angiotensin-converting enzyme (ACE) inhibitors

Standard dosage	Depends on choice of agent (*see manufacturer's current prescribing information*).
Contraindications	Angioedema, renal artery stenosis, pregnancy.
Main drug interactions	Hyperkalemia, synergistic with potassium-sparing diuretics.
Main side effects	Cough, renal impairment, angioedema (rare).

• For patients who develop cough on ACE inhibitors, direct angiotensin II inhibitors such as losartan at 25–50 mg daily are a useful alternative.

Calcium antagonists

Standard dosage	Depends on choice of agent (*see manufacturer's current prescribing information*).
Contraindications	Heart failure (relative).
Special points	Useful in black patients.
Main drug interactions	Bradycardia with diltiazem or verapamil and beta-blockers.
Main side effects	Edema, flushing.

Beta-blockers

Standard dosage	Depends on choice of agent (*see manufacturer's current prescribing information*).
Contraindications	Asthma, heart failure, heart block.
Special points	Less effective in elderly patients.
Main drug interactions	Bradycardia with diltiazem or verapamil.
Main side effects	Lethargy, fatigue, impotence.

Thiazide diuretics

Standard dosage	Low doses, depending on choice of agent (*see manufacturer's current prescribing information*).
Contraindications	Diabetes (relative).
Special points	Particularly beneficial in elderly patients [1–4].
Main drug interactions	Other diuretics.
Main side effects	Hypokalemia, glucose intolerance.

Alpha-blockers

Standard dosage	Depends on choice of agent (*see manufacturer's current prescribing information*).
Contraindications	Known hypersensitivity.
Special points	First-dose hypotension and tolerance may occur.
Main drug interactions	Few specific interactions.
Main side effects	Flushing, occasionally lupus-like syndrome.

Combination therapy

• Logical and synergistic combinations should be chosen, such as thiazides and ACE inhibitors; fixed-dose combinations are often a disadvantage.

Treatment aims

To reduce blood pressure to <140/90 mm Hg and to improve other cardiovascular risk factors.

Prognosis

• Prognosis is excellent if blood pressure is controlled (almost always possible).

Follow-up and management

• Follow-up must be for life.

Key references

1. Dahlöf B, *et al.*: Morbidity and mortality in the Swedish Trial in Old Patients with Hypertension (STOP-Hypertension). *Lancet* 1991, **338**:1281–1285.

2. MRC Working Party: Medical Research Council trial of treatment in older adults: principal results. *BMJ* 1992, **304**:405–412.

3. Mulrow CD, *et al.*: Hypertension in the elderly. *JAMA* 1994, **272**:1932–1938.

4. SHEP Co-operative Research Group: Prevention of stroke by antihypertensive drug treatment in older persons with isolated systolic hypertension. *JAMA* 1991, **265**:3255–3264.

Diagnosis

Symptoms

Weight loss, fatigue, sweating, heat intolerance, neck swelling.

Palpitations, shortness of breath.

Tremor, weakness, nervousness.

Increased frequency of bowel movements.

Staring, gritty eyes, swelling around eyes.

• Classic symptoms and signs may be absent in elderly patients.

Signs

Goiter: diffuse, with or without bruit, nodular, solitary nodule.

Fine tremor, proximal myopathy.

Lid retraction, lid lag, periorbital puffiness, chemosis, proptosis, corneal ulceration, ophthalmoplegia.

Sinus tachycardia, atrial fibrillation, cardiac failure.

Pretibial myxedema, palmar erythema, acropachy (finger clubbing).

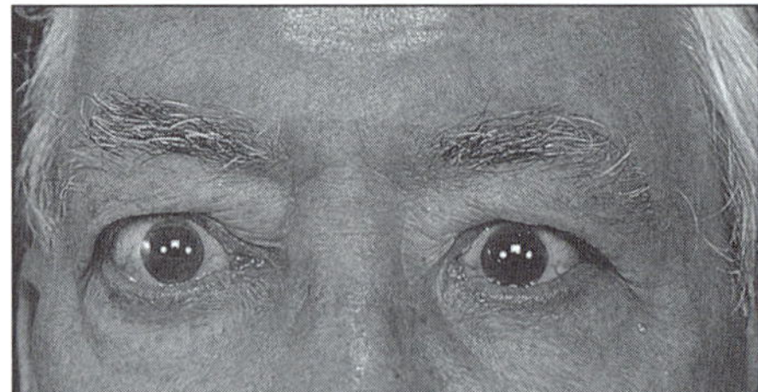

Periorbital edema, mild lid retraction and chemosis in a patient with Graves' ophthalmopathy. (*See* Color Plate.)

Investigations

Serum thyroid hormone measurements: free thyroxine (T_4) and total triiodothyronine (T_3) should be measured initially; T_3 may be elevated out of proportion to free T_4 in some patients (T_3-toxicosis).

Serum thyroid-stimulating hormone (TSH) measurement: undetectable in hyperthyroidism; normal value excludes primary hyperthyroidism.

Autoantibody tests: antithyroid peroxidase and antithyroglobulin antibodies are elevated in many forms of thyroid disease, including Graves' disease. Presence of anti-TSH receptor antibodies is diagnostic for Graves' disease.

Radioisotope scanning and uptake measurements: ^{99m}Tc scintigraphy distinguishes Graves' disease from toxic nodular goiter. Increased uptake of ^{131}I confirms hyperthyroidism, low uptake suggests thyroiditis.

Thyroid-releasing hormone stimulation test: rarely of use with advent of sensitive TSH assays.

Complications

Cardiac disease: especially atrial fibrillation and congestive cardiac failure (more common in elderly patients).

Reduced bone density and increased risk of osteoporotic fractures.

Graves' ophthalmopathy: may be progressive and occasionally sight-threatening because of corneal ulceration or optic nerve compression [1].

Treatment

Diet and lifestyle

• Increased iodine intake may precipitate hyperthyroidism in patients with euthyroid goiter.

• Cigarette smoking significantly increases the risk of ophthalmopathy in Graves' disease.

Pharmacological treatment [2]

Beta-adrenergic blockers

• Beta-andergenic blockers are recommended for patients with moderate or severe symptoms until serum thyroid hormones have returned to normal; often they are the only treatment needed for thyroiditis.

• They provide quick symptomatic relief of tremor and palpitations resulting from sympathetic overactivity.

Standard dosage	Propranolol, 20–80 mg 3 times daily (higher dose may be needed because of increased first-pass metabolism). Atenolol, 50–100 mg daily.
Contraindications	Asthma, obstructive pulmonary disease; caution in heart failure, even if induced by hyperthyroidism.
Main drug interactions	*See manufacturer's current prescribing information.*
Main side effects	*See manufacturer's current prescribing information.*

Thionamides [3]

• Both thionamide and radioactive iodine are acceptable therapies for Graves' disease.

• Thionamides can be used as first-line treatment in patients with Graves' hyperthyroidism or as short-term treatment before radioiodine treatment.

• They produce biochemical improvement and symptomatic relief within 2 months in most patients; a full course of 18 months is important to allow remission of disease.

Standard dosage	Methimazole, 30 mg single daily dose at diagnosis, reduced to maintenance dose of 5–10 mg. Propylthiouracil, 100 mg 2–3 times daily at diagnosis, reduced to maintenance dose of 50 mg 1–2 times daily.
Contraindications	Thionamide-induced agranulocytosis or other serious side effects.
Main drug interactions	No major interactions.
Main side effects	Agranulocytosis (rare; patients must be warned to stop treatment and seek an urgent complete blood count if they develop a fever, sore throat, or other infection); hepatitis, cholestatic jaundice, and lupus-like syndromes (rare but serious); skin rashes, nausea, and arthralgia (common but not serious).

Radioiodine

• Radioiodine treatment must be done under specialist supervision.

• It is often used as first-line therapy for Graves' disease and is the treatment of choice for patients who fail thionamide therapy. It can be used in patients with small toxic adenomas (<3 cm) and in some patients with toxic multinodular goiter.

Standard dosage	Radioiodine single dose initially; second dose after 4–6 months if hyperthyroidism not cured; larger initial doses for elderly patients or those with severe disease to produce rapid effect and induce hypothyroidism.
Contraindications	Pregnancy (standard of care is to avoid pregnancy for 6 months following treatment), breast-feeding, hyperthyroidism secondary to thyroiditis; caution in patients with active ophthalmopathy.
Special points	Thionamides should be withdrawn at least 4 days before treatment. They can be restarted 4 days after treatment. Can exacerbate hyperthyroidism and rarely induce "thyroid storm."
Main drug interactions	None.
Main side effects	Hypothyroidism (>50% within 10 years of treatment), may be intended outcome if larger dose of radioiodine used for thyroid ablation and thyroxine replacement.

Key references

1. Fells P: Thyroid-associated eye disease: clinical management. *Lancet* 1991, **338**:29–32.

2. Franklyn JA: The management of hyperthyroidism. *N Engl J Med* 1994, **330**:1731–1738.

3. Reinwein D, *et al.*: A prospective randomised trial of antithyroid drug dose in Graves' disease therapy. *J Clin Endocrinol Metab* 1993, **76**:1516–1521.

Diagnosis

Symptoms

• Patients may be asymptomatic.

Severe cardiac failure: in infants.

Premature unexpected death: may be presenting symptom in children or young adults [1].

Dyspnea on exertion: in ~50% of patients.

Chest pain: in ~50%; may be exertional or occur at rest.

Syncope: in 15–25%.

Dizziness, palpitations.

Signs

• In patients without outflow tract gradient, abnormalities may be subtle.

Rapid upstroke arterial pulse: best felt in carotid area.

Forceful left ventricular impulse: best appreciated on full held expiration in left lateral position.

Ejection systolic murmur: best heard at left sternal border; radiating toward aortic and mitral areas but not into neck.

Palpable atrial beat: reflecting forceful atrial systolic contraction.

Investigations

Two-dimensional echocardiography: important for assessing left ventricle structure and function, gradients, valvular regurgitation, and atrial dimensions.

ECG: may be normal in <5% of patients or show abnormalities reflecting left ventricular hypertrophy, atrial fibrillation, left axis deviation, right bundle branch block, and myocardial disarray (*e.g.*, ST- and T-wave changes, intraventricular conduction defects, abnormal Q waves); bizarre or abnormal findings in young patients should raise suspicion of hypertrophic cardiomyopathy, especially if a family member is also affected.

Chest radiography: may be normal or show evidence of left or right atrial or left ventricular enlargement.

Treadmill exercise test with maximum oxygen ventilatory capacity: simple and non-invasive; provides useful functional information; maximum oxygen ventilatory capacity often moderately reduced; one-third of patients have abnormal blood pressure response, with drops of 25–150 mm Hg from peak systolic recordings (probably of prognostic significance); ST segment changes of >2 mm documented in 25%, associated with symptoms of angina.

48-hour Holter monitoring: arrhythmias common during ECG monitoring; established atrial fibrillation in ~10% of patients, paroxysmal supraventricular arrhythmias in 30%, non-sustained ventricular tachycardia in 25%; ventricular tachycardia invariably asymptomatic during Holter monitoring, but most useful marker of risk of sudden death in adults; sustained supraventricular arrhythmias often symptomatic and predispose to thromboembolic complications.

Thallium scintigraphy: fixed and reversible perfusion defects common, useful in assessment of ischemia, particularly when resting ECG grossly abnormal and exercise changes uninterpretable.

Cardiac catheterization and left ventriculography: invasive evaluation not needed for diagnosis, but coronary arteriography often necessary in older patients with angina to exclude coronary artery disease; endomyocardial biopsy possibly necessary to exclude specific heart muscle disorder (amyloid, sarcoid) but has no other role in diagnosis because of patchy nature of myofiber disarray.

Complications

Atrial fibrillation.

Systemic embolism.

Infective endocarditis.

Sudden death.

Etiology

• Hypertrophic cardiomyopathy is an autosomal dominant heart muscle disorder.

• Mutations in the gene encoding contractile proteins cause disease in 50–60% of patients [2].

Pathology

Macroscopic: hypertrophied myocardium; thickened anterior leaflet of mitral valve; contact lesion upper anterior septum.

Histological: interstitial fibrosis; myofiber disorganization and whorling; myocyte hypertrophy.

Pathophysiology

Systolic: hyperdynamic contraction; left ventricular outflow tract gradient (30%; associated mitral regurgitation).

Diastolic: impaired relaxation; impaired filling; decreased compliance.

Epidemiology

• The male:female ratio is equal, although the disease tends to affect younger men and older women.

• In children and adolescents, myocardial hypertrophy often occurs during growth spurts; a negative diagnosis made before adolescent growth has been completed must be tempered by the proviso of subsequent reassessment.

• Myocardial hypertrophy does not ordinarily progress after adolescent growth is completed.

• The annual mortality from sudden death is 2.5% in adults and at least 6% in children and young adults.

• First-degree relatives of affected patients have a 50% chance of carrying the disease gene; they should be investigated by ECG and two-dimensional echocardiography.

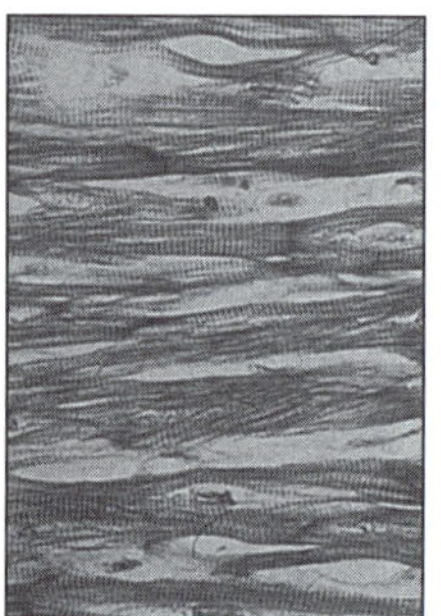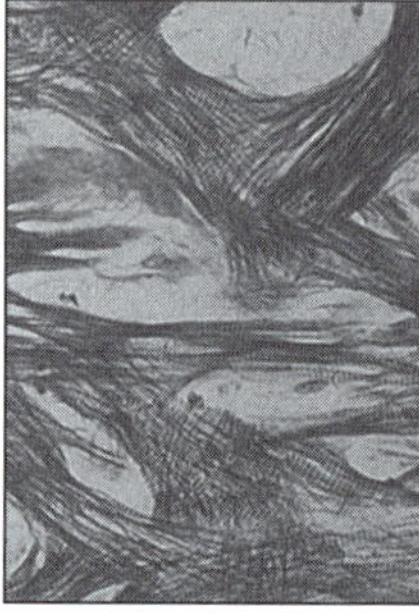

Myofibrillar stain from a normal person (*left*) and one with myocardial disarray (*right*). (*See* Color Plates.)

Treatment

Diet and lifestyle

• Competitive exercise is not recommended, especially in high-risk patients.

Pharmacological treatment

Beta-blockers

• Beta-blockers may reduce symptoms and increase exercise capacity, but they do not reduce the incidence of ventricular arrhythmia or risk of sudden death.

Standard dosage	Propranolol, 80–320 mg daily. Atenolol, 50–100 mg daily.
Contraindications	Conduction disease.
Main drug interactions	Other drugs that suppress impulse formation.
Main side effects	Other unwanted adrenergic blocking effects.

Calcium antagonists

• Calcium antagonism can improve hemodynamics and relieve symptoms but gives no reduction in risk of sudden death.

Standard dosage	Verapamil, 120–480 mg daily.
Contraindications	Outflow-tract gradient.
Special points	Verapamil fails to abolish ventricular arrhythmia.
Main drug interactions	Digoxin.
Main side effects	High-grade conduction block, negative inotropic effect.

Antiarrhythmics

• Antiarrhythmics are effective in short-term and long-term control of supraventricular and ventricular arrhythmias and can improve survival in adults with nonsustained ventricular tachycardia (low dose).

Standard dosage	Amiodarone, 100–200 mg daily.
Contraindications	Hyperthyroidism.
Special points	Plasma concentration should be maintained <1.5 mg/L.
Main drug interactions	Anticoagulants, digoxin.
Main side effects	Photosensitivity, sleep disturbance.

Other options

Anticoagulation: important in patients with paroxysmal or established atrial fibrillation.

Endocarditis prophylaxis: for patients with obstruction and valvular regurgitation (*see* Endocarditis *for details*).

Treatment aims

To improve symptoms.
To prevent complications.
To prevent sudden death.

Other treatments

Surgical myectomy [3]
• In patients with left ventricle outflow tract obstruction, this provides symptomatic and hemodynamic improvement.
• Perioperative mortality is high, at 5%–10%.

Dual-chamber permanent pacing
• Recently proposed for treatment of obstructions [4], this provides a reduction in outflow gradient and improvement in symptoms.
• Further assessment is needed.

Cardiac transplantation
• Transplantation is limited to patients who develop severe systolic impairment.

Prognosis

• Nonsustained ventricular tachycardia is the best marker of high risk in adults.
• Other patients at high risk are children and adolescents who have had recurrent syncope and patients with two or more siblings with hypertrophic cardiomyopathy who have died suddenly.

Follow-up and management

• Patients must be monitored for disease progression and risk of complications.

Key references

1. Maron BJ, *et al.*: Hypertrophic cardiomyopathy. *N Engl J Med* 1987, **316**:780–789.

2. Rosenzweig A, *et al.*: Preclinical diagnosis of familial hypertrophic cardiomyopathy by genetic analysis of blood lymphocytes. *N Engl J Med* 1991, **325**:1753–1760.

3. Seiler C, *et al.*: Long-term follow-up of medical vs. surgical therapy for hypertrophic cardiomyopathy. *J Am Coll Cardiol* 1991, **17**:634–642.

4. Fananapazir L, *et al.*: Impact of dual chamber permanent pacing in patients with obstructive hypertrophic cardiomyopathy with symptoms refractory to verapamil and beta-blocker therapy. *Circulation* 1992, **85**:2149–2156.

Diagnosis

Symptoms

Paresthesia: especially around face, hands, and feet.

Tetany: causing painful cramps culminating in hands going into tetanic spasm position.

Seizures.

Bone pain: common in vitamin D deficiency.

Signs

• Mild hypocalcemia may be asymptomatic; signs are due to neuromuscular irritability.

Twitching of local facial muscles: after tapping over facial nerve in front of and below ear; Chvostek's sign (positive in some normal people, rarely in those with hypokalemia).

Development of tetanic spasm (Trousseau's sign): after inflation of a sphygmomano-meter cuff on arm (a painful procedure and not recommended).

Proximal myopathy: common in vitamin D deficiency.

Obesity, "moon" face, shortened metacarpals and metatarsals: signs of pseudohypoparathyroidism.

Investigations [1]

Serum calcium measurement: low concentration.

Serum phosphorus measurement: low concentration in vitamin D deficiency, high in hypoparathyroidism, pseudohypoparathyroidism, and renal failure.

Serum creatinine measurement: raised concentration in renal failure.

Serum alkaline phosphatase measurement: often raised concentration in vitamin D deficiency.

Serum magnesium measurement: low concentration can cause hypocalcemia.

Serum parathyroid hormone measurement: raised concentration in vitamin D deficiency, pseudohypoparathyroidism, and renal failure; low concentration in patients with hypoparathyroidism.

Vitamin D level measurement.

Radiography: of wrists and knees in suspected rickets, chest and pelvis in suspected osteomalacia.

Complications

Epilepsy.

Cataracts and basal ganglia calcification: in longstanding hypocalcemia.

Differential diagnosis

Previous neck surgery.

Hypomagnesemia, especially if patient is an alcoholic, has extensive small-bowel disease or resection, or is on aminoglycoside drugs or cisplatinum.

Etiology [2]

Low plasma proteins (not true hypocalcemia).

Acute or chronic renal failure.

Vitamin D deficiency.

Hypoparathyroidism: rarely idiopathic, usually after neck surgery.

Pseudohypoparathyroidism.

Hypomagnesemia.

Severe acute pancreatitis.

Malabsorption.

Epidemiology

• Hypocalcemia is manifest most often at times of increased calcium shifts (*i.e.*, neonatal period, growth spurt, and pregnancy).

Treatment

Diet and lifestyle

• Patients should have an adequate calcium intake (800–2000 mg daily of elemental calcium).

• Low-dose vitamin D supplementation should be considered if exposure to sunlight is inadequate.

Pharmacological treatment [1]

For acute symptomatic hypocalcemia

Standard dosage	10% calcium gluconate, 10 mL i.v. slowly, followed by 50–100 mL i.v. in 1 L saline solution over 24 hours at a rate to relieve symptoms.
Contraindications	None.
Main drug interactions	None.
Main side effects	Tissue necrosis (if extravasation outside vein).

For hypoparathyroidism

Standard dosage	Calcitriol, 0.5–1.0 µg orally daily, plus adequate calcium intake.
Contraindications	None.
Special points	Regular serum calcium monitoring.
Main drug interactions	None.
Main side effects	Hypercalcemia.

For vitamin D deficiency

Standard dosage	Calciferol, 500–1000 U orally daily, plus adequate calcium intake.
Contraindications	None.
Main drug interactions	None.
Main side effects	None at this dose range.

For renal failure

Standard dosage	Calcitriol, 0.5–1.0 µg orally daily, plus calcium intake as appropriate.
Contraindications	None.
Special points	Hyperphosphatemia should be controlled.
Main drug interactions	None.
Main side effects	Hypercalcemia.

For hypomagnesemic hypocalcemia

• Patients with severe, symptomatic hypomagnesemia are best treated initially by an i.v. preparation: magnesium sulfate, 5–10 mg 50% solution in 1 L 5% dextrose over 3–4 hours.

• Daily infusions may be needed until serum magnesium is maintained within the normal range.

• If magnesium losses continue (*e.g.*, short bowel syndrome), this can be treated by intermittent infusions or oral therapy. Various oral preparations are available, all of which may cause diarrhea.

Key references

1. Tohme JF, Bilezikian JP: Hypocalcemic emergencies. *Endocrinol Metab Clin North Am* 1993, **22**:363–375.

2. Rude RK: Hypocalcemia and hypoparathyroidism. *Curr Ther Endocrinol Metab* 1997, **6**:546–551.

Diagnosis

Symptoms

Sweating, shaking, anxiety, feeling hot, nausea, palpitations, tingling lips: due to sympathetic and adrenergic response to low blood glucose concentration (autonomic).
Dizziness, tiredness, confusion, difficulty speaking, inability to concentrate, headache: due to impaired cerebral cortical function resulting from low blood glucose level.
Hunger, weakness, blurred vision.
Headache, malaise, confusion: posthypoglycemic.
• Patients with recurrent hypoglycemic attacks often present with symptoms of decreased cognitive function or conscious level of which they have no subjective awareness.
Fasting hypoglycemia: a concerning symptom that requires a thorough medical evaluation.
"Reactive" hypoglycemia (following a meal): less likely to represent significant pathology; however, some patients with early type II diabetes may have postprandial hypoglycemia.

Signs

Pallor, diaphoresis, tremor, tachycardia or occasionally bradycardia, increased pulse pressure, dilated pupils: autonomic.
Altered behavior, slurred speech, irritability, decreased level of consciousness, seizure, coma, transient focal neurological defects: neuroglycopenic.
• The formal diagnosis of hypoglycemia requires the following (Whipple's triad):
1. Symptoms consistant with neuroglycemia.
2. Low blood glucose during symptoms.
3. Resolution of symptoms with correction of hypoglycemia.

Investigations [1]
For all cases
Blood glucose measurement: <40 mg/dL, in treated diabetic patients ≤60 mg/dL.
• Glucose tolerance tests are rarely of value in the evaluation of hypoglycemia.

For nondiabetic patients
Plasma insulin and C-peptide analysis.
Blood and urine screening: for sulfonylureas.
Blood urea nitrogen, creatine, liver function, insulin antibody tests.

For diabetic patients
Thyroid and adrenal function tests, gastric emptying studies, growth hormone measurement.

For suspected insulinoma
Fasting glucose, insulin, and C-peptide measurement: repeated during 72-hour fast or until hypoglycemia documented; high C-peptide and insulin suggest insulinoma, sulfonylureas, or insulin autoantibodies (rare); high insulin with low C-peptide indicates exogenous insulin.

For noninsulinoma, nondiabetes-related hypoglycemia
08.00 hours cortisol and cosyntropin test, growth hormone, insulin-like growth factors, liver function tests.

For suspected "reactive" hypoglycemia
Home blood glucose monitoring: patients can be taught to perform home glucose monitoring during episodes for later laboratory estimates of blood glucose concentration.

Complications
Trauma: while patient is hypoglycemic.
Loss of subjective awareness of subsequent episodes.
Permanent neurological sequelae: usually only with large insulin overdosage.
Death.

Plasma insulin concentrations over 24 hours from a patient on twice-daily injections of mixed exogenous insulins and an approximation of the plasma insulin profile of a nondiabetic person eating 3 meals daily, showing times of risk of hypoglycemia.

Differential diagnosis

Acute
Other causes of coma or confusion, including the following:
Ketoacidosis, nonketotic hyperosmolar coma, intoxication or poisoning, uremia, epilepsy, stroke, intracranial hemorrhage, meningitis, head injury.

Recurrent
Epilepsy, arrhythmias, psychiatric disorder, pheochromocytoma.

Etiology [2]

Excess insulin action in diabetic patients [3]
Missed, small, or late meals, error in time or dose, exercise (effect may last several hours), alcohol (delayed effect), hypothyroidism, renal failure, gastroparesis: with pharmacological treatment of diabetes mellitus (insulin, sulfonylureas).
Vigorous insulin response to rapidly absorbed glucose or gastric surgery (dumping syndrome).
Insulinoma, nesidioblastosis.

Excess insulin action in nondiabetic patients
Tumors secreting insulin-like growth factor.
Surreptitious or malicious administration of insulin or sulfonylurea.

Increased insulin sensitivity
Cortisol deficiency.
Growth hormone deficiency.
Hypopituitarism and adrenal insufficiency (especially in children).

Defects of hepatic glucose production
Liver disease.
Alcohol toxicity.
Sepsis.
Congestive heart failure.
Glycogen storage diseases.
Ketotic hypoglycemia of childhood.
Prematurity.
Defective fatty acid oxidation.

Epidemiology

• 3% of the US population have diabetes mellitus; 4%–40% experience severe hypoglycemia.
• 10% of insulinomas are multiple, 10% are malignant, 9% with multiple endocrine neoplasia.

Treatment

Diet and lifestyle

• In "reactive hypoglycemia," patients should eat small, regular meals with high complex carbohydrates and should avoid simple sugars.

• In childhood disorders of metabolism, frequent high-carbohydrate, low-fat meals should be eaten.

• In patients with diabetes, regular meals and snacks are essential, with patient-led dosage adjustments for certain situations, *e.g.*, excessive exercise.

Pharmacological treatment [1]

For conscious patients

Rapidly absorbed carbohydrates (20 g, *e.g.*, 4 glucose tablets, a glass of skim milk, or ½ glass orange juice), then snack.

For confused or unconscious patients

50% glucose, 50 mL, or 20% glucose, 100–150 mL i.v.

In children: 20% dextrose, 2.5 mL/kg.

In infants: 10% dextrose, 2.5 mL/kg.

• Extravasation of glucose must be avoided.

• If hypoglycemia is due to sulfonylurea treatment, massive insulin overdose, or unknown cause, the patient should be admitted to hospital for observation and treatment. Insulin overdoses should be treated with i.v. glucose, whereas sulfonylurea-induced hypoglycemia often responds well to octreotide therapy [4].

Alternatively, glucagon, 1 mg i.m., followed by 30 g complex carbohydrate orally on recovery.

• Glucagon's effect is transient (<60 minutes), and more definitive therapy should be instituted after initial recovery.

• Patients requiring glucagon at home should be seen promptly by a physician.

• Glucagon may not be effective in very undernourished or very alcohol-intoxicated patients.

Treatment aims

To achieve recovery from acute event.

To prevent further episodes.

Other treatments

Surgery for insulinomas, tumors secreting insulin-like growth factor, nesidioblastosis.

Prognosis

• For diabetes, the prognosis is that of the underlying disease.

• For tumors secreting insulin-like growth factor, prognosis is poor.

Follow-up and management

Prevention of further episodes

• The diabetes regimen should be adjusted.

• Diazoxide can be given for insulinoma, after the diagnosis is established, pending definitive surgical management.

• Diet regimens should be followed for metabolic defects.

Key references

1. Service FJ: Hypoglycemic disorders. *N Engl J Med* 1995, **332**:1144–1152.

2. Amiel SA: Glucose counterregulation in health and disease: current concepts in hypoglycaemia recognition and response. *Q J Med* 1991, **293**:707–727.

3. Amiel SA: Hypoglycaemia in diabetes mellitus. *Med Int* 1993, **21**:279–280.

4. Boyle PJ, Justice K, Krentz AJ, *et al.*: Octreotide reverses hyperinsulinemia and prevents hypoglycemia induced by sulfonylurea overdoses. *J Clin Endocrinol Metab* 1993, **76**:752–756.

Diagnosis

Symptoms

• Symptoms may be due to an underlying cause (*e.g.,* tumor) or to hormone deficiencies. Hormone deficiencies have a gradual onset if secondary to an expanding pituitary lesion.

Impotence or amenorrhea, decreased libido: due to deficiency of gonadotropins.

Poor growth and development, hypoglycemia: in children, due to deficiency of growth hormone.

Cold intolerance, weight gain, tiredness, lethargy: due to deficiency of thyroid-stimulating hormone.

Dizziness, nausea, vomiting: due to deficiency of corticotropic hormone.

Urinary frequency, nocturia: due to deficiency of vasopressin (unusual with pituitary tumors).

Headache or visual disturbance: due to macroadenoma.

Galactorrhea: due to prolactinoma or pituitary stalk compression by lesion (in contrast to pituitary hormones, prolactin levels usually rise with pituitary enlargement).

Signs

Small soft testes, loss of pubic and axillary hair: due to deficiency of gonadotropins.
Short stature: in children, due to deficiency of growth hormone.
Cool skin, absent or slow reflexes: due to deficiency of thyroid-stimulating hormone.
Postural hypotension, shock: due to deficiency of corticotropic hormone.
Visual field defect, diplopia or cranial nerve palsies, papilledema, CSF rhinorrhea: indicating macroadenoma.
Signs of acromegaly.

Investigations

Cortisol measurement for adrenal axis: if 08.00 hours cortisol >20 µg/dL, significant deficiency improbable; if <2 µg/dL, corticotropic hormone (ACTH) deficiency very probable unless patient is taking steroids; intermediate values need cortrosyn stimulation test to assess adrenal function.
Thyroid tests: free thyroxine (T_4), thyroid-stimulating hormone (TSH); secondary hypothyroidism suggested by low T_4 or free T_4 index unaccompanied by raised TSH.
Sex hormone measurement for gonadal axis: *in men:* testosterone, sex hormone-binding globulin (high level can give rise to high total bound testosterone, while free level remains low), luteinizing hormone (LH) or follicle-stimulating hormone (FSH); gonadotropin deficiency suggested by low basal testosterone and no rise of LH/FSH; *in women:* estradiol, sex hormone-binding globulin, LH/FSH, progesterone on day 21 (normal concentration implies normal gonadal axis).
Prolactin test: on 2–3 occasions; hyperprolactinemia may suppress pulsatile gonadotropin secretion in either sex in absence of absolute deficiency.
Growth hormone (GH) measurement: basal values usually undetectable and therefore unhelpful; insulin tolerance or glucagon test used to assess GH reserve in children, but is usually unnecessary in adults [1].
Plasma and urine osmolality measurement for posterior pituitary: plasma osmolality >295 mOsm/L and urine : plasma osmolality ratio of <2 : 1 suggest diabetes insipidus.
Insulin tolerance test: to assess ACTH and GH reserve; must be done in a specialized unit; contraindicated in patients with ischemic heart disease, epilepsy, or unexplained blackouts; particular caution in children and elderly patients [2].
Releasing hormone tests: corticotropin-releasing, thyrotropin-releasing, and gonadotropin-releasing hormone tests only assess only "readily releasable" pool of anterior pituitary hormones and cannot be used to diagnose normality of physiological secretion of the hormone.
MRI or CT of pituitary gland: to visualize macroadenomas and most microadenomas.

Complications

Cardiovascular collapse: resulting from adrenocortical insufficiency.
Expanding pituitary mass: with optic chiasm compression and invasion of local structures.
Hydrocephalus: with third ventricular compression by tumor.
Temporal-lobe epilepsy: with temporal extension of tumor (unusual).

Treatment

Diet and lifestyle

• Patients need a steroid card, Medicalert bracelet or necklace, and emergency pack of parenteral hydrocortisone (for deficiencies of pituitary–adrenal axis).

Pharmacological treatment

For deficiencies of pituitary–adrenal axis

Standard dosage
Hydrocortisone, 20 mg on waking, 5 mg with evening meal (variable).

Contraindications
None.

Special points
Response monitored by clinical assessment.
For mild cold or sore throat, no change in dosage; with moderate illness manifested primarily with fever, double hydrocortisone dose; with severe illness, especially vomiting or diarrhea, or for perioperative cover, parenteral treatment is needed (hydrocortisone, 100 mg i.m. every 8 hours).

Main drug interactions
Estrogens increase cortisol-binding globulin and thus hydrocortisone concentration.

Main side effects
Iatrogenic Cushing's syndrome due to over-replacement.

For thyroid deficiencies

Standard dosage
Thyroxine, 100–150 µg daily (start with lower doses in the elderly and in patients with ischemic heart disease).

Contraindications
None.

Special points
Response monitored by clinical assessment and serum thyrotropin. Rule out (or treat) adrenal insufficiency before beginning thyroxine therapy.

Main drug interactions
Estrogens increase thyroid-binding globulin and raise total thyroxine; free thyroxine should be used for monitoring, along with thyrotropin.

Main side effects
None.

For growth hormone deficiencies [1]

• Children should be given growth hormone, 0.04 mg/kg daily.

• Growth hormone may be of some benefit in adults because it appears to improve psychological well-being and muscle strength and decrease adiposity. Expense remains a serious concern.

For deficiencies of pituitary–gonadal axis

Standard dosage
Men: testosterone enanthate or cypionate, 200 mg i.m. every 2 weeks or 300 mg every 3 weeks; transdermal testosterone patch daily.
Women: ethinyl estradiol, 30 µg daily, or conjugated equine estrogens, 0.125 mg daily. For intact uterus, medroxyprogesterone acetate, 5–10 mg for 10 days each month or 2.5–5.0 mg daily.

Contraindications
Prostatic cancer, breast cancer.

Special points
Response monitored by potency and serum testosterone, menses, and symptoms of estrogen deficiency.

Main drug interactions
Estrogen increases many binding globulins and thus total hormone concentrations.

Main side effects
Aggression may occur with initial testosterone replacement (rare).

For posterior pituitary deficiencies

Standard dosage
Desmopressin, 10–20 µg at night by intranasal spray; dose may also be needed in morning.

Contraindications
None.

Special points
Response monitored by plasma and urine osmolality.

Main drug interactions
None.

Main side effects
Dilutional hyponatremia due to over-replacement.

Key references

1. Cuneo RC, *et al.*: The growth hormone deficiency syndrome in adults. *Clin Endocrinol* 1992, **37**:387–397.

2. Jones SL, *et al.*: An audit of the insulin tolerance test in adult subjects in an acute investigation unit over one year. *Clin Endocrinol* 1994, **41**:123–128.

3. Littley MD, *et al.*: Hypopituitarism following external radiotherapy for pituitary tumors in adults. *Q J Med* 1989, **70**:145–160.

Diagnosis

Symptoms [1]

Weight gain, fatigue, cold intolerance, neck swelling, hoarseness.

Angina, shortness of breath.

Aches and pains, depression, carpal tunnel syndrome.

Dry skin.

Menorrhagia, infertility, galactorrhea secondary to hyperprolactinemia.

Constipation.

Poor growth, mental retardation, delayed puberty: in children.

Signs

Bradycardia, pericardial effusion (rare), cardiac failure.

Hoarseness, deafness, cerebellar ataxia, delayed relaxation of tendon reflexes, psychosis ("myxedema madness").

Anemia.

Goiter.

Dry skin, myxedema, vitiligo, yellowish discoloration, decreased sweating.

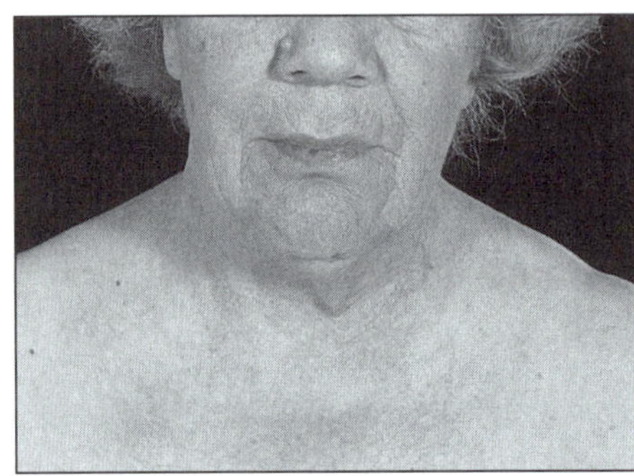

Hypothyroid appearance of an elderly patient with severe untreated Hashimoto's thyroiditis. (*See* Color Plate.)

Investigations [2]

Serum thyroid hormone measurement: reduction in free or total thyroxine indicates severity of hypothyroidism; serum triiodothyronine usually normal except in severely ill patients, so measurement not helpful.

Serum thyroid-stimulating hormone (TSH) measurement: elevation indicates primary thyroid failure; raised TSH with normal thyroxine is termed "subclinical" hypothyroidism; TSH within or below normal range, with low serum thyroxine, suggests secondary hypothyroidism (hypothalamic/pituitary; same picture seen in "nonthyroidal" illness and treatment by certain drugs, *e.g.*, glucocorticoids).

Autoantibody measurement: antithyroid peroxidase and antithyroglobulin antibodies often present in high titer in Hashimoto's thyroiditis.

Complications

Hypothermia and coma: in severely ill patients, typically in the elderly in cold weather.

Hyperlipidemia and ischemic heart disease: associated with longstanding hypothyroidism.

Treatment

Diet and lifestyle

• Long-term ingestion of iodine-containing compounds, *e.g.*, kelp preparations or expectorants, can result in hypothyroidism in adults.

Pharmacological treatment [3–5]

• Thyroxine for patients with symptomatic hypothyroidism; triiodothyronine is used occasionally in patients with myxedema coma to produce more rapid effect.

• Symptoms begin to resolve within 2–3 weeks of the beginning of treatment, but treatment at full dose for 8 weeks may be needed to restore serum thyroid-stimulating hormone to normal.

Standard dosage	Thyroxine, 100–150 µg daily as single dose. Triiodothyronine, 25 µg orally 2–3 times daily (rarely indicated).
Contraindications	Caution in severe ischemic heart disease (patient should be admitted to hospital and started on very low doses of thyroxine).
Main drug interactions	None.
Main side effects	Generally none; exacerbation of ischemic heart disease may follow initiation of treatment; can precipitate acute adrenal failure in patients with subclinical adrenal disease.

Treatment aims

To relieve symptoms.

To restore serum thyroid-stimulating hormone and thyroxine to normal values.

Prognosis

• Life expectancy is not adversely affected by long-term thyroxine treatment.

• Thyroxine treatment (in doses that reduce serum thyroid-stimulating hormone to below normal) may reduce bone density. However, no increased risk of osteoporotic fractures has been observed.

• Up to 25% of patients prescribed thyroxine have biochemical evidence of undertreatment that may be associated with hyperlipidemia and increased risk of ischemic heart disease.

Follow-up and management

• Serum thyroid-stimulating hormone should be measured 6 weeks after starting treatment to check whether the dose needs to be increased and should be measured annually in patients on established treatment.

• Treatment is for life, except in mild cases occurring within the first 6 months after radioiodine treatment, pregnancy, or partial thyroidectomy (possibly temporary) and in patients who are hypothyroid secondary to subacute or silent thyroiditis.

Key references

1. Anonymous: Hypothyroidism? *Lancet* 1990, **335**:1316.

2. Lazarus JH, Hall R (eds.): Hypothyroidism and goitre. *Ballières Clin Endocrinol Metab* 1988, **2**.

3. Toft AD: Thyroxine therapy. *N Engl J Med* 1994, **331**:174–180.

4. Utiger RD: Therapy of hypothyroidism. When are changes needed? *N Engl J Med* 1990, **323**:126–127.

5. Singer PA, *et al.*: Treatment guidelines for patients with hyperthyroidism and hypothyroidism. Standards of Care Committee, American Thyroid Association. *JAMA* 1995, **273**:808–812.

Diagnosis

Definition

• Infections in hematological malignancy are opportunistic infections that arise during the treatment of hematological malignancy due to the development of neutropenia. Patients are particularly vulnerable when the neutrophil count falls below 0.5×10^9/L.

Symptoms and signs

Fever: the only consistent indication of established infection.

Investigations

• Full examination should always be made, including mouth, pharynx, genitalia, perianal region, and central line sites.

• Surveillance cultures can be predictive of infection, *e.g.*, with *Pseudomonas aeruginosa*, allowing planning of empirical treatment for individual patients and monitoring of prophylaxis, as well as facilitating infection control.

• Stool should be screened, *e.g.*, for parasites, if patient comes from a high-risk area.

Blood cultures: from central line and peripheral vein, for bacteria and fungi.

Hickman swab: if inflamed or cutaneous discharge.

Specimens from clinically suspicious sites.

Urinalysis and culture.

Chest radiography.

CT of thorax: invaluable in invasive aspergillosis.

Bronchoalveolar lavage: especially in bone-marrow transplant patients with dry cough or chest radiography lesions early on.

Skin lesion aspiration: valuable in diagnosis of disseminated fungal infection.

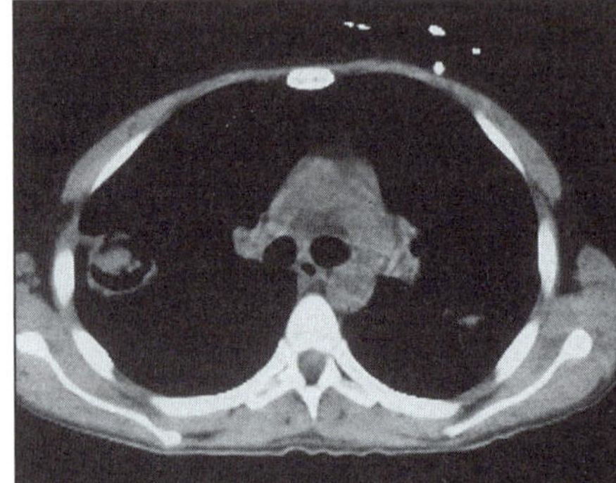
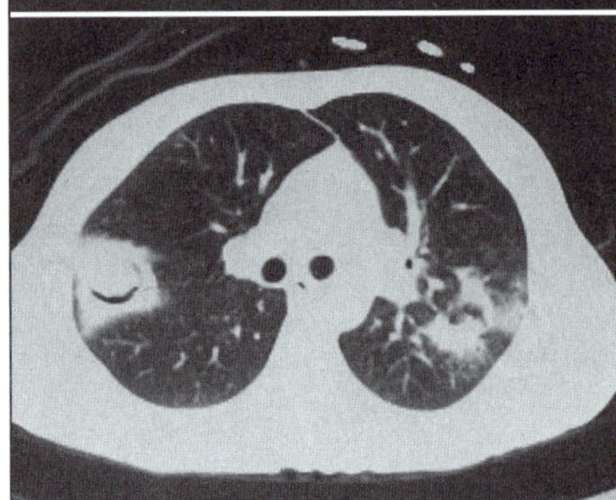

CT of lung with invasive aspergillosis. The mycotic lung sequestrum is usually pleural based and wedged shaped and often shows cavitation.

Complications

• Initially, complications may include those of septicemia, *e.g.*, acute tubular necrosis.

Increased risk of adult respiratory distress syndrome: in patients with *Streptococcus mitis* bacteremia.

Ecthyma gangrenosum in patients with local or disseminated *P. aeruginosa* infection.

Disseminated candidiasis: CT of liver or spleen can be helpful.

Pulmonary infarction or hemorrhage: especially in patients with invasive aspergillosis.

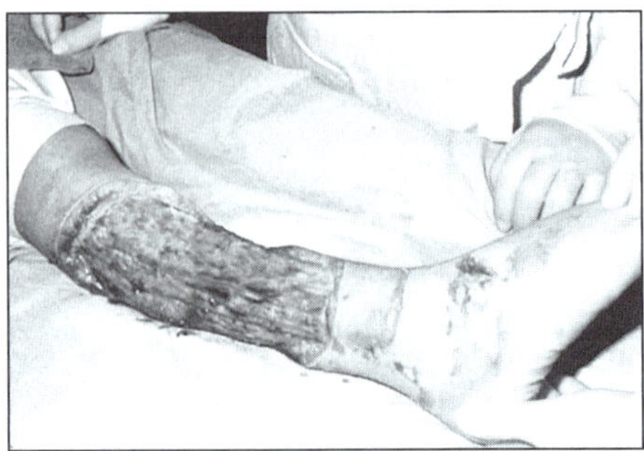

Extensive resection of necrotic tissue of the leg in a child with *Pseudomonas* septicaemia and Ecthyma gangrenosum. (*See* Color Plate.)

Treatment

Diet and lifestyle

• Neutropenic patients must eat a low-pathogen diet but maintain nutrition, *e.g.*, by parenteral route if needed.
• Patients should be given a dental review.
• Hygiene is important for patients and attendants, *e.g.*, hand-washing, cleaning of room and bedding, and i.v. catheter care.
• Water must be treated appropriately to prevent legionella infection.
• Patients must especially avoid exposure to measles and chickenpox; vaccination should be reviewed, but live vaccines must be avoided until immune recovery.

Pharmacological treatment [1–3]

Empirical treatment for pyrexia of unknown origin in neutropenia

• Patients with a fever of 38.5°C or 38°C for 2 hours should receive prompt empirical antibiotic treatment: *e.g.*, ceftazidime, or ceftazidime and aminoglycoside, or antipseudomonal penicillin and aminoglycoside. If aminoglycoside was not part of the original regimen and fever persists beyond 24–72 hours or clinical deterioration is apparent, add aminoglycoside after reculturing of all potential infection sites. Regardless of initial antibiotic regimen, if fever persists reculture and include vancomycin. Amphotericin B should be added if fever persists beyond 96 hours.

Standard dosage	Amphotericin B 1 mg/kg or AmBisome 3-5 mg/kg daily. Ceftazidine 2 g i.v. 8-hourly (adults). Gentamicin 1 mg/kg i.v. 3 times daily. Piperacillin 3–4 g i.v. every 4-6 hours. Vancomycin 500 mg i.v. every 6 hours or 1 g i.v. every 12 hours.
Contraindications	Hypersensitivity; caution in renal impairment; epilepsy, or known intracerebral lesion (imipenem).
Special points	Vancomycin and aminoglycoside dosages may need adjustment.
Main drug interactions	Ototoxicity when combined (uncommon with teicoplanin).
Main side effects	Nephrotoxicity (vancomycin, aminoglycosides, amphotericin). Ototoxicity (vancomycin, aminoglycosides).

Treatment of other specific infections

For most invasive fungal infection: amphotericin B, 0.5–1.5 mg/kg i.v. daily, possibly with 5-flucytosine, or liposomal amphotericin B 1–4 mg/kg daily.
For herpes simplex infection: acyclovir, 5 mg/kg 8-hourly for 7 days.
For varicella–zoster infection: acyclovir, 10 mg/kg 8-hourly for 7 days.
For cytomegalovirus infection: ganciclovir, 5 mg/kg i.v. 12-hourly for 2 weeks, maintained at 5 mg/kg daily for a further 2–3 weeks with immunoglobulin.
For *P. carinii* pneumonitis: co-trimoxazole, 120 mg/kg daily in divided doses, with steroids.

Prophylaxis [2]

For gram-negative bacteria: a 4-quinolone, *e.g.*, ciprofloxacin, 250–500 mg orally twice daily, with colistin, 1.5 MU orally.
For gram-positive bacteria: penicillin or macrolide antibiotic.
For mycobacteria (in cases of previous disease, family contact, endemic area): isoniazid 5 mg/kg daily or a 4-quinolone, *e.g.*, ciprofloxacin, 500 mg twice daily.
For legionella: a 4-quinolone, *e.g.*, ciprofloxacin, 500 mg twice daily.
For *Candida albicans* or *Cryptococcus neoformans*: fluconazole, 100–200 mg orally daily.
For *Candida glabrata*: amphotericin B suspension, 500 mg orally 6-hourly.
For aspergillosis: air filtration, itraconazole, or amphotericin B, 0.5–1 mg/kg i.v. daily.
For herpes simplex or varicella–zoster virus: acyclovir, 5 mg/kg 8-hourly.
For cytomegalovirus: possibly acyclovir, 10 mg/kg i.v. 8-hourly, ganciclovir (myelosuppression), or foscarnet.
For *P. carinii*: co-trimoxazole, 960 mg orally twice daily for 3 days weekly, or aerosolized pentamidine, 150 mg every 2 weeks.
For strongyloidiasis: thiabendazole, 25 mg/kg orally twice daily for 3 days.
For toxoplasmosis: pyrimethamine, 75 mg orally daily (loading dose, 100 mg), with folinic acid, 15 mg 3 times daily, and possibly sulfadiazine, 2 g i.v. or orally 3 times daily.

Key references

1. Rubin M, Walsh TJ, Pizzo P: Clinical approach to infections in the compromised host. In *Hematology Basic Principles and Practice.* Edited by Hoffman R, Benz E, Shattil S, *et al.*: New York: Churchill Livingstone; 1991:1063–1114.

2. Prentice HG, Kibbler CC, MacWhinney PH: Antimicrobial prophylaxis and treatment after chemotherapy or marrow transplantation. In *Recent Advances in Hematology*, vol 6. Edited by Hoffbrand AV, Brenner M. London: Churchill Livingstone; 1991.

3. Ramphal R, Gucalp R, Rotstein C, *et al.*: Clinical experience with single agent and combination regimens in the management of infection in the febrile neutropenic patient. *Am J Med* 1996, **100(suppl)**:835–895.

Diagnosis

Symptoms

Liquid stools: >3 movements and >200 mL per day.

Blood (dysentery): implies active mucosal inflammation.

Abdominal pain: variable and often predefecatory.

Tenesmus: suggests proctitis.

Fever.

Weight loss, malnutrition, dehydration: in prolonged cases.

Oily stools with malabsorbed food: common in giardiasis.

Signs

Pyrexia: suggests active mucosal inflammation.

Clinical evidence of dehydration or malnutrition.

Pallor: patients with chronic anemia or acute blood loss.

Anal rash or excoriation: nonspecific irritation from alkaline stool; however, may also be due to infection by *Enterobius vermicularis* or *Strongyloides stercoralis*.

Arthropathy: occasionally seen with gram-negative infections.

Borborygmi.

Splenomegaly, rose spots: due to *Salmonella typhi* or *paratyphi* infection.

Peritonitis: rare.

Investigations

• Diagnostic investigations are indicated in patients with severe symptoms or signs and in patients with disease processes lasting >1 week in duration.

Hematology: peripheral blood eosinophilia suggests invasive helminthic infection.

Fecal microscopy, parasitology, culture: fresh warm specimens yield highest positivity rate for *Entamoeba histolytica*, *Giardia lamblia*; stool should also be tested for *Clostridium difficile* toxin.

Upper gastrointestinal endoscopy, including duodenal biopsy: for morphology and parasitology in severe cases or when symptoms persist >2 weeks and stool studies are negative.

Giardia lamblia cysts. (Iodine stain.) (*See* Color Plate.)

Small-intestinal radiography: to check for ileocecal tuberculosis in patients at risk for tuberculosis or in those without diagnosis despite extensive evaluation.

Hydrogen breath test: to evaluate for bacterial overgrowth.

HIV serology: in patients with risk factors or otherwise negative evaluation [1].

Complications

Dehydration, electrolyte disturbance.

Renal failure: due to hypovolemia or sepsis-related acute tubular necrosis.

Anemia: due to hemorrhage.

Gram-negative septicemia: rare.

"Hyperinfection syndrome": due to *S. stercoralis* infection.

Ileal perforation, hemorrhage: due to salmonellosis.

Mesenteric adenitis or ileitis, nonsuppurative arthritis, ankylosing spondylitis, erythema nodosum, Reiter's syndrome: due to *Yersinia enterocolitica* infection.

Perforation, hemorrhage, Reiter's syndrome, hemolytic uremic syndrome: due to shigellosis.

Acute necrotizing colitis, appendicitis, ameboma, hemorrhage, stricture: due to amebic colitis.

Colonic necrosis: due to pseudomembranous colitis.

Differential diagnosis

Inflammatory bowel disease (usually ulcerative colitis).

Drug-induced diarrhea: laxatives, magnesium compounds, quinidine, prostaglandins.

Lactose intolerance.

Diabetic autonomic neuropathy.

Endocrine-associated diarrhea (*e.g.*, diabetes, hyperthyroidism).

Pheochromocytoma.

Other noninfective causes of bulky, fatty stools (malabsorption): Mediterranean lymphoma (alpha-chain disease), severe malnutrition, intestinal resection, chronic pancreatitis, chronic hepatocellular dysfunction, sprue [2], Whipple's disease.

Idiopathic diarrhea.

Bacterial overgrowth syndrome.

NSAID enteropathy.

Etiology

Bacteria: *Aeromonas* spp., *Campylobacter* spp., *C. difficile*, *Escherichia coli* (including 0157:H7), *Mycobacterium tuberculosis*, *Plesiomonas shigelloides*, *Salmonella* spp., *Shigella* spp., *Vibrio* spp., *Y. enterocolitica*.

Viruses: adenovirus, astrovirus, Norwalk virus, rotavirus, HIV.

Protozoa: *E. histolytica*, *G. lamblia*, *Isospora belli*, *Cryptosporidium* spp., *Mycobacterium avium-intracellulare*.

Helminths: *Capillaria philippinensis*, *E. vermicularis*, *Fasciolopsis buski*, *Schistosoma mansoni*, *Schistosoma japonicum*, *Strongyloides stercoralis*, *Taenia* spp., *Trichuris trichiuria*, *Ascaris* spp. [3,4].

Travelers' diarrhea: clinical syndrome with many causes including viruses, bacteria, and protozoa.

Food poisoning.

Postinfective malabsorption.

Immunosuppression.

Epidemiology

• Intestinal infection occurs worldwide.

• Fecal–oral transmission.

• Travelers' diarrhea occurs more often in people who have travelled to an area where socioeconomic standards and hygiene are compromised (including most tropical and subtropical countries), although great geographical variations are found in prevalence rates.

Treatment

Diet and lifestyle

- Food hygiene must be strictly observed: most intestinal infections result from a contaminated environment, commonly food or drink (especially drinking water).

- Avoidance of milk and dairy products is advised due to secondary hypolactasia complicating an intestinal infection of any cause.

- Aggressive intake of fluids while avoiding alcohol and caffeine is advised.

- Good handwashing must be stressed to avoid passage of the infection to others.

Pharmacological treatment

- Most infectious diarrheas are self-limiting and require no pharmacological management.

Indications

Travelers' diarrhea: prophylaxis with bismuth subsalicylate; hydration only for loose stools; ciprofloxacin for toxic patients (fever, dehydration) or dysentery, which may require treatment with metronidazole if entamoeba a consideration [5].

C. difficile infection: vancomycin, 125 mg every 6 hours for 10 days, or metronidazole, 500 mg 3 times daily for 10 days.

E. histolytica infection: metronidazole, 500 mg 3 times daily for 10 days.

G. lamblia infection: metronidazole, 250–500 mg 3 times daily for 7 days.

I. belli infection: trimethoprim-sulfamethoxazole, 160 mg/800 mg 3 times daily for 10 days, then twice daily for 3 weeks.

S. typhi or *paratyphi* infection: ciprofloxacin, chloramphenicol, trimethoprim-sulfamethoxazole, or amoxicillin.

S. mansoni, japonicum, mekongi, intercalatum, or *matthei* infection: praziquantel.

S. stercoralis infection: albendazole or thiabendazole.

Cholera, watery (enterotoxigenic) diarrheas: oral rehydration (i.v. in extreme cases, *e.g.,* infection by *Vibrio cholerae*).

Selected regimens

Amoxicillin, 500 mg 3 times daily for 14 days (in *S. typhi* infection, reduced after defervescence).

Ampicillin, 1g 4 times daily for 14 days.

Chloramphenicol, 50 mg/kg daily in 4 divided doses for 14 days.

Ciprofloxacin, 500–750 mg twice daily for 3 days for severe travelers' diarrhea; for 14 days for *Salmonella* spp.

Albendazole, 400 mg twice daily for 1–3 days; with *S. stercoralis* infection, 3-day course repeated after 3 weeks.

Mebendazole, 100 mg initially (for ascariasis second dose may be needed).

Thiabendazole, 25mg/kg twice daily for 3 days (longer in "hyperinfection syndrome").

Praziquantel, 40–50 mg/kg initially; for *S. japonicum* infection, 60 mg/kg in three divided doses on a single day.

See manufacturer's current prescribing information for further details.

Treatment aims

To relieve diarrhea, abdominal colic, and other intestinal symptoms.

To rehydrate patient as rapidly as possible, preferably orally.

To ensure bacteriological or parasitic cure.

To return patient's nutritional status to normal, especially when clinically overt malabsorption has accompanied infection.

To prevent recurrences, especially of *Salmonella typhi* or *paratyphi* infections.

To relieve symptoms in untreatable immunosuppressed patients.

Prognosis

- In some severe infections (*e.g.,* shigellosis, *E. histolytica* colitis), specific chemotherapy results in complete recovery in almost all patients.

- If surgery is necessary for complications, the prognosis is less favorable.

Follow-up and management

- Most intestinal infections are acute; follow-up is unnecessary.

- *S. typhi* or *paratyphi* infections should be followed up in order to establish that the carrier state has not ensued.

- Patients with overt malabsorption as a secondary manifestation of an intestinal infection should be followed up for maintenance therapy and ascertainment of ultimate cure.

Key references

1. Smith PD, *et al.*: Gastrointestinal infections in AIDS. *Ann Intern Med* 1992, **116**:63–77.

2. Gracey M (ed.): *Diarrhea*. Boca Raton, FL.: CRC Press; 1991.

3. Gorbach SL, Bartlett JG, Blacklow NR (eds.): *Infectious Diseases*. Philadelphia: WB Saunders; 1992.

4. Cook GC: *Parasitic Disease in Clinical Practice*. London: Springer-Verlag; 1990.

5. DuPont HL, Ericsson CD: Prevention and treatment of travelers' diarrhea. *N Engl J Med* 1993, **328**:1821–1827.

Diagnosis

Symptoms

Dyspnea: on exertion, progressive.

Cough: usually unproductive and irritating.

Signs

Clubbing: in many patients.

Fine late inspiratory crackles: at lung base, later throughout lungs.

Cyanosis.

Late right ventricular heave, right ventricular gallop, loud pulmonary second sound, raised jugular venous pulse, peripheral edema: signs of cor pulmonale.

Hypoxemia: especially with exertion.

Investigations [1–3]

Chest radiography: shows small lung fields, irregular nodular or reticulonodular opacities, often maximal in lower zones (classic "ground-glass" appearance); honeycombing in end-stage patients; pulmonary artery enlargement; and cardiomegaly with cor pulmonale.

High-resolution CT: sensitive; may detect disease when chest radiograph normal; characteristically shows subpleural area of increased density, with central sparing; distortion of bronchi and cystic air spaces in advanced disease.

Pulmonary function tests: restrictive ventilatory defect, with low lung volumes, decreased lung compliance, and reduced carbon monoxide transfer.

Arterial blood gas analysis: may be normal in patients with mild disease; partial oxygen pressure typically falls on exercise. Severe hypoxia in severe disease.

Bronchoalveolar lavage: increased cell counts in bronchoalveolar fluid; cell differention may give diagnostic clues. Useful in eliminating infectious causes.

Lung biopsy: open lung biopsy gold standard but inappropriate in very ill or elderly patients; transbronchial, percutaneous, or needle biopsy produces smaller specimens, limiting histological analysis.

Hematology and biochemistry: usually not helpful; ESR may be raised; globulin or immunoglobulin (one or more classes) concentrations often raised; 30% of patients positive for rheumatoid or antinuclear antibody.

Complications [4]

Death: ~60% of patients die as direct consequence of fibrosing lung disease (some with terminal infection, others from respiratory failure).

Pulmonary hypertension, right heart failure: clinically evident in some patients.

Lung cancer: apparent excess in patients with interstitial fibrosis (smokers and non-smokers).

Differential diagnosis

• Many conditions have a tendency to develop into interstitial fibrosis.

Fibrogenic dust inhalation: *e.g.*, silica, asbestos.

Granulomas: due to extrinsic allergic alveolitis, berylliosis, sarcoidosis.

Chronic exudates: *e.g.*, chronic left ventricular failure, drugs, chronic renal failure.

Etiology

• The cause of many interstitial lung diseases is unknown.

• Interstitial fibrosis is characterized by an inflammatory exudate of the alveolar wall, with a tendency to form fibrosis.

• Interstitial fibrosis can occur alone or be associated with connective tissue disorders of unknown cause, *e.g.*, systemic sclerosis, SLE, rheumatoid arthritis, polymyositis.

• Certain drugs, *e.g.*, bleomycin, methotrexate, and amiodarone, can produce a picture similar to that of interstitial fibrosis.

• Certain viral agents, *e.g.*, influenza A2 virus, have been reported as inducing interstitial fibrosis.

Epidemiology

• Interstitial fibrosis is manifest mostly in middle age, often between 50–70 years of age.

• The prevalence is estimated to be 3–5 in 100 000 population.

Treatment

Diet and lifestyle

- Morbidity is increased, with progressive restriction of daily activities.
- Diet has no effect.

Pharmacological treatment [3,5]

- Treatment depends on diagnosis.
- The following treatments may be considered for idiopathic pulmonary fibrosis:

Corticosteroids

- 30%–50% of patients have some symptomatic benefit, at least short-term, from steroids; no more than 20% show objective radiographic or physiological improvement.

Standard dosage	Prednisone, 60 mg daily for 2–3 months; reduced slowly to maintenance dose if condition responsive.
Contraindications	Uncontrolled hypertension, diabetes mellitus, infection, severe osteoporosis.
Main drug interactions	None.
Main side effects	Weight gain, edema, bruising, purple striae in skin (especially of abdomen), moon face, osteoporosis, collapse of vertebrae, diabetes mellitus, hypertension, myopathy (especially proximal girdle muscles), hirsutism, menstrual disturbances, psychotic reactions, cataracts, withdrawal phenomena.

Cyclophosphamide

- Many patients fail to respond to high-dose steroids alone; in patients who continue to deteriorate, low-dose prednisone can be combined with cyclophosphamide, an immunosuppressant drug.

Standard dosage	Cyclophosphamide, 2 mg/kg daily with prednisone.
Contraindications	Severe renal impairment, porphyria.
Special points	Clinical improvement not expected within 2 months of starting treatment.
Main drug interactions	Muscle relaxants.
Main side effects	Hemorrhagic cystitis, bone-marrow suppression, alopecia.

Other drugs

- D-Penicillamine, azathioprine, colchicine, and methotrexate have proved disappointing.

Supportive treatment

Supplemental oxygen for patients with arterial oxygen tension of <55 mm Hg.

Diuretics for heart failure.

Opiates for suppression of cough and alleviation of breathlessness.

Pneumococcal and influenza vaccines: should be administered.

Treatment aims

To improve quality of life by preventing deterioration of lung function.
To relieve symptoms.
To give maximum supportive care, including counseling, when symptomatic relief not possible.

Other treatments

- Lung transplantation is indicated for patients with rapidly progressive disease and young patients who do not respond to conventional treatment.

Prognosis [6]

- Mortality within 5 years of diagnosis is 50%.
- Probable responders usually have a more cellular histological response.
- Improved survival may be achieved if the disease is detected early and more precise predictors of progression are developed to prevent high-risk patients, in whom more aggressive treatment would be justified.
- The 1-year survival rate after single-lung transplantation is 50%.

Follow-up and management

- The response should be assessed by clinical, subjective, and objective changes in chest radiography and pulmonary function tests.

Key references

1. Schwartz DA, *et al.*: Determinants of progression in idiopathic pulmonary fibrosis. *Am J Respir Crit Care Med* 1994, **149**:444–449.

2. Terriff BA, *et al.*: Fibrosing alveolitis: chest radiography and CT as predictors of clinical and functional impairment at follow-up in 26 patients. *Radiology* 1992, **184**:445–449.

3. Schwarz MI, King TE Jr (eds.): *Interstitial Lung Disease*. St. Louis: Mosby-Yearbook, 1993.

4. Panos R, *et al.*: Clinical deterioration in patients with idiopathic pulmonary fibrosis: causes and assessment. *Am J Med* 1990, **88**:396–404.

5. Schwarz MI: The acute (noninfectious) interstitial lung diseases. *Compr Ther* 1996, **22**:622–630.

6. Schwartz DA, *et al.*: Determinants of survival in idiopathic pulmonary fibrosis. *Am J Respir Crit Care Med* 1994, **149**:450–454.

Diagnosis

Symptoms

Headache, nausea, vomiting, drowsiness: due to raised intracranial pressure.

Seizure: due to lobar hematoma, in 28%–30% of patients.

Diplopia, gaze impairment, hiccoughs, dysarthia, facial hyperesthesia: due to brain stem hematoma.

Signs

Confusion, coma, papilledema: due to raised intracranial pressure.

Hemiplegia, aphasia, homonymous visual-field defects: due to cortical or subcortical hematomas.

Vertical-gaze palsy, skew deviation of eyes, miotic unreactive pupils: due to thalamic hematoma.

III nerve palsy, skew deviation of eyes: due to midbrain hematoma.

Horizontal-gaze palsy, pin-point reactive pupil, hyperpyrexia: due to pontine hematoma.

Ipsilateral V–VII nerve palsy, ataxia or nystagmus: due to cerebellar hematoma.

Investigations [1]

• Laboratory tests are not diagnostic but may identify underlying abnormalities.

Hematology profile: to identify bleeding disorders.

Clotting profile: to identify disorders of coagulation.

ESR and antinuclear antibody measurement: to identify vasculitic disorders.

CT of brain with bone windows: to identify skull fractures, hemorrhage, hydrocephalus, or edema; after
2 weeks, may be indistinguishable from infarct.

MRI of brain: examination of choice for cavernous angiomas; may help in identifying multiple lesions in patients with intracerebral metastasis.

Four-vessel angiography: to identify aneurysms (causing subarachnoid hemorrhage) or arteriovenous malformations; four-vessel because, in 20%–25% of patients, several aneurysms may be present.

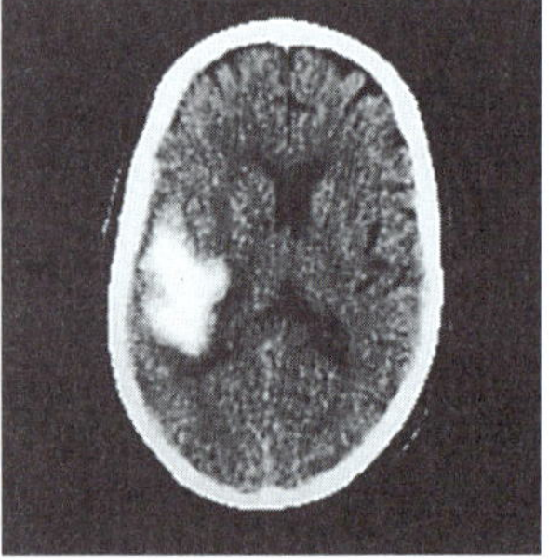
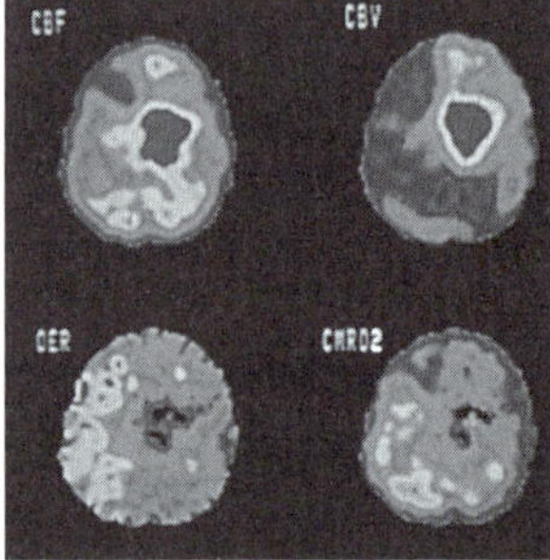

Intracerebral hemorrhage (*left*); fractional images of large arteriovenous malformation (*right*; *see* Color Plate).

Complications

Tentorial herniation: with large supratentorial hematoma; herniation from below may occur rarely with large brain stem or cerebellar hematoma.

Foramen magnum herniation: preterminal event with large hematoma.

Hydrocephalus: with ventricular extension of hemorrhage from extrinsic pressure on CSF pathways, especially at aqueduct level and in cerebellar, caudate (75%), and thalamic hemorrhages.

Hyperpyrexia: usually in preterminal pontine hemorrhage.

Seizures: subcortical hematoma, which isolates strip of cortex.

Rebleed and vasospasm: in subarachnoid hemorrhage, risk of bleeding again is 35% within 1 month, with 42% mortality; vasospasm causing cerebral ischemia occurs ~5 days after subarachnoid hemorrhage and may last ≥2 weeks.

Differential diagnosis

Hemorrhagic infarction: usually maximal neurodeficit from onset, raised intracranial pressure improbable, source of emboli present, CT showing mottled attenuation with minimal mass effect.

Subarachnoid hemorrhage: sudden (thunderclap) headache often preceded by warning (sentinel) headache (30%–60%), meningism with possible neck stiffness, photophobia, III (posterior communicating artery aneurysm) or VI nerve palsies, confusion and emotional lability (anterior communicating artery aneurysm).

Hemorrhage into brain tumor: papilledema, multiple-site hemorrhages, mass effect, noncontrasted CT showing high-density hemorrhage surrounding low-density center.

Etiology

Hypertensive intracerebral hemorrhage.

Vascular malformations.

Bleeding into intracranial tumor.

Anticoagulant treatment (8%–11% increased risk) and hemorrhagic disorders.

Sympathomimetic drugs (amphetamine, phenylpropanolamine).

Trauma.

Cerebral amyloid angiopathy (history of dementia in 10%–30%, rare before 55 years).

Granulomatous vasculitis of CNS.

Necrotizing systemic vasculitis.

Epidemiology [2]

• Intracerebral hemorrhage accounts for 10% of all strokes.

• Putaminal hemorrhage is the most usual variety of intracerebral hemorrhage (35%).

• Other common sites include the globus pallidus and pons.

Treatment

Diet and lifestyle

• No special precautions are necessary.

Pharmacological treatment

• Lack of prospective data on intracerebral hemorrhage treatment has led to most patients being treated nonsurgically. A national trial of surgical vs. medical management is currently underway.

For hypertension [3]

• Severe hypertension should be treated to maintain mean arterial pressure between 60 and 70 mm Hg.

• Intravenous beta-blockers with additional alpha-blocking action (labetalol) and diuretics are useful.

• Nitroprusside, hydralazine, and calcium antagonists should be avoided in the first week; these are cerebral vasodilators and may worsen intracerebral pressure.

Standard dosage	Labetalol, 2 mg/min i.v. infusion, 50–200 mg total.
Contraindications	Asthma, heart block.
Special points	Upright position must be avoided for 3 hours after infusion.
Main drug interactions	Antiarrhythmics.
Main side effects	Postural hypotension.

For seizures

• Routine prophylaxis is not justified.

• Tonic–clonic convulsions need urgent control.

Standard dosage	Diazepam, 10–20 mg i.v., and phenytoin, 1 g i.v. over 30–45 minutes, with cardiac monitoring.
Contraindications	None of importance.
Special points	May precipitate in 5% glucose solution.
Main drug interactions	None of importance.
Main side effects	Nausea, vomiting, mental confusion.

For coagulopathies

• Patients should be given fresh frozen plasma, vitamin K, or platelet infusion.

For raised intracerebral pressure

• If facilities permit, intracerebral pressure can be monitored, and cerebral perfusion pressure (blood pressure minus intracerebral pressure) can be measured.

• Current techniques for measuring intracerebral pressure are invasive and have a 2%–8% risk of intracranial infection.

• Intracerebral pressure should be maintained <20–25 mm Hg.

Standard dosage	Mannitol, 0.5 g/kg i.v. initially, with furosemide or subsequent albumin infusion.
Contraindications	Congestive cardiac failure, pulmonary edema.
Special points	Mannitol should not be used when serum osmolality is >320 mOsm/L.
Main drug interactions	None of importance.
Main side effects	Chills, fever.

• Hyperventilation is indicated to maintain arterial carbon dioxide concentration at 3.5 kPa; excessive hyperventilation may produce cerebral ischemia.

• Corticosteroids have no role in the management of raised intracerebral pressure caused by hemorrhage.

Treatment aims

To reverse neurodeficit.
To prevent complications.

Other treatments

• Direct evacuation of hematoma, ventricular drainage for hydrocephalus, or surgical obliteration for aneurysm is indicated for the following:
Cerebellar hemorrhage if signs of tegmental compression, hematoma 3 cm in diameter (on CT), hydrocephalus or obliteration of quadrigeminal cisterns.
Lobar hemorrhage (hematoma volume 20–40 mL), with progressive deterioration (100% mortality with medical treatment).
Acute hydrocephalus.
Subarachnoid hemorrhage: direct clipping aneurysms, thrombosis for giant aneurysms.
Hemorrhage from arteriovenous malformation: pre- and intraoperative embolization and staged resection.

Prognosis

• Large hematoma with progressive neurological deficits, coma at presentation, or ventricular extension has poor prognosis (overall mortality, 25%–60%).

• Large pontine hemorrhage is usually fatal within 24–48 hours.

• Caudate hemorrhage usually has a benign outcome despite ventricular extension and hydrocephalus.

Follow-up and management

• In patients needing anticoagulation after surgical treatment, aspirin can be started a few days after surgery, warfarin probably after 1 month unless mechanical valve necessitates earlier treatment.

• CT is mandatory if neurological deterioration occurs.

Key references

1. Kase CS: Intracerebral hemorrhage. In *Neurology in Clinical Practice.* Edited by Bradley WG, *et al.* Oxford: Butterworth Heinemann; 1991:940–954.

2. Thompson DW, Furlam AJ: Clinical epidemiology of stroke. *Neurosurg Clin North Am* 1997, **8**:265–269.

3. Adans RF, Powers WJ: Management of hypertension in acute intracerebral hemorrhage. *Crit Care Clin* 1997, **13**:131–161.

Diagnosis

Symptoms

• Criteria for irritable bowel syndrome are continuous or recurrent symptoms for at least 3 months consisting of abdominal pain and disturbed defecation (*i.e.*, at least two of the following: altered stool frequency, form, or passage; passage of mucus).

Abdominal pain: often intermittent, crampy lower abdominal pain; relieved by defecation or passage of flatus; associated with change in frequency or consistency of stool.

Straining, urgency, passage of mucus, feeling of incomplete evacuation.

Loose stools: often in morning or after meals.

Constipation: small, hard stools, difficult to pass.

Abdominal distension: bloating worse after meals and at end of day, relieved by defecation or passage of flatus.

• Passage of blood, weight loss, or nocturnal symptoms that awaken the patient from sleep suggest an alternative diagnosis.

Signs

Variable abdominal tenderness: often over palpable sigmoid colon; frequently present but nonspecific.

• Structural abnormalities such as a mass, ascites, or organomegaly suggest an alternative diagnosis.

Investigations

• Irritable bowel disease is diagnosed on the basis of symptoms, signs, and the clinical course; diagnostic investigations should be aimed at evaluating other competing diagnoses.

Assessment of mental health: a history of previous physical or sexual abuse is relatively common, particularly in women with functional abdominal complaints; anxiety, depression, and personality disorders are frequently identified in these patients and adverse life events may precede symptoms.

Complete blood count: anemia or leukocytosis suggests an alternative diagnosis.

Liver chemistry tests: abnormal tests suggest an alternative diagnosis.

Thyroid function tests: for myxedema manifest as constipation, or thyrotoxicosis as diarrhea.

Colonic imaging: barium enema or colonoscopy; for new or different symptoms in patients aged >40 years to exclude colonic carcinoma or inflammatory bowel disease. The barium enema or colonoscopy should be normal in patients with irritable bowel syndrome.

Small-bowel contrast studies, gastroscopy, abdominal ultrasonography or CT, duodenal or jejunal biopsy, or aspiration: in selected cases to exclude Crohn's disease, peptic ulcer, biliary or pancreatic disease.

Colonic biopsy: may be useful in patients with diarrhea predominantly to exclude collagenous colitis and laxative abuse.

Plain abdominal radiography, colonic transit timing, full-thickness colonic biopsy, or defecography: of occasional use in patients with severe constipation to exclude megacolon, idiopathic slow-transit constipation, neuromuscular gut disorders, obstructed defecation.

Complications

Increased incidence of colonic diverticulosis: caused by prolonged constipation.

Major physical and psychological morbidity: this often leads to "doctor shopping" for a cure and, often, excessive testing.

Dependency on narcotics or benzodiazepines.

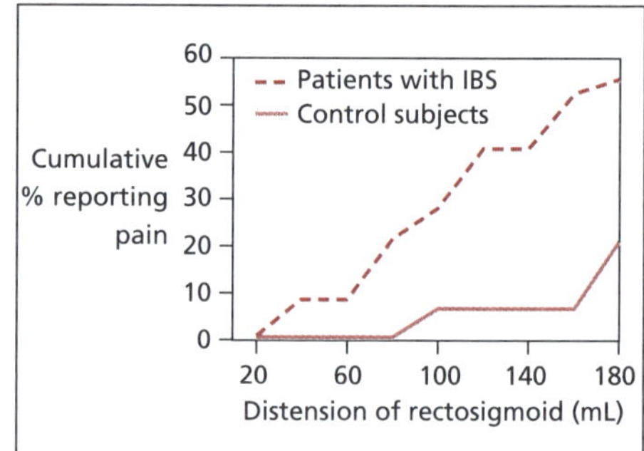

Irritable bowel syndrome. Heightened visceral sensitivity to balloon distention of the sigmoid colon in patients with irritable bowel syndrome (IBS) (*n*=25), using a latex balloon, compared with healthy persons (*n*=20). A sensitive gut is found more often in patients with diarrhea-predominant IBS. Gut sensitivity is not caused by a nonspecific intolerance to pain, because pain tolerance to noxious stimuli such as immersion in ice-cold water is normal in IBS.

Treatment

Diet and lifestyle

• A thorough explanation of the intermittent nature of the symptoms, despite therapy, must be stressed with the patient to achieve realistic expectations for future results.

• Patients should be encouraged to maintain a high-fiber diet and exercise regularly.

• A food-intake diary may identify certain foods that often aggravate symptoms.

Pharmacological treatment

• Placebo response rates are high (range, 20%–70%).

• Few drugs have been proved to be of unequivocal benefit; many patients, however, find drugs helpful in controlling symptoms, often preferring "as-required" medication to long-term usage [1,2].

• Treatment should be targeted to the predominant complaint.

Bulking agents

• These are useful mostly for constipation-predominant symptoms and supplementation with a cathartic (*e.g.,* lactulose) maybe of help.

• The full effect may not be apparent for several days.

Standard dosage	Bran ispaghula husk, or psyllium titrated to achieve ~1 bowel movement each day. Lactulose, 15 mL twice daily, increased as needed for patients with a major component of constipation; stimulant laxatives are rarely needed for intractable cases.
Contraindications	Intestinal obstruction.
Special points	Patients must take adequate fluid.
Main drug interactions	None.
Main side effects	Distension, flatulence, abdominal pain.

Antispasmodics

• Antispasmodics, either with anticholinergic properties or direct muscle relaxants, are given for pain relief with variable results. They should be discontinued if the patient doesn't note a significant benefit.

Standard dosage	*Anticholinergics:* dicyclomine, 10–20 mg up to 3 times daily, or scopolamine, 20 mg up to 4 times daily. *Direct relaxants:* peppermint oil, 1 capsule up to 3 times daily.
Contraindications	Paralytic ileus, ulcerative colitis. *Anticholinergics:* glaucoma.
Special points	Dosage times should be varied to suit the individual.
Main drug interactions	*Anticholinergics:* disopyramide, cisapride, antidepressants.
Main side effects	*Anticholinergics:* dry mouth, blurring of vision, palpitations, constipation. *Direct relaxants:* heartburn.

Antidiarrheal drugs

• The diarrhea must be confirmed (not pseudodiarrhea or fecal retention with overflow).

Standard dosage	Loperamide, 2–16 mg daily in divided doses or diphenoxylate and atropine, 2 tablets 3–4 times daily; dose adjusted to control symptoms.
Contraindications	Intestinal obstruction, inflammatory bowel disease.
Special points	Night-time dosage might prevent morning diarrhea.
Main drug interactions	*Diphenoxylate/atropine:* anxiolytics and hypnotics.
Main side effects	*Diphenoxylate/atropine:* constipation, dependence.

Other options

Motility stimulants: prostaglandins may be useful in constipation.

Antidepressants: tricyclic antidepressants (*e.g.,* amitriptyline, 25–50 mg at night) can be helpful, but side effects and excess sedation limit use; 5-HT uptake inhibitors (*e.g.,* fluoxetine, 20 mg daily) are also effective and less sedating.

Treatment aims

To control or cure the most intrusive complaint.

To treat associated psychological disorders [3].

Other treatments

• Behavioral therapy (hypnotherapy, psychotherapy, relaxation techniques) is effective for some intractable cases.

• Younger patients or those with identifiable psychological disease appear to benefit most.

• Behavioral therapy is relatively ineffective for older patients or constant or chronic pain sufferers [4].

Prognosis

• This is a chronic relapsing condition.

• >75% of patients respond to treatment over 1 year.

• Response is better in men, constipation-predominant sufferers, and those with a short history or symptoms after acute diarrhea.

Follow-up and management

• Follow-up is not needed for mild or moderate cases.

• Patients must be monitored for change in symptoms; new or different complaints should be investigated; persistent symptoms do not need further tests.

• Regular, brief review of intractable cases may reduce inappropriate investigation and further referral.

Key references

1. Lynn RB, Friedman LS: Irritable bowel syndrome. *N Engl J Med* 1993, **329**:1940–1945.

2. Thompson WG: Irritable bowel syndrome: pathogenesis and management. *Lancet* 1993, **341**:1569–1572.

3. Camilleri M, Prather CM: The irritable bowel syndrome: mechanisms and a practical approach to management. *Ann Intern Med* 1992, **116**:1001–1008.

4. Heaton KW, *et al.*: Symptoms of irritable bowel syndrome in a British urban community: consulters and non-consulters. *Gastroenterology* 1992, **102**:1962–1967.

Diagnosis

Symptoms

Mucocutaneous
Painless purplish patches.

Lymphatic
Lymphadenopathy and edema.

Pulmonary
Dyspnea, cough.
Hemoptysis, chest pain (pleuritic or dull ache).

Gastrointestinal
Anorexia, abdominal pain, hematemesis, melena.

Signs

Mucocutaneous
Violacious macule, plaque, or nodule, surrounding edema.

Lymphatic
Firm or indurated lymphadenopathy.
Edema of dependent limbs.
Compression of adjacent structures.

Pulmonary
Pulmonary nodules or effusion.

Gastrointestinal
Palpable mass, tenderness.

Other signs
Organomegaly.

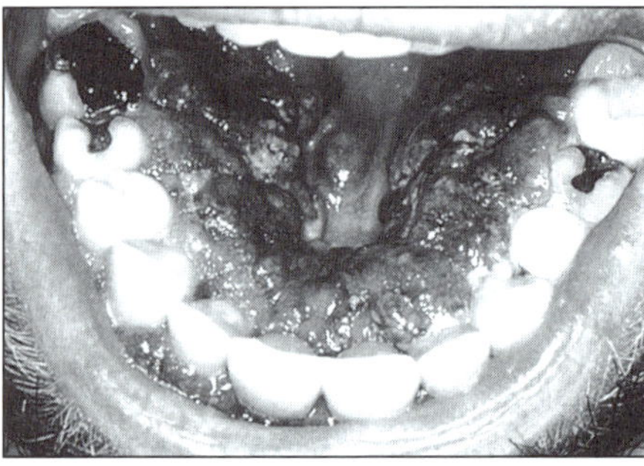

Oral Kaposi's sarcoma in HIV disease. (*See* Color Plate.)

Investigations

General
Lymphocyte subset analysis: Kaposi's sarcoma can occur at any stage.
Complete blood count: to assess anemia; neutrophil and platelet count needed before chemotherapy.
Biopsy of involved organ: required for confirmation.

Pulmonary
Chest radiography: may be normal or reveal infiltrates, nodules, or pleural effusion.
Fiberoptic bronchoscopy: for visualization and biopsy.

Gastrointestinal
Fiberoptic endoscopy or sigmoidoscopy: for visualization and biopsy.
Ultrasonography or CT: with guided biopsy, if disease is not seen by endoscopy.

Complications

Ulceration, infection, immobilization edema.

Gastrointestinal obstruction, hemorrhage.

Respiratory failure.

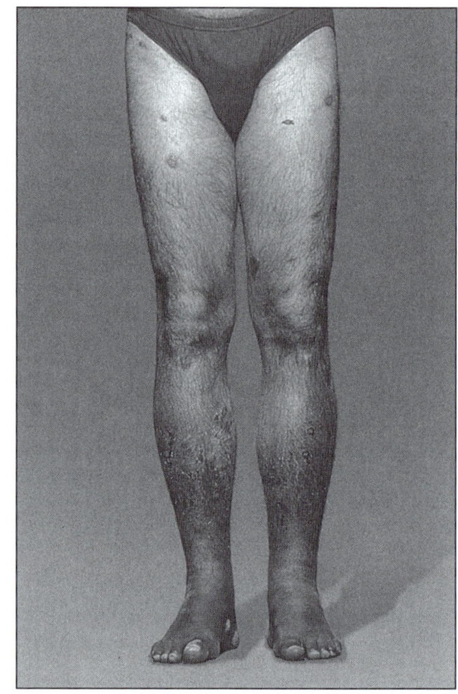

Generalized cutaneous Kaposi's sarcoma. (*See* Color Plate.)

Treatment

Diet and lifestyle

• No special precautions are necessary.

Pharmacological treatment

• All treatment must be given under specialist supervision.

Intralesional chemotherapy

• Intralesional chemotherapy is indicated for limited mucocutaneous disease.

Standard dosage	Vinblastine into lesion until blanching occurs.
Contraindications	Infection at site.
Main drug interactions	None of importance.
Main side effects	Local pain and ulceration.

Interferon

• Interferons are indicated for good-prognosis Kaposi's sarcoma.

Standard dosage	Interferon-α, i.m. or s.c. daily, possibly with zidovudine.
Contraindications	Bone-marrow suppression, renal or hepatic impairment.
Special points	Lesions may recur after treatment stops.
Main drug interactions	None of importance.
Main side effects	Influenza-like symptoms, neutropenia, anemia.

Bleomycin and vincristine

• These are the first-line chemotherapy in the United States for patients with visceral disease or rapidly progressive cutaneous disease.

Standard dosage	Vincristine (or vinblastine if neuropathy develops) and bleomycin every 2 weeks, with hydrocortisone.
Contraindications	Pregnancy and lactation (all), severe lung impairment (bleomycin); caution if patient has a neuropathy.
Main drug interactions	Increased phenytoin concentrations.
Main side effects	*Bleomycin*: rashes, increased skin pigmentation, Raynaud's phenomenon, hypersensitivity reaction, dose-related progressive pulmonary fibrosis. *Vincristine*: alopecia, peripheral and autonomic neuropathy. *Vinblastine*: myelotoxic, neurotoxic (less than vincristine).

Liposomal daunorubicin and doxorubicin

• Liposomal daunorubicin and doxorubicin are currently available within clinical trials or for compassionate use only; they are fairly widely used in the United States.

Treatment aims

To achieve cosmetic improvement (limited disease).

To control new lesion development and to treat existing lesions (advancing disease).

To reduce tumor bulk and to treat pain, immobility, and infection (advanced disease).

Other treatments

• Radiotherapy under specialist supervision is the treatment of choice unless control of new lesion is required; it is often combined with chemotherapy.

• Side effects include erythema, increased pigmentation.

Prognosis

• Prognosis is extremely variable; survival may be for months or years.

• Death is often due to other AIDS-defining illnesses.

• Factors indicating poor prognosis include the following:

CD4 count $<200 \times 10^6$/L.

Previous opportunistic infections.

"B" symptoms.

Tumor-associated edema.

Nonnodal visceral Kaposi's sarcoma.

Follow-up and management

• Complete blood count must be monitored.

• Patients with limited disease must be followed up every 3 months.

• Patients with extensive disease must be followed up every 1–2 weeks.

General references

Anonymous: Kaposi's sarcoma and its management in AIDS patients: recommendations from a Scandinavian study group. *Scand J Infect Dis* 1997, **29**:3–12.

Krown SE: Acquired immunodeficiency syndrome–associated Kaposi's sarcoma: biology and treatment. *Med Clin North Am* 1997, **81**:471–494.

Schaty U, Bogner JR, Gaebel FD: Kaposi's sarcoma: is the hunt for the culprit over now? *J Mol Med* 1997, **75**:28–34.

Diagnosis

Symptoms

Pain: various locations—anterior, medial, lateral, posterior.

Locking.

Buckling/"giving-way."

Instability.

Popping.

Tearing.

Swelling.

Stiffness.

Limitation of flexion or extension.

Signs

Swelling (effusion, soft tissue).

Deformity.

Erythema.

Heat.

Muscular atrophy.

Tenderness to palpation (exact location).

Provocative maneuvers: Lachmann's test (best), Drawer sign, McMurray test, etc.

Investigations

Physical examination: of paramount importance; skillful examination by experienced musculoskeletal specialist may exceed the diagnostic accuracy of MRI, ultrasound, or arthrography.

Arthrocentesis.

Ultrasound.

MRI.

Arthrography.

Arthroscopy.

Complications

Atrophy.

Weakness.

Swelling.

Deformity.

Chronic pain.

Chronic arthritis.

Instability.

Locking.

Falling.

Gait disturbance.

Exercise limitation.

Chronic impairment.

Differential diagnosis

Hemarthrosis
Meniscal tears.
Ligamentous injuries.
Osteochondral fractures.
Patellar dislocation.

Locking
Bucket handle tear of meniscus.
Loose body.
Anterior cruciate ligament (ACL) tear.
Suprapatellar plica.

"Popping" noise
• ~70% of patients with ACL tear heard a "pop."
Immediate onset of effusion.
Unable to continue to participate in activity.

Timing of effusion
• Acute bleeding results in effusion within 1 hour of injury.
Ligamentous injuries.
Peripheral meniscal tears.
Osteochondral fractures.
• Late effusions (12–18 hours) are more typical for meniscal tears.

Etiology

Trauma of various types
Acute athletic injuries.
Chronic (repetitive, overuse).
Falling.
Multifactorial (*e.g.*, degenerative plus falling).

Mechanism of injury
• Internal or external rotation is most common.
• Contact is not required.
"Cutting" maneuvers.
Impact or collision.
Overuse.

Specific anatomical injuries
ACL tears.
Posterior cruciate ligament tears.
Meniscal tears.
Medical collateral ligament tears.
Sprains.
Patellar dislocation.
Fractures.

Proposed etiologies
Genetic predisposition.
"Q angle."
Inadequate pre-athletic competition conditioning.
Inadequate proprioceptive training.

Epidemiology

•Knee injuries are among the most common disabling injuries in all walks of life, especially among athletes (both casual/recreational and competitive/elite).
•Collision and contact sports are responsible for many knee injuries.
•An estimated 50% of high school football players will experience a knee injury per year.

Treatment

Diet and lifestyle

• Individualized treatment programs must consider patient preferences and activity expectations.

• Sports psychology strategies may be critical.

Pharmacological treatment

• Analgesic with acetaminophen, NSAIDs, codeine, and hydrocodone may be necessary.

• Attention to accurate diagnosis and early rehabilitation may help limit habituation.

Nonpharmacological treatment

• Conservative therapy involves the following:

RICE—*R*est, *I*ce, *C*ompression, *E*levation.

Early range-of-motion exercises.

Immobilization vs. ambulation.

Functional bracing.

Hamstring strengthening.

Rehabilitation: closed-chain kinetic exercises are best.

• Surgical therapy is another option.

• Other therapeutic options include arthroscopy and reconstructive surgery.

Treatment aims

To relieve pain.

To reduce swelling.

To restore full range of motion.

To prevent or reverse muscular atrophy.

To allow safe return to participation in previous activities.

Prognosis

• Prognosis varies widely depending on the specific structural injury and severity.

• ACL reconstruction may have a 50% failure rate.

• ACL-deficient knee may be complicated by degenerative changes in 40% of cases.

• Posterior cruciate ligament injury management is controversial: 5%–8% progress to arthritis; worse prognosis for combination injury; only moderate stability is currently achievable with surgery.

General references

Baker CL: *The Hughston Clinic Sports Medicine Book*. Baltimore: Williams and Wilkins; 1995.

Bergfeld JA: *Injuries of the Athlete's Knee*. Phoenix: American College of Rheumatology; 1996.

Birrer RB: *Sports Medicine for the Primary Care Physician*. Boca Raton, FL: CRC Press; 1994.

Garrick JG, Webb DR: *Sports Injuries: Diagnosis and Management*. Philadelphia: WB Saunders; 1990.

Mellion MB: *Sports Medicine Secrets*. Philadelphia: Hanley and Belfus; 1994.

Diagnosis

Symptoms and signs

• Any organ or tissue can be infected, so the clinical picture can vary enormously.

• The disease follows a biphasic course: the incubation period lasting 7–12 days (range, 2–20 days) is followed by the septicemic phase lasting 4–7 days, which precedes the immune phase lasting 4–30 days.

Anicteric leptospirosis

• This occurs in 90% of patients.

• Onset is abrupt.

Fever, headache, myalgia, malaise, prostration.

Abdominal pain, nausea, vomiting, occasionally diarrhea.

Excruciating headache: usually heralds meningitis in immune stage.

Joint pains, myalgia, conjunctival suffusion, rashes, lymphadenopathy: common findings.

Lymphocytic meningitis: usually lasting a few days, never fatal.

Icteric leptospirosis (Weil's syndrome)

• This form occurs in 10% of patients.

Impaired renal and hepatic function: with anuria and deepening jaundice.

Hepatosplenomegaly, severe hemorrhages into skin, pleura, peritoneum, or gastrointestinal tract.

Vascular collapse and alterations in consciousness.

Myocarditis, hemorrhage, adult respiratory distress syndrome, multiorgan failure: causing death in 10%–20% of icteric patients.

Investigations

• Diagnosis is confirmed by isolation of the organism or detection of a rise in antibody titers.

Isolation: special media needed; organisms isolated from blood or CSF during septicemic phase and from urine during third week in untreated patients.

Serology: slide agglutination tests unreliable; antibodies appear in 6–12 days, reach maximum in 4 weeks, can be suppressed by antibiotic treatment; enzyme-linked immunosorbent assay IgM test detects antibodies from day 5 of illness; microagglutination test is specific and identifies infecting serotype.

Complete blood count and coagulation screen: to identify bleeding disorder and thrombocytopenia.

Liver function tests: usually normal except for raised bilirubin.

Serum creatinine measurement: to identify degree of renal impairment.

CSF analysis: to confirm lymphocytic meningitis.

Complications

Uveitis 6–12 weeks after original illness and chronic persistent leptospiruria: extremely rare.

Transplacental transmission, with fetal death and abortion: has occurred.

Differential diagnosis

Influenza-like illness, viral infections, aseptic meningitis, encephalitis.

Enteric-fever–like illness.

Infective hepatitis, other causes of jaundice.

Rickettsioses, brucellosis, malaria.

Septicemia, nephritis.

Leukemia, thrombocytopenic purpura, meningococcal disease.

Etiology

• In the United States, prevalent serotypes of pathogenic leptospires, *Leptospira interrogans*, are *icterohaemorrhagiae*, *australis*, *autumnalis*, and *canicola*.

• Wild and domestic animals, especially rats (*icterohaemorrhagiae*) and cattle.

• Contact of mucous membranes or abraded skin with infected animal tissue or urine or contaminated water or soil can lead to transmission.

Epidemiology

• People at risk include farmers, dairy-workers, abattoir workers, veterinarians, and those working or engaged in recreational pursuits on or in natural inland waters.

Treatment

Diet and lifestyle

- Rodents must be controlled in and around human habitations.
- Contamination of living, working, and recreational areas by infected urine should be prevented.
- Cuts should be covered by waterproof dressings and protective clothing worn.
- Immersion in natural inland waters should be avoided.
- Participants should shower after swimming, canoeing, windsurfing, or waterskiing.
- Safety cards should be issued to people at risk to show medical staff if illness occurs.
- Patients should be educated on modes of transmission and preventive measures.
- Domestic animals, especially cattle and dogs, should be immunized.

Pharmacological treatment

Antibiotics

- Antibiotics may influence the course of the disease only if given in the first week.
- Treatment may be needed for severe infections; efficacy unproven.

Standard dosage	Penicillin G, 900 mg; ampicillin, 1 g; or erythromycin, 500 mg, all parenterally 4 times daily for 1 week. Amoxicillin, 500 mg orally 3 times daily, or doxycycline, 100 mg twice daily for 1 week.
Contraindications	Hypersensitivity; oral agents should be avoided in pregnancy, infancy, and childhood.
Special points	*Penicillin:* can induce a short-lived exacerbation with pyrexia and hypotension: this Jarisch-Herxheimer reaction is regarded as a sign of leptospiral lysis.
Main drug interactions	*Penicillins:* inactivate aminoglycoside in syringe. *Erythromycin:* potentiates digoxin, warfarin, and carbamazepine. *Doxycycline:* affects anticoagulant treatment.
Main side effects	*Parenteral agents:* anaphylactic reaction, gastrointestinal reactions (rare). *Amoxicillin:* erythematous rash in patients with glandular fever. *Doxycycline:* photosensitivity (rare), permanent teeth discoloration.

For symptoms

Prompt correction of electrolyte imbalance.

Fresh blood, platelets, or clotting factors for hemorrhage.

Meperidine or morphine for severe pain.

Diazepam and phenytoin for seizures.

Steroids for thrombocytopenia.

Hemodialysis for renal failure.

Treatment aims

To alleviate symptoms.

Prognosis

- Most cases are mild and often undiagnosed; patients recover spontaneously.
- In Weil's syndrome with hepatorenal involvement, mortality is 10%–20%.
- No ill effects are seen after renal or hepatic involvement in surviving patients.
- Death without jaundice is extremely rare.
- Reinfection by a different serotype is possible.

Follow-up and management

- Supportive treatment includes analgesics, sedation, and antiemetics.
- Renal and cardiac function must be monitored daily.

General references

Ferguson IR: Leptospirosis surveillance: 1990–1992. *Commun Dis Rep* 1993, **3**:R47–R48.

Ferguson IR: Leptospirosis update. *BMJ* 1991, **302**:128–129.

Hill MK, Sanders CV: Leptospiral pneumonia. *Semin Respir Infect* 1997, **12**:44–49.

Diagnosis

Symptoms

• Usually, acute lymphoblastic leukemia has a short history of 2–3 months.

Tiredness and dyspnea: due to anemia.

Recurrent infections: due to leukopenia.

Bruising and bleeding: due to thrombocytopenia.

Symptoms of hyperviscosity: if leukocyte count is very high (*e.g.*, $>200 \times 10^9$/L).

Joint and bone pain: less common than in children.

Signs

• Often no physical signs are manifest.

Pallor.

Evidence of infection.

Purpura or bruising.

Lymphadenopathy or hepatosplenomegaly.

Investigations

General

Full blood count (with Romanowsky's or Wright-Giemsa stained film): diagnosis may be evident from careful morphological examination; leukemic blasts not always seen in peripheral blood; platelet count and hemoglobin may be low or normal.

Bone-marrow aspiration: blasts should be >30% to make the diagnosis.

Blood urea nitrogen, creatinine, electrolytes, calcium, phosphate, urate measurement: important initial investigations before starting treatment, particularly if leukocyte count is high.

Chest radiography: to look for mediastinal mass, seen in 70% of patients with T-cell acute lymphoblastic leukemia (ALL; high risk of tumor lysis syndrome if this is present).

Lumbar puncture with CSF cytology: important initial investigation to detect CNS involvement (unusual at presentation).

Special

• These tests help to confirm the diagnosis; confirming that blasts are lymphoid in origin is occasionally difficult on light microscopy.

• They also help to categorize the disease more fully, giving additional prognostic information.

Cytochemistry: helps to differentiate ALL from acute myeloblastic leukemia (*e.g.*, negative reaction with Sudan black).

Immunophenotyping: identifies origin of blast cell using panel of cell-surface "markers"; useful markers include TdT (all subtypes positive except B ALL), CD10 (identifies common ALL antigen), CD19 (positive in B-lineage ALL), CD2 (positive in T-lineage ALL).

Cytogenetics: direct examination of chromosomes at metaphase can identify translocations in ~70% of patients with ALL; this can identify poor-risk patients, *e.g.*, those with t(9,22) or Philadelphia-positive ALL, which has bad prognosis; may provide a marker that can be used to detect early relapse.

Complications

• Most complications are related to bone-marrow failure (cytopenia) due to the disease or, more often, to the intensive treatment needed.

Differential diagnosis

Acute myeloid leukemia:

Aplastic anemia: diagnosis of acute lymphoblastic leukemia might not be obvious initially if presenting leukocyte count is low and bone-marrow aspirate "dry."

Lymphoblastic lymphoma: predominantly lymphomatous presentation, with <25% blasts in bone marrow; distinction may be arbitrary in adults because treatment is often the same.

Etiology

• The cause of acute lymphoblastic leukemia is unknown; it is presumed to be due to genetic mutations, the risk of which is increased by DNA damage, *e.g.*, due to radiation or DNA repair defects.

• Victims of exposure to ionizing radiation have a higher incidence of leukemia, but this is more often myeloid than lymphoid in origin.

Epidemiology

• Acute lymphoblastic leukemia is uncommon in adults, particularly in those aged >30 years.

• Patients aged >15 years are defined as adults because they constitute a separate group with much poorer remission and survival rates.

Classification [1]

Morphological

• Based on appearance on light microscopy, the French–American–British (FAB) classification divides ALL into L1, L2, and L3.

• This has little correlation with prognosis or immunophenotype, except L3 morphology with B-cell ALL.

Immunological

• On the basis of expression of surface antigens by the blast cells, ALL is divided into T lineage (early T precursor and T cell ALL) and B lineage (early B precursor, common ALL, pre-B ALL, and B cell ALL).

Treatment

Diet and lifestyle

- Nutrition must be maintained.
- Psychological support should be provided to patients and their relatives, especially if a young family is involved; financial support should be considered if earnings are disrupted.
- Patients must take precautions against infection during neutropenia.

Pharmacological treatment [2]

Principles

- Treatment should be given under specialist supervision, within the context of a clinical trial if possible to allow adequate evaluation and the development of new treatments.
- Initial treatment involves several blocks of inpatient treatment.

Induction: remission (*i.e.*, <5% blasts in bone marrow) can be achieved in ~80% of adults usually within 1 month of starting treatment; agents include steroids, vincristine, and anthracyclines.

Consolidation: usually follows quickly after induction, and new chemotherapeutic agents should be introduced; optimum duration and intensity of treatment have not yet been established.

CNS-directed treatment: often described as "CNS prophylaxis"; CNS leukemia occurs in ~37% of patients in hematological remission if no specific treatment directed at the CNS is given; possible treatments include cranial irradiation, intrathecal methotrexate, or high-dose i.v. methotrexate (which crosses the blood–brain barrier).

Maintenance therapy: continuous treatment for ~2 years improves outcome; usual treatment involves weekly methotrexate and 6-mercaptopurine, with monthly courses of vincristine and steroids.

Supportive treatment: particularly important in the early stages of treatment; includes allopurinol, adequate hydration, blood-product support, and timely use of antimicrobial treatment.

General complications of treatment

Myelosuppression (inevitable).

Hair loss.

Compromise or loss of fertility.

Infection, particularly during neutropenia: empirical treatment is often needed for bacterial, viral, or fungal infection.

Nausea and vomiting: may be easy to control.

Complications of specific drugs

Vincristine: extravasation injury, alopecia, muscle and jaw pain, urinary retention, dysphagia, peripheral neuropathy.

Prednisone: Cushing's syndrome and other steroidal side effects (including psychiatric).

L-Asparaginase: thrombotic episodes, pancreatitis, anaphylaxis.

Daunorubicin: extravasation injury, cardiomyopathy, bone-marrow suppression, vomiting, gut toxicity.

Cytarabine: gut and bone-marrow toxicity, erythema, cerebellar toxicity in high doses.

Thioguanine: hepatic and bone-marrow toxicity, rashes.

VP16 epipodophyllotoxin: gut and bone-marrow toxicity.

Methotrexate: renal, hepatic, and gut dysfunction; bone-marrow suppression; mucositis (depending on dose and mode of treatment); affects intellect.

Mercaptopurine: bone-marrow suppression, rashes, hepatic dysfunction.

Key references

1. Bain BJ: *Leukaemia Diagnosis: A Guide to the FAB Classification.* London: Gower Medical Publishing; 1990.

2. Copelan EA, McGuire EA: The biology and treatment of acute lymphoblastic leukemia in adults. *Blood* 1995, **85**:1151–1168.

3. Bruserud O (ed.): Lymphoblastic leukemia. *Leukemia* 1997, **11(suppl 4)**:1395–1597.

Diagnosis

Symptoms

• A constellation of symptoms is seen, many nonspecific and related to bone-marrow failure.

Easy bruising, bone pain, fevers, pallor, lethargy, anorexia, malaise: due to bone-marrow failure.

Abdominal distention: due to hepatosplenomegaly.

Shortness of breath, facial swelling: due to mediastinal mass; unusual.

Headache, vomiting: due to CNS disease; unusual.

Overt bleeding: due to bone-marrow failure; unusual.

Signs

Pyrexia, mucosal bleeding, skin purpura, pallor, congestive heart failure (rare): due to bone-marrow failure.

Hepatosplenomegaly, lymphadenopathy, upper trunk and facial edema with distended superficial veins, skin infiltrates, testicular enlargement: due to leukemic "mass."

Cranial nerve palsies (III, V, VI, VII), papilledema, fundal hemorrhages, leukemic infiltrates: due to CNS disease (rare).

Investigations

Full blood count: shows pancytopenia, normal counts, or isolated raised leukocyte count.

Blood film: shows possible presence of leukemic blasts.

Bone-marrow morphology: confirms diagnosis in conjunction with cytochemistry and immunophenotyping (mature B cell varieties treated on lymphoma-type protocols).

Chest radiography: for mediastinal mass.

Lumbar puncture: for CNS disease.

Blood urea nitrogen, creatine, electrolytes, and urate analysis.

Liver function tests: for liver failure (rare).

Complications

Early

• Early complications are usually related to drug side effects or further bone-marrow suppression.

Tumor lysis syndrome, associated with hyperkalemia, hyperuricemia, hyperphosphatemia, renal dysfunction.

Infection of all types.

Bleeding.

Anemia.

Vomiting, hair loss, peripheral neuropathy and myopathy, mucositis.

Late

Learning difficulties: *e.g.*, problems with short-term memory or concentration; due to cranial radiation.

Cardiotoxicity: due to anthracycline treatment.

Cataracts, sterility, growth and hormone problems: due to cyclophosphamide treatment and total body irradiation for bone-marrow transplantation.

Secondary malignancies: due to epipodophyllotoxins.

Differential diagnosis

Lymphadenopathy

Infections: *e.g.*, infectious mononucleosis.

Lymphomas or other tumors.

Hepatosplenomegaly

Leishmaniasis.

Macrophage, metabolic, storage, or auto-immune disorders.

Lymphomas.

Bone-marrow failure

Aplastic anemia.

Myelodysplasia.

Macrophage disorders.

Autoimmune disorders.

Bone-marrow tumor: *e.g.*, neuroblastoma.

Infections: *e.g.*, tuberculosis, visceral leishmaniasis.

Etiology [1]

• The cause is unknown but is presumed to be a genetic mutation.

• Increased risk is associated with the following:

Down syndrome.

Fanconi's anemia.

Bloom syndrome.

Ataxia telangiectasia and various immuno-deficiency disorders.

• The effects of irradiation or electro-magnetic fields are unconfirmed.

Epidemiology [1]

• Acute lymphoblastic leukemia is the most common malignant disease of childhood.

• A peak incidence at 2–5 years accounts for 20% of all leukemia.

• Slightly more boys than girls are affected.

• 85% of childhood leukemia is acute lymphoblastic.

Treatment

Diet and lifestyle

• Specialist support is needed for children and their families, including siblings, both in hospital during treatment and after discharge.

• Maintenance of nutrition is important.

Pharmacological treatment

• Treatment should be given under specialist supervision, in the context of a clinical trial if possible to allow adequate evaluation and the development of new treatments.

Treatment choice [2–6]

For high-risk patients (slow remitters, near haploid, Philadelphia-chromosome positive, older boys with high leukocyte counts, usually $>100 \times 10^9$/L): transplantation in first remission.

For patients at high risk of CNS disease relapse (leukocyte count $>50 \times 10^9$/L): cranial irradiation or high-dose i.v. methotrexate or cytosine arabinoside or triple-drug therapy.

For lower-risk patients (leukocyte count $<50 \times 10^9$/L): continuing intrathecal or high-dose methotrexate or cytosine arabinoside.

For patients with CNS disease at diagnosis: craniospinal or cranial irradiation and continuing intrathecal methotrexate.

For infants <6 months: intensive multiagent treatment.

Principles

Induction: usually vincristine, asparaginase, steroids; remission in 97% of patients.

Consolidation: intensive treatment with some different drugs from induction course to eradicate "resistant clones."

CNS-directed treatment: to eradicate disease in CNS sanctuary site.

Consolidation: as for second step; two or three consolidations may be needed.

Continuation of treatment up to 2 years: to eradicate minimal residue disease.

Complications of specific drugs

Vincristine: extravasation injury, alopecia, muscle and jaw pain, urinary retention, dysphagia, peripheral neuropathy.

Prednisone: Cushing's syndrome and other steroidal side effects (including psychiatric).

L-Asparaginase: thrombotic episodes, pancreatitis, anaphylaxis.

Daunorubicin: extravasation injury, cardiomyopathy, bone-marrow suppression, vomiting, gut toxicity.

Cytarabine: gut and bone-marrow toxicity, erythema, cerebellar toxicity in high doses.

Thioguanine: hepatic and bone-marrow toxicity, rashes.

VP16 epipodophyllotoxin: gut and bone-marrow toxicity.

Methotrexate: renal, hepatic, and gut dysfunction, bone-marrow suppression, mucositis (depending on dose and mode of treatment); affects intellect.

Mercaptopurine: bone-marrow suppression, rashes, hepatic dysfunction.

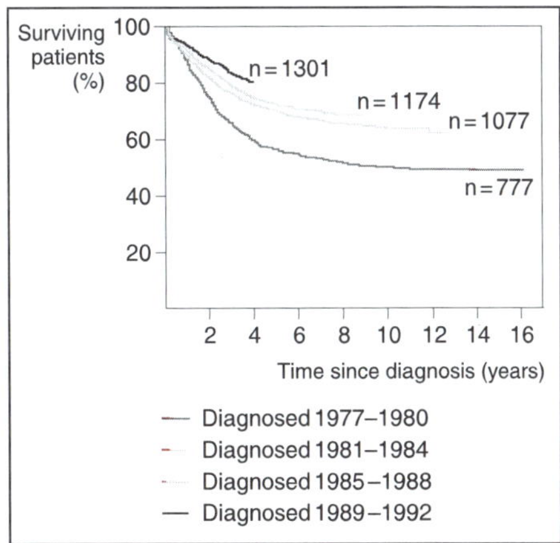

Survival rates of patients with acute lymphoblastic leukemia 1977–1992.

Key references

1. Greaves MF: Speculations on the cause of childhood acute lymphoblastic leukemia. *Leukemia* 1988, **2**:120–125.

2. Chessell JM: Treatment of childhood acute lymphoblastic leukemia: present issues and future prospects. *Blood Rev* 1992, **6**:193–203.

3. Eden OB, *et al.*: Report to the MRC: results of MRC UKALL VIII. *Br J Haematol* 1990, **78**:187–196.

4. Hann IM: CNS directed therapy in childhood. *Br J Haematol* 1992, **82**:2–5.

5. Hann IM, *et al.*: UKCCSG MACHO chemotherapy for B stages IV NHL & B-ALL. *Br J Haematol* 1990, **76**:359–364.

6. Pinkel D, Woo S: Prevention and treatment of meningeal leukemia in children. *Blood* 1994: **84**:355–366.

Diagnosis

Symptoms

• Some patients are symptom-free.

Lethargy, irritability, fatigue, reduced exercise tolerance: symptoms of anemia.

Infection: due to leukopenia.

Spontaneous bleeding or bruising: symptom of thrombocytopenia.

Signs

Pallor, infections, bruises, petechiae.

Lymphadenopathy or hepatosplenomegaly: occasionally.

Gum hypertrophy, skin infiltration: features of monocytic leukemia.

Hemorrhagic manifestations: feature of promyelocytic leukemia.

Investigations

Complete blood count: often shows reduced hemoglobin; thrombocytopenia frequent; leukocyte count $>100 \times 10^9$/L unusual, associated with poor response to treatment; presentation with count $<3.0 \times 10^9$/L common; differential leukocyte count usually abnormal, with neutropenia and presence of "blast cells" (large cells, ~1.5–2 times diameter of erythrocytes; usually have large nuclear:cytoplasmic ratio [less common with acute myeloid leukemia]; nucleus may contain at least one nucleolus [usually large single nucleus in monoblast]; blasts may show features of maturation, *e.g.*, cytoplasmic granulation, Auer dies, or monocytic features); numerical thrombocytopenia confirmed morphologically.

Bone-marrow analysis: increased proportion of blast cells; conventionally, >30% of bone-marrow cellularity to distinguish from the blastic forms of myelodysplasia.

Cytochemistry: useful to confirm myeloid or monocytic origin of blast cells; Sudan black, chloroacetate esterase, or myeloperoxidase stains.

Immunophenotyping: most reliable method of determining hematopoietic lineage of origin; expression of CD33 or CD15 indicates some myeloid maturation; CD34 and HLA DR earlier nonlymphoid markers, providing important objective methods for distinguishing myeloid from lymphoid leukemia; antigens are expressed on normal cells, but "leukemia-specific" or aberrant phenotypes have been identified that will probably be useful for monitoring remission status when normal antigens are inappropriately expressed on leukemic cells.

Cytogenetics: many structural chromosome abnormalities have been described; relationship between prognosis and cytogenetic abnormality, *e.g.*, better prognosis with French–American–British (FAB) M3 (usually has 15:17 translocation), some M2s (8:21 translocation), and inverted 16; worse prognosis with abnormalities or deletions of chromosomes 5 and 7.

Molecular genetics: molecular probes for the 15:17 and 8:21 translocations now available; polymerase chain reaction detection of minor cell populations therefore possible; such technology will be important in assessing quality of remission.

Complications

Overwhelming infection.

Bleeding: especially intracranial in promyelocytic leukemia.

Differential diagnosis

Any cause of pancytopenia.

Etiology

• The risk is increased in the following:

Radiation exposure.

Chemotherapy for cancer, *e.g.*, Hodgkin's disease.

Chronic myeloproliferative disorders or myelodysplasia.

Epidemiology

• Acute myeloid leukemia is the most common form in adults.

• The median age of presentation is ~60 years.

• The male:female ratio is equal.

• The prevalence increases with age (*e.g.*, 1 in 10^5 in children, up to 3 in 10^5 in patients aged >70 years).

Classification

• Based on morphological appearance, acute myeloid leukemia is divided into FAB types M0–7.

• The M3 type (promyelocytic) has a high chance of remission and a lower risk of relapse.

• Although valuable in standardizing terminology, this classification has limited prognostic power.

Treatment

Diet and lifestyle

• Nutrition must be maintained.

• Psychological support should be provided to patients and their relatives, especially if a young family is involved; financial support should be considered if earnings are disrupted.

• Patients must take precautions against infection during neutropenia.

Pharmacological treatment

Supportive

• Infection can be prevented by expert nursing care; isolation in a single room with air filtration; mouth care; vigilance of temperature, mucous membranes, perineum, and central-line site.

• Infection can be treated, after appropriate bacteriological, fungal, and viral samples have been taken, by rapid introduction of i.v. antibiotics (usually aminoglycoside and ceftazidime or penicillin with anti-pseudomonal activity).

• If a response occurs within 48 hours, treatment should be continued for 3–5 days; in cases of no or incomplete response and no bacteriological guidance, vancomycin should be added; if further failure, i.v. amphotericin should be added. (*See* Infections in hematological malignancy *for details*.)

For coagulopathy

• Coagulation factor deficiency should be corrected by appropriate blood products or vitamin K supplements.

• Severe coagulopathy, including disseminated intravascular coagulation, can be a dominant feature in promyelocytic leukemia (FAB M3), needing specific attention.

• All-*trans*-retinoic acid (ATRA) can be effective in correcting the defect (usually within 2–3 days).

• Blood-product support is essential, but fibrinolytic inhibition (tranexamic acid) and heparin have become less widely used.

Chemotherapy [1–3]

• Treatment should be given under specialist supervision.

• If induction of remission and consolidation phases are sufficiently intense, maintenance should be of no benefit.

• Drugs include anthracyclines, cytosine arabinoside, thioguanine, and etoposide; side effects include cardiotoxicity.

• Intensive supportive care is needed during remission induction, but most patients achieve complete remission with one course.

• An extra course may be needed for less intensive approaches, and more supportive care may be needed overall in all patient groups.

Treatment aims

To restore normal bone-marrow function. To establish prolonged remission or cure.

Other treatments

Allogeneic bone-marrow transplantation

• The risk of relapse is reduced from 60% to 15%.

• Treatment-related mortality of 30% is due to toxicity, infection, pneumonitis, and graft-versus-host disease.

• Treatment may result in infertility and late cataracts (in 10%–15% of patients).

• Allogeneic transplantation is available only to 10%–15% of patients.

Autologous bone-marrow transplantation

• Autologous transplantation is indicated for patients aged <55 years without a sibling donor.

Advantages: less toxicity, no graft-versus-host disease, available to more patients, low procedure-related mortality (6%–8%).

Disadvantages: potential for the harvested marrow to be contaminated, lack of graft-versus-leukemia effect.

Prognosis [1–3]

• Current schedules achieve remission in 80% of patients aged <55 years (range, 90% in children to 70% in those in fifth decade); in older patients, remission rates of 60% should be achieved.

• 30%–40% of patients aged <55 years treated by chemotherapy alone and 20% of older patients remain in remission at 5 years.

• Allogeneic bone-marrow transplantation cures 50%–60% of recipients; autologous transplantation cures 45%–55% of recipients.

• Treatment failure >5 years is rare after bone-marrow transplantation but occurs in chemotherapy patients, although at a much lower rate than in the first 2–3 years.

Follow-up and management

• 2–3 weeks after recovery from hypoplasia induced by chemotherapy, the bone marrow should be checked for remission status.

Key references

1. Burnett AK, Lowenberg B: Treatment options for remission in acute myeloid leukemia. In *Hematological Oncology*, vol 1. Cambridge: Cambridge University Press; 1991.

2. Foon KA, Gale RP: Therapy for acute myelogenous leukemia. *Blood Rev* 1992, **6**:15–25.

3. Zittoun RA, Mondelli F, Willemze R, *et al.*: Autologous or allogeneic bone marrow transplantation compared with intensive chemotherapy in acute myelogenous leukemia. *N Engl J Med* 1995, **332**: 217–223.

Diagnosis

Symptoms

• 70% of patients are asymptomatic, the diagnosis being made on incidental blood count.

Enlarged lymph nodes or discomfort in left upper quadrant of abdomen: in 20%.

Symptoms of anemia: uncommon.

Bruising or bleeding: rare.

Weight loss, fever unassociated with infection, night sweats: "B" symptoms; very unusual and often signal transformation to high-grade lymphoma.

Signs

Lymphadenopathy in cervical, axillary, or inguinal regions: in 30% of patients.

Mild to moderate splenomegaly: in 10%.

Hepatomegaly: rare.

Anemia: unusual.

Purpura: rare.

Investigations [1]

Complete blood count: shows lymphocytosis $>5 \times 10^9$/L, mature monomorphic small lymphocytes with smear cells.

Lymphocyte marker analysis: shows sparse surface immunoglobulin of a single light chain (κ or λ); CD5⁺, CD19⁺, CD20⁺, CD23⁺, CD37⁺, CD3⁻, CD10⁻, CD22⁻.

Serum immunoglobulin measurement: reduced concentration in all classes; IgM paraprotein in 5% of patients.

Direct antiglobulin test: positive in 10%.

Bone-marrow trephine analysis: interstitial, nodular, or diffuse infiltration by small lymphocytes.

Karyotyping: trisomy 12 in 30%, deletion 13q14 in 25%.

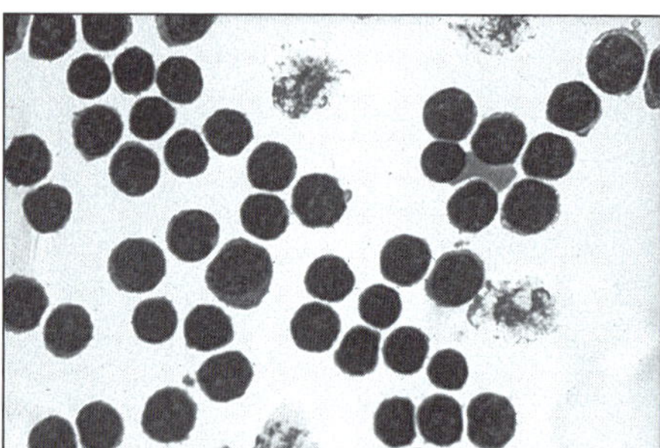

Leukapheresis specimen from chronic lymphocytic leukemia with Romanowsky's stain, showing small monomorphic lymphocytes with occasional prolymphocytes and smear cells. (*See* Color Plate.)

Complications

Autoimmune hemolytic anemia: in 10% of patients, more in stage C.

Autoimmune thrombocytopenia, neutropenia, pure erythrocyte aplasia: in <2%.

Infection: due to hypogammaglobulinemia in a few patients.

Shingles: in 25%.

Transformation to prolymphocytic leukemia or high-grade lymphoma: in 10% and 2% (Richter's syndrome), respectively.

Pneumococcal pneumonia.

Treatment

Diet and lifestyle

• Patients should be encouraged to lead a normal life.

Pharmacological treatment

• All treatment should be given under specialist supervision.

• Stage A patients should not receive chemotherapy.

Alkylating agents

• Chlorambucil is the mainstay of treatment.

• The response rate is 50%.

Standard dosage	Chlorambucil, continuous oral dose or intermittently every 4 weeks. Cyclophosphamide, orally or i.v. every 2–3 weeks.
Contraindications	None.
Main drug interactions	None established.
Main side effects	Nausea and bone-marrow suppression, drug rash (in 5% of patients on chlorambucil), alopecia (cyclophosphamide).

Nucleoside analogues

• Fludarabine is a purine analogue that produces responses in up to 50% of patients resistant to chlorambucil.

• 2-Chlorodeoxyadenosine is a similar agent.

Standard dosage	Fludarabine, i.v. daily for 5 days every 28 days.
Contraindications	None.
Special points	Less bone-marrow suppression than chlorambucil, but profound T lymphocytopenia, which predisposes to infection by viruses, fungi, or protozoa.
Main drug interactions	None established.
Main side effects	Bone-marrow suppression, immunosuppression.

Other options

Prednisone: for patients with autoimmune complications; effects a redistribution of lymphocytes from tissue to blood and may be useful in thrombocytopenic patients beginning treatment with alkylating agents.

CHOP chemotherapy (cyclophosphamide, doxorubicin, vincristine, prednisone): may be more effective than chlorambucil in stage C cases.

Immunoglobulin replacement therapy: for patients with recurrent infections whose serum immunoglobulin concentration is <4 g/L.

Currently under investigation

Bone-marrow transplantation: for younger patients with HLA matched sibling donor. Results appear promising [3].

Treatment aims

To relieve symptoms.
To prolong life in stage B or C patients.

Other treatments

• Leukapheresis may be used to prevent or treat hyperleukocytosis in patients with very high leukocyte counts (>500 × 10⁹/L) or to control the leukocyte count in drug-resistant patients.

Prognosis

• Stage A patients have the same prognosis as age- and sex-matched controls.
• Median survivals achieved with chlorambucil are 12 years for stage A, 5 years for stage B, and 2 years for stage C patients.

Follow-up and management

• Patients should be observed to determine whether the disease is progressive; patients whose disease is static and who are asymptomatic may safely be observed.
• Progressive disease should be treated by chlorambucil.
• All patients need long-term follow-up, the frequency being determined by the pace of the disease.

Key references

1. Litz CE, Brunning RD: Chronic lympho-proliferative disorders: classification and diagnosis. *Clin Haematol* 1993, **6**:767–783.

2. Binet JL: Treatment of chronic lymphocytic leukaemia. *Clin Haematol* 1993, **6**:867–878.

3. Michallet M, Arrbimbaud E, Bandini G, Rowlings PA: HLA-identical sibling bone marrow transplantation in younger patients with chronic lymphocitic leukemia. *Ann Intern Med* 1996, **124**:311–315.

Diagnosis

Symptoms

- 25% of patients are asymptomatic.

Fatigue, weight loss, weakness: in 25%.

Bruising or infections: in 25%.

Abdominal fullness or discomfort: in 25%.

Signs

Moderate to massive splenomegaly: in 75% of patients.

Lymphadenopathy: rarely.

Hepatomegaly: occasionally.

Signs of infection, bleeding, or bruising.

Investigations

Complete blood count: shows normochromic, normocytic anemia, neutropenia, monocytopenia, thrombocytopenia, "hairy" leukocytosis. Hairy cells are large lymphocytes with open nucleus, with loose, lacy chromatin and one or two distinct nucleoli; the cytoplasm is pale blue-grey, with fine, hair-like projections; usually few are found in blood, but they number $>10 \times 10^9$/L in 10% of patients.

Bone-marrow trephine: shows diffuse or patchy infiltration of leukemic cells, characteristic pale halos of cytoplasm surrounding monotonous, bland nuclei.

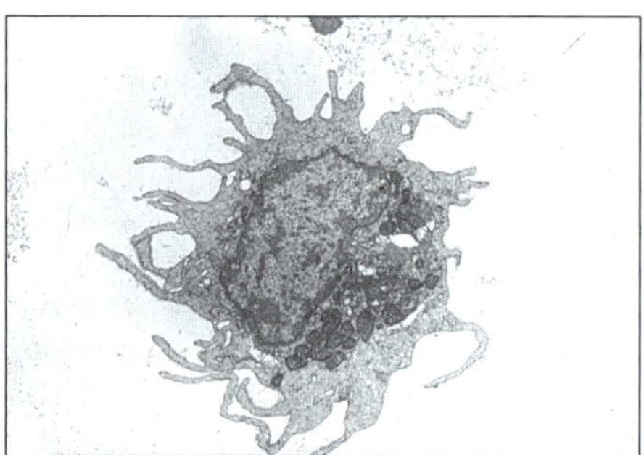

Hairy cell on transmission electron microscopy.

Cell marker analysis: moderately positive for surface immunoglobulin of a single light chain class; CD11c$^+$, CD19$^+$, CD20$^+$, CD25$^+$, CD37$^+$, CD3$^-$, CD15$^-$, CD10$^-$; tartrate-resistant acid phosphatase positive.

Complications

Infections: neutropenia and monocytopenia render patients susceptible to infection, so both bacterial and more atypical infections are seen; fungal, protozoan, and mycobacterial organisms are implicated.

Vasculitis: microscopic polyarteritis in 5% of patients.

Treatment

Diet and lifestyle

• Patients should be encouraged to live as normal a life as possible.

Pharmacological treatment [1]

• Treatment should be given under specialist supervision.

2-Chlorodeoxyadenosine

Standard dosage   0.1 mg/kg/day by continuous infusion for 7 days.

Main side effects   Fever and infection during the first month following therapy, decline in the neutrophil and platelet counts, which generally reverse by the end of the fourth week.

• This is currently the drug of choice in the United States.

• It may be capable of producing long-term complete remissions [2].

• Side effects include myelotoxicity (intense hematological support needed early in treatment to prevent death from hemorrhage or infection), and the risk of fungal, viral, or protozoan infection due to $CD4^+$ T-cell suppression (similar to 2′deoxycoformycin).

Additional agents

α-Interferon

Standard dosage   α-Interferon, 3 MU 3 times weekly usually for 2 years, is effective in 80% of patients.

Contraindications   Hypersensitivity, severe renal failure, hepatic or myeloid dysfunction.

Special points   Early in treatment, cytopenias may be exacerbated, with risk of hemorrhage or infection.
Antibodies to interferon-α occur in 50% of patients but only occasionally cause treatment failure.

Main drug interactions   No information available.

Main side effects   Mild influenza-like symptoms (improve with time).

2′Deoxycoformycin

• This inhibitor of adenosine deaminase produces a higher rate of complete remissions than interferon (up to 80%); early studies suggest that most remissions are prolonged beyond 4 years.

Standard dosage   2′Deoxycoformycin, 4 mg/m² weekly for 3 weeks, then on alternate weeks for 6 weeks.

Contraindications   Low glomerular filtration rate; caution in renal dysfunction.

Main drug interactions   No information available.

Main side effects   Risk of fungal, viral, or protozoan infections due to $CD4^+$ T-cell suppression.

Treatment aims

To allow patient to lead symptom-free life.
To attempt, particularly in younger patients, long-term remission, albeit at some early risk from increased pancytopenia.

Other treatments

• Splenectomy was the mainstay of treatment before effective drugs were available; it is still used in patients with the following: Important splenomegaly and cytopenias. Relatively little bone-marrow involvement. Intolerance of pharmaceutical intervention. Laparotomy for other reasons.

Prognosis

• With modern treatment, most patients have a normal lifespan.

• Only a few patients achieve complete remission after interferon treatment, but most achieve sufficient hematological improvement to make their disease of no consequence to them.

• Relapse occurs progressively 1–2 years off treatment with interferon [2].

• Progression-free survival 83% for 4 years for patients with complete remission.

Follow-up and management

• All patients should be followed up indefinitely.

• Treatment should be reintroduced if symptoms or blood count warrants it.

Key reference

1. Jeiyesimi IA, Kantarjian HM, Estey EH: Advances in therapy for hairy cell leukemia: a review. *Cancer* 1993, **72**:5–16.

2. Tallman MS, Hakimian D, Rademaker AW, *et al.*: Relapse of hairy cell leukemia after 2-chlorodeoxyadenosine. *Blood* 1996, **88**:1954–1959.

Diagnosis

Symptoms

Lethargy, nausea, vomiting: prodromal symptoms of viral hepatitis.

Abdominal pain, hematemesis: common after acetaminophen overdose.

Drowsiness or confusion: in grades 1 and 2 encephalopathy.

Restlessness, agitation: possibly aggressive; in grade 3.

Unresponsiveness: in grade 4.

Signs

Jaundice: common but not always manifest at presentation.

Encephalopathy of varying severity: asterixis, fetor hepaticus late features.

Liver size: typically normal, although hepatomegaly may be seen in severe hepatitis, Budd–Chiari syndrome.

Ascites: late finding.

Systemic hypertension, decerebrate posturing, hyperventilation: indicating cerebral edema.

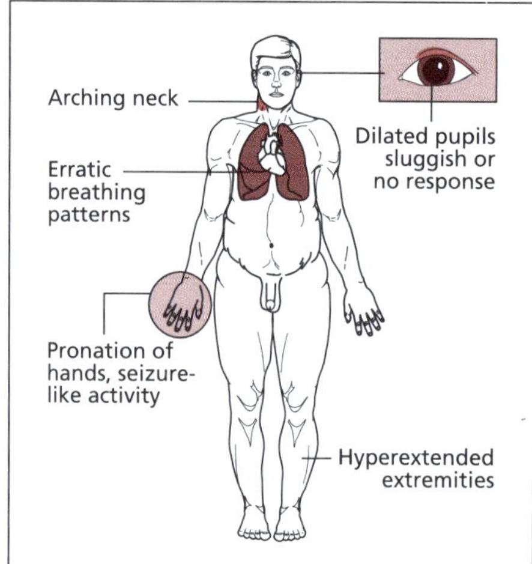

Physical findings in patients with fulminant liver failure.

Investigations

History: of toxin (amanita mushrooms, carbon tetrachloride) or drug exposure (*e.g.*, acetaminophen, isoniazid, NSAIDs).

Prothrombin time or INR measurement: prolongation (in the absence of disseminated intravascular coagulation or vitamin K deficiency) indicates severe hepatic dysfunction.

Hemoglobin measurement: hemolytic anemia suggests Wilson's disease.

Serum bilirubin measurement: prognostic significance in non–acetaminophen-induced cases.

Serum creatinine measurement: urea underestimates renal impairment; prognostic significance in acetaminophen-induced cases.

Glucose measurement: hypoglycemia indicates poor prognosis.

Acetaminophen measurement.

Hepatitis A serology: to detect IgM anti-hepatitis A virus.

Hepatitis B and D serology: to detect IgM anti-core, hepatitis B surface antigen, anti-hepatitis D virus.

Hepatitis C antibody: often negative in fulminant non-A, non-B viral hepatitis.

Ceruloplasmin and 24-hour urinary copper excretion: low and high, respectively, in Wilson's disease.

Cytomegalovirus, Epstein-Barr serology.

Ultrasonography: to assess liver size and texture.

Complications

• All of the following are late complications, mainly occurring in patients with advanced encephalopathy.

Hypoglycemia.	**Cerebral edema [1].**	**Respiratory failure.**
Renal failure.	**Bleeding, infection.**	**Hypotension.**

Differential diagnosis

Acute decompensation of chronic liver disease.

Reye's syndrome.

Other metabolic encephalopathy.

Etiology

Acetaminophen ingestion.

Hepatitis A, B, B/D, or E virus infection, seronegative hepatitis (non-A, non-B, non-C), halothane hepatitis, idiosyncratic drug reactions.

Pregnancy-related, Budd–Chiari syndrome, autoimmune liver disease, malignancy, mushroom poisoning [2,3].

Epidemiology

• Fulminant liver failure complicates 0.1%–4.7% of hospitalized patients with viral hepatitis, depending on the cause.

Classification

Fulminant liver failure

Acute liver failure with encephalopathy in a patient presumed to have a normal liver within 8 weeks of the onset of illness.

Hyperacute liver failure

Encephalopathy within 7 days of onset of jaundice, characterized by high incidence of cerebral edema; despite this, many patients survive with medical management.

Subacute liver failure

Encephalopathy 8–12 weeks after onset of jaundice, low incidence of cerebral edema and less severe prolongation of prothrombin times, but poor prognosis [4,5].

Treatment

Diet and lifestyle

- Referral to a liver transplant center is required.
- Parenteral or enteral nutritional support is usually needed.
- Survivors return to a normal diet and lifestyle, unless they are recipients of liver grafts, in which case they need lifelong follow-up and immunosuppressive treatment.

Pharmacological treatment

N-acetylcysteine

- Administration should begin as soon as possible and optimally within 12 hours of ingestion of acetaminophen [6].

Standard dosage	*N*-acetylcysteine, 140 mg/kg loading dose, followed by maintenance dose of 70 mg/kg orally every 4 hours.
Contraindications	Hypersensitivity.
Main drug interactions	None.
Main side effects	Occasional hypersensitivity reactions; vomiting and aspiration should be watched for.

Gastric protection

- H_2 antagonists or sucralfate reduce the incidence of gastrointestinal bleeding.

Standard dosage	Ranitidine, 50 mg i.v. 8-hourly. Sucralfate, 1 g orally 6-hourly.
Contraindications	Hypersensitivity.
Main drug interactions	None relevant.
Main side effects	*Ranitidine:* thrombocytopenia.

Lactulose

- This is often ineffective and recommended only in patients with grade 1 or 2 encephalopathy.

Standard dosage	Lactulose, 30 mL 8-hourly; doses titrated to three bowel movements daily.
Contraindications	Gastrointestinal obstruction.
Main drug interactions	None relevant.
Main side effects	Nausea, flatulence, abdominal discomfort.

King's College criteria for liver transplantation in fulminant liver failure

PT >100 seconds (irrespective of grade of encephalopathy) or any of the following criteria:

   Age <10 or >40 years

   Period of jaundice to encephalopathy >7 days

   PT >50

   Bilirubin >17 mg/dL

   Etiology: viral hepatitis, halothane, drug reaction, Wilson's disease

For acetaminophen-induced liver failure

pH <7.3 (irrespective of grade of encephalopathy) or all three of the following:

   Grade III-IV encephalopathy

   PT >100

   Serum creatinine >3.4 mg/dL

Treatment aims

To anticipate and treat complications.

Other treatments

- Liver transplantation must be considered early in patients with progressive fulminant hepatitis (*see* table) [7].

Prognosis

- Most patients who do not progress beyond grade 2 encephalopathy survive.
- Survivors make complete recoveries; progression to chronic liver disease is unusual.

Follow-up and management

- Long-term medical follow-up is rarely needed, except in liver-graft recipients.
- Psychiatric and social support is important in overdose cases.

Key references

1. Blei AT, *et al.*: Complications of intracranial pressure monitoring in fulminant hepatic failure. *Lancet* 1993, **341**:157–158.
2. Lee WM: Acute liver failure. *N Engl J Med* 1993, **329**:1862–1872.
3. Fingerote RJ: Fulminant hepatic failure. *Am J Gastroenterol* 1993, **88**:1000–1010.
4. O'Grady JG, Schalm SW, Williams R: Acute liver failure: redefining the syndromes. *Lancet* 1993, **342**:273–275.
5. Devlin J: Pretransplantation clinical status and outcome of emergency transplantation for acute liver failure. *Hepatology* 1995, **21**:1018–1024.
6. Harrison PM, *et al.*: Improvement by *N*-acetylcysteine of hemodynamics and oxygen transport in fulminant hepatic failure. *N Engl J Med* 1991, **324**:1853–1857.
7. Lee WM: Management of acute liver failure. *Semin Liver Dis* 1996, **16**:369–378.

Diagnosis

Symptoms

Back pain: acute, <7 days' duration; chronic, >30 days' duration.

Morning stiffness.

Leg pain.

Limitation of motion.

Functional impairment.

Signs

Loss of lumbar lordosis.

Muscle spasm: visible, palpable.

Thoracolumbar scoliosis.

Pelvic tilt.

Antalgic gait.

"Foot drop" gait.

"Listing gait."

Limitation of lumbar motion: flexion, extension, lateral bending.

Soft-tissue tenderness.

Straight leg raising test.

Great toe extension weakness.

Ankle dorsiflexion weakness.

Diminished ankle strength reflexes.

Sensory deficit.

Calf wasting.

Sciatica.

Investigations

Complete blood count, alkaline phosphatase, prostate-specific antigen.

Plain radiographs.

CT/MRI imaging.

Electromyography.

Serum protein electrophoresis.

Myelography.

Cybex muscle strength testing.

Complications

Sensory deficit.

Motor deficit.

Gait disturbance.

Work impairment.

Narcotic dependence.

Foot drop.

Bowel/bladder incontinence.

Paresis.

Atrophy.

Differential diagnosis

Osteoarthritis.

Herniated nucleus pulposus.

Infection (osteomyelitis).

Seronegative spondyloarthropathy (ankylosing spondylitis).

Compression fracture.

Spinal stenosis.

Neoplasm.

Radiculopathy.

Etiology

Muscle spasm.

Herniated nucleus pulposus.

Spondylolisthesis.

Bony spurring.

Spinal stenosis.

Degenerative disk disease.

Infection (vertebral body or disk).

Seronegative spondyloarthropathy.

Ankylosing spondylitis.

Psoriatic arthritis.

Reiter's syndrome.

Enteropathic arthritis.

Epidemiology

- 25% of patients are 30–50 years of age.
- The most common cause of disability in people aged <45 years.
- 60% of patients have recurrence within 1 year.
- Low back pain accounts for ~10% of family practice visits annually.
- Risk factors for low back pain include occupation, anxiety, depression, pregnancy, and cigarette smoking.
- Back pain is among the top 10 most common symptoms seen by internists.
- Back pain is the second most common reason for surgery in the United States.
- Costs are estimated at $25 billion in direct medical care costs annually (1995).
- Associated costs are >$40 billion (includes lost productivity, compensation, litigation).

Treatment

Diet and lifestyle

• Patients should discontinue smoking.

• Weight reduction and a regular exercise regimen are important in the treatment of low back pain.

• Patient education and participation in their own rehabilitation is important in maintaining back health and preventing back pain recurrence ("back school").

• Job modification may be necessary.

• Physiatry referral may be helpful.

Pharmacological treatment

NSAIDs: ibuprofen, 400–800 mg 4 times daily; piroxicam, 20 mg daily.

• NSAIDs are of modest benefit.

• Analgesics and narcotics are best avoided or used only in short-term strategy.

• The use of muscle relaxants is controversial.

Nonpharmacological treatment

Chronic pain management techniques, visual imagery, meditation, relaxation techniques.

Electrical stimulation.

Transcutaneous electrical nerve stimulation unit: controversial.

Physical therapy (ultrasound, massage).

Extension exercises.

Flexion exercises.

Activity restriction.

Treatment aims

To restore range of motion.

To improve comfort.

To improve sleep.

To improve function.

Prognosis

• Prognosis is highly variable.

• 90% of back pain sufferers experience recurrences.

Follow-up and management

• A multidisciplinary approach may be very helpful.

General references

Borenstein DG: Chronic low back pain. *Rheum Dis Clin North Am* 1996, **22**:439–456.

Cavanaugh JM, Ozaktay AC, Yamashita T, *et al.*: Mechanisms of low back pain: a neurophysiologic and neuroanatomic study. *Clin Orthop* 1997, **335**:166–180.

Diagnosis

Symptoms

Visible red blood per rectum (*i.e.,* hematochezia).

Rectal urgency.

Orthostatic light-headedness.

Abdominal pain: relief most common with defecation.

Burning perianal pain with defecation: suggestive of a perianal fissure.

Signs

Hematochezia (occasionally melena).

Tachycardia, orthostatic hypotension: indicates significant blood loss.

Occult blood in stool.

Investigations

Complete blood testing: to determine the presence of anemia.

• Microcytic anemia suggests chronic blood loss in the absence of other explanations; thrombocytopenia should also be excluded.

• Iron deficiency requires a thorough evaluation of the lower gastrointestinal mucosa (*i.e.*, colonoscopy) and, if normal, studies of the small bowel or upper gastrointestinal tract in patients with upper gastrointestinal symptoms or weight loss.

Colonic imaging: usually required to exclude the presence of malignancy; lower gastrointestinal bleeding in the setting of clinical infection in patients <50 years of age can usually be managed without colonic imaging, however, careful observation for inflammatory bowel disease is warranted and a high suspicion for pseudomembranous colitis maintained.
Anoscopy: to evaluate symptoms of perianal bleeding (*i.e.*, blood only on the toilet paper or surface of formed stool) in relatively young patients without a family history of gastrointestinal malignancies if a bleeding source is readily identified.
Colonscopy: to evalute patients >50 years of age with lower gastrointestinal bleeding, particularly if a drop in the hemoglobin was observed; signs and symptoms of obvious perianal disease alone in patients with a negative family history for gastrointestinal cancer may be evaluated with flexible sigmoidoscopy alone with close clinical follow-up.
Air contrast barium enemas: relatively poor sensitivity for etiologies of lower gastrointestinal bleeding, particularly of the rectosigmoid and perianal regions.

Stool studies: for *Clostridium difficile* and *Entamoeba histolytica*, infectious causes of lower gastrointestinal bleeding that respond to antibiotics (*e.g.*, metronidazole, 500 mg every 8 hours), that may be lethal if missed.

Nuclear medicine scans: tagged erythrocyte scans for patients with unexplained recurrent blood loss; Meckel's scan for patients with possible Meckel's diverticulum.

Complications

Exsanguination.

Cardiac or cerebrovascular ischemia.

Metabolic acidosis.

Prerenal insufficiency.

Etiology

Slow or brisk bleeding most commonly from the colon but occasionally from the small intestine.

Epidemiology

More common in the elderly.

Differential diagnosis

Diverticular bleeding.

Arteriovenous malformations/angiodysplasia.

Hemorrhoids.

Perianal fissure.

Inflammatory bowel disease (ulcerative colitis > Crohn's disease; acute self-limited colitis).

Infectious colitis/enteritis (*e.g.*, *E. histolytica, Campylobacter jejuni, Shigella* spp., *Salmonella* spp., *Escherichia coli, C. difficile.*)

Ischemic colitis, radiation colitis.

Colonic malignancies (*e.g.*, adenocarcinoma, lymphoma, carcinoid).

NSAID enteropathy.

Upper gastrointestinal bleeding with rapid transit.

Meckel's diverticulum.

Treatment

Diet and lifestyle

• Patients should seek medical advice promptly.

• Patients must maintain proper hydration.

• Patients should refrain from inhibitors of platelet function (*i.e.*, aspirin, other NSAIDs).

• High-fiber diet and sitz baths are recommended for patients with perianal disease (*i.e.*, fissures, hemorrhoids).

Pharmacological treatment

• *See* Anal fissures, Hemorrhoidal disease, Diverticular disease of the colon, Colorectal cancer, and Inflammatory bowel disease.

Iron replacement

• Patients with gastrointestinal blood loss and iron deficiency anemia typically benefit from iron replacement therapy, *e.g.*, ferrous sulfate.

Standard dosage	325 mg 3 times daily on an empty stomach.
Contraindications	Hypersensitivity.
Main drug interactions	Antacids, tetracycline impair the absorption of iron and should not be taken within 2 hours.
Main side effects	Nausea, abdominal discomfort, and constipation; parenteral iron therapy may be required if side effects of oral iron are intolerable.
Special points	Inform patient that iron supplements will result in black-colored stool that may be confused with (or mask) gastrointestinal bleeding; iron supplements compromise visualization of the mucosa during colonoscopy and as such should be discontinued at least 5 days prior to the procedure.

• Intra-arterial vasopressin via selective catheterization of the bleeding vessel may be effective in the control of bleeding from diverticula or angiodysplasia.

• Chronic anemia from angiodysplasia despite the use of iron supplements may respond to daily estrogen therapy (*e.g.*, Ovcon 50 = norethindrone + ethinyl estradiol); use with caution in men or patients with cardiovascular disease.

Treatment aims

To identify source of bleeding.

To treat underlying disease process to achieve cessation of bleeding.

To prevent complications from anemia or hypovolemia.

Other treatment options

Therapeutic colonoscopy or enteroscopy with cautery of identified bleeding sites.

Angiographic embolization of bleeding vessels.

Surgical resection of bleeding site (identified by endoscopy, radionuclide scans, or angiography).

Prognosis

Highly dependent on the source of bleeding and degree of blood loss.

Follow-up and management

Highly dependent on the source of bleeding; an explanation for gastro-intestinal blood loss must always be sought.

General references

Elta GH: Approach to the patient with gross gastrointestinal bleeding. In *Textbook of Gastroenterology*, edn 2. Edited by Yamada T. Philadelphia: JB Lippincott; 1995:685–691.

Richter JM, Hedberg SE, Athanasoulis CA, *et al.*: Angiodysplasia: clinical present-ation and colonoscopic diagnosis. *Dig Dis Sci* 1984, **29**:481–485.

Wagner HE, Stain SC, Gilig M, *et al.*: Systematic assessment of massive bleeding of the lower part of the gastrointestinal tract. *Surg Gynecol Obstet* 1992, **175**:445–449.

Diagnosis

Symptoms

Cough, hemoptysis, breathlessness, hoarseness.

Chest pain, lymphadenopathy.

Weight loss, general malaise.

Intellectual impairment, headache, focal neuropathy, tremor.

Signs

• Signs are not always manifest.

Lung nodule or mass.

Lobar or lung collapse, consolidation, pleural effusion, monophonic wheeze.

Cervical lymphadenopathy, hepatomegaly, local chest-wall tenderness, Horner's syndrome, neurological deficit.

Finger clubbing, cerebellar degeneration, peripheral neuropathy.

Investigations [1]

For diagnosis

Chest radiography: shows mass, collapse, distal infection, abscess, adenopathy, metastases.

Sputum cytology: shows malignant cells.

Bronchoscopy: tumor often directly visible; operability can be assessed, and samples obtained for cytology and histology.

Pleural aspiration and biopsy: primary test if effusion present; malignant cells indicate inoperable tumor.

For staging

Bronchoscopy: to assess presence of central disease.

CT of thorax: to assess presence of hilar or mediastinal adenopathy.

Mediastinoscopy: to evaluate lymphadenopathy.

Biochemistry: may indicate bone or liver involvement; sodium and calcium disturbance may occur without metastasis.

Liver ultrasonography: disease often spreads to liver.

CT of brain: disease often spreads to brain.

Pulmonary function tests: to assess ability to tolerate lung resection.

Complications

Lobar collapse, obstruction of superior vena cava.

Pneumonia, abscess.

Pain, pleural effusion.

Pericardial effusion, direct invasion.

Metastases: especially bone, brain, liver, adrenal glands.

Local neurological invasion, neuropathies.

Cushing's syndrome, inappropriate antidiuretic hormone secretion, hypercalcemia.

Recurrent venous thrombosis.

Clubbing, hypertrophic osteoarthropathy.

Differential diagnosis

Simple pneumonia.

Benign tumor or cysts.

Tuberculosis.

Pulmonary metastases.

Other causes of lung abscess.

Other causes of pleural effusion.

Etiology [2]

• Causes include the following:

Cigarette smoking: lung cancer was rare in the 19th century, and its increase is closely linked to the increasing popularity of cigarettes in the 20th century.

Atmospheric pollution: increased rates in urban areas.

Radioactivity: radon, uranium.

Manufacturing: chromate, asbestos, nickel, arsenic, hematite.

Epidemiology

• Lung cancer is the most common fatal cancer in men and women in the United States.

• The rate of lung cancer mortality is increasing.

Treatment

Diet and lifestyle

• Anorexia is a common feature; no specific diet is needed.

• Patients should be encouraged to be active.

• Most patients stop smoking after diagnosis, but this does not alter prognosis significantly.

Pharmacological treatment [3,4]

• Chemotherapy is the treatment of choice for small-cell cancer; various regimens are available.

• No satisfactory regimen has yet been found for large-cell tumors (*i.e.*, adenocarcinoma, squamous-cell or anaplastic tumors).

• The local oncology service should be consulted.

Nonpharmacological treatment [3,4]

Surgical resection

• Surgical resection is possible in only a few patients.

• It is limited by the frequent involvement of mediastinal nodes and central structures.

• Adequate lung function is needed (forced expiratory volume in 1 second >1.2 L for lobectomy, >1.5 L for pneumonectomy).

• Surgical resection is rarely appropriate for small-cell lung cancer (usually has extensive central disease, even if endoscopically resectable).

Radiotherapy [5]

• Palliative radiotherapy is useful in the management of hemoptysis and bony deposits.

• Radiation therapy can achieve local control of primary tumor and may improve survival.

• "Local" (endobronchial) radiotherapy, a novel experimental treatment, has yet to show any superiority to palliative external beam radiotherapy.

Endobronchial laser resection [6]

• This is a palliative procedure for tracheal or main bronchus disease.

• It is available in only a few specialist centers.

Treatment aims

To identify patients who can be treated surgically.

To identify patients with small-cell cancer and treat them by chemotherapy.

To provide palliative treatment, guided by symptoms, to the remaining patients.

Prognosis

• Prognosis is generally poor unless the tumor is resectable.

• When disease is technically resectable, the 5-year survival rate is ~28%.

Follow-up and management

• Surgical cure is possible in 5%–10% of patients.

• In patients who are inoperable, the main goal is palliation.

• Local symptoms are usually best treated by radiotherapy.

Key references

1. Lillington G: Management of solitary pulmonary nodules. *Dis Mon* 1991, **37**:279–318.

2. Sethi T: Science, medicine, and the future: lung cancer. *BMJ* 1997, **314**:652–655.

3. Murren J, Buzaid A: Chemotherapy and radiation for the treatment of non–small-cell lung cancer. *Clin Chest Med* 1993, **14**:161–200.

4. Burn PA, Corney DN: Overview of chemotherapy for small cell lung cancer. *Semin Oncol* 1997, **24(suppl 7)**:S7–S74.

5. Hazuka MB, Bunn PA: Controversies in the nonsurgical treatment of stage III non-small cell lung cancer. *Am Rev Resp Dis* 1992, **145**:967–977.

6. Pierce RJ: Lasers, brachytherapy and stents—keeping airways open. *Resp Med* 1991, **85**:263–265.

Diagnosis

Symptoms

• Patients may be asymptomatic.

Acute disease

• Symptoms occur 3–32 days after tick bite.

Influenza-like illness: malaise, pyrexia, myalgia, arthralgia, sore throat.

Rash.

Stiff neck.

Photophobia.

Chronic disease

• Symptoms occur weeks or months later.

Headache, stiff neck, photophobia, confusion, concentration and memory impairment.

Chest pain.

Joint pain and swelling.

Abdominal pain, tenderness, diarrhea.

Rashes.

Signs

Acute disease

Pyrexia, tender muscles or joints, inflamed throat.

Erythema chronicum migrans: characteristic rash (~5 cm), red macule or papule at site of tick bite, enlarges peripherally with central clearing over several weeks; metastatic lesions may develop; can last months.

Lymphadenopathy.

Meningism.

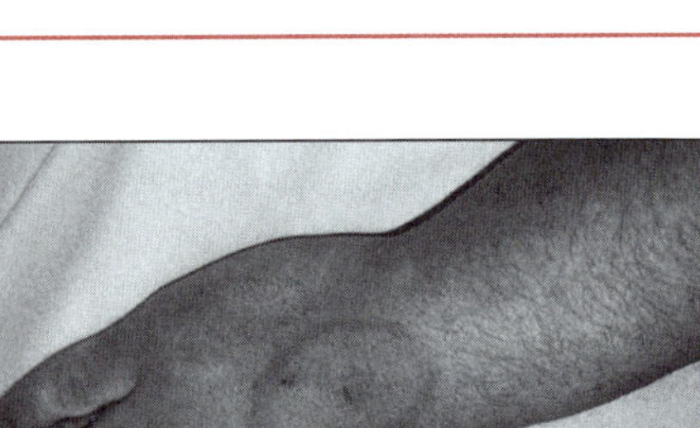

Erythema chronicum migrans. (*See* Color Plate.)

Chronic disease

Meningitis, encephalitis, cranial neuritis (especially Bell's palsy), radiculoneuritis, peripheral neuropathies.

Atrioventricular block, myopericarditis.

Arthritis.

Hepatomegaly, splenomegaly.

Acrodermatitis chronica atrophicans: vivid red lesions becoming sclerotic or atrophic.

Acrodermatitis chronicum atrophicans.

Investigations

Microscopy, histopathology, and culture: lack sensitivity and not widely available but may be diagnostic.

Serological tests: widely available but not diagnostic (support clinical diagnosis); IgM tests positive 3–6 weeks after infection, may persist for many months, but may not be reproducible; IgG tests positive 6–8 weeks after infection, may remain positive for years, but more reproducible so are mainstay of diagnosis; immunofluorescence tests and enzyme-linked immunosorbent assays most widely available.

• False-negative antibody results may occur early in illness, with antibiotic treatment, or due to immune complexes; a negative antibody test does not exclude the diagnosis. False-positive results are due to other spirochete infections, other infections, or the test; Western blotting may distinguish true- from false-positive results.

Complications

CNS abnormalities.

Cardiac conduction disturbances.

Oligoarthitis.

Differential diagnosis

Erythema chronicum migrans

Erythema marginatum.

Erythema multiforme rheumaticum.

Granuloma annulare.

Lymphadenopathy

Infectious mononucleosis.

Cytomegalovirus.

Toxoplasmosis.

Neurological symptoms

Infectious diseases.

Toxoplasmosis.

Guillain–Barré syndrome.

Multiple sclerosis.

Cardiac symptoms

Infectious diseases.

Chronic heart disease.

Digitalis use.

Arthritis

Rheumatoid arthritis.

Reactive arthritis.

Other dermatological symptoms

Erythema nodosum.

Circulatory insufficiencies.

Lymphoma.

Etiology

• Infection is transmitted by tick bites, usually *Ixodes scapularis* in the United States.

• The causative organism is *Borrelia burgdorferi*, a spirochete.

Epidemiology

• Lyme disease is found in the United States, Europe, Russia, China, Japan, and Australia.

• Occurrence parallels distribution and infection in ticks (0%–25%).

• In forested areas, 5%–10% of the population have antibodies.

• Infection peaks in June and July.

• It is found in patients of all ages but especially in the most active and those exposed to ticks.

Treatment

Diet and lifestyle

• No special precautions are necessary.

Pharmacological treatment

Criteria for treatment

• The risk depends on infected tick attachment: <24 hours, little risk; 48 hours, 50% risk; 72 hours, almost certain infection.

• Infection occurs in ~10% of people bitten by infected ticks, so empirical treatment is not justified in areas where infected ticks are rare.

• Erythema chronicum migrans must be treated; acute disease with positive serology and chronic disease when other causes are excluded warrant treatment.

• Treatment should be considered in anxious patients with possible infection but without high expectation of success.

• Asymptomatic individuals with positive serology probably should not be treated.

For acute disease

Standard dosage	Doxycycline, 200 mg orally daily for 14 days. Amoxicillin, 500 mg 3 times daily for 14 days.
Contraindications	*Doxycycline:* pregnancy, lactation, children aged <12 years, SLE, porphyria. *Amoxicillin:* penicillin hypersensitivity.
Main drug interactions	*Doxycycline:* anticoagulants, antiepileptics, oral contraceptives. *Amoxicillin:* anticoagulants, oral contraceptives.
Main side effects	*Doxycycline:* nausea, vomiting, diarrhea, headache. *Amoxicillin:* nausea, diarrhea, rashes.

• Erythromycin and clarithromycin are less effective but can be used in penicillin-sensitive children.

For chronic disease

• Chronic disease may be cardiac, neurological, or rheumatological.

Standard dosage	Ceftriaxone, 2 g i.v. or i.m. daily for 14–21 days. Penicillin G, 3 g i.v. 4 times daily for 14–21 days.
Contraindications	*Ceftriaxone:* hypersensitivity to cephalosporin. *Penicillin:* hypersensitivity.
Main drug interactions	*Ceftriaxone:* anticoagulants, probenecid. *Penicillin:* anticoagulants, oral contraceptives.
Main side effects	*Ceftriaxone:* gastrointestinal complaints, allergic reactions, rashes, hematological disturbance, liver dysfunction. *Penicillin:* sensitivity reactions, especially urticaria, angioedema, anaphylaxis.

Treatment aims

To kill organism.

To prevent disease progression.

To alleviate symptoms.

Prognosis

• Despite antibiotic treatment, symptoms recur in 50% of patients, although severity and duration are greatly reduced; occasionally, recurrent symptoms may last several years.

• Acute Lyme disease and carditis have good prognosis.

• Cranial nerve palsies and meningitis have good prognosis; radiculoneuritis, peripheral neuropathy, encephalitis, and encephalomyelitis usually have a favorable outcome, but a tendency toward chronic or recurrent disease is seen.

• Arthritis often resolves, but response may be slow, often needing further treatment.

• In chronic disease, recurrence is not usual.

Follow-up and management

• Patients may need careful monitoring for months or years, depending on the severity of the symptoms.

General references

Halperin JJ (ed.): Lyme disease. *Semin Neurol* 1997, **17**:1–77.

Hofmann H: Lyme borreliosis: problems of serological diagnosis. *Infection* 1996, **24**:470–472.

Lutwick LI: Postexposure prophylaxis. *Infect Dis Clin North Am* 1996, **10**:899–915.

Magid D, *et al.*: Prevention of Lyme disease after tick bites. *N Engl J Med* 1992, **327**:534–541.

Nagi KS, Joshi R, Thakur RK: Cardiac manifestations of Lyme disease: a review. *Can J Cardiol* 1996, **12**:503–506.

Rahn DW, Malawista SE: Recommendations for diagnosis and treatment. *Ann Intern Med* 1991, **114**:472–481.

Weber K, Pfister H: Clinical management of Lyme borreliosis. *Lancet* 1994, **343**:1017–1020.

Diagnosis

Symptoms and signs [1,2]

Delayed puberty and hypogonadism [3]

Failure to gain sufficient weight: in children.

Weight loss: in adults.

Poor virilization, tall stature with long limbs, gynecomastia; diminished libido, reduction in nocturnal emissions or masturbation; small firm testes, partial puberty, azoospermia: suggests Klinefelter's syndrome.

Hypergonadotropic gonadism, progressive decline in sperm count: azoospermia within months, with subsequent decline in Leydig cell function; may follow testicular irradiation or chemotherapy.

Anosmia: indicating Kallmann's syndrome.

History of pituitary tumor or past pituitary surgery, multiple hormonal deficiencies, absence of secondary sexual hair: suggests pituitary failure.

Mild hypogonadism with Turner's features, pulmonary stenosis: suggests Noonan's syndrome.

Obesity, micropenis, hypotonia, mental retardation, moderate hypogonadism: suggests Prader-Willi syndrome.

Adult male infertility [4]

Diminished sperm count, defective sperm motility.

Absent or obstructed epididymis or vas deferens, postepididymitis or seminal vesiculitis: suggests obstruction.

History of orchitis, torsion, or incomplete testicular descent: may result in tubular damage.

Swelling: sometimes painful; empties on lying down; suggests varicocele; however, tumors should be ruled out in patients with unilateral testicular enlargement.

Male pseudohermaphroditism

Normal female genitalia, primary amenorrhea: suggests failure of testis to develop.

Inguinal testes, female external genitalia with short, blind vagina, female breasts at puberty, scant secondary sexual hair: suggests defective androgen receptor (testicular feminization).

Investigations [1]

Hormone tests: serum luteinizing hormone, follicle-stimulating hormone, prolactin and testosterone; raised follicle-stimulating hormone with oligo- or azoospermia suggests primary testicular damage; dynamic endocrine testing is usually unnecessary.

Serum oestradiol measurements: for gynecosmastia.

Karyotyping: for Klinefelter's syndrome in hypergonadotropic hypogonadism.

Semen morphology, count, motility, and postcoital test: for infertility evaluation.

Testicular biopsy: not often indicated.

Ultrasonography: for testicular masses or prostatic disease.

MRI: for possible pituitary or hypothalamic tumors.

Complications

Delayed puberty and hypogonadism

Major psychological damage: if untreated at puberty.

Long-term increased risk of fracture: due to osteoporosis.

Androgen deficiency

Infertility.

Impotence.

Male pseudohermaphroditism

Psychological damage: without effective and sympathetic handling at outset.

Malignancy: in XY patients with streak gonads.

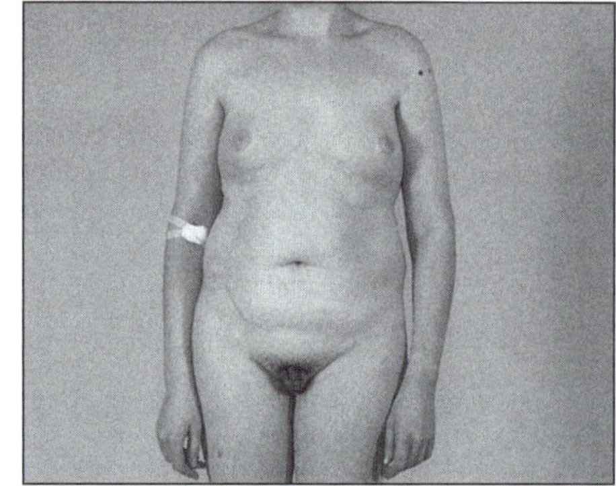

26-year-old man with untreated Kallmann's syndrome. (*See* Color Plate.)

Treatment

Diet and lifestyle

• Most phenotypic female patients with androgen-receptor disorders (male pseudohermaphroditism, testicular feminization, pure XY gonadal dysgenesis) are raised as females.

Pharmacological treatment [1,2]

• For each patient, the relative importance of androgen deficiency vs. infertility as well as the practicability of treatment must be defined clearly.

For androgen deficiency

Standard dosage	Testosterone enanthate or cypionate, 200 mg i.m. every 2 weeks; or testosterone patch daily. *For gonadotropin deficiency, when fertility is desired*: pulsatile gonadotropin-releasing hormone, 15 µg s.c. every 90 minutes by pump, or human chorionic gonadotropin, 2000 IU s.c. twice weekly or 5000 IU s.c. weekly, with subsequent menotropin, 225 IU 3 times weekly.
Contraindications	Caution if history of violent behavior.
Special points	*Gonadotropin replacement*: should be done in coordination with an infertility specialist; sperm may be stored in sperm bank for future use.
Main drug interactions	None.
Main side effects	Secondary sexual characteristics, balding, stimulation of prostatic hyperplasia; gynecomastia with human chorionic gonadotrophin therapy.

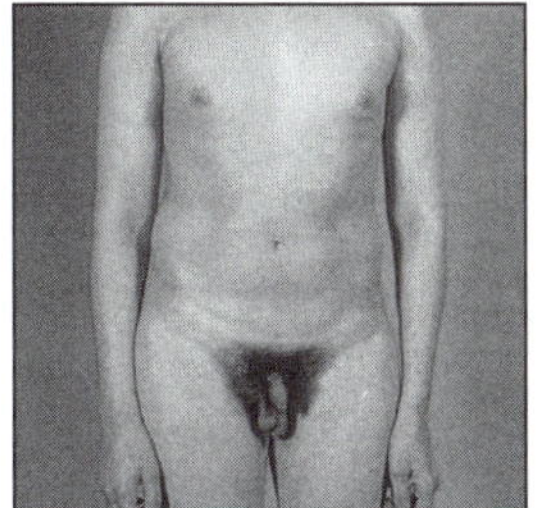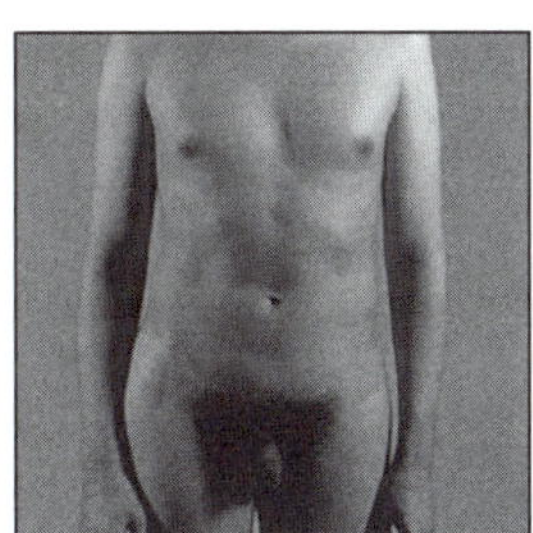

Hypogonadal patient with partial gonadotrophin deficiency (fertile eunuch syndrome) before (*left*) and after (*right*) 1 year's treatment with twice-weekly human chorionic gonadotropin. (*See* Color Plates.)

Key references

1. Griffen JE, Wilson JD: Disorders of the testes and male reproductive tract. In *Williams Textbook of Endocrinology*, edn 8. Edited by Wilson JD, Foster DW. Philadelphia: WB Saunders; 1992:799–852.

2. Grumbach MM, Conte FA: Disorders of sex differentiation. In *Williams Textbook of Endocrinology*, edn 8. Edited by Wilson JD, Foster DW. Philadelphia: WB Saunders; 1992:853–951.

3. Anderson DC: Endocrine diseases. In *Textbook of Medicine*, edn 2. Edited by Souhami RL, Moxham J. London: Churchill Livingstone; 1994:706–718.

4. Anderson DC, Large DM: Endocrine function of the testis: normal and abnormal. In *Scientific Foundation of Urology*, edn 3. Edited by Chisholm GD, Fair WR. Oxford: Heinemann; 1990:379–390.

Diagnosis

Symptoms

Impotence: the inability to obtain and sustain an erection to orgasm during ≥75% of attempts.

Erectile dysfunction: sexual dysfunction of any degree related to achieving adequate erection with associated satisfactory performance; includes flaccidity, loss of erection, semirigid erection, loss of nocturnal erection, anorgasmia, unsatisfied sexual partner, loss of libido, marital/relationship discord, anxiety, depression.

• Patients are frequently reluctant to express symptoms without direct questioning.

Signs

• Direct signs of impotence/erectile dysfunction are infrequently elicited in the office, even in specialized clinics.

• Indirect signs of possible contributing factors include evidence of peripheral vascular disease (audible bruits, palpable thrills), signs of peripheral neuropathy, or central nervous system disease/injury including absence of a normal bulbocavernosus reflex.

Investigations

All patients
Serum testosterone, serum prolactin, glycohemoglobin level: screen for hypogonadism, hyperprolactinemia, diabetes as contributors.

Selected patients
Nocturnal penile tumescence, postage stamp test, Rigi-scan: to determine presence or absence of any erectile function.

Cavernosography, cavernosometry, ultrasonagraphy: specialized examination to rule out venous leak as cause.

Pelvic electromyography: advised when neurogenic cause is possible but not clearly demonstrable on examination.

Complications

• These relate mainly to the deterioration of quality of life, with possible reactive psychiatric sequlae and loss of self-esteem.

Treatment

Diet and lifestyle

- The centerpiece of managing this condition is involvement of the patient and his sexual partner.

- Alcohol intake should be restricted.

- Adequate, quality sleep time and absence of excessive fatigue improve management.

Pharmacological treatment

Not cause-specific.

- Most cases of impotence/erectile dysfunction respond to prostaglandin E_1 (PGE_1) therapy; although other treatments are used (yohimbine, papavernine), PGE_1 is the only pharmacologic treatment with Food and Drug Administration approval for impotence/erectile dysfunction; failure to respond suggests venous leak as the cause of impotence/erectile dysfunction.

- Treatment of associated/underlying causes is necessary and helpful (*e.g.*, hypogonadism).

Standard dosage	Alprostadil (PGE_1) (intracavernosal prostaglandin [Caverject]), 2.5 µg increased to 5 µg, then increased by increments of 5–10 µg until adequate tumescence occurs and lasts 1 hour (doses should be titrated in the physician's office). Intrauerthral prostaglandin (Muse), dose range 125–1000 µg until adequate response achieved and lasts ~1 hour; full detumescence should occur before discharge from the office (doses should be titrated in the physician's office).
Contraindications	*Intracavernosal and intraurethral:* condition predisposing to priapism (*e.g.*, sickle-cell disease), anatomical deformation of the penis (*e.g.*, Peyronie's disease). *Intraurethral only:* abnormal urethral anatomy, intercourse with pregnant woman.
Special points	*Prostaglandin (intracavernosal and intraurethral):* priapism, erection lasting >6 hours, requires emergency urologic referral, and occurs in <1% of cases. *Prostaglandin (intracavernosal):* use with caution in patients on anticoagulation.
Main drug interactions	*All agents:* none known.
Main side effects	*Prostaglandin (intraurethral and intracavernosal):* penile pain, prolonged erection. *Prostaglandin (intraurethral):* urethral burning.

Other treatment options

- Referral is recommended if suspected cause is venous leak or psychological, or if implantable prosthesis is the preferred treatment option.

Sex therapy

- Sex therapy is a strongly recommended adjunct to any successful intervention.
- The drawback is limited availability of qualified experts.

Vacuum erection device

- This is indicated regardless of cause.

Implantable penile prosthesis

- This is indicated regardless of cause and is very effective.
- The drawback is expense, and surgical revision is required in 10%-50% of cases.

Treatment aims

To ensure patient and sexual partner satisfaction with sexual performance. To improve quality of life. To limit effects from treatment.

Prognosis

- Response rates are high for one or more of available treatment options. Patients' and their partners' satisfaction rates are 70% with vacuum erection device, 80% with injection therapy, and 90% with inflatable prosthesis.

Follow-up and management

- Priapism resulting from PGE_1 therapy is a medical emergency and deserves immediate referral to a well-qualified urologic surgeon.

- Reassurance and indicating concern are reason enough for frequent follow-up with the patient and sexual partner after treatment has been prescribed.

Key references

1. Impotence. *NIH Consensus Statement* (http://odp.od.nih.gov/consensus/) 1992, **10**:1–31.

2. Dewire DM: Evaluation and treatment of erectile dysfunction. *Am Fam Physician* 1996, **53**:2101–2106.

3. Perring M, Moran J: Holistic approach to the management of erectile disorders in a male sexual health clinic. *Br J Clin Pract* 1995, **3**:140–144.

Diagnosis

Symptoms

Fever: for 3–4 days.
Rash.
Systemic upset; "misery."

Unproductive cough.
Catarrh.
Conjunctivitis.

Signs

Prodromal period before rash

Fever.

Enanthema, Koplik's spots: pathognomic small greyish-white spots on reddened mucous membranes, notably the buccal mucosa.

Rash: maculopapular, blotchy, not itchy; starts on face and behind ears; spreads downwards over a few days; lasts ~5 days; almost invariably stains (persisting discoloration that does not blanch on pressure) from erythrocyte leakage during active rash.

Associated with development of rash

Reddened throat.
Bronchitic cough.
Conjunctivitis.
Lymph-node enlargement.

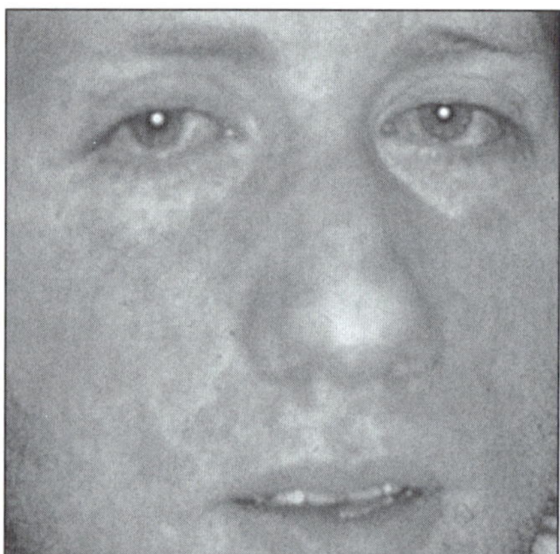

Blotchy rash of measles and conjunctivitis. (*See* Color Plate.)

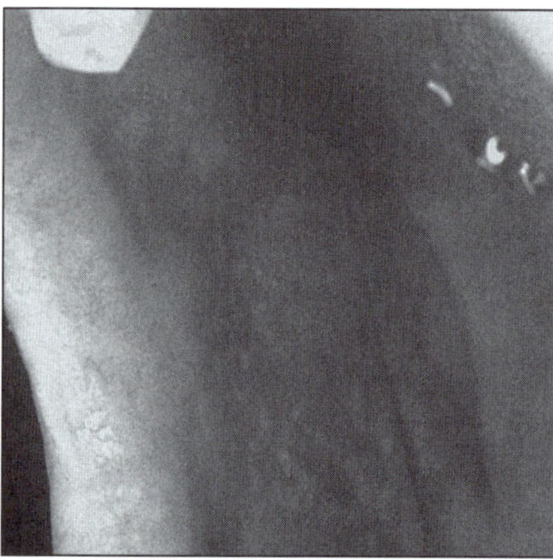

Koplik's spots in measles. (*See* Color Plate.)

Investigations

• The clinical picture is usually diagnostic.

Throat swab or nasopharyngeal aspirate: measles virus may be grown (technically difficult).
Immunofluorescent staining of throat secretions: may identify measles virus.
Serology: measles-specific IgM may be present in blood early in illness.
Paired sera examination: may show diagnostic rises in antibody (about fourfold).

Complications

• Complications are more severe in old or very young patients.

Measles bronchiolitis: when rash heaviest on trunk.
Secondary bacterial pneumonia and otitis media: in ~15%, especially children.
Febrile convulsions: in children, especially during prodrome.
Post–acute measles encephalitis: immune-mediated, at about day 6 of illness.
Subacute sclerosing panencephalitis: caused by persisting measles virus infection in nervous system, usually fatal; develops several years after acute infection.
Gastroenteritis: in malnourished children can lead to kwashiorkor and acute vitamin A deficiency.
Thrombocytopenia.
Giant-cell pneumonia or measles encephalitis: progressive in immunocompromised patient.

Treatment

Diet and lifestyle

• Patients should be isolated during the period of infectivity, which usually lasts from the onset of symptoms until the rash has stained.

Pharmacological treatment

Symptomatic

Analgesics, *e.g.*, acetaminophen.

Antibacterial drugs for bacterial complications.

Prophylactic

Vaccination by live virus preparation in second year of life as MMR: may cause mild measles-like illness.

Pooled human immunoglobulin: protective if given shortly after exposure.

• Vaccination and pooled human immunoglobulin can be given together if vaccination of vulnerable patients (*e.g.*, those with cystic fibrosis) is desired.

• Vitamin A deficiency (clinical or subclinical) increases the severity, complications, and risk of death from measles.

• In countries where the measles fatality rate is 1% or more, vitamin A should be given in all cases; elsewhere, it should be given in severe cases.

General references

Hutchins S, Markowitz L, Atkinson W, *et al.*: Measles outbreaks in the United States, 1987 through 1990. *Pediatr Infect Dis J* 1996, **15**:31–38.

Lutwick LI: Postexposure prophylaxis. *Infect Dis Clin North Am* 1996, **10**:899–915.

Makhene MK, Diaz PS: Clinical presentations and complications of suspected measles in hospitalized children. *Pediatr Infect Dis J* 1993, **12**:836–840.

de Quadros CA, Olive JM, Hersh BS, *et al.*: Measles elimination in the Americas: evolving strategies. *JAMA* 1996, **275**:224–229.

Diagnosis

Symptoms

Headache.
Neck and back pain and stiffness.
Vomiting.
Photophobia.

Fever.
Altered level of consciousness.
Seizures.

• Atypical clinical manifestations may occur in very young, elderly, or immunocompromised patients (highest-risk groups).

Signs

Nuchal rigidity: on flexion only, not on lateral rotation.

"Meningeal cry": high-pitched, in infants.

Kernig's sign: pain and hamstring spasm on passive knee extension with hip flexed.

Brudzinski's sign: spontaneous knee and hip flexion on attempted neck flexion.

Cranial nerve palsies and other focal signs.

Deteriorating level of consciousness: in up to 25% of patients.

Papilledema, bulging fontanelle in infants: indicating raised intracranial pressure.

Fever, tachycardia, shock, evidence of primary source of infection: *e.g.*, pneumonia, endocarditis, sinusitis, otitis media.

Rash: in ~50% of patients with meningococcal infections, sometimes briefly erythematous before becoming petechial or purpuric.

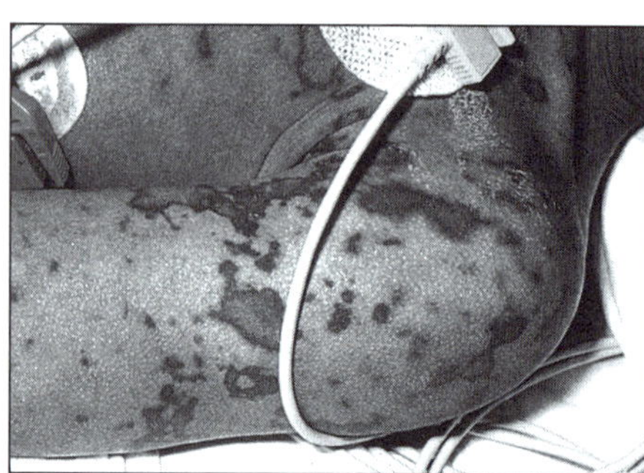

Purpuric rash of meningococcal meningitis. (*See* Color Plate.)

Investigations

Lumbar puncture: in untreated acute bacterial meningitis, reveals turbid CSF under raised pressure, neutrophilic pleocytosis (hundreds or thousands of cells/μL), protein concentration usually >1 g/L, glucose concentration low. Specific tests for causative organisms include Gram stain, culture, sensitivity testing, fungal and tubercular microscopy and culture, and bacterial antigen immunoassay. Contraindications include papilledema, deteriorating level of consciousness, and focal neurological signs; prepuncture cranial CT is needed in such patients to exclude mass lesion.

Complete blood count: to detect neutrophil leukocytosis.

Coagulation screen and fibrin degradation product analysis: for disseminated intravascular coagulation.

Electrolyte analysis: to detect hyponatremia.

Blood culture: may be positive when CSF sterile.

Chest and skull (sinus) radiography: to identify primary source of infection.

Complications

Seizures, focal CNS signs, raised intracranial pressure, subdural effusion, cerebral or subdural abscess formation, hydrocephalus (obstructive or communicating).

Septic shock, disseminated intravascular coagulation with adrenal hemorrhage: Waterhouse–Friderichsen's syndrome, complication of meningococcal meningitis.

Inappropriate antidiuretic hormone secretion: in <10% of patients.

Arthritis: septic or immune complex, in <10% of meningococcal infections.

Behavioral disturbances, mental retardation, hearing loss, epilepsy, cranial nerve palsies, visual and motor deficits: long-term complications (more usual in *Streptococcus pneumoniae* infections; <30% of patients).

Differential diagnosis

• Few patients, even with severe headache and fever, have meningitis.

Viral meningitis, especially enteroviruses, mumps.

Intercurrent infections, especially influenza A and B with meningism.

Cranial infections: cerebral abscess, sinusitis, throat infections.

Noninfective meningitis: subarachnoid hemorrhage, leukemic infiltration, Mollaret's meningitis (recurrent fever, meningeal signs, and CSF pleocytosis).

Autoimmune diseases, vasculitis.

Chemical meningitis, *e.g.*, intrathecal drugs.

Etiology

• 70%–90% of cases of bacterial meningitis are due to one of three organisms:
Neisseria meningitidis.
Haemophilus influenzae (type b).
S. pneumoniae.

• Other organisms found in specific at-risk groups include the following:

Enterobacteriaceae, group B streptococci in neonates.

Listeria monocytogenes in neonates and immunocompromised patients.

Mycobacterium tuberculosis in patients from developing countries and immunocompromised patients.

Staphylococci in patients with head trauma or neurosurgical shunts.

Epidemiology

• The incidence of bacterial meningitis is ~5–10 in 100 000 annually in developed countries.

• The three common organisms have characteristic patterns of occurrence: *N. meningitidis* in epidemics, *H. influenzae* in children aged <5 years, *S. pneumoniae* in patients aged >40 years (especially alcoholic, splenectomized, and sickle-cell anemic patients).

Treatment

Diet and lifestyle

• No special precautions are necessary.

Pharmacological treatment

General management

• Bacterial meningitis may prove fatal within hours; successful treatment depends on early diagnosis and i.v. administration of appropriate antibiotics in appropriate doses; agents that penetrate CSF and cover likely pathogens should be used (*e.g.*, ampicillin and ceftriaxone).

• If lumbar puncture is delayed by the need for prepuncture CT, antibiotic treatment should be started before the scan, after blood cultures.

• Treatment should ideally be bactericidal with a high therapeutic ratio, the drug penetrating the CSF in adequate concentrations; very high i.v. doses may be needed despite damage to the blood–brain barrier in meningitis.

• Adjunctive corticosteroids are indicated when bacterial organisms are present on Gram stain or in the setting of increased intracranial pressure.

Against *N. meningitidis*, *S. pneumoniae*, and *H. influenzae*

Standard dosage	*Adults:* ceftriaxone, 2 g every 12 hours for 10 days.
Contraindications	Cephalosporin hypersensitivity; caution in renal impairment, history of allergy.
Special points	Other options include cefotaxime, ceftriaxone, and chloramphenicol.
Main drug interactions	None.
Main side effects	Sensitivity reactions.

Against penicillin-susceptible pneumococcus or established meningococcus

Standard dosage	*Adults:* penicillin G, 14.4 g (24 MU) i.v. daily in divided doses (usually 4 MU initially, then 2 MU 2-hourly; can be relaxed to 4- or 6-hourly regimen with evidence of clinical improvement, usually within 48–72 hours); treatment should continue for 7 days after the patient has become afebrile. *Children and infants:* penicillin G, 100–300 mg/kg daily depending on age, according to manufacturer's current prescribing information.
Contraindications	Penicillin hypersensitivity; caution in renal impairment, history of allergy.
Special points	Other options include cefotaxime, ceftriaxone, and chloramphenicol.
Main drug interactions	None.
Main side effects	Sensitivity reactions.

Prevention

• Chemoprophylaxis (using rifampicin or ciprofloxacin) is indicated for household contacts and index patients before hospital discharge.

• Immunization against *H. influenzae* infection (using *H. influenzae* type b vaccine) is recommended routinely for children at the ages of 2, 3, and 4 months.

Treatment aims

To secure survival and prevent persistent neurological complications.

To reduce the of recurrence by treating any predisposing cause.

To prevent spread to close contacts.

Prognosis

• Mortality is ~10% overall, 5%–10% from *H. influenzae* infection, 5%–10% from *N. meningitidis* infection, and 10%–30% from *S. pneumoniae* infection.

• Long-term sequelae are 9%–22%, 4%–6%, and 14%–40%, respectively.

Follow-up and management

• Repeat lumbar puncture to monitor treatment is not necessary if the patient is improving.

• Bacteriological relapse needs immediate reinstitution of treatment.

• Adults should be reviewed at 3 months, children at 6–12 months, and neonates for longer to detect any long-term sequelae.

Causes of treatment failure

Wrong diagnosis: *e.g.*, tuberculosis, abscess.

Wrong drug: poor CSF penetration, antimicrobial resistance.

Wrong route: intraventricular instillation needed for ventriculitis with "resistant" infections.

Poor-risk patient: extremes of age, immunocompromise.

Unrecognized complication: treatable raised intracranial pressure, abscess or ventriculitis, subdural effusion or abscess (treatable); vasculitis, cerebritis (less treatable).

Shock.

General references

Miller LG, Choi C: Meningitis in older patients: how to diagnose and treat a deadly infection. *Geriatrics* 1997, **52**:43–55.

Quagliarello V, Scheld WM: Bacterial meningitis: Pathogenesis, pathophysiology and progress. *N Engl J Med* 1992, **327**:864–872.

Segreti J, Harris AA: Acute bacterial meningitis. *Infect Dis Clin North Am* 1996, **10**:797–809.

Tunkel AR, Wispelwey B, Scheld M: Bacterial meningitis: recent advances in pathophysiology and treatment. *Ann Intern Med* 1990, **112**:610–623.

Diagnosis

Symptoms

• Symptoms are usually chronic, usually <3 weeks, but can be acute.

Immunosuppression: with CD4 counts $<100 \times 10^9$/L.

Headache: in 81% of patients.

Fever: in 77%.

Nausea or vomiting: in 44%.

Photophobia: in 27%.

Seizures: in 5%; can be the presenting feature.

Signs

• No signs are reported in >50% of patients.

Abnormal mental status: in 28%. Nuchal rigidity uncommon.

Focal neurological signs and papilledema: rare; may be present if the patient has cryptococcomas.

Extraneural involvement: in 20%, with pulmonary infiltrates, skin lesions, and prustatic involvement.

Investigations

• Cryptococcal antigen in blood is positive in 90% of patients.

CT or MRI: should be performed before lumbar puncture to exclude a mass lesion if focal neurological signs are present; usually shows no abnormality or cerebral atrophy; communicating hydrocephalus infrequent; low-density lesions, scattered and symmetrical, sometimes seen, attributed to cryptococci.

CSF analysis: to establish diagnosis; usually shows minimum pleocytosis (<20 leukocytes) and raised protein; glucose may be low. The CSF may be entirely normal; India-ink preparation may show cryptococci; cryptococcal antigen (>1:16) positive in 95% of patients.

Other investigations: cryptococcus can be cultured from other sites (sputum, blood, bone marrow). Abnormal liver function, low albumin concentration, or hyponatremia in 20%; lymphopenia common in peripheral blood.

Complications

Death: during the acute illness despite treatment (up to 30% of patients); increased intracranial pressure or progression of the meningitis with seizures, cranial nerve palsies, stupor, and coma.

Cerebral cryptococcomas: *i.e.*, cryptococcal abscesses; rare.

Differential diagnosis

Viral and tuberculous meningitis.

Cerebral toxoplasmosis.

Cerebral lymphoma.

Benign headaches (migraine, tension, depression).

Meningitis due to hysteria.

Etiology

• Cryptococcus is a yeast present in high quantities in the environment.

• Infection is acquired by inhalation.

• The spread to the CNS is hematogenous.

Epidemiology

• Most cases of cryptococcal meningitis are AIDS-related.

• Cryptococcal meningitis is found in 2%–12% of AIDS patients in different clinical series.

• It is the most frequent cause of meningitis.

Treatment

Diet and lifestyle

• No special precautions are necessary.

Pharmacological treatment

Initial treatment

• The established initial treatment is by amphotericin B and flucytosine.

• Treatment of the first episode fails in 20%–40% of patients.

Standard dosage	Amphotericin B, 0.75 mg/kg i.v. daily. Usual course is 15 mg/kg total.
Contraindications	Renal failure, pregnancy, breast-feeding, old age.
Special points	Hepatic and renal function, blood count, electrolytes, and drug concentrations must be monitored.
Main drug interactions	*Amphotericin B:* increased risk of nephrotoxicity with cyclosporine, aminoglycosides; antagonizes miconazole.
Main side effects	*Amphotericin B:* nausea, vomiting, fever, nephrotoxicity. *Flucytosine:* diarrhea, bone-marrow suppression.

Adjunctive 5-fluorocytosine

• This agent may improve the outcome when added to amphotericin.

Standard dosage	5F-C, 100 mg/kg daily.
Contraindications	Hepatitis, vomiting.
Main drug interactions	None.
Main side effects	Vomiting, hepatitis, bone-marrow suppression. Serum levels should be monitored.

Maintenance treatment

• ~50% of HIV-seropositive patients with cryptococcal meningitis relapse without maintenance treatment.

• The relapse rate can be markedly reduced with fluconazole.

Standard dosage	Fluconazole, 200 mg orally daily for life.
Contraindications	Possibly breast-feeding, pregnancy, children.
Special points	Can be used for initial treatment i.v. or orally at 400 mg daily in mildly ill patients who are not obtunded. Itraconazole is a useful alternative.
Main drug interactions	Enhances warfarin, phenytoin, theophylline, cyclosporine, sulfonylureas; reduces rifampin.
Main side effects	Diarrhea, bone-marrow suppression.

Treatment aims

To eradicate cryptococcal infection.

Prognosis

• 30%–50% of patients do not respond to treatment.

Follow-up and management

• Patients should be closely followed, particularly for the first year when relapses are more common.

General references

Chuck SL, Sande MA: Infections with *Cryptococcus neoformans* in the acquired immunodeficiency syndrome. *N Engl J Med* 1989, **321**:794–799.

Sharkey PK, Graybill JR, Johnson ES, *et al.*: Amphotericin B lipid complex compared with amphotericin B in the treatment of cryptococcal meningitis in patients with AIDS. *Clin Infect Dis* 1996, **22**:315–321.

van der Horst CM, Saag MS, Cloud GA, *et al.*: Treatment of cryptococcal meningitis associated with the acquired immuno-deficiency syndrome. *N Engl J Med* 1997, **337**:15–21.

Weinke T, *et al.*: Cryptococcosis in AIDS patients: observations concerning CNS involvement. *J Neurol* 1989, **236**:38–42.

Diagnosis

Symptoms [1]

• Symptoms are primarily due to estrogen deficiency.

Shortened, irregular, or absent menstrual periods: menstrual cycle normally shortens during the perimenopause due to a reduced follicular phase.

Vasomotor symptoms ("hot flashes"): affect about half of all women in the first 2 years of menopause; sudden onset of vasodilation, heat, and perspiration in the upper body; typically lasts several minutes; can be debilitating, however symptoms decrease with time in most women.

Vaginal atrophy and dyspareunia.

Urethral syndrome: symptoms of urinary tract infection without evidence of infection (controversy exists as to whether these symptoms are secondary to estrogen deficiency, aging, or both).

Fractures: due to loss of bone mineral density (*see* Osteoporosis *for further details*).

Psychological symptoms: Incidence of depression does not increase during menopause; however, stress associated with menopause may exacerbate underlying problems.

Signs

• Symptoms predominate over signs in most women.

Genitourinary complications: pale, atrophic, friable vaginal mucosa; vagina, cervix, and uterus may decrease in size; increased incidence of cystoceles and rectoceles (may be related to aging).

Investigations

• Menopause and hypoestrogenism are primarily clinical diagnoses.

Serum estradiol levels: <20 pg/mL (in the setting of an elevated follicle-stimulating hormone) is consistent with ovarian failure.

Follicle-stimulating hormone levels: elevated in ovarian failure; may be low or normal with other causes of hypogonadism.

Bone densitometry: useful for women at risk of osteoporosis; some women find this information helpful in deciding whether or not to begin hormone replacement therapy.

Lipid panel: loss of cardiovascular protective effects of estrogen at menopause increases the importance of diagnosing and treating hyperlipidemia.

Complications

Premenopausal hypogonadism

Failure to achieve predicted peak bone mass: increases risk of subsequent osteoporosis and fractures.

Early loss of cardioprotective effects of estrogen.

Infertility.

Menopause

• Most complications are related to symptoms and signs discussed above, including osteoporotic fractures and coronary artery disease.

Senile dementia (Alzheimer's disease): recent evidence suggests an association with estrogen deficiency.

Treatment

Diet and lifestyle

• The importance of weight-bearing exercise, healthy diet, smoking cessation, and adequate intake of calcium and vitamin D should be reviewed with the postmenopausal patient.

• Women with athletic amenorrhea should be encouraged to alter their exercise and diet to facilitate the return of normal menses.

• Physicians should inquire about eating disorders in young, thin, amenorrheic women.

Pharmacological treatment

Estrogen replacement therapy

• Estrogen replacement remains the therapy of choice in suitable women due to its beneficial effects on bone density, coronary heart disease, and overall mortality. It may also decrease the incidence of senile dementia [4].

Standard dosage	*Anovulatory premenopausal women*: low-dose oral contraceptives, containing <35 µg/day of ethinyl estradiol. *Postmenopausal women*: ethinyl estradiol, 5–10 µg daily; Estrace, 1–2 mg daily; Ogen, 0.625 daily; Premarin, 0.625–0.9 mg daily; estrogen patches.
Contraindications	Patients with estrogen-responsive tumors or strong family history of breast cancer, pregnancy, abnormal vaginal bleeding, history of thromboembolic disease.
Special points	If the uterus is present, progestational therapy is also required to reduce the incidence of endometrial cancer. This can be given as a cyclic regimen (medroxyprogesterone, 10 mg daily for 10 days of each month) or continuously (medroxyprogesterone, 2.5–5.0 mg daily). Estrogen patches avoid first-pass metabolism through the liver, and may be useful in women with a history of thromboembolic disease who wish to be on estrogen.
Main drug interactions	May increase requirements for thyroxine in women on thyroid hormone replacement.
Main side effects	Breast swelling and tenderness, weight gain.

Nonhormonal therapies for vasomotor symptoms [5]

Clonidine: dosages range from 50–400 µg daily. Increased incidence of side effects at higher doses (insomnia, orthostatic hypotension).

Medroxyprogesterone: 20–40 mg daily. Effective at treating hot flashes, but with detrimental effects on lipids.

• If indicated, patients should also be treated for osteoporosis and hyperlipidemia.

Treatment aims

Menopause
To alleviate or reduce symptoms of estrogen deficiency.
To maintain a favorable lipid profile.
To prevent the rapid loss of bone mass associated with menopause.

Premenopause
To restore normal estradiol levels, either by the resumption of normal menses or by estrogen replacement therapy.

Prognosis
• Menopause is a normal part of the aging process and does not have a specific prognosis.
• The deleterious effects of estrogen deficiency (in both premenopausal and postmenopausal women) can be effectively treated, with good prognoses.

Follow-up and management
• Estrogen doses may be titrated upward in women with persistent vasomotor symptoms.
• All women should be encouraged to have regular Papanicolaou smears and, if indicated, mammograms. This is particularly important in postmenopausal women on estrogen replacement therapy.
• Patients should receive ongoing assessment of bone density and lipid profile, as clinically indicated.

Key references

1. Greendale GA, Sowers M: The menopause transition. *Endocrinol Metab Clin North Am* 1997, **26**:261–277.

2. Hergenroeder AC: Bone mineralization, hypothalamic amenorrhea, and sex steroid therapy in female adolescents and young adults. *J Pediatrics* 1995, **126**:683–689.

3. Grodstein F, Stampfer MJ, Colditz GA, *et al.*: Postmenopausal hormone therapy and mortality. *N Engl J Med* 1997, **336**:1769–1775.

4. Paganini-Hill A, Henderson VW: Estrogen replacement therapy and risk of Alzheimer disease. *Arch Intern Med* 1996, **156**:2213–2217.

5. Ravnikar VA: Alternate therapies for vasomotor symptoms and osteoporosis in the menopausal patient. In *Treatment of the Postmenopausal Woman: Basic and Clinical Aspects*. Edited by Lobo RA. Philadelphia: Lippincott-Raven; 1996:307–312.

Diagnosis

Definition

Migraine with aura (classic migraine): characterized by aura followed by episodic unilateral throbbing headache, with nausea, photophobia, and phonophobia; auras usually last 10–20 minutes but can persist for up to 1 hour; laterality of neurological disturbance not related to side of ensuing headache.

Migraine without aura (common migraine): characterized by episodic unilateral or bilateral headache, gastrointestinal upset, photo- or phonophobia, but no aura.

• Migraine headaches are paroxysmal, lasting from a few hours up to 3 days, but with periods of complete relief between attacks.

Cluster headache: 90% of sufferers men; paroxysmal very severe unilateral periorbital pain lasting 0.5–2 hours, once or twice daily (often at night) for weeks, with months or years of relief between bouts; usually associated with Horner's syndrome, lacrimation and nasal stuffiness ipsilateral to pain.

Ophthalmoplegic migraine: recurrent attacks of III or VI cranial-nerve palsies associated with headache; resolution of deficit may be delayed by several days.

Retinal migraine: monocular visual loss involving scotoma or altitudinal defect followed by headache.

Hemiplegic migraine: recurrent attacks of hemiparesis of rapid onset followed by headache; weakness may last hours.

• Migraine variants are diagnoses of exclusion; other more serious causes of the clinical picture (*e.g.,* stroke, aneurysmal leak, transient ischemic attack) must be excluded, especially if the pain is severe, before the diagnosis is accepted.

Symptoms

• The aura of classic migraine may be visual (in 50% of patients) or sensory (in 30%) or occasionally may involve dysphasia or motor deficit.

Visual auras: teichopsia, fortification spectra, fragmentation, scotoma, homonymous hemianopia.

Transient tingling or numbness: sensory symptoms; upper limbs more frequently involved than lower limbs.

Signs

• Common migraine may have no signs.

• The scotomas, hemianopia, and sensorimotor phenomena of classic migraine may be detected if the aura is still present at the time of examination.

• Prolonged deficit requires exclusion of other causes.

Investigations [1,2]

• Investigation is not needed if the diagnosis of migraine is well founded; it is needed when the diagnosis is in doubt and in patients with residual neurological deficit after migraine.

• Investigation including the following is aimed at excluding alternative diagnoses:

ESR measurement: for temporal arteritis.

Radiography, MRI: for cervical spondylosis.

CT or MRI: for tumor, vascular malformation, hydrocephalus.

CSF analysis: for subarachnoid bleed, arteritis.

Angiography: for aneurysmal bleeding.

Complications

Complicated migraine: rarely, residua from migraine auras continue as permanent deficits or stroke.

Dehydration.

Migrainous infarction: rare, usually posterior parietal or occipital.

Treatment

Diet and lifestyle

• Dietary precipitants, *e.g.*, chocolate, cheese, coffee, red wine, should be avoided in sensitive patients.

• Stress is a common precipitant of migraine: appropriate measures may reduce the frequency of attacks.

• Oral contraceptives are best avoided; they are contraindicated in migraine with focal neurological deficits.

Pharmacological treatment

• Many patients treat attacks satisfactorily with rest, darkness, and simple analgesics, including naproxen, Midrin, ketorolac.

For migraine with and without aura: acute

• Patients with gastrointestinal disturbance and more severe headache may benefit from a combination of analgesic and antiemetic; the antiemetic not only reduces vomiting but increases gastric emptying, thereby improving absorption of the analgesic.

• More severe attacks unresponsive to this treatment may be treated by sumatriptan or ergotamine.

Standard dosage	Sumatriptan, 25–100 mg orally at onset or 6 mg s.c. by autoinjector. Ergotamine in varying doses according to route.
Contraindications	*Sumatriptan:* patients aged >65 years or with history of coronary disease; to be avoided in children or hemiplegic migraine. *Ergotamine:* vascular disease, active infection, hemiplegic migraine.
Special points	*Sumatriptan:* effective in 60% at 2 hours and 80% at 4 hours. *Ergotamine*: maximum dose of preparation must not be exceeded because of risk of vasospasm.
Main drug interactions	*Sumatriptan:* ergotamine, monoamine oxidase inhibitors, lithium. *Ergotamine:* beta-blockers, methysergide, and sumatriptan all increase risk of vasospasm.
Main side effects	*Sumatriptan:* chest pain or tightness, light-headedness, transient pain at site of injection. *Ergotamine:* nausea, vomiting, headache (possibly due to overuse), tingling, chest tightness. *Zolmitriptan*: under development.

For common and classic migraine: prophylactic [4]

• Beta-blockers or 5-HT antagonists should be considered for ≥2 attacks a month; 6–12 months' effective treatment may allow withdrawal at original frequency.

Standard dosage	Propranolol, 60–160 mg long-acting daily (or nadolol or metaprolol). Tricyclic antidepressants: amitriptyline, nortriptyline.
Contraindications	*Beta-blockers:* asthma, cardiac failure, heart block.
Main drug interactions	*See manufacturer's current prescribing information.*
Main side effects	*Beta-blockers:* bradycardia, heart failure, bronchospasm, fatigue, depression. *Tricyclic antidepressants:* dry mouth, orthostasis, fatigue, weight gain.

• Other agents that may be helpful include nonsteroidals (naproxen sodium, ketorolac tromethamine), valproic acid, calcium channel blockers, or methysergide.

For cluster headache: acute

Sumatriptan or ergotamine.
Oxygen (>40%), if not contraindicated.
Prednisolone, 60 mg (occasionally helpful).

For cluster headache: prophylactic

Short-term sumatriptan or ergotamine before predicted onset of attack.
Lithium and methysergide in refractory patients: regular monitoring of lithium concentrations and checking of thyroid function needed; methysergide used intermittently (no longer than 6 months) to reduce risk of retroperitoneal fibrosis.

Key references

1. Dalessio DJ: Diagnosing the severe headache. *Neurology* 1994, **44(suppl 3)**:S6–S12.

2. Pryse-Phillips WE, Dodick DW, Edmeads GW, *et al.*: Guidelines for the diagnosis and management of migraine in clinical practice. *Can Med Assoc J* 1997, **156**:1273–1287.

3. Baumel B: Migraine. *Neurology* 1994, **44 (suppl 3)**:S13–S17.

4. Tfelt-Hansen P: Prophylactic pharmacotherapy of migraine: some practical guidelines. *Neurol Clin* 1997, **15**:153–165.

Diagnosis

Symptoms [1]

• Symptoms are often mild or absent.

Dyspnea: due to pulmonary congestion.

Fatigue: due to low cardiac output.

Palpitation: due to atrial fibrillation.

Fluid retention: in late-stage disease.

Signs

Irregular pulse: if patient is in atrial fibrillation.

Low-amplitude pulse pressure.

Raised venous pressure.

Parasternal heave: right ventricular hypertrophy and systolic left atrial expansion.

Laterally displaced and hyperdynamic apical impulse.

Pansystolic murmur.

Third heart sound.

Loud pulmonary second sound: if patient has pulmonary hypertension.

Investigations

ECG: shows broad bifid P wave (P mitrale), atrial fibrillation.

Chest radiography: shows pulmonary congestion, left atrial enlargement, cardiac enlargement, pulmonary artery enlargement (if severe and long-standing).

Echocardiography and Doppler ultrasonography: large left atrium, large left ventricle, increased fractional shortening, regurgitant jet (Doppler), leaflet prolapse (floppy valve or flail leaflet).

Transesophogeal echocardiography: may give better visualization of valve apparatus.

Cardiac catheterization: large "V" wave in wedge trace, angiographic evidence of mitral regurgitation.

Complications

Systemic embolism.

Pulmonary hypertension, right heart failure.

Endocarditis.

Differential diagnosis

Floppy mitral valve: late systolic murmur and midsystolic click [2].

Hypertrophic cardiomyopathy: ECG and echocardiographic evidence of left ventricular hypertrophy.

Etiology

Rheumatic disease.

Floppy mitral valve.

Chordal rupture.

Papillary muscle dysfunction or rupture.

"Functional" disorder, *i.e.*, secondary to dilated, poorly contracting left ventricle.

• Floppy valve and chordal rupture are associated with connective tissue abnormalities, papillary muscle dysfunction and rupture with coronary artery disease.

Epidemiology

• The increasing availability of echocardiography may result in more patients with mitral regurgitation being found.

Treatment

Diet and lifestyle

• Patients should avoid being overweight, stop smoking, and maintain normal activities, if possible.

Pharmacological treatment

Digoxin

• If the patient is in atrial fibrillation, digoxin is indicated for control of ventricular rate (less easy than with mitral stenosis).

Standard dosage	Digoxin, 0.5 mg loading dose, repeated after 8 hours; maintenance dose usually 0.25 mg daily.
Contraindications	Caution in patients who are elderly, relatively small, or renally impaired (reduced dosage).
Main drug interactions	Diuretic-induced hypokalemia enhances effect of digoxin.
Main side effects	Nausea, vomiting, diarrhea, yellow discoloration to vision (xanthopsia), bradycardia.

Diuretics

• Diuretics are indicated to relieve pulmonary congestion.

Standard dosage	Furosemide, 20–80 mg daily with potassium supplements or potassium-sparing agent (particularly if patient is also taking digoxin).
Contraindications	None.
Special points	May precipitate attacks of gout in susceptible patients and may interfere with diabetic control.
Main drug interactions	Digoxin.
Main side effects	Hypokalemia, dehydration.

Vasodilators

• Vasodilatation is used to reduce regurgitant factor by reducing afterload unless systemic blood pressure is low.

Standard dosage	Angiotensin-converting enzyme (ACE) inhibitors, *e.g.*, enalapril, 5–20 mg twice daily, or captopril, 12.5–50 mg 3 times daily. Calcium antagonists, *e.g.*, long-acting preparations of nifedipine, 30–120 mg daily. Hydralazine, 12.5–75 mg 3 times daily. Initially given at night to avoid immediate hypotensive effects.
Contraindications	Hypotension.
Special points	*ACE inhibitors*: treatment best started in hospital if patient taking large dose of diuretic or other vasodilator at same time.
Main drug interactions	*ACE inhibitors:* potassium-sparing diuretics or supplements.
Main side effects	*ACE inhibitors*: hypotension, renal dysfunction, dysgeusia (taste dysfunction), rashes, dry unproductive cough. *Calcium antagonists:* flushing, headache, fluid retention. *Hydralazine:* hypotension, headache, lupus-like syndrome (rare).

Beta-adrenergic blockers

• For patients in atrial fibrillation who have effort-related tachycardia despite digitalis, beta-blockers are helpful in reducing tendency to extreme tachycardia.

Standard dosage	Atenolol 25–100 mg daily or metoprolol 50–200 mg daily to control heart rate.
Contraindications	Asthma, heart failure, bradycardia, heart block.
Main drug interactions	Bradycardia when combined with digitalis or calcuim channel blockers. Low doses are usually the rule when used with digitalis.

Treatment aims

To achieve normal functional capacity.

To perform surgical repair prior to development of left ventricular dysfunction owing to chronic volume overload.

• Recent studies suggest that early surgical repair for flail leaflet when symptoms begin or noninvasive tests indicate significant left ventricular volume overload result in optimal long-term outcome. Delays in surgery may lead to permanent left ventricular dysfunction and reduced survival [3].

Other treatments

Surgical mitral valve repair or replacement [4,5].

• When possible, repair is preferable to replacement.

Prognosis

• Prognosis is good unless pulmonary artery pressures have been chronically high or left ventricle is severely impaired.

Follow-up and management

• Drug treatment needs regular review to ensure that it has not become inadequate.

Key references

1. Braunwald E: Mitral regurgitation: physiological, clinical, and surgical considerations. *N Engl J Med* 1969, **281**:425–432.

2. Devereux RB, *et al.*: Mitral valve prolapse: causes, clinical manifestations, and management. *Ann Intern Med* 1989, **111**:305–317.

3. Ling LH, *et al.*: Clinical outcome of mitral regurgitation due to flail leaflet. *N Engl J Med* 1996, **335**:1417–1423.

4. Cohn LH: Surgery for mitral valve regurgitation. *JAMA* 1988, **260**:2883–2887.

5. Galloway AC, *et al.*: Long-term results of mitral valve reconstruction with Carpentier techniques. *Circulation* 1988, **78(suppl I)**:I-97–105.

Diagnosis

Symptoms

Fatigue: insidious onset; due to low cardiac output [1].

Dyspnea, orthopnea: due to pulmonary congestion.

Palpitation: due to atrial fibrillation.

Signs

Irregular pulse: in atrial fibrillation.

Loud (palpable) first heart sound.

Opening snap: if valve is mobile.

Mitral diastolic murmur: long if severe.

Raised venous pressure.

Parasternal heave: right ventricular hypertrophy.

Loud pulmonary second sound.

Investigations

ECG: shows broad bifid P wave (P mitrale), usually atrial fibrillation if disease advanced.

Chest radiography: shows left atrial enlargement, pulmonary congestion, prominent pulmonary arteries (in pulmonary hypertensive patients).

Echocardiography and Doppler ultrasonography: show thickened mitral valve with reduced movement, large left atrium, reduced left ventricular filling rate, reduced mitral valve area.

Cardiac catheterization: shows raised right heart pressures and an end-diastolic gradient from pulmonary artery wedge pressure (or left atrium if transseptal puncture done) to left ventricle.

Complications

Systemic embolism: from left atrium.

Pulmonary hypertension, right heart failure.

Endocarditis: unusual.

Differential diagnosis

Left atrial myxoma: physical signs may be identical (echocardiography confirms diagnosis).

Etiology

Rheumatic disease.
Congenital abnormality (rare).

Epidemiology

• The occurrence of mitral stenosis is decreasing in developed countries as a result of the declining incidence of rheumatic fever.

Treatment

Diet and lifestyle

• Patients should avoid being overweight, give up smoking, and maintain normal activities, if possible.

Pharmacological treatment

Digoxin

• If the patient is in atrial fibrillation, digoxin is indicated for control of ventricular rate.

Standard dosage	Digoxin, 0.5 mg loading dose, repeated after 8 hours; maintenance dose usually 0.25 mg daily, adjusted according to serum digoxin concentration.
Contraindications	Caution in patients who are elderly, relatively small, or renally impaired (reduced dosage).
Main drug interactions	Diuretic-induced hypokalemia enhances effect of digoxin.
Main side effects	Nausea, vomiting, diarrhea, yellow discoloration to vision (xanthopsia), bradycardia.

Diuretics

• Diuretics are indicated for dyspnea or fluid retention.

Standard dosage	Furosemide, 20–80 mg daily with potassium supplements or potassium-sparing agent (particularly if patient is also taking digoxin).
Contraindications	None.
Special points	May precipitate attacks of gout in susceptible patients and may interfere with diabetic control.
Main drug interactions	Digoxin.
Main side effects	Hypokalemia, dehydration.

Anticoagulants

• Anticoagulants are mandatory if the degree of stenosis is high, even if the patient is still in sinus rhythm.

Standard dosage	Warfarin, 10 mg daily for 3 days; maintenance dose depends on regular checks of INR.
Contraindications	Bleeding tendency.
Main drug interactions	Any drug that displaces warfarin from protein-binding sites or increases liver enzyme activity may cause alteration in INR and thus necessitate dose adjustment.
Main side effects	Increased bleeding tendency.

Beta-adrenergic blockers

• For patients in atrial fibrillation who have effort-related tachycardia despite digitalis, beta-blockers are helpful in reducing tendency to extreme tachycardia.

Standard dosage	Atenolol, 25–100 mg daily, or metoprolol, 50–100 mg daily to control heart rate.
Contraindications	Asthma, heart failure, bradycardia, heart block.
Main drug interactions	Bradycardia when combined with digitalis or calcium channel blockers. Low doses are usually the rule when used with digitalis.

Treatment aims

To achieve normal exercise capability and normal functional capacity.

Other treatments

Balloon valvuloplasty if valve is mobile and not heavily calcified [2].
Surgical valvotomy or replacement.

Prognosis

• The prognosis is good unless pulmonary hypertension is chronic.

Follow-up and management

• Restenosis may occur after valvotomy or valvuloplasty.

• Drug treatment may become inadequate and indicate intervention eventually.

• Patients should have prophylactic treatment against endocarditis (*see* Endocarditis *for details*).

Key references

1. Wood P: An appreciation of mitral stenosis. *BMJ* 1954, **1**:1051–1055.

2. Abascal VM, *et al.*: Echocardiographic evaluation of mitral valve structure and function after percutaneous mitral valvuloplasty. *J Am Coll Cardiol* 1988, **12**:606–615.

Diagnosis

Definition

• Motor neuron disease is one of many motor neuron disorders. The term covers amyotrophic lateral sclerosis (the most common form), progressive muscular atrophy, and progressive bulbar palsy (thought to be variants of the same disorder).
• The disorder is progressive and is characterized by degeneration of cortical, brain stem, and spinal-cord motor neurons.

Symptoms [1]

Cramps or fasciculations: may precede other symptoms by months.
Asymmetrical painless weakness or wasting of proximal or distal upper limb muscles: presenting symptom in 40%–60% of patients with upper limb involvement and 20% with lower limb involvement (unilateral foot drop common).
Dysarthria: presenting complaint in 25%–30%, usually followed by limb involvement; 70%–80% presenting with limb involvement develop dysarthria, culminating in anarthria.
Dysphagia: accompanying dysarthria.
Shortness of breath: usually due to diaphragmatic weakness.
Minor sensory symptoms: occasionally.
Changes in character and behavior: in 5%–10%.
Frontal-lobe dementia: rarely.

Signs

Typical disease

Fasciculations, wasting, depressed reflexes: lower motor neuron signs.
Spasticity, slowing of alternating movements, brisk tendon reflexes, Babinski responses: upper motor neuron signs.

• Typical motor neuron disease has lower and upper motor neuron signs in several regions (cranial nerves, arms, legs), with evidence of disease progression.
• Signs are usually asymmetrical in the early stages, with no evidence of sensory signs or bladder or bowel involvement.

Bulbar involvement

Emotional lability, with inappropriate laughter and crying, brisk jaw jerk, spasticity of facial muscles, spastic dysarthria, dysphagia, spasticity of tongue: indicating upper motor neuron involvement (pseudobulbar palsy).
Wasting of facial and jaw muscles, fasciculation and wasting of tongue, nasal speech, dysphagia, bovine cough: indicating lower motor neuron involvement (bulbar palsy).

Investigations

• Laboratory results are usually normal (creatine kinase activity may be 2–3 times normal).

Electromyography: shows widespread anterior horn cell damage; nerve conduction studies usually normal; electrophysiology supports clinical diagnosis and excludes root and plexus lesions or motor neuropathy; characteristic abnormalities include fibrillation potentials and positive sharp waves, fasciculations, abnormal motor units of increased amplitude and duration.
MRI or myelography: may be needed to exclude spinal cord or root compression; MRI may show altered signal in posterior limb of internal capsule in region of degenerating corticospinal tract fibers.
Muscle biopsy: sometimes needed to exclude other diagnoses in atypical cases; confirms denervation, with small angular fibers and prominent fiber type grouping.

Complications

Depression: social and emotional isolation, especially in patients with severe dysarthria.
Dysphagia: leading to weight loss, malnutrition, dehydration, and aspiration.
Bronchopulmonary infections: related to aspiration and ventilatory muscle weakness.
Venous thrombosis and pulmonary embolism.
Constipation: due to pelvic and abdominal wall weakness and poor fluid intake.
Ventilatory failure: usual cause of death.

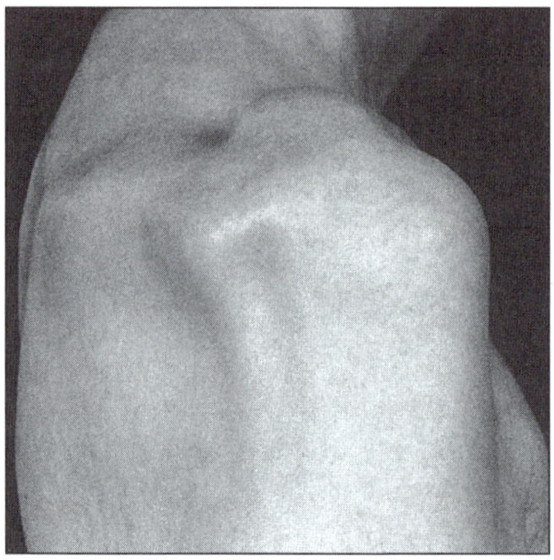

Marked muscle wasting around the shoulder girdle in a patient with motor neuron disease. (*See* Color Plate.)

Treatment

Diet and lifestyle

• Dietary advice is needed for patients with dysphagia and those who are being treated by percutaneous endoscopic gastrostomy.

Pharmacological treatment

Symptomatic medications

Glycopyrrolate, hyoscine (orally or transdermal patches), amitriptyline for drooling.

Quinine for cramps.

Baclofen, tizanidine, diazepam for spasticity.

Amitriptyline, dothiepin, fluoxetine for depression and emotional lability.

Fibercon, Colace, Mylanta, glycerine suppositories for constipation (with increased fluid intake).

Opiates, diazepam for symptomatic relief of anxiety related to dyspnea.

• The antiglutamate agent riluzole prolongs survival modestly.

To slow progression and prolong survival

• Riluzole's action is through inhibition of glutamate release [4].

Standard dosage	Riluzole, 100 mg/day orally. Gabapentin, 800 mg 3 times daily orally.
Contraindications	*Riluzole:* hepatic dysfunction, pregnancy. *Gabapentin:* pregnancy.
Special points	*Riluzole:* check liver function monthly for 3 months then every 3 months. *Gabapentin:* approved for epilepsy; early trials in ALS show a trend toward slower progression of weakness.
Main side effects	*Riluzole:* asthenia, nausea, dizziness, elevated hepatic enzymes. *Gabapentin:* tremor, dizziness, sedation.

•Other drug trials with insulin-like growth factor 1 show some promise.

Nonpharmacological treatment

Physical therapy.

Counseling for depression.

Percutaneous endoscopic gastrostomy for dysphagia (best considered early).

Radiotherapy to the parotid glands for excess saliva.

Assisted ventilation for respiratory failure: techniques available include nasal intermittent positive airway pressure ventilation, a rocking bed, a cuirasse, or, in exceptional circumstances, a tracheostomy and intermittent positive pressure ventilation.

Treatment aims

To maintain patient's independence and quality of life.
To alleviate symptoms.

Prognosis

• 80%–90% of patients develop upper and lower motor neuron signs at some stage.

• 10% show only lower motor neuron signs (progressive muscular atrophy).

• The median survival is 4 years (2 years for bulbar onset).

• 5%–10% of patients survive for 5 years or more; a few live for 15 years or more.

• Patients with only lower motor neuron signs tend to have a better prognosis than those with typical motor neuron disease.

Follow-up and management

• A multidisciplinary neuro-care team approach is recommended; the team comprises neurologist, physical therapist, occupational therapist, speech therapist, dietitian, social worker, and other relevant health care workers. Each patient may be allocated a "key worker" to integrate the activities of the team.

• Communication and other aids should be provided, and the home adapted.

• Patients might require referral to a hospice.

Patient support

Amyotrophic Lateral Sclerosis Association, 21021 Ventura Blvd., Suite 321 Woodland Hills, CA 91364; phone (818) 340-7500 or (800) 782-4747.

Key references

1. Miller RG, Sufit R: New approaches to the treatment of ALS. *Neurology* 1997, **48(suppl 4)**:S28–S32.

2. Leigh PN, Ray-Chaudhuri K: Motor neurone disease. *J Neurol Neurosurg Psychiatry* 1994, **57**:886–896.

3. Rosen DR, *et al.*: Mutations in the Cu/Zn superoxide gene are associated with familial amyotrophic lateral sclerosis. *Nature* 1993, **362**:59–62.

4. Miller RG, *et al.*: Clinical trials of riluzole in patients with ALS. ALS/Riluzole Study Group II. *Neurology* 1996, **47(suppl 2)**: S86–S90.

Diagnosis

Symptoms

• Up to 10% of patients are asymptomatic.

Anorexia, weight loss.

Bone pain, back pain, pathological fracture.

Anemia, purpura, infection: symptoms of bone-marrow failure.

Polyuria, nocturia, pruritus: symptoms of renal failure.

Abdominal pain, anorexia, polyuria, polydipsia, constipation: symptoms of hypercalcemia.

Infection: due to hypogammaglobulinemia.

Visual symptoms, confusion, dyspnea, bleeding manifestations, polyneuropathy: symptoms of hyperviscosity.

Cardiac failure and edema: due to increased plasma oncotic pressure or viscosity.

Signs

Anemia, purpura.

Bony tenderness: over sites of lytic deposits.

Infections: especially skin, respiratory tract, and urinary tract.

Skin and soft-tissue deposits: particularly in IgD myeloma.

Proteinuria.

Peripheral neuropathy: due to paraprotein deposition.

Hepatosplenomegaly and lymphadenopathy: rare; suggest an IgM paraprotein or amyloidosis.

• Diagnosis requires the presence of >10% abnormal plasma cells in bone marrow and one of the following: bone lesions, serum paraprotein, and urine paraprotein.

Investigations [1]

Complete blood count: to check for anemia or bone-marrow failure.

ESR measurement: characteristically raised, often exceeds 100 mm/h.

Complete biochemical screening: including creatinine, creatinine clearance, serum calcium (alkaline phosphatase usually normal), albumin.

Skeletal survey: preferred to isotope bone scan, to show osteolytic lesions, vertebral collapse or osteoporosis.

Serum protein electrophoresis, immunoelectrophoresis, serum and urine analysis: to measure immunoglobulin concentrations, paraprotein quantification, and urinary Bence Jones protein.

β_2**-Microglobulin and CRP measurement:** to assess prognosis.

Bone-marrow aspiration and trephine biopsy: to show infiltration by malignant plasma cells and to assess normal bone-marrow reserve.

Microbiological cultures: if signs of infection.

Plasma cell labeling index, immunophenotype analysis, cytogenetic and DNA studies: if available, for further characterization of disease and prognosis.

MRI: a sensitive indicator of skeletal disease, especially good for detecting deposits around spine.

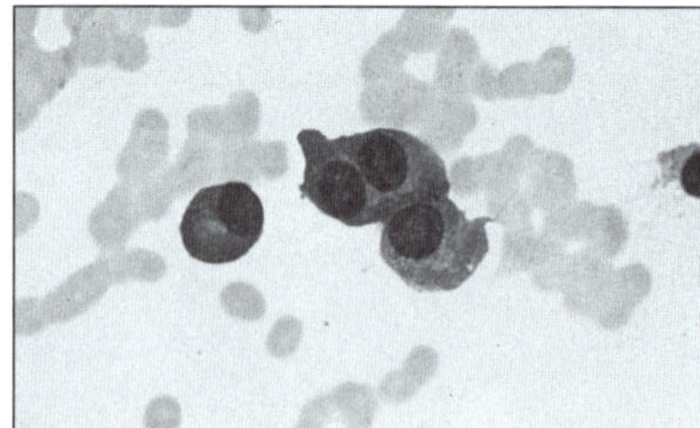

Plasma cells infiltrating bone marrow. (*See* Color Plate.)

Complications

Renal failure, hypercalcemia, hyperviscosity syndrome.

Infection: most common cause of death.

Pathological fracture and spinal-cord compression.

Polyneuropathy, cardiac and renal failure, macroglossia, skin infiltration: in 5%–10% of patients, caused by amyloidosis.

Differential diagnosis

Metastatic carcinoma: hypercalcemia, lytic lesions, but normal alkaline phosphatase differentiates.

Polymyalgia rheumatica, temporal arteritis: anemia, high ESR, but no paraprotein.

Other causes of renal failure.

Benign monoclonal gammopathy: but paraprotein is <30 g/L, with normal concentrations of other immunoglobulins, anemia, renal failure, lytic lesions all absent, little or no Bence Jones proteinuria and no progression on follow-up.

Solitary plasmacytoma, primary amyloidosis, other lymphoproliferative disorders (*e.g.*, Waldenström's macroglobulinemia, non-Hodgkin's lymphoma).

Etiology [1]

• The cause is largely unknown, but risk factors include the following:
Ionizing radiation, organic chemical exposure, chronic antigenic stimulation, chronic inflammatory disease.

Genetic predisposition: acquired genetic mutations to oncogenes may promote tumor growth, and certain cytokines (*e.g.*, interleukin-6) may function as growth factors.

Epidemiology [1]

• Multiple myeloma forms ~1% of all malignancies, 10%–15% of all hematological malignancies.

• The median age at diagnosis is 71 years.

• The disease occurs more often in blacks.

• The male:female ratio is ~5:3.

Staging [1]

Stage I: hemoglobin >10 g/dL, normal calcium, normal skeletal survey or solitary plasmacytoma, low paraprotein (IgG <50 g/L, IgA <30 g/L, urinary Bence Jones protein <4 g/24 h).

Stage II: neither stage I nor stage III.

Stage III: hemoglobin <8.5 g/dL, hypercalcemia, advanced skeletal disease, high paraprotein (IgG >70 g/L, IgA >50 g/L, urinary Bence Jones protein >12 g/24 h).

Subclassification: A, normal creatinine; B, raised creatinine.

Treatment

Diet and lifestyle

- Patients may need a diet appropriate for the degree of renal failure.
- Cooked food is needed for severely neutropenic patients.
- Patients should avoid bone damage, *e.g.*, heavy lifting.

Pharmacological treatment

Supportive treatment

- Careful supportive care is important, *e.g.*, the following:

Hydration and promotion of diuresis in renal failure and before chemotherapy.

Appropriate antibiotics or antifungal agents.

Adequate analgesia.

Blood component support.

Treatment of hypercalcemia (*e.g.*, biphosphonates): pamidronate may also reduce progression of bone disease and relieve pain.

Chemotherapy [2,3]

- Oral chemotherapy is the simplest protocol and involves melphalan and prednisone for 4–7 days every 4–6 weeks.

- Intravenous combination chemotherapy generally leads to a more rapid response, with higher complete remission rates, but the survival advantage over melphalan and prednisone is marginal and probably occurs only in patients aged <70 years. Current regimens include the following:

ABCM (doxorubicin, BCNU, cyclophosphamide, melphalan).
VBMCP (vincristine, BCNU, melphalan, cyclophosphamide, prednisone).
VAD (vincristine, doxorubicin by continuous i.v. infusion over 4 days with oral dexamethasone; standard for relapsed patients, also has a place in induction).

- α-Interferon, s.c. 3 times weekly, may improve combination therapy response rates and may prolong remission ("plateau" phase) and overall survival.

- Relapsed patients can be given cyclophosphamide orally or i.v. weekly, high-dose steroids (dexamethasone or methylprednisolone), and melphalan, single i.v. dose (high or intermediate).

- VAD gives responses in up to 40% of patients, and cyclosporine (to block multiple drug resistance) combined with VAD may be even more effective. High-dose cyclophosphamide with etoposide and granulocyte–macrophage colony-stimulating factor is valuable in VAD-resistant myeloma.

Complications of treatment

- Chemotherapy is immunosuppressive and myelotoxic.

- Growth factor support (granulocyte- and granulocyte–macrophage colony-stimulating factor) elevates the leukocyte count to reduce infective complications due to leukopenia, but also causes bone pain.

- Recombinant erythropoietin reduces erythrocyte transfusion requirement, particularly in renal failure.

- VAD and cyclophosphamide are preferred in renal failure because they are metabolized primarily by the liver.

- Antibacterial and antifungal prophylaxis with blood component support (principally platelets) is needed for myeloablative and intensive chemotherapy regimens.

- Hair loss, nausea, vomiting, mucositis (i.v. melphalan); bone demineralization (prednisone); and fatigue, fever, and anorexia (interferon-α) also occur.

- NSAIDs may accelerate renal failure if used for pain relief.

Treatment aims

To achieve normal immunoglobulin and blood counts and to relieve bone pain.

Other treatments [4]

- The following are indicated for primary nonresponders, relapsed patients, or those with local complications.

Radiotherapy: relieves pain from lytic lesions; systemic activity against tumor but often leads to prolonged pancytopenia. Internal fixation of pathological fractures.

Allogeneic bone-marrow transplantation: after conditioning by high-dose cyclophosphamide and total-body radiotherapy; for patients aged <50 years with histocompatible sibling.

Autologous bone-marrow transplantation or peripheral blood stem cell infusion: intensive treatment for patients aged <60 years, after high-dose chemotherapy.

Plasma exchange: for hyperviscosity syndrome.

Dialysis.

Prognosis

- In untreated patients, the median survival is <1 year; with treatment, it rises to 3–4 years.

- β_2-Microglobulin concentrations correlate well with prognosis (<6 mg/L good, 6–12 mg/L intermediate, >12 mg/L poor prognosis).

- Raised CRP, poor response to treatment, age >75, skin or soft-tissue involvement, and advanced stage indicate poor prognosis.

- Disappearance of paraprotein and restoration of normal immunoglobulin (complete remission) or normal blood counts with stable paraprotein ("plateau" phase) are achieved after 4–6 cycles of chemotherapy in >85% of patients.

Follow-up and management

- Complete blood count, renal function, β_2-microglobulin and serum and urine paraprotein concentrations should be assessed regularly (every 1–2 months) to monitor the disease and the effects of treatment.

- Patients should be checked for opportunistic infection and new skeletal abnormalities.

Key references

1. Barlogie B, ed: Multiple myeloma. *Hematol Oncol Clin North Am* 1992, **6**:211–484.

2. Alexanian R, Dimopoulos M: The treatment of multiple myeloma. *N Engl J Med* 1994, **330**:484–489.

3. Bataille R: New insights in the clinical biology of multiple myeloma. *Semin Hematol* 1997, **34**:23–28.

4. Kovacsovics T, Delaly A: Intensive treatment strategies in multiple myeloma. *Semin Hematol* 1997, **34(suppl 1)**:49–60.

Diagnosis

Symptoms

Relapsing and remitting
• 90% of patients initially have relapses and remissions of neurological disturbance attributable to CNS white matter lesions, including the following:

Visual loss.	**Weakness.**	**Urinary urgency.**
Diplopia.	**Incoordination.**	**Pain.**
Vertigo.	**Paresthesia.**	**Impotence.**

Progressive
• Progressive disease takes two forms.

Primary, in 10%: progressive from onset without remission.

Secondary, in 50%: progressive after an initially relapsing and remitting course.

Signs

• Signs are variable but include the following:

Optic atrophy.

Ophthalmoplegia.

Nystagmus.

Weakness: hemiparesis or paraparesis.

Sensory loss.

Spasticity.

Investigations

• The diagnosis is primarily clinical and depends on the demonstration of two or more necessarily separate CNS lesions in a patient with a history of two characteristic episodes.

• Investigations provide invaluable support, but none of the abnormalities is specific to multiple sclerosis.

Evoked potentials: especially visual and somatosensory, to detect subclinical involvement and provide evidence for demyelination.

MRI: to detect subclinical involvement and the characteristic pattern of lesions.

CSF analysis: for electrophoresis to show oligoclonal IgG, present in 90% of patients; CSF can be useful in making the diagnosis in patients with only a single clear flare of disease.

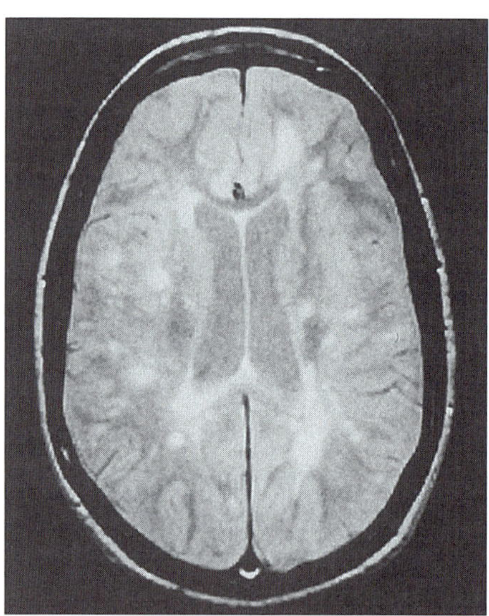

T_2-weighted MRI showing areas of abnormal signal in the cerebral hemispheres in a patient with multiple sclerosis.

Differential diagnosis

Relapsing and remitting
Collagen vascular disease.

Neurosarcoidosis.

Lyme disease.

Progressive
Compression: *e.g.*, tumor, craniocervical anomaly.

Spinocerebellar degeneration.

Motor neuron disease.

Etiology [1]

Genetic predisposition: HLA association, but probably additional factors.

Extrinsic factor: probably infective, possibly viral.

Epidemiology [2]

• 60 in 100 000 population in the United States are affected by multiple sclerosis.

• 20% of patients have an affected relative.

• Multiple sclerosis is diagnosed in patients aged <10 years or >40 years in only 13% of cases.

Complications

Visual loss, paresis, tremor, incontinence: due to persistent neurological deficit.

Significant cognitive impairment: may occur late.

Treatment

Diet and lifestyle

• Patients should be assessed for functional limitations to determine appropriate modifications in lifestyle (neurorehabilitation, physical therapy, occupational therapy).

• Exposure to heat or fever worsens the motor symptoms temporarily.

Pharmacological treatment [3]

For symptoms

Standard dosage	*For spasticity:* baclofen initially, 5 mg 3 times daily; maximum 100 mg daily. *For urinary frequency, urgency, and incontinence:* oxybutynin, 5 mg 2–3 times daily.
Contraindications	*Baclofen:* peptic ulceration. *Oxybutynin:* bladder outflow obstruction, glaucoma.
Main drug interactions	*Baclofen:* muscle relaxants. *Oxybutynin:* antimuscarinics.
Main side effects	*Baclofen:* weakness, sedation enhanced by alcohol. *Oxybutynin:* antimuscarinic effects.

• For impotence, patients should be referred to a urologist.

For relapse

• Steroids are indicated when functional impairment is significant.

Standard dosage	Methylprednisolone, 1 g in 250 mL normal saline solution i.v. over 30 minutes daily for 3 days, often followed by oral taper.
Contraindications	Hypertension, diabetes, peptic ulceration, systemic infection, history of tuberculosis, osteoporosis, history of psychiatric disorder.
Special points	Frequent use should be avoided.
Main drug interactions	Other drugs causing hypokalemia, drugs inducing liver enzymes.
Main side effects	Fluid retention, hypokalemia, depression, psychosis, hypertension, glucose intolerance, peptic ulceration, osteoporosis.

For prophylaxis-rr

Standard dosage	Interferon-β 1b, 8 million IU s.c. every other day or interferon-β 1a, weekly i.m., or copaxone 20 mg daily s.c. to reduce relapses in some patients with relapsing-remitting disease.
Contraindications	Hypersensitivity.
Main side effects	Fatigue, malaise, flu-like symptoms, injection site reactions, sometimes depression with interferon-β 1b.

• Several agents (*e.g.*, linomide, oral myelin) have recently failed trails, whereas others are still under investigation (*e.g.*, chadribine).

• In chronic progressive multiple sclerosis, there are no clearly proven agents; interferons-β are in trials, and weekly oral methotrexate may improve upper extremity function slightly.

Treatment aims

To alleviate symptoms.

To control relapse.

To modify course.

Prognosis

• Prognosis is very variable, ranging from death in a few months to survival without disability for 50 years.

• At least one-third of patients have little disability after 15 years.

Follow-up and management

• Follow-up depends on the condition of the patient.

• In complete remission, regular follow-up is not needed.

• When significant disability is present, assessment in a comprehensive neurological rehabilitation clinic is useful as the condition changes.

Patient support

National Multiple Sclerosis Society, 733 3rd Ave., New York, NY 10017-3240; phone (212) 986-3240 or (800) FIGHT-MS

Key references

1. Sowcer S, Goodfellow PN, Compston A: The genetic analysis of multiple sclerosis. *Trends Genet* 1997, **13**:234–239.

2. Matthews WB, *et al.* (eds.): *McAlpine's Multiple Sclerosis.* Edinburgh: Churchill Livingstone; 1991.

3. McDonald WI: New treatments for multiple sclerosis. *BMJ* 1995, **310**:345–346.

Diagnosis

Symptoms

Painless muscle weakness increasing with exercise ("fatigue").

Drooping eyelids (one or both) and double vision.

• Weakness may characteristically also affect smiling, swallowing, chewing, speaking, neck muscles, arm elevation, elbow extension, hand movements, walking, and breathing.

• Symptoms are worst at the end of the day.

Signs

Fatiguable ptosis.

Variable limitation of eye movement.

Impaired eye closure.

Transverse smile.

Nasal speech.

Fatiguable weakness of affected muscles.

Wasting: rare.

Hypoactive tendon reflexes.

Investigations

Serum acetylcholine receptor (AChR) antibody analysis: raised titer specific for myasthenia gravis.

Edrophonium (Tensilon) test: double-blind test showing transient improvement.

Clinical electrophysiology: increased decrement to repetitive motor nerve stimulation; increased jitter on single fiber study.

CT of chest: for thymoma, lung tumor.

Striated muscle antibody analysis: positive in 90% of patients with thymoma, 50% of patients with generalized myasthenia gravis.

Complications

Myasthenic crisis: acute respiratory or bulbar symptoms.

Cholinergic crisis: due to excess anticholinesterase treatment; causing hypersalivation, lacrimation, increased sweating, vomiting, and miosis; can also cause weakness and respiratory failure.

Local or pleural spread of thymoma.

Differential diagnosis

Lambert–Eaton myasthenic syndrome.
Congenital myasthenia gravis.
Chronic fatigue syndrome.

Etiology

• Antibodies to muscle AChRs cause receptor loss.

• Immune response genes influence susceptibility.

• Penicillamine may induce AChR antibodies and typical myasthenia gravis.

• Placental transfer of AChR antibodies causes neonatal myasthenia gravis in the offspring of 12% of mothers with the disease [1].

• "Seronegative" myasthenia gravis is antibody-mediated: the antigenic target is not known.

Epidemiology

• The prevalence is 8–9 in 100 000 people.

• The annual incidence is 0.4 in 100 000.

• All races are susceptible; restricted ocular myasthenia gravis is more frequent in Asian patients.

• The disease is manifest from infancy to extreme old age.

Clinical classification

• The clinical subgroup influences treatment selection; typical features are shown below.

Early onset (50%)
Symptom distribution: generalized.
Age at onset: <40 years.
Thymus pathology: hyperplasia.
AChR antibody titer: high.

Late onset (25%)
Symptom distribution: generalized or ocular.
Age at onset: >40 years.
Thymus pathology: atrophy/normal.
AChR antibody titer: low.

Seronegative (15%)
Symptom distribution: ocular or generalized.
Age of onset: any.
Thymus pathology: atrophy/normal.
AChR antibody titer: absent.

Thymoma (10%)
Symptom distribution: generalized.
Age at onset: any.
Thymus pathology: thymoma.
AChR antibody titer: intermediate.
Increased frequency of striated muscle antibody.

Treatment

Diet and lifestyle

• No special precautions are necessary.

• Elevated body temperature can worsen weakness.

Pharmacological treatment [2,3]

Management strategy

• The following treatments are helpful, usually in this order:

Anticholinesterase for immediate symptom control.
Plasma exchange in some cases (*see* Other treatments).
Thymectomy in some patients (*see* Other treatments).
Prednisone.
Azathioprine.
Intravenous immunoglobulin.
Other immunosuppressive treatment (cyclosporine, cyclophosphamide).

Drugs to be avoided

Antiarrhythmics (quinidine), antibacterials (aminoglycosides, clindamycin, lincomycin, and polymyxins), antimalarials (chloroquine), beta-blockers (propranolol), lithium, muscle relaxants.

Anticholinesterase

• This provides symptomatic relief in all patients.

Standard dosage	Pyridostigmine, 30–120 mg 5 times daily. Glycopyrrolate, 1 mg up to 3 times daily, if necessary, to control adverse gastrointestinal effects.
Contraindications	Intestinal or urinary obstruction.
Main drug interactions	*See* Drugs to be avoided.
Main side effects	Diarrhea, abdominal cramps, increased salivation, nausea and vomiting.

Prednisone

• For generalized disease of moderate severity unresponsive to other treatments (inpatients).

Standard dosage	*Outpatients:* prednisone, 5-mg single dose on alternate days, increased by 5 mg at weekly intervals to controlling dose or 0.75–1 mg/kg/day, whichever is lower. *Inpatients:* prednisone, or solumedrol burst, usually with simultaneous plasmaphoresis. In both groups, dose should be tapered by 5 mg/month when remission is established and adjusted to define effective minimal dose.
Contraindications	Osteoporosis, diabetes.
Main drug interactions	Antibacterials, *e.g.*, rifampicin, antiepileptics.
Main side effects	Initial exacerbation of myasthenic symptoms, adrenal suppression, diabetes, osteoporosis, avascular necrosis of femoral head, mental disturbance, weight gain, cushingoid features, cataracts.

Azathioprine

• Azathioprine is indicated in combination with prednisone for generalized moderate or severe disease; often takes months to be effective.

Standard dosage	Azathioprine, 2.5 mg/kg/day orally.
Contraindications	Myelosuppression.
Special points	Full blood count and liver function tests weekly for 8 weeks, every 1–3 months thereafter.
Main drug interactions	Allopurinol enhances toxic effect.
Main side effects	Myelosuppression, hepatotoxicity, gastrointestinal symptoms, rashes, B-cell lymphoma (very rare).

Key references

1. Shillito P, Vincent A, Newsom-Davis J: Congenital myasthenic syndromes. *J Neuromusc Dis* 1993, **3**:183–190.

2. Verma P, Oger J: Treatment of acquired autoimmune myasthenia gravis. *Can J Neurol Sci* 1992, **19**:360–375.

3. Younger DS: Advances in the diagnosis, pathogenesis, and treatment of myasthenia gravis. *Neurology* 1997, **48(suppl 5)**:S1–S81.

Diagnosis

Symptoms

• Symptoms of disseminated *Mycobacterium avium* or *M. intracellulare* infection may be difficult to distinguish from those of other opportunistic infections associated with HIV infection.

• Disseminated infection may be asymptomatic.

Systemic

Fever: with or without sweats.

Anorexia and malaise.

Weight loss: often associated with anemia and neutropenia.

Gastrointestinal

Chronic diarrhea and abdominal pain: resulting from *M. avium-intracellulare* invasion of the colon or small bowel or bulky retroperitoneal lymph nodes infected by *M. avium-intracellulare.*

Signs

Weight loss, oral candidiasis, cutaneous Kaposi's sarcoma: evidence of underlying HIV infection and other HIV-associated complications.

Weight loss, anemia, hepato(spleno)megaly: indicating disseminated disease.

Localized or cutaneous abscesses, endophthalmitis, arthritis.

Investigations

Blood culture: using lysis/centrifugation or radiometric technique, yield increased (from 60% to almost 100%); 5–50 days needed for blood cultures to become positive.

Biopsy: diagnosis of disseminated *M. avium-intracellulare* infection made by isolation or culture from any normally sterile site (blood, bone-marrow, lymph-node, and liver biopsy best); negative blood cultures unusual with positive histology from lymph-node, liver, or bone-marrow biopsy; stains may show acid-fast bacilli before blood cultures become positive, thus suggesting diagnosis.

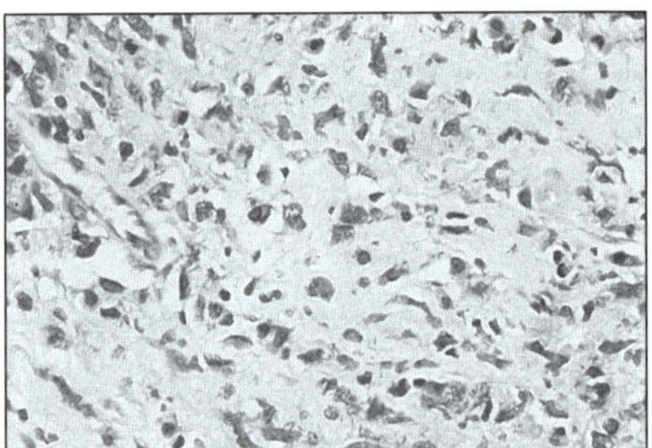

Lymph-node biopsy. Numerous clumps of acid-fast bacilli are seen within the tissue. There is no granulamatous response. Magnification × 400. (*See* Color Plate.)

• Isolation of *M. avium-intracellulare* from sputum and bronchoalveolar lavage may occur but is not diagnostic of disseminated infection.

Complications

None.

Differential diagnosis

Progression of HIV or other systemic opportunistic infection.

Etiology

• Two closely related species, *M. avium* and *M. intracellulare*, known as *M. avium* complex, cause widely disseminated infection in AIDS patients: up to 30% have disseminated infection diagnosed before death, and about 50% are found to have it at postmortem examination.

• Disseminated infection occurs exclusively in patients with advanced HIV disease and CD4 counts $<75 \times 10^6$/L.

• The host defect in AIDS patients allowing dissemination is probably macrophage dysfunction.

• The source of invasion in AIDS patients may be gastrointestinal; large numbers of mycobacteria within macrophages of the small bowel lamina propria suggest that the bowel is the portal of entry.

Epidemiology

• *M. avium-intracellulare* is ubiquitous in the environment, being found in water, soil, animals, and dairy products.

Pathogenesis and pathology

• Almost all AIDS patients with disseminated *M. avium-intracellulare* have positive blood cultures (in contrast to those with stool, urine, or respiratory secretion colonization).

• Mycobacteremia usually ranges from 10^1 to 10^4 colony-forming units/mL blood.

• In patients with disseminated infection, the liver, spleen, and lymph nodes are found at postmortem examination to contain up to 10^{10} colony-forming units/g tissue.

• Histology of involved organs reveals absent or poorly formed granulomata and mycobacteria within macrophages. Little tissue destruction is seen, despite heavy mycobacterial load.

Treatment

Diet and lifestyle

• No special precautions are necessary.

Pharmacological treatment

• *M. avium-intracellulare* is resistant to many antituberculous drugs at concentrations achievable in plasma, yet >50% of strains can be inhibited by achievable concentrations of amikacin, azithromycin, ciprofloxacin, clarithromycin, clofazimine, cycloserine, ethambutol, ethionamide, or rifabutin.

• Single-agent treatment (*e.g.*, by clarithromycin) is of temporary benefit only: fever, anorexia, and mycobacteremia return rapidly; combination therapy is more effective.

• A two-drug regimen with clarithromycin and ethambutol is recommended.

• Additional agents may be used if the standard two- or three-drug regimens have failed or have resulted in toxicities.

Standard dosage	Ethambutol, 15 mg/kg orally once daily, with clarithromycin, 500–1000 mg orally twice daily. Ciprofloxacin, 500 mg orally twice daily, and clofazimine, 100 mg orally once daily can be added. Ciprofloxacin and rifabutin are used in case of toxicities or failure. Amikacin, 7.5 mg/kg i.v. once daily, may be added for patients with refractory fever or anorexia. Treatment is given for 2–4 weeks.
Contraindications	Previous drug hypersensitivity. *Rifabutin*: jaundice, porphyria. *Ethambutol*: renal impairment, optic neuritis. *Clarithromycin*: porphyria, hepatic or renal failure.
Special points	Drug levels must be monitored. Palliative glucocorticoids (oral prednisolone, 1–2 mg/kg daily) may be given to patients with very advanced HIV disease who have profound anorexia and weight loss, without adversely affecting prognosis.
Main drug interactions	*Rifabutin:* induces hepatic microsome enzyme activity and so increases metabolism of azole drugs; interacts with fluconazole or clarithromycin to produce uveitis in 30% of patients if >300 mg of rifabutin are given daily. If steroids are given with an antibacterial regimen containing rifampin or rifabutin, the dose should be doubled to take into account the hepatic microsome-inducing effects of the drugs.
Main side effects	*Rifabutin*: nausea and vomiting, diarrhea, anorexia; body fluids become orange-red. *Ethambutol*: optic neuritis, red–green color blindness, peripheral neuritis. *Ciprofloxacin*: nausea and vomiting, abdominal pain, diarrhea, headache, photosensitivity, arthralgia, myalgia. *Clarithromycin*: nausea and vomiting, abdominal pain, diarrhea. *Clofazimine*: nausea, giddiness, headache, diarrhea; skin and urine colored terracotta red.

• Rifabutin, 300 mg orally once daily given as primary prophylaxis reduces the risk of developing *M. avium-intracellulare* bacteremia by half but does not improve survival. It is indicated for persons with CD4 cell counts <100/mm^3.

Treatment aims

To reduce mycobacteremia or fever and transfusion requirements.
• Cure is not achievable.

Prognosis

• Survival in AIDS patients with disseminated *M. avium-intracellulare* infection is shorter (median, 4.1 months) than in comparable patients (with similar CD4 counts) without disseminated infection (median, 11 months).
•The presence of *M. avium-intracellulare* in gastrointestinal secretions strongly predicts the subsequent development of disseminated infection.

Follow-up and management

• Treatment is for life.

General references

Fordham von Reyu C, Arbeit RD, Tostesum AN, *et al.*: The international epidemiology of disseminated *Mycobacterium avium* complex infection in AIDS. *AIDS* 1996, **10**:1025–1032.

Jacobson MA: Mycobacterial disease. In *The Medical Management of AIDS*, edn 3. Edited by Sande MA, Volberding PA. Philadelphia: WB Saunders; 1992:284–296.

Masur H: Recommendations on prophylaxis and therapy for disseminated *Mycobacterium avium* complex disease in patients infected with the human immuno-deficiency virus. *N Engl J Med* 1993, **329**:898–904.

Diagnosis

Symptoms

• Chronic myeloid leukemia is usually manifest in chronic phase; it transforms spontaneously to an accelerated phase and then to an acute blastic phase normally within 3–6 years of diagnosis (range, 0–10 years).

• Polycythemia vera, essential thrombocythemia, and primary myelofibrosis are manifest more insidiously and evolve more slowly.

• Symptoms are an incidental finding in many patients.

Abdominal pain and distention: also due to renal occlusive disease in polycythemia vera.

Spontaneous bleeding: including hematuria, bruising, visual disturbances.

Sweats, weight loss.

Priapism: in chronic myeloid leukemia.

Pruritus: in chronic myeloid leukemia.

Symptoms of hyperviscosity syndrome: in polycythemia vera.

Gout.

Peptic ulceration and hypertension: in polycythemia vera.

Signs

Splenomegaly.

Ecchymoses, retinal hemorrhages.

Weight loss.

Hepatomegaly: occasionally.

Investigations

Complete blood count: raised leukocyte count (20 to >500 × 10⁹/L); increased numbers of blasts, promyelocytes, neutrophils, eosinophils, basophils; low neutrophil alkaline phosphatase content in chronic myeloid leukemia; variable anemia; thrombocytosis especially in essential thrombocythemia; raised hemoglobin, packed-cell volume, and erythrocyte mass in polycythemia vera.

Bone-marrow analysis: hypercellular, loss of fat spaces; increased megakaryocyte count, especially in essential thrombocythemia; variable amounts of fibrosis in chronic myeloid leukemia; increased reticulin and collagen in myelofibrosis; in chronic myeloid leukemia, all dividing cells have a Philadelphia chromosomal translocation, designated t (9;22) (q34;q11), bringing into apposition parts of the *bcr* gene normally on chromosome 22q with the bulk of the *abl* proto-oncogene normally present on chromosome 9q.

Biochemistry: uric acid raised, especially in myelofibrosis; increased vitamin B_{12} and vitamin B_{12}-binding protein.

Complications

"Blast" transformation: in chronic myeloid leukemia; blast cells may be myeloid or lymphoid.

Changes between groups: *e.g.*, polycythemia vera to myelofibrosis.

Vascular or thrombotic complications: in polycythemia vera.

Gout: especially in myelofibrosis.

Renal tubular obstruction.

Splenic infarction: in chronic myeloid leukemia.

Retinal hemorrhages: in chronic myeloid leukemia.

Gonadal failure: due to busulfan.

Treatment

Diet and lifestyle

• Patients may live normal lives during the chronic phase of chronic myeloid leukemia.

Pharmacological treatment [1]

• Drug treatment is indicated for polycythemia vera (hydroxyurea, radioactive phosphorus [^{32}P]), myelofibrosis (hydroxyurea, busulfan), and essential (primary) thrombocythemia (hydroxyurea, busulfan, Anagrelide [imidazole-2,1-b, quinazolin-2-1 is currently undergoing phase II and III FDA investigations, but is available for compassionate purposes], ^{32}P, supportive measures, *e.g.*, dipyridamole, aspirin).

• α-Interferon (given daily or on alternate days by injection) controls hematological features in 70%–80% of patients with CML and induces some degree of Philadelphia chromosome negativity in the bone-marrow in 10%–20%; it is the drug of first choice [2].

• Hydroxyurea is easier to tolerate.

• Busulfan should not be used in patients aged <50 years but can be used for older patients or those who cannot take hydroxyurea.

Nonpharmacological treatment

Bone-marrow transplantation [3]

• Transplantation is indicated for chronic myeloid leukemia; if applicable, it should be done within 1 year of diagnosis.

• Allogeneic bone-marrow transplantation is indicated for patients aged <55 years with HLA-identical siblings (~15% of all patients).

Other Treatments

Polycythemia vera: venesection.

Myelofibrosis: splenic irradiation, splenectomy (in selected patients).

Treatment aims

To cure the patient.

To prolong life without cure.

To prevent or alleviate symptoms.

To maintain leukocyte count in normal range.

To re-establish Philadelphia chromosome-negativity with interferon treatment.

Prognosis

• The median duration of chronic phase CML is 4 years and of survival with conventional treatment is 4.3 years.

• A few patients survive >10 years in chronic phase.

• The 5-year disease-free survival after bone-marrow transplantation is about 65%; most of these patients are cured; the procedure-related mortality is 15%–20%, and the relapse rate 10%–15%.

Follow-up and management [1]

• Regular follow-up is needed if the patient is on chemotherapy or interferon.

• Bone marrow must be checked annually for progressive fibrosis or cytogenetic evolution.

• Patients should have the usual follow-up for bone-marrow transplantation.

Key references

1. Goldman JM: Management of chronic myeloid leukemia. *Blood Rev* 1994, **8**:21–29.

2. Kantarjian HM, *et al.*: Chronic myelogenous leukemia: a concise update. *Blood* 1993, **82**:691–703.

3. Soutar RL, King DJ: Bone-marrow transplantation. *BMJ* 1995, **310**:31–36.

Diagnosis

Symptoms

Chest pain: typically precordial, often with radiation to left or right arm, throat, lower jaw, epigastrium, or back; usually severe; crushing or vice-like; pain often described as indigestion-like, may be relieved by belching.

Breathlessness: common, often without cardiac failure.

Malaise, nausea, vomiting, syncope, apprehension, sweating.

Signs

• Few cardiovascular signs may be apparent on acute presentation.

Malaise, pallor, sweating, restlessness.

Pyrexia: usually developing the day after infarction.

Unexpectedly slow or rapid pulse.

Raised jugular venous pressure: only with significant right ventricular failure.

Third or fourth heart sounds, dyskinetic apical impulse: indicating significant myocardial dysfunction.

Chest crackles: may indicate left ventricular failure.

New murmurs or pericardial rub: may be heard in patients with complications.

• Many patients present with sudden cardiac death.

Investigations

12-lead ECG: often sufficient to establish diagnosis; adjunctive tests may be necessary for confirmation if infarction is minor or if ECG shows pre-existing abnormalities, *e.g.*, previous infarction, conduction abnormalities (especially left bundle branch block).

Chest radiography: to check for pulmonary congestion.

Cardiac enzymes evaluation: creatine kinase, aspartate transaminase, and lactate dehydrogenase rise characteristically after myocardial infarction; creatine kinase MB cardiospecific isoenzyme may be helpful with skeletal muscle damage. New enzyme assays such as troponin I or T also are frequently used.

Echocardiography: to assess wall motion abnormalities, ventricular septal defect, regurgitation, and mural thrombus.

Complications

Left ventricular failure.

Cardiogenic shock.

Bradyarrhythmias.

Tachyarrhythmias.

Cardiac rupture.

Pericarditis.

Acute ventricular septal defect.

Acute mitral regurgitation.

Systemic emboli.

Aneurysm formation.

Differential diagnosis

Angina without infarction.

Pericarditis.

Esophageal or gastrointestinal pain.

Aortic dissection.

Pulmonary embolus.

Musculoskeletal or nonspecific chest pain.

Etiology

Causes

Thrombotic occlusion of a coronary artery, related to rupture of an atherosclerotic plaque and subsequent intraluminal hemorrhage.

Risk factors

Smoking.

Increasing age.

Family history.

Hypertension.

Diabetes mellitus.

Lack of exercise.

Male gender.

Hyperlipidemia.

Thrombotic tendency (fibrinogen).

Obesity.

Surgical menopause at young age.

Epidemiology

• 10–17 in 1000 men aged 40–69 years sustain myocardial infarctions.

• In the United States >500 000 myocardial infarctions occur per year.

Treatment

Diet and lifestyle
• Patients must give up smoking, reduce weight, take up regular exercise, and achieve low-fat, low-cholesterol diet.

Pharmacological treatment

Immediate treatment
Analgesia: i.v. morphine sulfate.
Oxygen.
Aspirin: 325 mg orally initially, then maintenance dose 75–325 mg daily.
Nitrates: particularly in patients with continuing ischemia.
Beta-blockade: atenolol or metoprolol i.v. and then orally, except in patients with left ventricular failure, pulse rate <70/min, or blood pressure <100 mm Hg.

Thrombolytic treatment
• Treatment should be given as soon as possible, unless contraindicated.

• It is indicated for all suitable patients within 12 hours of onset of symptoms.

• Maximum benefit is with large myocardial infarction and early administration (especially <4 hours).

• The value is proven for patients with acute myocardial infarction and ST elevation or bundle branch block; no benefit has been shown in patients with ST depression or normal ECG.

• Recombinant tissue plasminogen activator (rt-PA) is more effective than streptokinase but is much more expensive; it should be used in patients for whom streptokinase is unsuitable and particularly for patients presenting within 4–6 hours of symptom onset and large infarction such as those with anterior infarction, hypotension, and/or persistent sinus tachycardia. Recent data suggest reteplase (rPA) has similar mortality benefit to rt-PA.

Standard dosage	Streptokinase, 1.5 MU over 1 hour. rt-PA, 15-mg bolus, then 50 mg in 30 minutes, then 40 mg in 60 minutes, followed by i.v. heparin [1].
Contraindications	Possible aortic dissection, active peptic ulceration, recent surgery, hemorrhagic diathesis, possible pregnancy, subarachnoid hemorrhage, cardiovascular accident with residual defect, recent transient ischemic attack, unconscious patient, severe hypertension, systemic thrombus (*e.g.*, aortic aneurysm, left atrial clot), prolonged or traumatic resuscitation, recent central venous or arterial puncture. Few contraindications are absolute.
Special points	Streptokinase should be avoided in patients with known allergy or those who have been treated between 5 days and 1 year previously.
Main side effects	•Hemorrhage (treated by tranexamic acid, 1 g slow i.v. injection, and fresh frozen plasma to restore clotting factor).

Nonpharmacological treatment

Primary coronary angioplasty (PCA) [2]
• May be more effective than thrombolytic therapy in establishing antegrade coronary flow and relieving fixed coronary obstruction.

• Should be performed only when:
Experienced interventional team can be readily mobilized.
Cardiac surgical back-up is available.
Perceived time delay from presentation to open artery will not exceed 60–90 minutes.
It can be done at cardiac center of excellence with high-volume interventional program.

• Primary PCA is a reasonable option only in a small minority of US hospitals because few have a catheterization laboratory, cardiac surgery is performed only at a few, and most lack a sufficient volume of experience.

Follow-up treatment
• Secondary prevention is needed for all patients.

• Statin therapy for patients with elevated LDL cholesterol improves survival and reinfarction risk [3].

Beta-blockers: *e.g.*, atenolol, 25–50 mg twice daily, or metoprolol, 50–100 mg daily.

Angiotensin-converting enzyme inhibitors: *e.g.*, captopril titrated to maximum tolerated dose, if possible 50 mg 3 times daily (12.5 mg 3 times daily by hospital discharge); indicated for all patients with left ventricular ejection fractions <40% or myocardial infarction complicated by congestive heart failure [4].

Key references

1. GUSTO Investigators: An international randomized trial comparing four thrombolytic strategies for acute myocardial infarction. *N Engl J Med* 1993, **329**:673–682.

2. Grines CL: A comparison of immediate angioplasty with thrombolytic therapy for acute MI. *N Engl J Med* 1993, **328**:673–679.

3. Scandinavian Simvastatin Survival Study Group: Randomized trial of cholesterol lowering in 4444 patients with coronary heart disease (4S). *Lancet* 1994, **344**:383–389.

4. Pfeffer MA, *et al.*: Effect of captopril on mortality and morbidity in patients with left ventricular dysfunction after myocardial infarction. *N Engl J Med* 1992, **327**:669–677.

5. DAVIT-II: Effect of verapamil on mortality and major events after acute myocardial infarction. *Am J Cardiol* 1990, **66**:779–785.

Diagnosis

Symptoms

Weakness: principally affecting proximal muscles in arms and legs; 15%–30% of these patients have associated arthralgias, Raynaud's phenomenon, or myalgia; painless weakness is common [1].

Unusual, severe manifestations: interstitial lung disease, pulmonary hypertension, ventilatory failure, heart block or arrhythmias, dysphagia [2].

Skin rashes.

• Patients with dermatomyositis, especially men aged >45 years, may have an accompanying tumor, causing various symptoms, *e.g.*, weight loss [3].

Signs

Muscle wasting: principally of proximal muscles.

Loss of muscle reflexes: in late-stage disease.

Heliotrope rash: lilac discoloration around eyelids.

Gottron's papules: small raised reddish plaques over knuckles.

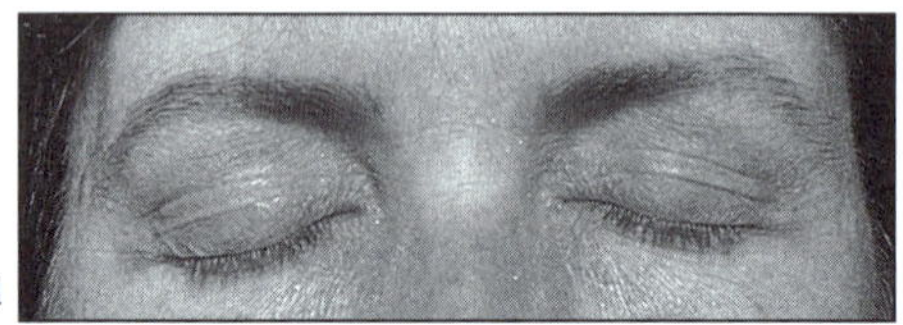

Classic heliotrope rash on the eyelids of a patient with dermatomyositis. (*See* Color Plate.)

Erythematous rash: over face, upper chest, and arms, usually on extensor surfaces.

Investigations

Key investigations

Creatine kinase, aldolase measurement: concentration 5–30 times upper limit of normal but not disease-specific; concentrations higher in many patients with muscular dystrophy [4] and hypothyroidism.

Electromyography: to check for insertional irritability and small polyphasic potentials.

Muscle biopsy: needle or open surgical technique; classic changes are inflammation, with mononuclear cell infiltrate composed mainly of lymphocytes (some macrophages and plasma cells), with muscle-fiber necrosis, and, in chronic cases, replacement of muscle fibers by fat and fibrous tissue; changes often patchy, and up to 20% of patients may have relatively normal appearance.

Other investigations

Measurement of other enzymes: *e.g.*, transaminase concentrations may be raised [4].

24-hour urine creatine excretion measurement: may be high; more sensitive but less specific than raised creatine kinase.

Myoglobin measurement: appears to reflect disease activity.

Autoantibody analysis: weak positive antinuclear antibody reaction in 60%–80% of patients with myositis; antibodies to transfer RNA synthetase enzymes have been found to be virtually disease-specific, notably the anti-Jo-1 antibody.

Thyroid stimulating hormone (TSH).

Complications

Interstitial lung fibrosis, arthritis, Raynaud's phenomenon: in patients with Jo-1 antibody.

Cardiac or respiratory failure: rare; caused by rapidly progressive myositis.

Underlying neoplasm: muscle disease often intractable until tumor identified and treated.

Recurrent falls and danger of major internal trauma: caused by an unusual, steroid-resistant form of myositis, associated with inclusion bodies.

Differential diagnosis

Muscular dystrophy.
Osteomalacia.
Rhabdomyolysis.
Drug-induced inflammatory disease (including D-penicillamine).
Metabolic myopathies (*e.g.*, McArdle's disease).
Inclusion body myositis [1].
Hypothyroidism.

Etiology

• Inflammatory muscle diseases are part of the family of autoimmune rheumatic diseases.

• Causes include the following:
Hormonal component.
Immunogenetic predisposition: HLA B8 and DR3 associated with myositis, principally in whites; DR3 linked to Jo-1 antibody.
Environmental factors: increased risk of developing myositis at different times of year found in one study.
Viruses, *e.g.*, picornaviruses and retroviruses: may be triggering factors; link between myositis and HIV has been suggested.

Epidemiology

• The annual incidence of myositis is 5 in one million population.
• The prevalence is 5–8 in 100 000.
• The female:male ratio is 2–3:1 overall and 9:1 in patients with an associated autoimmune rheumatic disease.

Factors suggesting malignancy [1,3]

Dermatomyositis in male patients.
Age >45 years.
Weight loss.
Poorer than expected response to treatment.
Absence of autoantibodies.
Unexplained historical, physical, or laboratory abnormalities.

Dermatomyositis or polymyositis? [1]

Dermatomyositis
Onset: childhood to old age.
Skin rash, microvascular injury.
Perifascicular atrophy common.
Endomysial infiltration less common.
Surrounded and invaded fibers less than in polymyositis.
Anti-Jo-1 in 5%, other antisynthetases at least as much as in polymyositis.

Polymyositis
Onset: adulthood.
No skin rash or microvascular injury.
Perifascicular atrophy uncommon.
Endomysial infiltration common.
Surrounded and invaded fibers frequent.
Anti Jo-1 in 30%.

Treatment

Diet and lifestyle

• Exercise and activity are limited during the inflammatory period. Rehabilitative efforts must be limited until muscle enzymes return to nearly normal.

• No special diet is necessary.

Pharmacological treatment

Corticosteroids

• After the diagnosis has been established, treatment should be initiated quickly [1,2,5,6].

Standard dosage	Prednisone, 1 mg/kg daily initially (usually 60–80 mg); continued until creatine kinase returned to near normal (usually 1–3 months); then reduced to 5–10 mg daily over following 3 months.
Contraindications	Severe osteoporosis.
Main drug interactions	None.
Main side effects	Osteoporosis, increased risk of infection, diabetes, hypertension.

Other immunosuppressants

• These are indicated in patients who have not shown a response to high-dose steroids after 1 month or who cannot tolerate them [5].

Standard dosage	Azathioprine, 2–3 mg/kg. Methotrexate, up to 15 mg weekly.
Contraindications	*Methotrexate:* abnormal liver function, major renal disease, porphyria.
Main drug interactions	*Methotrexate:* many analgesics and antibacterials.
Main side effects	Bone-marrow suppression, liver damage.

Other options [6]

• Oral or occasionally i.v. cyclophosphamide has been used in severely affected patients, occasionally combined with steroids and methotrexate or azathioprine.

• Reports of the use of cyclosporine in myositis are conflicting, and it is not widely used in this disease.

• Intravenous gammaglobulin may be used.

Nonpharmacological treatment

Plasmapheresis.

Total lymph-node irradiation and thoracic duct drainage in severe cases.

Physical therapy and hydrotherapy.

Treatment aims

To control disease as soon as possible.
To maintain reasonable degree of mobility.
To reduce treatment to smallest dose needed after 3–4 months of aggressive therapy to avoid side effects (*e.g.*, intercurrent infection or osteoporosis).

Prognosis

• ~20% of patients recover fully.
• 10%–20% die as a direct result of the disease or as a consequence of its treatment.
• Most patients are left with some muscle weakness.
• Patients who respond most slowly to initial treatment have the poorest prognosis.

Follow-up and management

• Patients must be followed for several years.
• Regular clinical examination, creatine kinase measurement, and formal muscle strength testing are needed.
• Physical therapy and hydrotherapy help to keep the range of joint movement normal and to maintain muscle power.

Key references

1. Dalakas MC: Polymyositis, dermatomyositis, and inclusion-body myositis. *N Engl J Med* 1992, **325**:1487–1498.

2. Targoff IN: Polymyositis and dermatomyositis: adult onset. In *Textbook of Rheumatology*. Edited by Maddison P, *et al.* Oxford: Oxford University Press; 1993:794–821.

3. Sigurgeirsson B, *et al.*: Risk of cancer in patients with dermatomyositis or polymyositis. *N Engl J Med* 1992, **326**:363–367.

4. Bohlmeyer TJ, *et al.*: Evaluation of laboratory tests as a guide to diagnosis and therapy of myositis. *Rheum Dis Clin North Am* 1994, **20**:845–856.

5. Joffe MM, *et al.*: Drug therapy of the idiopathic inflammatory myopathies: predictors of response to prednisone, azathioprine and methotrexate in a comparison of their efficacy. *Am J Med* 1993, **94**:379–387.

6. Villalba L, Adams EM: Update on therapy for refractory dermatomyositis and polymyositis. *Curr Opin Rheumatol* 1996, **8**:544–551.

Diagnosis

Symptoms

Nasal obstruction.

Hyposmia and/or hypogeusia.

Dry mouth.

Snoring.

Signs

Glistening, yellow-tan mass in middle meatus or nasal cavity.

Pharyngeal mass (choanal polyp).

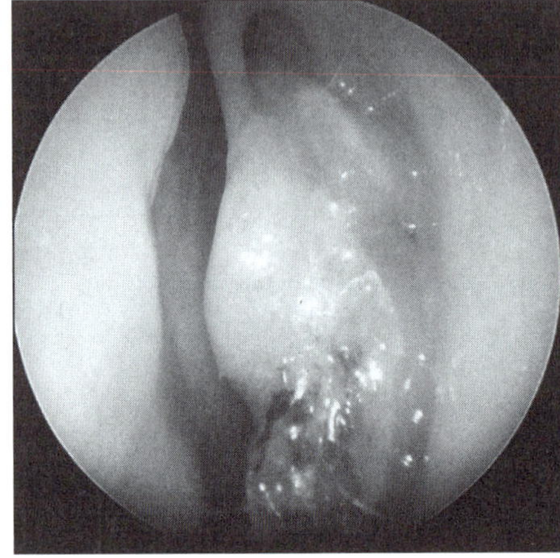

Nasal polyp. (*See* Color Plate.)

Investigations

CT: to rule out invasive process, tumor, fungal disease, encephalocele and to define potential extent of associated sinusitis.

MRI: rarely indicated except for instances of tumors or encephaloceles to define soft-tissue involvement. Otherwise MRI shows bony architecture of sinuses poorly and is overly sensitive to mucosal changes.

Sweat chloride: indicated in some young patients with polyposis to rule out cystic fibrosis.

Complications

Chronic sinusitis due to sinus obstruction, poor mucociliary clearance.

Sleep apnea secondary to obstruction.

Broadening of nasal bones.

Exacerbation of asthma: especially in triad asthma patients.

Aspirin hypersensitivity triad (polyposis, asthma, aspirin intolerance)

• Typical onset is after age 20 years.

• Common first symptom is profuse watery rhinorrhea.

• Patients then develop nasal congestion, hyposmia indicative of hyperplasia of the mucosa.

• Polyps typically develop early in disease.

• Aspirin sensitivity may develop years later.

• Aspirin intolerance is characterized by profuse rhinorrhea, rash, abdominal complaints, followed by asthma attack, which is typically severe.

• Patients will have cross-sensitivity to all NSAIDs, which should be avoided. Acetaminophen in routine doses is rarely problematic.

• Patients typically have chronic purulent sinusitis, which exacerbates the asthma.

• In patients refractory to steroid and antibiotic therapy, surgery is indicated.

Differential diagnosis

Nasal tumor: must be suspected in unilateral nasal mass or if bony erosion on CT scan. Inverted papilloma most common tumor; has high recurrence rate and 5%–10% chance of malignant degeneration. Encephalocele: must be ruled out in patients with unilateral nasal polyps, meningitis and polyps, or unilateral clear rhinorrhea and polyps. Turbinate hypertrophy.

Etiology and associated conditions

Triad asthma (aspirin sensitivity, asthma, nasal polyps).

Allergic rhinitis.

Chronic sinusitis (bacterial or fungal).

Cystic fibrosis.

Kartagener's syndrome.

Mucosal diseases (Wegener's disease, sarcoidosis, Churg-Strauss syndrome, Young's syndrome).

Epidemiology

• Nasal polyps occur in 7% of asthmatics, 36% of patients with aspirin intolerance, and 90% of patients with asthma and sinusitis; 70% of patients with polyps have associated asthma.

Treatment

Diet and lifestyle

• Patients should avoid allergens, irritants, and smoke.

• Saline irrigations with Ocean Spray or similar saline sprays are recommended.

• Bulb syringe saline irrigations (1 teaspoon salt in 2 cups water mixed daily) are recommended for patients with stasis of secretions and bacterial crusting or suprainfections.

Pharmacological treatment

Prednisone

Standard dosage	40–60 mg daily divided twice daily with rapid taper over 7–12 days.
Contraindications	Caution should be used in patients with diabetes, hypertension, peptic ulcer disease, history of tuberculosis, other infections that may be masked.
Special points	Steroids will be most effective for watery, acutely inflamed polyps than for more mature fibrotic polyps; polyps will typically return with repeated infectious, inflammatory, or allergic exacerbations; surgery may be indicated for patients with recurrent symptomatic polyps after steroids.
Main side effects	Cushingoid features, osteoporosis, easy bruisability, weight gain, growth retardation in children, hypertension, aseptic necrosis of bone, glucose intolerance, hyperlipidemia, cataracts, gastritis.

Topical nasal steroid sprays

Special points	Used for daily maintenance therapy; patients must be sure to aim toward turbinate, not septum, to avoid atrophy of mucosa, dryness, crusting, bleeding, and subsequent septal perforation; adrenal suppression rare except for dexamethasone preparations.
Contraindications	Atrophic rhinitis, epistaxis, septal perforation.

Treatment aims

To minimize symptoms of obstruction and hyposmia.
To prevent or minimize the occurrence of sinusitis.

Other treatments

Antibiotics for 3–6 weeks if associated purulent sinusitis (*see* Sinusitis).
Antihistamine–decongestants as needed.
• Endoscopic sinus surgery is effective for symptomatic polyps after medical therapy; typically performed for nasal obstruction and/or chronic rhinosinusitis; prognosis is excellent, although polyps will eventually return in many patients; short course of moderate-dose steroids postoperatively assists with healing.
• Allergy testing and possibly immunotherapy are indicated for patients with severe seasonal or perennial allergic rhinitis not responsive to avoidance therapy, steroid sprays, and antihistamine therapy.

Prognosis

• If polyps are large and mature, steroid therapy will not cause complete involution of polypoid disease and recurrence is eventually likely. Many will benefit from surgical removal.
• Endoscopic sinus surgery will typically yield longer symptom-free periods than will medical treatment, but polyps will recur in many patients.
• After medical or surgical therapy, aspirin-sensitive patients will typically have substantial improvement in nasal and asthma symptoms but tend to have recurrent polyps sooner than patients without aspirin sensitivity.

Follow-up and management

• Follow-up should be as needed based on patient symptoms and the frequency and severity of complications such as sinusitis.
• Consider a referral to an otolaryngologist if surgical treatment is needed.
• Watch for symptoms of aspirin sensitivity; the triad of polyposis, asthma, and aspirin intolerance may develop late in the course of the disease.

General references

Lumry WR, Curd JG, Zeiger RS, *et al.*: Aspirin sensitive rhinosinusitis: the clinical syndrome and effects of aspirin administration. *J Allergy Clin Immunol* 1987, **80**:788–790.

Settipane GA, Settipane RA: Nasal polyposis: clinical spectrum and treatment approaches. In *Diseases of the Sinuses*. Edited by Gershwin ME. Totowa, NJ: Humana Press; 1995.

Diagnosis

Symptoms and signs

Acute interstitial nephritis

• This is usually manifest as acute (potentially reversible) nonoliguric renal failure, less often as acute on chronic renal failure.

• The clinical picture may be dominated by the disease process for which an offending drug was administered or by features of extrarenal infection.

Fever, skin rash, and eosinophilia: in the majority of cases associated with beta-lactam antibiotics (the most common medication other than NSAIDs causing acute interstitial nephritis).

• NSAIDs are typically not associated with a hypersensitivity syndrome, but instead present with acute renal failure and often nephrotic range proteinuria.

Arthralgias and lymphadenopathy.

Anterior uveitis and granulomatous infiltration of other organs: in a small group of patients with idiopathic disease.

Chronic interstitial nephritis

• This usually manifests insidiously as chronic (irreversible) renal failure.

• The clinical picture may be dominated by features of an underlying disease process or by the condition for which analgesics were taken.

• No specific features allow differentiation from other causes of chronic renal failure.

Investigations

Complete blood count: with differential for eosinophilia in acute interstitial nephritis.

Blood urea nitrogen, creatinine clearance, 24-hour urinary protein excretion measurement: to quantify renal function.

Blood cultures and other specific serological tests: if systemic infection, connective tissue disease, or vasculitis suspected (casts, eosinophiluria).

Microscopy and culture of midstream urine.

Urinary Bence Jones protein and serum protein electrophoresis: to screen for myeloma.

Ultrasonography of urinary tract and plain abdominal radiography: in all patients.

Renal biopsy: in all patients with renal impairment and normal-sized, nonhydronephrotic kidneys on ultrasonography, except those in whom diagnosis is apparent from clinical features (*e.g.*, prerenal cause of acute tubular necrosis) or previous investigations (*e.g.*, i.v. urographic diagnosis of reflux nephropathy or papillary necrosis); renal biopsy is dangerous in patients with small kidneys—a careful history provides more reliable diagnostic clues in these.

Complications

Acute interstitial nephritis

• The major complications are those of acute renal failure.

Chronic interstitial nephritis

• The major complications are those of chronic renal failure.

Salt wasting, renal tubular acidosis, occasionally Fanconi's syndrome.

Symptomatic anemia inappropriate to level of renal function: in patients with analgesic nephropathy.

Differential diagnosis

Acute interstitial nephritis
Other causes of acute renal impairment, especially rapidly progressive glomerulonephritis (either idiopathic or associated with systemic vasculitis).

Chronic interstitial nephritis
All other causes of chronic renal failure.

Etiology

Causes of acute interstitial nephritis
Drug hypersensitivity: beta-lactam antibiotics (*e.g.*, methicillin, ampicillin), other antibiotics (*e.g.*, sulfonamides, rifampicin), NSAIDs (*e.g.*, fenoprofen, indomethacin), diuretics (*e.g.*, thiazides, furosemide), and other miscellaneous drugs (*e.g.*, phenindione, phenytoin, allopurinol).
Infections: complicating urinary tract infection (especially in diabetic patients) or complicating extrarenal infection (*e.g.*, with streptococci, legionella, brucella, tuberculosis, leptospira, mycoplasma, *Toxoplasma* spp., infectious mononucleosis, hantavirus).
Immunological disorders: interstitial lesions sometimes overshadow glomerular (*e.g.*, lupus polyarteritis nodosa).
Idiopathic.

Causes of chronic interstitial nephritis
Toxic and metabolic: analgesics, lithium, cisplatinum, lead, cadmium, hypercalcemia.
Granulomatous: sarcoidosis, tuberculosis, drugs.
Immunological: associated with primary glomerular disease, Sjögren's syndrome, transplant rejection, rheumatoid arthritis.
Miscellaneous: reflux nephropathy, postobstructive, myeloma, sickle cell disease, radiation nephritis, Balkan nephropathy, hereditary.

Causes of papillary necrosis
Analgesic nephropathy, sickle cell disease, diabetes mellitus, obstruction with infection, tuberculosis, cryoglobulinemia.

Epidemiology

• The true incidence of acute interstitial nephritis is unknown.

• Renal biopsy studies suggest that it accounts for up to 8% of cases of acute renal failure; this is almost certainly an underestimate.

• 20%–40% of patients being treated for end-stage renal failure have primary tubulointerstitial disease.

Treatment

Diet and lifestyle

• Patients who habitually abuse analgesics may benefit from psychological support and counseling.

• Occupational health measures have helped to limit industrial exposure to heavy metals.

• Patients with chronic renal failure have accelerated atherogenesis; smoking should be discouraged, and a diet low in saturated fat recommended.

• Patients with drug-related interstitial nephritis should be advised never to take the same or a related drug in the future.

Pharmacological treatment

• Patients may present with features of severe uremia and need stabilization by urgent dialysis before definitive investigation and treatment can safely be carried out.

For acute interstitial nephritis

Drug-associated: withdrawal of offending drug; prednisolone, 40 mg daily, with rapid tapering according to response, may hasten resolution.

Infection-associated: antibiotic treatment tailored to causative organism; steroids not indicated at least until infection is controlled.

Idiopathic disease associated with uveitis: steroids as for drug-associated disease dramatically improve renal and ocular lesions.

For chronic interstitial nephritis

Toxin-induced: withdrawal of causative agents.

Reflux nephropathy: childhood urinary tract infection must be eradicated by appropriate antibiotics; this should be followed by long-term low-dose chemoprophylaxis until reflux is resolved or renal growth complete.

Sarcoidosis: long-term steroid treatment, using minimum dose to maintain stable renal function (*see* Sarcoidosis *for details*).

Tuberculosis: antituberculous chemotherapy; concurrent use of low-dose steroids may limit renal scarring (*see* Tuberculosis, extrapulmonary *for details*).

Myeloma: referral to hematologist or oncologist recommended for institution of appropriate treatment regimen; hypovolemia must be avoided; allopurinol to prevent acute urate nephropathy (*see* Multiple myeloma *for details*).

For analgesic nephropathy

Withdrawal of offending drugs.

Provision of psychological support.

Monitoring and treatment of the following:
Hypertension: antihypertensive agents (diuretics often inappropriate).
Salt wasting: oral slow sodium may improve glomerular filtration rate.
Renal tubular acidosis: oral sodium bicarbonate.
Inappropriate anemia (gastrointestinal blood loss): misoprostol, iron supplements.
Early renal osteodystrophy: alpha calcidol and calcium carbonate.
Frequent urinary tract infection: prolonged treatment for upper tract infections.
Obstruction due to sloughed papillae: nephrostomy or double-J stents.
Increased incidence of urothelial tumors: regular urine cytology.
Increased atheromatous renovascular disease.

General references

Bennett WM, Henrich WL, Stoff JS: The renal effects of nonsteroidal anti-inflammatory drugs: summary and recommendations. *Am J Kidney Dis* 1996, **28(suppl 1):**S56–S62.

Mayer HB, *et al.*: Epstein-Barr virus-induced infectious mononucleosis complicated by acute renal failure: case report and review. *Clin Infect Dis* 1996, **22:**1009–1018.

Murray KM, Keane WR, *et al.*: Review of drug-induced acute interstitial nephritis. *Pharmacotherapy* 1992, **12:**462–467.

Singh AK, Ucci A, Madias NE: Predominant tubulointerstitial lupus nephritis. *Am J Kidney Dis* 1996, **27:**273–278.

Viero RM, Cavallo T: Granulomatous interstitial nephritis. *Hum Pathol* 1995, **26:**1347–1353.

Diagnosis

Definition

• Acute herpetic neuralgia merges into postherpetic neuralgia. The most widely accepted definition seems to be persisitent pain 1 month after skin eruption.

Symptoms

• Pain may precede the eruption by days to weeks and may persist months to long-term. It may be continuous, paroxysmal, or lancinating and is generally dermatomal.

Signs

Depigmented scars.

Sensory: Local decreased sensation over scars; hyperalgesia and allodynia in other areas of dermatome.

Weakness: Very rare, if virus spreads to other parts of CNS segment.

Investigations

• No investigation is needed in most patients.

• In younger patients, shingles, either isolated or with generalized zoster, may be a symptom of immunosuppression, particularly associated with lymphoma or leukemia; HIV and cancer are also associated. Appropriate investigation of patients at risk is needed.

Complications

Depression: common, sometimes severe.

Weakness in a limb: when an appropriate dermatome is affected.

Differential diagnosis

Other causes of sensory ganglion and root disease, including diabetes, Sjögren's disease.

Etiology

• Reactivation of dormant herpes varicella zoster virus in dorsal root ganglion causes acute shingles.

• Corticosteroid treatment for an unrelated condition sometimes precipitates shingles.

• Histopathology in postherpetic neuralgia shows damage to peripheral nerve, dorsal root ganglion, sensory root, and dorsal horn atrophy [1].

Epidemiology

• The female:male ratio is 3:2.

• The overall incidence of postherpetic neuralgia at 1 year is 3%–10% of all patients with acute shingles.

• The most common sites are the mid-thoracic dermatomes and the ophthalmic division of the trigeminal nerve: it may occur in any dermatome.

• Postherpetic neuralgia becomes more common with increasing age.

Treatment

Diet and lifestyle

- No special precautions are necessary.

Pharmacological treatment

- Prednisone bursts and antiviral therapy (acyclovir, 800 mg 5 times daily, or famciclovir, 750 mg 3 times daily for 7 days) lessen acute pain.

- Some studies do report a decrease in incidence in postherpetic neuralgia after acute treatment with antivirals, but this remains controversial.

Local

- Possibilities for local treatment must always be exhausted because simple measures may give partial relief and avoid the side effects so often seen with systemic drug treatment in this mainly elderly patient population.

- Treatments include the following:

Local anesthetic ointment (5% lidocaine) 3 times daily: sometimes effective.

Capsaicin, 0.075% ointment 3 times daily: causes initial burning but helps a few patients significantly [2].

Systemic

Standard dosage	Amitriptyline or nortriptyline, 10–25 mg at night, gradually increased, as tolerated.
Contraindications	Recent myocardial infarction, heart block, mania, porphyria.
Special points	Up to maximum tolerated doses have been consistently shown in controlled trials to provide partial relief of postherpetic neuralgia.
Main drug interactions	Sedation enhanced by other sedatives.
Main side effects	Drowsiness, constipation, urinary hesitancy, dry mouth, blurred vision, postural hypotension, tachycardia, sweating, tremor.

- Anticonvulsants may be useful for lancinating pain, and opioids may be helpful in refractory cases.

Treatment aims

To relieve pain.

Other treatments

Local measures

- Cold packs applied for 15–20 minutes several times daily may produce partial analgesia, sometimes lasting a few hours after a single application.

- Transcutaneous electrical nerve stimulation and biofeedback may each be helpful in some patients.

- Local anesthetic, peripheral nerve or root blocks, and sympathetic blocks (occasionally) may temporarily relieve postherpetic neuralgia but has no long-term benefit.

Psychological measures

- Counseling by a clinical psychologist about coping strategies may help some patients.

Prognosis

- Most patients with troublesome postherpetic neuralgia at 1 year have the condition lifelong, although some patients slowly improve over long periods.

- After acute shingles, persistent, troublesome neuralgia gradually decreases over months.

Follow-up and management

- ~50% of patients with postherpetic neuralgia benefit from regular long-term follow-up; the role of a sympathetic doctor who is prepared to listen should not be underestimated, even when all treatment options have apparently been exhausted.

- Many patients can be discharged from follow-up when treatment leads to partial relief of pain.

Key references

1. Bennett GJ: Hypotheses on the pathogenesis of herpes zoster associated pain. *Ann Neurol* 1994, **35(suppl)**:S38–S41.

2. Kost RG, Straus SE: Drug therapy: postherpetic neuralgia. *N Engl J Med* 1996, **335**:32–43.

Diagnosis

Symptoms

Pain: unilateral shooting, shock-like, usually along zygomatic arch; rare in ophthalmic division; paroxysmal, lasting <1 minute but may occur frequently; occurs spontaneously but often triggered by innocuous facial or oral stimulation, *e.g.*, wind, touching face, washing or shaving, brushing teeth, eating, talking, and drinking; bouts last weeks to months, with remissions of months to years; may become chronic in some patients; rarely develops on contralateral side; in chronic trigeminal neuralgia, some patients complain of background aching pain.

Signs

• Idiopathic trigeminal neuralgia has no signs.

Trigeminal sensory impairment: caused by a compressive lesion of the trigeminal root; such lesions may rarely lead to trigeminal neuralgia.

Investigations

• Investigation is not usually needed.

CT or MRI: in patients being considered for surgical treatment (V nerve decompression) or in whom sensory impairment is present.

Complications

Depression.

Treatment

Diet and lifestyle

• No special precautions are necessary.

Pharmacological treatment

Carbamazepine

• Carbamazepine is the drug of choice.

Standard dosage	Carbamazepine, 100 mg twice daily initially, increased to a dose that controls pain or to maximum tolerated dose.
Contraindications	Hypersensitivity.
Special points	Blood level monitoring often helpful.
Main drug interactions	Sedation enhanced by other sedatives.
Main side effects	Drowsiness, nausea, ataxia, hypersensitivity rash, neutropenia.

Other drugs

• Phenytoin, tricyclic antidepressants, and baclofen are also often helpful.

General references

Gonda JJ, Brown JA: Atypical facial pain and other pain syndromes: differential diagnosis and treatment. *Neurosurg Clin North Am* 1997, **8**:87–100.

Loeser JD: Tic douloureux and atypical face pain. In *Textbook of Pain,* edn 3. Edited by Wall PD, Melzack R. Edinburgh: Churchill Livingstone; 1994:699–710.

Diagnosis

Symptoms

General
Distal numbness.

Paresthesia, burning, lancinating pain.

Progressive distal weakness and wasting.

Foot and hand deformities, neuropathic ulcer, neuropathic arthropathy.

Of autonomic neuropathy
Impotence, orthostatic hypotension, dry eyes or mouth, urinary or fecal incontinence, nausea and vomiting, constipation or diarrhea.

Signs

General
Stocking-glove sensory loss.

Muscle weakness and wasting.

Reduced or absent tendon reflexes.

Sensory ataxia, neuropathic tremor.

Nerve thickening.

Of autonomic neuropathy
Anhidrosis, unreactive or asymmetric pupils, postural hypotension (fall of 30 mm Hg in systolic and 15 mm Hg in diastolic pressure).

Investigations

All patients
Complete blood count.

ESR measurement.

Glucose tolerance test: if random and fasting samples give equivocal results.

Liver and renal function tests.

Measurement of thyroid-stimulating hormone, vitamin B_{12} (folate), serum protein electrophoresis, autoantibodies.

Urinalysis: for glucose, Bence Jones protein, porphyrins.

CSF analysis: elevated protein concentration in inflammatory neuropathies.

Nerve conduction studies: diagnosis confirmed by slowing of motor or sensory conduction velocities (moderate in axonal type, marked in demyelinating type) and reduction in sensory action potential amplitude (small in axonal neuropathy).

Electromyography: characteristic pattern in denervated muscle.

Sometimes indicated
DNA analysis: for hereditary demyelinating neuropathies; chromosome 17 duplication in a subgroup of patients with HMSN type 1 (HMSN 1A); chromosome 17 deletion associated with hereditary liability to pressure palsies (tomaculous neuropathy).

Sensory threshold recording: thermal (useful in patients with small-fiber neuropathy).

Imaging: screening for malignancy in patients with suspected paraneoplastic neuropathy; skeletal survey for suspected myeloma; chest radiography for suspected sarcoidosis.

Nerve biopsy: done in operating room under strict aseptic conditions using local anesthetic; fascicular biopsy limits degree of sensory loss; full thickness biopsy indicated for suspected vasculitis; used to discover cause of progressive neuropathy not revealed by detailed investigation or to confirm presence of vasculitis, leprous neuropathy, or inflammatory infiltrates; sensory nerves (sural, superficial peroneal, superficial radial) usually undergo biopsy.

Bone-marrow biopsy: for myeloma.

Formal autonomic function tests, endoscopy, colonoscopy, barium studies, urodynamic studies: for autonomic neuropathy.

Complications
Burns, cuts, bruising, neuropathic ulcers: unnoticed when sensory loss is severe.

Distal weakness.

Treatment

Diet and lifestyle

- Patients with alcoholic neuropathy should abstain from drinking alcohol.
- Postural hypotension can be improved by wearing support stockings.
- Examine feet daily, use night light, remove obstacles to reduce foot injury.

Pharmacological treatment

For focal and multifocal neuropathies

For vasculitis: prednisone, 60 mg daily orally; azathioprine or cytoxan can be introduced to enable dose of steroids to be reduced; degree of immunosuppression and duration of treatment depend on clinical response.

For protection against peptic ulceration: H_2 antagonists.

For alcoholic neuropathy: vitamin B supplements.

For herpes zoster infection: acyclovir, 800 mg orally 5 times daily for 1 week.

- Leprosy should be treated under specialist supervision.

For autonomic neuropathy

For postural hypotension: fludrocortisone, 100–400 mg, or ephedrine, 15–60 mg daily.

For gastroparesis: erythromycin, 125 mg daily; cisapride, 10 mg 3 times daily; domperidone, 10–20 mg 3 times daily; or metoclopramide, up to 10 mg 3 times daily.

For diarrhea: diphenoxylate (Lomotil), loperamide (Imodium), codeine phosphate.

For impotence: penile intracavernous papaverine injection.

For painful neuropathy

- Treatment is extremely difficult and often unsatisfactory.

Regular simple analgesic, *e.g.*, acetaminophen, 1 g 4 times daily.

For burning diffuse pain and paresthesia: amitriptyline, 25–75 mg at night; gabapentin, 300–600 mg 3 times daily.

For shooting pain: carbamazepine, 100 mg at night, increasing slowly to 600 mg daily in divided doses; mexiletine, 100–400 mg daily may be worth trying.

For postherpetic neuralgia or diabetes: topical capsaicin, 0.075% after lesions have healed.

For chronic inflammatory demyelinating polyradiculoneuropathy

For acute disorder: *see* Guillain–Barré syndrome.

For mild to moderate disease: prednisone, 60 mg/day, tapering as possible; azathioprine may be added for steroid-sparing effect.

For progressive disease or relapses: i.v. plasmaphoresis or immunoglobulin, 0.4 g/kg/day for 5 days and possible replacement of azathioprine with either cyclosporine titrated to leukocytes or cyclophosphamide [3].

Treatment aims

- Treatment aims depend on the type of neuropathy.

To treat underlying illness.

To treat dysesthesias or pain, orthostasis.

Other treatments

For focal and multifocal neuropathies
Conservative: wrist and foot support, elbow pad.

Surgical decompression:
Median and ulnar nerve entrapment with evidence of wasting or weakness of denervated muscles.
For persistent sensory symptoms when conservative measures have failed.

For chronic inflammatory demyelinating polyradiculoneuropathy
Plasma exchange for progressive neuropathy unresponsive to immunoglobulin.

Prognosis

- Prognosis depends on the underlying cause of the neuropathy.

Follow-up and management

- Regular follow-up is needed to assess progression.
- Patients requiring immunosuppression need frequent follow-up.

Key references

1. Lupski JR, *et al.*: DNA duplication associated with Charcot–Marie–Tooth disease type 1A. *Cell* 1991, **66**:219–232.

2. Chance PF, *et al.*: DNA deletion associated with hereditary neuropathy with liability to pressure palsies. *Cell* 1993, **72**:143–151.

3. van Doorn PA, *et al.*: High dose intravenous immunoglobulin treatment in chronic inflammatory demyelinating neuropathy: a double blind, placebo controlled, crossover study. *Neurology* 1990, **40**:212–214.

General references

Dyck PJ, Thomas PK: *Peripheral Neuropathy*, edn 3. Philadelphia: WB Saunders; 1993.

Wokke JH, van Dijk GW: Sensory neuropathies including painful and toxic neuropathies. *J Neurol* 1997, **244**:209–221.

Diagnosis

Symptoms

Lymph node in neck, axilla, or groin, noticed by patient as unexplained "lump": the most common presenting symptom.

• The disease may be seen in multiple sites at presentation.

• Systemic symptoms (*e.g.*, the "B" symptoms of Hodgkin's disease) are less common than in Hodgkin's disease.

• Symptoms may relate to the anatomical site of disease, *e.g.*, superior vena cava obstruction due to mediastinal nodes or to primary lymphomas at extranodal sites (*e.g.*, CNS, gastrointestinal tract).

• Primary extranodal non-Hodgkin's lymphoma occurs much more often than extranodal Hodgkin's disease.

Signs

Palpable lymphadenopathy: careful examination of all nodal areas essential.

Hepatomegaly and splenomegaly: possibly.

Signs of other organ involvement: *e.g.*, pleural effusion as a result of pulmonary parenchymal involvement, skin involvement (rarely).

Investigations

• Initially, investigations must be directed at confirming the diagnosis.

• A good sample of tissue that has not been placed in formalin is needed.

• The diagnosis may be apparent on routine staining with hematoxylin-eosin or Giemsa.

• Immunohistochemistry, especially markers for T and B lymphocytes and leukocyte common antigen, is vital in subclassification and may help to distinguish undifferentiated lymphomas from carcinoma.

• Subsequent investigations must be systematic and thorough to enable accurate localization of disease and if possible to estimate disease volume.

Complete blood count: usually normal.

Urine and electrolyte analysis: as a baseline.

Liver function tests: may be abnormal if liver is involved.

Lactate dehydrogenase measurement: useful marker of disease bulk and activity.

Chest radiography: to rule out hilar or mediastinal nodes or intrapulmonary disease.

CT of chest and abdomen: to rule out node or organ involvement.

Bone-marrow examination: trephine is particularly important.

Examination of postnasal space and tonsillar fossa.

Lumbar puncture with cytology: in high-grade disease only.

Complications

Recurrent or atypical infections.

Autoimmune hemolysis and thrombocytopenia.

Bone-marrow failure.

Gastrointestinal bleeding or perforation: obstructive jaundice.

Differential diagnosis

Other causes of lymphadenopathy: *e.g.*, Hodgkin's disease.

Infective causes: *e.g.*, toxoplasmosis, glandular fever, Epstein–Barr virus.

Etiology

• The cause is unknown, but the following may have a role:

Epstein–Barr virus: associated with endemic Burkitt's lymphoma in Africa.

Adult T-cell leukemia–lymphoma: associated in all cases with human T-cell lymphotropic virus.

HIV infection: particularly primary CNS non-Hodgkin's lymphoma (rare in other settings).

Epidemiology

• The median age of onset is 50 years.

• Intermediate- or high-grade disease is more common in younger patients.

Classification [1]

• Non-Hodgkin's lymphomas constitute a diverse group of disorders arising from different cell types, usually T and B lymphocytes; the wide spectrum of disease biology is reflected by the varying clinical presentations, responses to treatment, and overall outcomes.

• Various schemes for classification have been proposed and developed; the most useful are those that can be used to predict clinical behavior and prognosis.

• Classifications include the following:
Rappaport.

Lukes-Collins.

Lennert: the Kiel classification.

The Working Formulation (used here): an international attempt to provide a translation from one classification to another, now widely used in its own right; non-Hodgkin's lymphoma is divided into low, intermediate, and high grades, each having different treatment and prognosis.

Staging

• Patients may be staged I–IV according to the Ann Arbor system originally developed for Hodgkin's disease (*see* Hodgkin's disease).

• Staging is less useful than for Hodgkin's disease because, with the exception of stage 1 disease, all patients with non-Hodgkin's lymphoma should receive chemotherapy.

Treatment

Diet and lifestyle

• Many patients maintain a fairly normal lifestyle during treatment, but some are unwell and need multiple hospital admissions.

Pharmacological treatment

• Treatment should take place in the context of a clinical study whenever possible.

• It should be given by a specialist hematologist or oncologist.

For intermediate-grade non-Hodgkin's lymphoma

• Treatment should begin as soon as investigation is completed.

• These lymphomas are usually sensitive to many chemotherapy drugs, and many effective combination regimens may be curative.

• Stage 1 disease may be treated successfully by radiotherapy alone, but localized disease is very unusual in non-Hodgkin's lymphoma.

• The standard treatment is by CHOP (cyclophosphamide, doxorubicin, vincristine, prednisone), usually given on a monthly cycle for 6 months; other regimens including additional drugs, *e.g.*, PACEBOM (prednisone, doxorubicin, cyclophosphamide, etoposide, bleomycin, vincristine, methotrexate), are given more intensively, reducing total time taken for treatment, but none has been shown to be superior to CHOP [2].

• Allopurinol, 300 mg daily, should be given for at least the first month.

• Main side effects include hair loss, nausea (often preventable), and myelosuppression (for which dose reductions may be needed during subsequent cycles).

For low-grade non-Hodgkin's lymphoma

• These lymphomas are also sensitive to chemotherapy, but, although they usually do not behave aggressively clinically, they are usually considered incurable by standard treatment.

• A conservative approach is often advocated, particularly in elderly asymptomatic patients, because early treatment has no survival advantage.

• 50% of patients may avoid treatment for up to 3 years.

• In truly localized low-grade disease, radiotherapy may give long-term remission.

• Patients may respond well to treatment and often may have considerable periods when no treatment is needed.

• Initial treatment is usually by oral chlorambucil, best used cyclically rather than continually.

• Combination chemotherapy, *e.g.*, cytoxan with prednisone, vincristine, and possibly anthracycline, is sometimes used but has no proven advantage over chlorambucil initially.

• The new agents fludarabine and 2-chlorodeoxyadenosine may be of value in relapsed disease [3].

• Interferon-α has just been licensed for low-grade disease, but its indications and benefits are not yet clear.

• Monoclonal antibody therapy for lymphomas is currently a promising new therapy for low-grade lymphomas, available under research protocol in some centers [4,5].

• Main side effects of chlorambucil include myelosuppression and mild nausea.

For high-grade non-Hodgkin's lymphoma

• Lymphoblastic and Burkitt's lymphomas are very aggressive clinically and often manifest with widespread disease, including bone-marrow and CNS involvement; they need intensive leukemia-style treatment, usually involving very myelosuppressive inpatient regimens and CNS-directed prophylaxis.

Treatment aims
To cure patient, with minimum toxicity.
To palliate if cure is not possible.

Other treatments
• High-dose treatment and autologous bone-marrow transplantation are indicated for the following:
Intermediate grade: age <60 years, relapsed disease still sensitive to chemotherapy.
Low grade: criteria difficult to define because long-term follow-up is needed to assess benefit because of the indolent nature of the disease.
• Allogeneic transplantation may have a role for young patients with high-grade disease.

Prognosis
Low grade
• At 5 years, ~70% of patients are still alive, but few are in complete remission; most patients eventually die of their disease.
• In many patients, the disease ultimately transforms to high grade and becomes refractory to chemotherapy.

Intermediate and high grades
• The complete remission rate is ~85% in patients with limited disease, ~55% with extensive disease.
• Overall disease-free survival is ~40% and depends on several factors; poor prognostic factors include stage III or IV disease, high lactate dehydrogenase concentration, failure to attain complete remission on first-line treatment, and older age.

Follow-up and management
• During treatment, regular follow-up is needed, including examination and full blood count before each course of chemotherapy; toxicity must be monitored, and complications treated.
• After treatment is completed, full restaging should take place: if the patient is in complete remission, regular follow-up should be continued to detect early relapse.

Key references

1. Falzon M, Isaacson PG: Histological classification of the non-Hodgkin's lymphoma. *Blood Rev* 1990, **4**:111–115.

2. Armitage JO: The place of third generation regimens in the treatment of adult aggressive non-Hodgkin's lymphoma. *Ann Oncol* 1991, **2(suppl 1)**:37–41.

3. Cheson B: New chemotherapeutic agents in the treatment of low grade non-Hodgkin's lymphomas. *Semin Oncol* 1993, **20**:96–110.

4. Renner C, *et al.*: Monoclonal antibodies in the treatment of non-Hodgkin's lymphoma: recent results and future prospects. *Leukemia* 1997, **11(suppl 2)**:S555–S559.

5. Kaminski MS, *et al.*: Radioimmunotherapy of B cell lymphoma with [131] anti-B, (anti-CD 20) antibody. *N Engl J Med* 1993, **329**:459–465.

Diagnosis

Symptoms

- Many patients are asymptomatic.
- Women have more symptoms than men.
- Symptoms occur more frequently in large, weight-bearing joints.
- They are often phasic and are not always progressive; muscle weakness and psychological status are often better predictors of symptoms or functional impairment than structural damage [1].

Pain: typically on use.

Stiffness after inactivity: "gelling" phenomenon common.

Functional impairment: particularly of gait; a major problem.

Signs

- Signs are often discordant with symptoms.

Bony swelling, deformity, crepitus, restriction of movement: bony swelling may be marked in interphalangeal joints (Heberden's and Bouchard's nodes).

Joint-line tenderness.

Local heat, effusion: occasional inflammatory features, particularly in crystal-related osteoarthritis or developing finger nodes.

Investigations

- Osteoarthritis is principally a clinical diagnosis. Often occuring in middle-aged or elderly patients, the question is not usually whether it is present but whether it is the cause of current symptoms; only clinical examination can answer this.

General
Radiography: may show structural change, *e.g.*, loss of joint space (cartilage), osteo-phytosis, sclerosis, cysts, osteochondral bodies.

Premature osteoarthritis
- Onset occurs before the age of 55 years [1].

Ferritin measurement: for hemochromatosis.

Calcium, phosphate, alkaline phosphatase measurement: for hyperparathyroidism.

Urine homogentisic acid measurement: if ochronosis suspected.

Lateral spine radiography: for spondyloepiphyseal dysphasia.

Pituitary studies: if acromegaly suspected.

Acute flare
Synovial fluid examination: for sepsis and crystals.

"Locking" of knee
- *See* Knee injuries *for details*.

Arthroscopy or MRI: for loose bodies (osteochondral), meniscal lesions.

Complications

Acute crystal synovitis: mainly calcium pyrophosphate crystals.

Septic arthritis.

Loose-body formation.

Avascular necrosis.

Differential diagnosis

- Periarticular lesions may coexist and may be the prime source of symptoms.

Polyarticular osteoarthritis
Inflammatory arthropathies.
Gout.

Poor bone response and destruction
Charcot's arthropathy.
Sepsis.

Acute crystal-related oligoarthritic osteoarthritis
Sepsis.
Gout.
Inflammatory arthropathy.

Etiology

- Osteoarthritis probably has many causes; recognized factors include the following:
Obesity.
Age.
Occupational trauma.
Genetics: nodal osteoarthritis, (spondylo-) epiphyseal dysplasia, type II collagen abnormalities.
Metabolic or endocrine disorders: hemo-chromatosis, hyperparathyroidism, ochronosis, acromegaly [1].
Previous joint disease or damage.

Epidemiology

- Osteoarthritis is strongly age-related.
- It is the most common cause of locomotor disability.
- Nodal osteoarthritis may manifest with florid polyarticular disease and Heberden's nodes in menopausal women.

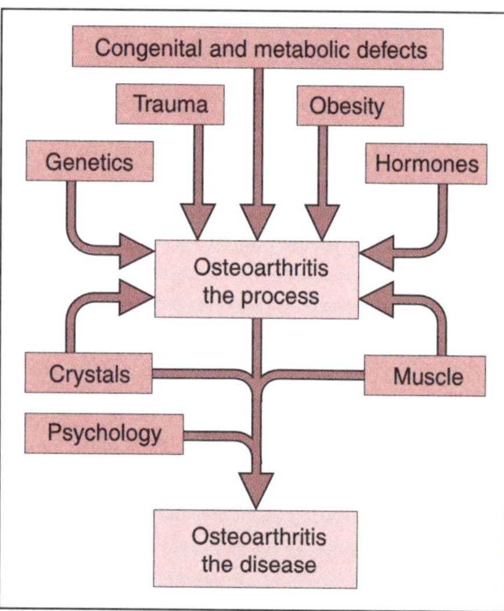

Factors leading to progression of osteoarthritis.

Treatment

Diet and lifestyle

- Patients should be encouraged to take control of the condition.
- Physical activity should be encouraged, *e.g.*, aerobic fitness and muscle strengthening.
- Biomechanical factors, *e.g.*, obesity, varus knee deformity, should be tried (wedge insoles, shock-absorbing footwear, use of cane).
- Caloric reduction may improve osteoarthritis of the hip or knee.

Pharmacological treatment

Topical antirheumatics

- These include NSAIDs and capsaicin ointment.
- Their role is controversial, but they are probably effective.
- Contraindications include sensitive or broken skin.

Analgesics

- These are often sufficient [2].
- Compound preparations with opiates may only increase adverse effects, without improving symptom control.

Standard dosage	Acetaminophen, 1 or 2 650-mg tablets orally every 6–8 hours, as required [2].
Contraindications	Liver disease.
Main drug interactions	None.
Main side effects	Rare, except in overdosage when hepatic failure may ensue.

NSAIDs

- NSAIDs may be tried [1,3,4].
- Use should be regularly reviewed.

Standard dosage	Depends on agent; lowest dose needed for benefit.
Contraindications	Active peptic ulceration, hypersensitivity, renal impairment (relative).
Special points	Patients show marked variation in response to different drugs.
Main drug interactions	Warfarin.
Main side effects	Gastrointestinal ulceration, anemia, renal dysfunction, skin rashes.

Intra-articular steroids

- Local corticosteroids are indicated for short-term relief of inflammatory episodes or coexistent periarticular lesions.

Standard dosage	Depends on agent and joint; in large joints, generally no more than 3-monthly; in small joints, yearly.
Contraindications	Septic arthritis, hypersensitivity (rare).
Special points	Longer-acting steroids provide more benefit.
Main drug interactions	None.
Main side effects	Occasional facial flushing, deterioration of diabetic control.

Nonpharmacological treatment

- Arthroplasty is particularly helpful for patients with disease of hips, knees. Indications include exercise/activity limitation, sleep disturbance, poor quality of life secondary to joint pain.
- Physical therapy (heat, cold, range-of-motion exercises, joint protection, pacing of activities, splinting, assistive devices) may be more helpful than medication.

Treatment aims

To relieve pain.
To maintain functional ability.

Other treatments

Arthroplasty: for patients with persistent pain or marked functional impairment.

Prognosis

- Many patients show phasic symptoms, and some improve with time.
- Symptoms may remain static for years.

Follow-up and management

- Follow-up is usually in a primary care setting.
- The aims are to determine the need for further intervention as a result of deterioration in symptoms or function and to monitor treatment, particularly by NSAIDs, to assess the need for continued use and the development of adverse effects.

Key references

1. Brandt K: The pathogenesis of osteoarthritis. *Rheumatol Rev* 1991, **1**:3–11.

2. Bradley JD, *et al.*: Comparison of an anti-inflammatory dose of ibuprofen, an analgesic dose of ibuprofen, and acetaminophen in the treatment of osteoarthritis of the knee. *N Engl J Med* 1991, **325**:87–91.

3. Brandt KD: NSAIDs in the treatment of osteoarthritis. Friends or foes? *Bull Rheum Dis* 1993, **42**:1–4.

4. Kraus VB: Pathogenesis and treatment of osteoarthritis. *Med Clin North Am* 1997, **81**:85–112.

Diagnosis

Symptoms

• Most patients will be asymptomatic.

Loss of height.

Fractures with minimal trauma: especially Colles', vertebral, hip, and rib fractures.

Kyphosis.

Symptoms of menopause in women, hypogonadism in men.

Signs

• There are few other specific signs for osteoporosis; *see* Symptoms.

Inadequate calcium intake.

Early menopause, including surgical.

Longstanding amenorrhea or oligomenorrhea.

Signs of Cushing's syndrome (endogenous or exogenous).

Investigations

Bone densitometry: several methods are available; dual emission x-ray absorptiometry (DEXA) of the hip and spine is emerging as the test of choice.

Gonadal function: Follicle-stimulating hormone and estradiol in women, follicle-stimulating hormone and testosterone in men.

Chemistry panel (including liver function tests), thyroid function tests, serum protein electrophoresis, urinalysis, urinary calcium, intact parathyroid hormone, vitamin D level analysis: to rule out secondary causes of osteoporosis.

Glucocorticoids [1], dilantin, phenobarbitol, heparin, gonadotropin- releasing hormone analog: to identify medications associated with bone loss.

Tests for other illnesses associated with bone loss: *see* Etiology.

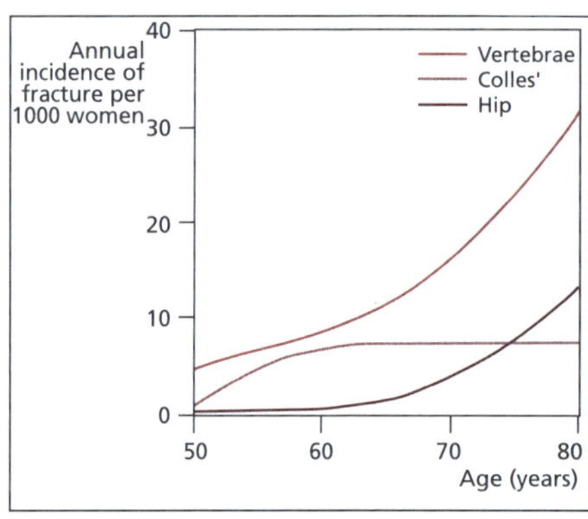

Incidence rates for vertebral, Colles', and hip fractures in women.

Complications

Fractures in the elderly: associated with significant mortality and frequent nursing home placement.

Fractures in younger patients: can cause significant pain and loss of mobility.

Loss of height.

Differential diagnosis

Metastatic disease.

Fracture in otherwise normal bone.

Etiology

Most common: postmenopausal women, older women and men, anovulatory women (*e.g.*, competitive athletes), hypogonadal men.

Less common: Cushing's syndrome, thyrotoxicosis, liver disease, rheumatoid arthritis, diabetes, alcoholism.

Epidemiology

• Health care costs resulting from osteoporotic fractures exceed $13 billion annually.

• One-third of women >65 years of age will have one or more vertebral fractures.

• One-third of women >80 years of age will have a hip fracture.

• 25% of all hip fractures occur in men.

Other information

• DEXA scores are reported as T-scores and Z-scores. T-scores compare bone mass with that of young persons (matched for gender) and are reported in standard deviations above or below the mean. Z-scores compare bone mass of persons of the same age and gender. T-scores are more predictive of fracture risk.

• Osteopenia is defined as a T-score of -1.0 to -2.5. Osteoporosis is defined as a T-score of >-2.5.

Treatment

Diet and lifestyle

• Patients should be encouraged to intake 1000–1500 mg of elemental calcium through diet (preferably) or calcium supplementation.

• Fall hazards should be removed from the home.

• Patients should be encouraged to perform weight-bearing exercises.

Pharmacological treatment [2]

Calcium

• Calcium supplementation is recommended for all patients (*see* Diet and lifestyle *for guidelines*).

Standard dosage	Calcium carbonate, 40% elemental calcium by weight (1250-mg tablet contains 500 mg calcium). Calcium citrate, 21% elemental calcium by weight (950-mg tablet contains 200 mg calcium).
Special points	Supplements should be taken with meals to enhance absorption and reduce the incidence of nephrolithiasis.

Vitamin D$_3$

• Vitamin D$_3$ is recommended for all patients.

Standard dosage	400–800 U daily.
Special points	Most multivitamins contain 400 U; activated forms of vitamin D (*e.g.*, calcitriol and dihydrotachysterol) are rarely required.

Estrogen replacement therapy [3]

• This remains the therapy of choice in suitable women due to its beneficial effects on bone density, coronary heart disease, and overall mortality. (*See* Menopause and hypoestrogenism *for further details.*)

Androgen replacement therapy

Standard dosage	*Hypogonadal men*: testosterone enanthate, 200 mg i.m. every 2 weeks; Androderm patch, 5 mg daily.
Contraindications	Contraindicated in patients with prostate cancer; use with caution in men with symptomatic prostatic hypertrophy.
Special points	Rule out prostate cancer with rectal examination and prostate-specific antigen in men aged >50 years before beginning testosterone therapy; no evidence that testosterone therapy improves bone mass in eugonadal men.
Main side effects	Increased libido; priapism with initial dose (very rare).

Nasal calcitonin (Miacalcin)

Standard dosage	One squirt (200 IU) daily, alternating nostrils.
Special points	*Pros*: extensive experience with calcitonin, excellent safety profile, easy administration; may reduce pain associated with vertebral compression fractures. *Cons*: only modest increases in bone density; minimal data on fracture prevention.

Alendronate (Fosamax) [4]

Standard dosage	Treatment of existing osteoporosis: 10 mg daily. Prevention of osteoporosis: 5 mg daily. Correct administration is critical because alendronate is poorly absorbed and can cause esophagitis: take on an empty stomach with a full glass of water; must then remain upright and take nothing by mouth for 30 minutes.
Contraindications	Esophageal lesions, including dysmotility; inability to take alendronate as described above.
Special points	*Pros*: gives greater increases in bone density than estrogen or calcitonin; reduces hip and vertebral fractures in well-controlled prospective trials. *Cons*: effectiveness frequently limited by difficulties in administration; not suitable for bedridden patients; little long-term safety data.

Key references

1. Canalis E. Clinical review 83: mechanisms of glucocorticoid action in bone: implications to glucocorticoid-induced osteoporosis. *J Clin Endocrinol Metab* 1996, **81**:3441–3447.

2. Kleerekoper M: Extensive personal experience: the clinical evaluation and management of osteoporosis. *J Clin Endocrinol Metab* 1995, **80**:757–763.

3. Kiel DP, Felson DT, Anderson JJ, *et al.*: Hip fractures and the use of estrogen in postmenopausal women. *N Engl J Med* 1987, **317**:1169–1174.

4. Black DM, Cummings SR, Karpf DB, *et al.*: Randomised trial of effect of alendronate on risk of fracture in women with existing vertebral fractures. *Lancet* 1996, **348**:1535–1541.

5. Adachi JD, Bensen WG, Brown J, *et al.*: Intermittent etidronate therapy to prevent corticosteroid-induced osteoporosis. *N Engl J Med* 1997, **337**:382–387.

Diagnosis

Symptoms [1]

Primary or secondary amenorrhea: erratic menstruation or oligomenorrhea in earliest phases.

Delayed puberty.

Primary or secondary infertility.

Hot flashes, vaginal dryness and dyspareunia, thin skin, and scalp hair loss: symptoms or estrogen deficiency.

Signs [1]

• Few signs are manifest, particularly shortly after onset of amenorrhea.

Incomplete pubertal maturation: indicating primary amenorrhea.

Atrophic vaginal mucosa.

Short stature, webbed neck: if secondary to Turner's syndrome.

Investigations

For the disorder

Serum follicle-stimulating hormone (FSH) measurement: persistently raised concentration (>40 IU/L); in women with possible incipient ovarian failure (erratic cycles and moderately raised serum FSH [10–40 IU/L]), care must be taken to ensure sampling was not done during a preovulatory gonadotropin surge (risk of false-positive results) [2].

• Absence of menstrual bleeding following progesterone therapy (progesterone-induced withdrawal bleeding) suggests an anovoluntary state. This is *not* an indication of ovarian failure, but is consistent with the diagnosis.

For the underlying cause

Autoimmune profile: including antiovarian antibodies.

Chromosome analysis: to check for aneuploidy (45XO, 47XXX, 46XY).

Laparoscopy: if streak ovaries present, possibility of conception is ruled out; if ovaries "normal," then biopsy unhelpful because conception has been reported in women with no follicles on histology.

For assessment of bone state

Radiography for bone age: if delayed in girls with primary amenorrhea, ultralow-dose estrogen should be used to achieve maximum height (ethinyl estradiol, 2 μg daily).

Bone densiometry: to assess degree of bone loss.

Complications

Infertility: usually permanent, but spontaneous pregnancies have been reported.

Osteoporosis or atraumatic fractures: resulting from estrogen deficiency [3].

Cardiovascular disease: effect of estrogen deficiency on lipid state.

Gonadal neoplasia: in women with gonadal dysgenesis and 46XY karyotype.

Differential diagnosis

Gonadotropin-secreting pituitary adenomas (with elevated FSH) are rare; the distinguishing feature is estrogenization.

Spurious elevation of FSH.

Polycystic ovarian syndrome.

Etiology

Autoimmune: antiovarian antibodies.

Idiopathic premature menopause.

Gonadal dysgenesis: *e.g.*, Turner's syndrome, pure gonadal dysgenesis.

Infection: mumps.

Irradiation or chemotherapy.

Extensive ovarian surgery: for endometriosis or recurrent cysts.

Treated galactosemia.

17α-hydroxylase deficiency (non–salt wasting congenital adrenal hyperplasia).

Epidemiology

• The lifetime risk (before age 40 years) is 0.6%.

• ~5% of cases of anovulation, 10% of amenorrhea, and 2% or oligomenorrhea are due to ovarian failure.

Treatment

Diet and lifestyle

• Advice about increasing dietary calcium and the risk of atraumatic fractures should be given to women with long-standing untreated amenorrhea.

• Women not wishing to conceive should be warned of the small risk of conception.

Pharmacological treatment

• Sex-steroid therapy alleviates symptoms of estrogen deficiency and prevents osteoporosis and cardiovascular disease.

• Estrogen is the active agent; progestogens are used to prevent endometrial neoplasia.

• Standard hormone replacement preparations are not contraceptive; women who wish to avoid the small risk of conception should use low-dose combined oral contraceptive.

Standard dosage	Depends on patient's needs.
Contraindications	Undiagnosed abnormal menstruation.
Special points	*Transdermal estradiol patches:* poor absorption in young women because of thick skin.
Main drug interactions	Anticonvulsants, warfarin, troglitazone.
Main side effects	*Estrogen:* nausea (avoided by slow introduction). *Progestogen:* premenstrual symptoms.

Treatment aims

To avoid general health risks.
To achieve conception.

Other treatments

For infertility [4]

• Ovarian failure represents end-organ failure for which the chances of resumption of ovulation (spontaneous or induced) are small and difficult to predict.

• Several methods of inducing ovulation have been described, but, for most women, in-vitro fertilization with donated oocytes offers the best chance of pregnancy.

• Fostering, adoption, and surrogacy should also be considered.

Prognosis [4]

• The results from one trial of estrogen and human menopausal gonadotropin treatment in 91 women with hypergonadotropic amenorrhea are as follows:
34 patients ovulated.
19 conceptions.
10 miscarriages (53% of conceptions).
1 stillbirth.
8 live births.

Key references

1. Rebar RW, *et al.*: Clinical features of young women with hypergonadotrophic amenorrhea. *Fertil Steril* 1990, **53**:804–810.

2. Cahill DJ, *et al.*: Spurious elevation of follicle-stimulating hormone. *Acta Obstet Gynecol Scand* 1992, **71**:388–389.

3. Davies MC, *et al.*: Bone mineral loss in young women with amenorrhea. *BMJ* 1990, **301**:790–793.

4. Check JH, *et al.*: Ovulation induction and pregnancies in 100 consecutive women with hypergonadotrophic amenorrhea. *Fertil Steril* 1990, **53**:811–817.

Diagnosis

Symptoms

Weight loss: in 90% of patients.

Pain: in 80%.

Anorexia: in 60%.

Lethargy: in 40%.

Pruritus: in 40%.

Diabetes mellitus: in 15%.

Acute pancreatitis: in 5%.

Acute cholangitis: in 2%.

Deep-vein thrombosis: in 1%.

Signs

Jaundice: in 85% of patients, often painless.

Cachexia: in 70%.

Hepatomegaly: in 60%.

Palpable gallbladder: Courvoisier's sign in 40%.

Epigastric mass: in 15%.

Ascites: in 10%.

Abdominal tenderness: in 5%.

Trousseau's syndrome: migratory thrombophlebitis in <1%.

Virchow's node: firm fixed node in left supraclavicular fossa in <1%.

Splenic-vein thrombosis: gastric fundus varices in <1%.

Investigations

Complete blood count: to detect anemia or leukemoid reaction.

Clotting studies: prothrombin time may be prolonged but should correct after vitamin K, 10 mg i.m.

Liver chemistry tests: to confirm "obstructive" jaundice; alkaline phosphatase often elevated and albumin low.

Ultrasonography: to confirm dilated bile ducts and to localize disease (75% accuracy); increased detection of small tumors with endoscopic ultrasonography (90% accuracy).

Endoscopic retrograde cholangiopancreatography: 90%–95% accuracy; brush or pancreatic juice cytology positive in 60%–70% of cases [1].

Contrast-enhanced CT: 80%–90% accuracy [2].

Laparoscopy: to detect small metastatic lesions otherwise missed [3].

Percutaneous biopsy: 80%–93% accuracy; should not be used in patients with potentially resectable tumors.

Serum marker analysis: *e.g.*, CA-19-9, CA-125; may be influenced by jaundice and have poor sensitivity for "early" pancreatic cancer [3].

Complications

• The symptoms and signs are complications in themselves, pruritis.

Massive gastrointestinal hemorrhage: caused by erosion into duodenum.

Gastric outlet obstructions/gastroparesis.

Differential diagnosis [4]

Obstructive jaundice

Bile-duct stones, ampullary tumor, tumors of the biliary tract, benign bile duct strictures, metastatic disease, duodenal cancer.

Hepatic jaundice

Chronic hepatitis, sclerosing cholangitis, congestive heart failure.

Cachexia

Gastric, colorectal, or ovarian cancer.

Other pancreatic disease

Chronic pancreatitis (may coexist), nonfunctioning endocrine tumors, metastases to pancreas.

Etiology

• The cause is largely unknown, but the following may have a role:

Smoking: relative risk, ~2.0 (compared with relative risk of lung cancer, ~20).

Diets high in total or animal fat.

Genetic predisposition (rare): familial colonic and pancreatic cancer, hereditary chronic pancreatitis, familial adenomatous polyposis, Peutz–Jeghers disease, von Hippel–Lindau disease, Lynch II, ataxic telangiectasia.

Long-standing chronic pancreatitis.

Epidemiology

• The incidence varies widely according to country and ethnicity, the highest incidences being in central and northern Europe, North America, and Australasia.

• The incidence standardized by age is 8–11 in 100 000 women and 10–12.5 in 100 000 men.

• Pancreatic cancer occurs less in premenopausal women, but the difference between men and women decreases with age.

• The mean age of presentation is 67 years for women and 63 years for men.

Pathology

• 70%–80% of pancreatic cancers arise in the head of the gland, the rest in the body or tail or diffusely located; <6% are multicentric.

Duct cell origin: 95%.

Acinar cell origin: 2%.

Uncertain histogenesis: 2%.

Nonepithelial tumors: 1%.

Treatment

Diet and lifestyle
• No special precautions are necessary.

Pharmacological treatment

Before surgery or endoscopy
• The following are needed initially before resection or relief of jaundice (surgical or nonsurgical):

Correction of anemia, optimization of nutritional status.

Vitamin K, 10 mg i.m. daily for 3 days.

Crystalloid solution, 1–2 L i.v. for at least 24 hours before any procedure.

Antibiotic cover for any procedure requiring instrumentation of the biliary tract.

For pain
• In up to 30% of patients, the disease is so advanced that conservative management is most appropriate (*i.e.*, pain relief and palliative care).

• NSAIDs may precipitate acute renal failure.

• Patients can be given morphine slow-release orally, i.v., or by epidural infusion using a portable pump; this may cause constipation, nausea, and drowsiness.

Nonpharmacological treatment
• The choice of treatment to relieve jaundice depends on age, tumor burden, and local expertise.

• In-hospital mortality figures are comparable for the different techniques, although endoscopic methods are probably superior.

• Patients who are potential surgical candidates must be appropriately staged (endoscopic ultrasonography, CT, laparoscopy, or angiography), with the help of a radiologist and surgeon.

Surgical resection
• Resection is possible in 10%–15% of patients, with a hospital mortality of 3%–10% [5].

Endoscopic stents
• Stents are most useful in patients with symptoms caused by biliary tract obstruction (*i.e.*, pruritis).

• Expandable metal stents need fewer changes and are recommended for patients with an expected better survival rate [6].

Percutaneous internal stenting
• The complication rate is higher than for endoscopic stents.

Surgical bypass
• Duodenal bypass (gastrojejunostomy) may be used to avoid obstruction from growth into duodenum (10%–15%).

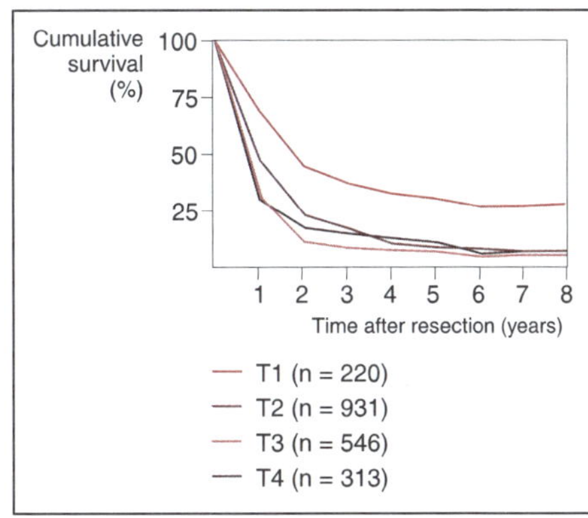

Survival rates after resection for pancreatic cancer stages T1–T4, based on data from the Japanese Pancreatic Cancer Registry.

Key references

1. Zerby AL III, Lee MJ, Brugge WR, Mueller PR: Endoscopic sonography of the upper gastrointestinal tract and pancreas. *AJR Am J Roentgenol* 1996, **166**:45–50.

2. Raptopoulos V, Steer ML, Sheiman RG, *et al.*: The use of helical CT and CT angiography to predict vascular involvement from pancreatic cancer: correlation with findings at surgery. *AJR Am J Roentgencol* 1997, **168**:971–977.

3. Gattani AM, Mandeli J, Bruckner HW: Tumor markers in patients with pancreatic carcinoma. *Cancer* 1996, **78**:57–62.

4. Warshaw AL, Fernandez-del Castillo C: Pancreatic carcinoma. *N Engl J Med* 1992, **326**:455–465.

5. Sperti C, Pasquali C, Piccoli A, Pedrazzoli S: Survival after resection for ductal adenocarcinoma of the pancreas. *Br J Surg* 1996, **83**:625–631.

6. Howden CW, Woods BL: Self-expanding metal stents for palliative treatment of malignant biliary and duodenal stenoses. *Gastrointest Endosc* 1995, **42**:104–105.

7. Ahlgren JD: Chemotherapy for pancreatic carcinoma. *Cancer* 1996, **78(suppl)**:654–663.

Diagnosis

Symptoms

Epigastric pain: sudden onset; radiation into back (relative relief obtained by sitting forward or curling into a "fetal position"); may become increasingly severe.

Anorexia, nausea, vomiting.

Fever: less common.

Signs

Tachycardia, diaphoresis, peritoneal signs, hypotension, tachypnea: suggestive of more severe disease.

Turner's sign, Cullen's sign: ecchymosis on flanks and periumbilically, respectively; rare but classic signs of intra-abdominal hemorrhage secondary to pancreatitis.

Peripheral fat necrosis: uncommon (more frequent in alcohol-induced pancreatitis).

Jaundice: especially in gallstone-induced pancreatitis.

Tetany: secondary to hypocalcemia.

Investigations

Amylase measurement: abnormal serum concentration (*e.g.*, >100 IU/dL); elevated lipase more specific and sensitive (both may be falsely elevated in renal failure).

Serum transaminase, alkaline phosphatase, and bilirubin measurement: elevations raise the possibility of biliary pancreatitis.

Complete blood count: to evaluate for anemia and systemic evidence of inflammation.

Serum creatinine, serum calcium: in toxic patients.

Serum lipids: in patients with unexplained pancreatitis.

Ultrasonography: to determine as soon as possible whether gallstones are causative (~80% sensitive); useful in following course of acute fluid collections (*i.e.*, pseudocysts and abscesses).

Arterial blood gases: in patients with tachypnea, shock; hypoxia indicates poor prognosis.

Contrast-enhanced CT: extent of necrosis accurately determined in 85%–90% of cases; only for clinically severe or suspected "silent" pancreatitis.

Fine-needle aspiration: to sample necrotic tissue for Gram stain and culture to ascertain presence of infected tissue.

Endoscopic retrograde cholangiopancreatography (ERCP): acutely for patients with biliary pancreatitis to remove obstructing stones from the bile duct or ampulla of patients suspected of having traumatic rupture of the pancreatic duct and traumatic pancreatitis. ERCP may aggravate acute pancreatitis and should be performed with caution to ascertain presence of gallstones of choledocholithiasis requiring endoscopic extraction and other causes in biliary tree or pancreas; in severe pancreatitis, disruption of main pancreatic duct suggests significant central necrosis; also indicated in cases of pancreatic trauma.

Complications

• At least one systemic complication occurs in 25%–30% of patients [1].

Cardiovascular, respiratory, and renal failure.

Uremia, hyperglycemia, hypocalcemia.

Disseminated intravascular coagulation, major hematological abnormalities: in 1%–5%.

Acute fluid collections: occur early, in 30%–50% with severe disease and often in patients with mild disease; only 33%–50% of these become clinically significant pseudocysts.

Pancreatic necrosis: clinically significant in 3%–5%; up to 70% are infected necrosis; lesser degrees (<30% of the gland) often occur in clinically mild pancreatitis.

Hemorrhage: splenic artery aneurysm (an uncommon but particularly serious complication).

Treatment

Diet and lifestyle

• During acute illness, patients should not ingest liquids or solids.

• Once pancreatitis has resolved, patients must eat regular meals; prolonged starvation followed by large meals must be avoided; clinical symptoms, rather than serum amylase or lipase levels, should determine when the patient may begin eating.

• Refraining from alcohol must be stressed to patients with alcohol-related pancreatitis.

Pharmacological treatment

• Supportive care involves the following:

Intravenous fluid: crystalloid and colloid (up to 12 L may be sequestered outside of the vascular compartment in the first 24–48 hours).

Pain relief with narcotics such as meperidine (50–100 mg i.m. every 4–6 hours).

Calcium supplementation as needed for patients with hypocalcemia and tetany.

Monitoring and treatment of diabetes mellitus as needed.

Pressor support: if systolic blood pressure <90 mm Hg or renal perfusion inadequate despite fluid replacement.

Antibiotics: for patients with gallstone pancreatitis.

• Glucagon, antiproteases (*e.g.*, aprotinin), somatostatin, are probably of no value in the setting of severe pancreatitis.

Nonpharmacological treatment

Nasogastric suction only for symptomatic relief of nausea and vomiting.

Oxygen administration: if oxygen saturation in arterial blood <90%; large pleural effusions should be drained.

Hemodialysis: for renal failure refractory to fluid replacement and inotropic support.

Endoscopic retrograde cholangiopancreatography and endoscopic sphincterotomy: for patients with severe pancreatitis in whom biliary tract disease (*i.e.*, biliary pancreatitis) is suspected.

Infected necrosis is a strong indication for surgery; patients who fail to improve or who deteriorate over 5–10 days of conservative therapy should undergo CT scanning with needle aspiration of any regions suspicious for infection.

Drainage: for large pseudocysts (>6 cm), persisting in size, expanding, or causing symptoms; repeated percutaneous tapping increases risk of infection and abscess; percutaneous or endoscopic drainage can be used, although surgical internal drainage is preferred in many patients; abscess or infected necrosis must be treated early and aggressively preferably with surgical drainage [3,4].

Treatment aims

To provide supportive care.

To prevent further attacks.

To reduce complications and underlying disorders (*e.g.*, hyperlipidemia).

Prognosis

• The mortality can be as high as 10%, particularly in patients with underlying medical problems or biliary pancreatitis.

• Most patients recover after management in hospital with fluid replacement.

• Recurrent attacks are highly probable if alcohol abuse continues or if hyperlipidemia is not treated.

• Unless cholecystectomy or endoscopic sphincterotomy is performed in patients with gallstones, 10%–40% suffer recurrent attacks [2].

Follow-up and management [5]

• Further attacks can be prevented by laparoscopic cholecystectomy (for gallstones) or endoscopic sphincterotomy, stopping alcohol intake, treating hyperlipidemia and other underlying disorders.

• Follow-up is needed only in patients in whom the cause has not been identified or treated or in those who have had extensive surgery for necrosis.

Key references

1. Bradley EL III: A clinically based classification system for acute pancreatitis. *Arch Surg* 1993, **128**:586–590.

2. Steinberg W: Acute pancreatitis. *N Engl J Med* 1994, **330**:1198–1210.

3. Poston GJ, Williamson RCN: Surgical management of acute pancreatitis. *Br J Surg* 1990, **77**:5–12.

4. Fernandez del Castillo C, Rattner DW, Warshaw AL: Acute pancreatitis. *Lancet* 1993, **342**:475–479.

5. Steinberg WM, *et al.*: Controversies in clinical pancreatology. *Pancreas* 1996, **13**:219–225.

Diagnosis

Symptoms

• Chronic pancreatitis usually evolves over 5–20 years; symptoms, signs, and complications vary during this period [1].

Abdominal pain: in 90% of patients; often worse with eating.

Weight loss: in 80%.

Diarrhea or steatorrhea: in 40%.

Recurrent polyphagia, polydipsia of diabetes mellitus: in 40%.

Acute pancreatitis: in 40%.

Signs

Marked weight loss: in 40% of patients.

Greasy stool: in 10% on rectal examination.

Epigastric mass: in 10%.

Anemia.

Jaundice: suggests biliary stricture from chronic pancreatitis.

Investigations

Serum amylase, lipase measurement: concentrations raised in acute exacerbation of pancreatitis; however, often normal in chronic pancreatitis.

Ultrasonography: for parenchymal changes, duct dilatation, calcification, pseudocysts, ascites; endoscopic ultrasonography is particularly good at rendering a diagnosis of chronic pancreatitis.

Abdominal radiography: pancreatic calcification has high specificity for chronic pancreatitis but limited sensitivity.

72-hour fecal fat collection: excretion of >6 g fecal fat/24 hours in patients ingesting at least 100 g of fat per day in the absence of other causes of malabsorption is highly suggestive of chronic pancreatitis.

Contast-enhanced CT: highly sensitive for calcification; also useful to evaluate for inflammatory mass, ductal dilation, pseudocysts, ascites.

Pancreatic function tests: collection of pancreatic secretions via a nasogastric tube following stimulation by i.v. secretin or cholecystokinin; reduced lipase, bicarbonate, proteolytic enzymes confirms the presence of exocrine pancreatic insufficiency.

Blood glucose measurement and glucose tolerance test: at least 20% of functional parenchyma is required for euglycemia.

Endoscopic retrograde cholangiopancreatography: for changes in main duct and side branches ("minimal change pancreatitis"), stones (calcified and noncalcified) and protein plugs in duct, pseudocysts, fistulas.

Complications

Pancreatic exocrine insufficiency.

Pancreatic endocrine insufficiency.

Duodenal ulcer.

Common bile duct obstruction: secondary biliary cirrhosis (rare).

Duodenal obstruction.

Pseudocysts: pancreatic, intra-abdominal, mediastinal.

Pancreatic ascites.

Pleural effusion.

Pancreatic abscess.

Pancreatic pseudoaneurysm.

Splenic vein thrombosis: gastric fundus varices.

Pancreatic adenocarcinoma.

Narcotic dependency.

Differential diagnosis

Recurrent acute pancreatitis without chronic pancreatitis.

Idiopathic hypertrophy of head of pancreas.

Secondary pancreatic inflammation (duodenal ulceration).

Pancreatic cancer (increased risk in chronic pancreatitis).

Celiac disease.

Bacterial overgrowth of small bowel.

Etiology

Alcohol in 60%–80% of patients.

Obstruction in 10%: ampullary stenosis, pancreas divisum, annular pancreas, stricture (trauma, tumor), irradiation, pancreatitis.

Idiopathic in 10%.

Hereditary (chronic familial pancreatitis).

Malnutrition (tropical pancreatitis).

Cystic fibrosis.

Hypercalcemia.

Epidemiology

• In industrialized countries, the incidence largely depends on alcohol consumption (other factors have a modifying effect): 1–10 in 100 000 population are affected annually.

• Chronic pancreatitis occurs more often in men than in women; the ratios vary from 10 : 1 to 2 : 1.

• The incidence is increasing in all countries.

Treatment

Diet and lifestyle

• Patients should eat regular meals and abstain from alcohol.

• Use of medium-chain triglycerides is occasionally helpful for patients with malnutrition and extensive fat malabsorption.

Pharmacological treatment

• When possible, therapy should be directed at the underlying cause.

For exocrine insufficiency: pancreatic enzyme therapy consisting of 28,000 IU of lipase administered over a 4-hour postprandial period and titrated to control symptoms (steatorrhea, weight loss), concomitant H_2-receptor antagonists (*i.e.*, cimetidine, ranitidine, nizatidine, famotidine) may improve the activity of enzyme supplements [2].

For endocrine insufficiency: insulin therapy is usually required.

For pain

• Self-titration of pancreatic supplements containing proteases may reduce mild or moderate pain (despite the absence of overt steatorrhea) [3].

• Simple analgesics or NSAIDs can be used; however, patients often require management with narcotics.

• Celiac plexus block with steroids can be considered, repeated if necessary.

Nonpharmacological treatment

Main pancreatic duct drainage

• Endoscopic sphincterotomy and stone extraction are suitable in only a few patients; stenting of strictures or pancreatic sphincterotomy may be helpful in select cases [4].

• Pancreaticojejunostomy or transduodenal sphincteroplasty are alternatives to endoscopic treatment; draining alone is usually insufficient in the presence of extensive parenchymal calcification, inflammation, and pain [5–8].

Surgery for pain

• Surgery is a consideration in patients with intractable pain.

• For nondiabetic patients or those having an operation for the first time, treatment should be conservative and only "dominant" disease resected.

• For patients with diabetes or previous surgery, extensive surgery may be required.

• Preservation of the stomach, pylorus, duodenum, and spleen is almost always possible.

Treatment aims

To eliminate the underlying cause.
To relieve pain.
To delay disease progression (duct drainage).
To treat malabsorption.

Prognosis [4]

• The disease is not always progressive.

• Pain and calcification occur after 5–10 years, and both may subsequently regress, but this is unpredictable.

• The long-term survival may be poor: up to 50% of patients die within 7 years.

• Preservation of the quality of life and chronic pain management are the biggest challenges of dealing with this group of patients.

Follow-up and management

• All patients must be followed up to monitor endocrine and exocrine function and pain and to ascertain the need for operation or reoperation.

Key references

1. Steer ML, *et al.*: Chronic pancreatitis. *N Engl J Med* 1995, **332**:1482–1490.

2. Gold EB, Cameron JL: Chronic pancreatitis and pancreatic cancer. *N Engl J Med* 1993, **328**:1485–1486.

3. Ihse I, Permerth J: Enzyme therapy and pancreatic pain. *Acta Chir Scand* 1990, **156**:281–283.

4. Ammann RW, *et al.*: Course of alcoholic chronic pancreatitis. *Gastroenterology* 1996, **111**:224–231.

5. Malfertheiner P, Dominquez-Munoz JE, Büchler M: Diagnosis and staging of chronic pancreatitis. In *Standards in Pancreatic Surgery*. Edited by Beger HG, *et al.* Berlin: Springer-Verlag; 1993:297–313.

6. Nealon WH, Thompson JC: Progressive loss of pancreatic function in chronic pancreatitis is delayed by main pancreatic duct decompression. *Ann Surg* 1993, **217**:458–466.

7. Watanapa P, Williams RC: Pancreatic sphincterotomy and sphincteroplasty. *Gut* 1992, **33**:865–867.

8. Beger HG, Büchler M, Bittner R: The duodenum preserving resection of the head of the pancreas (DPRHP) in patients with chronic pancreatitis and an inflammatory mass in the head. *Acta Chir Scand* 1990, **156**:309–315.

Diagnosis

Symptoms

Panic

Recurrent attacks of severe unprovoked anxiety: starting suddenly, reaching a peak within a few minutes, and lasting at least 20 minutes, with at least four of the following:

Palpitations.
Stomach churning.
Hot or cold flushes.
Shaking or trembling.
Choking or difficulty breathing.
Fear of dying.
Feelings of unreality.
Fear of losing control.
Sweating.
Chest pain or discomfort.
Feeling dizzy, unsteady, lightheaded, or faint.
Paresthesias (numbness or tingling sensations).

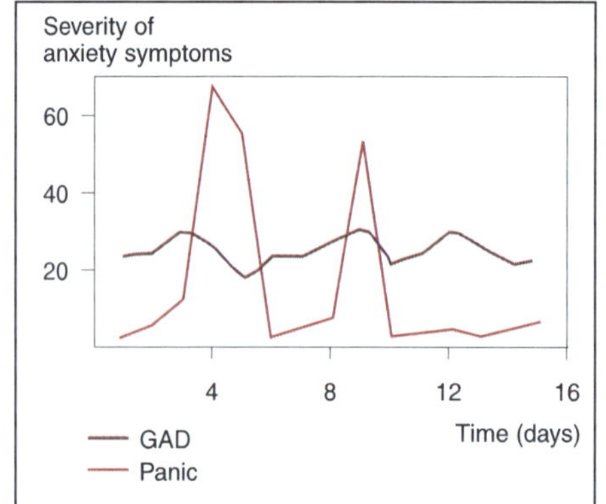

Course of pure panic disorder and pure generalized anxiety disorder (GAD).

Generalized anxiety disorder

Relatively persistent anxiety: at least 6 months, associated with worrying and apprehension about events and other matters that do not justify excessive worry; the anxiety and worry are associated with at least three of the following symptoms:

Restlessness: feeling keyed up or on edge.
Being easily fatigued.
Difficulty concentrating or mind going blank.
Irritability.
Muscle tension.
Sleep disturbance: difficulty falling or staying asleep or restless, unsatisfying sleep.

Signs

Panic

• Physicians seldom see a panic attack in vivo because patients usually feel more secure in a medical setting. Features present on examination include the following:

Fear of having a panic attack.
Reassurance that a heart attack or other physical catastrophe is not imminent.
Wish to be physically examined.
Physiological evidence of anxiety: usually no different from generalized anxiety disorder.

Generalized anxiety disorder

Furrowed brow, hunted look, lack of confidence: evidence of long-standing anxiety.
Tachycardia: pulse 80–100 beats/min.
Sweating.
Dilated pupils.
Observed tremor.

Investigations

• Investigations should not be entered into lightly in patients with anxiety disorders because they may cause hypochondriacal concern and increased anxiety. If, however, anxiety appears for the first time in middle age or later, it may have an organic cause.

Thyroid function tests, complete blood screening, neurological assessment: may sometimes be indicated if anxiety is episodic, diurnally varied, or linked to specific somatic symptoms persistently; epilepsy and pheochromocytoma are rare but remediable causes of anxiety.

Complications

Alcohol dependence: with persistent anxiety (alcohol provides temporary relief).
Hypochondriasis: due to anxiety about bodily complaints.
Agoraphobia: due to persistent severe anxiety, particularly after panics in public places.
Social phobia: due to self-consciousness of anxiety attacks.

Differential diagnosis

Adjustment disorder, pheochromocytoma, thyrotoxicosis: anxiety related to physical disease.

Posttraumatic stress: anxiety due to major unusual event (*e.g.*, rape, major disaster).

Hypochondriasis, somatoform disease: anxiety due entirely to fear of disease or preoccupation with bodily symptoms.

Organic psychoses, schizophrenia, affective psychoses: anxiety due to psychotic symptoms, *e.g.*, delusions or hallucinations.

Agoraphobia, social or simple phobias: anxiety due to specific stimuli, accompanied by avoidance of the stimuli.

Mixed anxiety and depressive disorder, depressive episode: anxiety due to depressive symptoms.

Substance abuse disorders: anxiety due to alcohol or drug abuse.

Etiology

• The immediate cause of anxiety in panic and generalized anxiety disorder is unknown.

• The episodes of anxiety are unfocused or "free-floating" (generalized anxiety disorder) or spontaneous (panic).

• Both disorders are associated with life changes and events and may sometimes be a delayed reaction to the events.

• A genetic component is possible.

Epidemiology

• Panic attacks are most frequent in the 15–24-year age range and have an annual prevalence of ~2% in this group, with ~1% in the total population.

• Generalized anxiety disorder is much more common, with an annual prevalence of ~6%.

• Major depression coexists with generalized anxiety disorder and panic disorder in up to 60% of patients.

Treatment

Diet and lifestyle

• A good square meal is sometimes said to be the best tranquillizer in the world; unsurprisingly therefore, some anxious people resolve their anxiety by overeating and getting fat. This may relieve their anxiety (good studies show that fat people are less anxious generally than thin people) but does not improve their health overall.

• Because anxious people fear trouble around every corner, they often restrict their lifestyles; this is seen to its extreme in the housebound agoraphobic.

Pharmacological treatment

• The patient's view must be taken into account: some refuse drug treatment, others are equally negative about psychological treatment.

• Less effective treatments, *e.g.*, beta-blockade and relaxation training, should be avoided in patients with panic disorder.

• Combined drug and psychological treatments are acceptable and may even be more effective than individual treatments alone.

• Patients must be warned against self-medication with alcohol for anxiety and pain: it provokes worse symptoms in the longer term.

• The duration of treatment should be set in advance, whenever possible.

Standard dosage	Benzodiazepines, *e.g.*, diazepam, 2–10 mg daily; alprazolam, 0.25–6.0 mg daily. Buspirone, 10–60 mg daily. Beta-blockers, *e.g.*, propranolol, 40–120 mg daily. Heterocyclic antidepressants, *e.g.*, clomiprimine, 100–150 mg daily [1]. Specific 5-HT reuptake inhibitors, *e.g.*, paroxetine, 20–60 mg daily [2].
Contraindications	*Benzodiazepines:* caution with previous or present evidence of dependent personality or behavior.
Special points	*Benzodiazepines:* rapid and more effective in short term than other treatments, but tolerance and dependence makes them generally unsuitable for regular treatment; may interfere with success of behavior therapy. *Beta-blockers:* useful if somatic symptoms of anxiety are prominent but not severe (more useful in generalized anxiety disorder). *Heterocyclic antidepressants:* more effective than benzodiazepines when given for more than 4 weeks, but slow onset of antianxiety effects. *Serotonin reuptake inhibitors:* recent trials suggest that these agents are at least as effective and better tolerated than benzodiazepines and tricyclic antidepressants [2].
Main drug interactions	Additive effects with alcohol.
Main side effects	Sedation (not beta-blockers).

Nonpharmacological treatment

Psychological treatments [3]

Relaxation training: of some value (but less than other more intensive therapies) and can be very cheap.

Cognitive therapy: effective in both disorders, may be superior to other psychological treatments; substantially decreases relapse rates after medication taper; aimed at altering unproductive dysfunctional thinking that helps to generate and maintain anxiety; patients with panic disorders learn to decatastrophize thinking, so that attacks are avoided.

Behavior therapy: effective in treating maladaptive behaviors associated with anxiety, mainly by gradual exposure to more adaptive situations.

Combination therapies: cognitive behavior therapy, anxiety management training.

Hypnosis and alternative therapies (yoga, meditation): sometimes useful but not as effective as cognitive and behavior therapies.

Key references

1. Modigh K, Westberg P, Eriksson E: Superiority of clomiprimine over imiprimine in the treatment of panic disorder: a placebo-controlled trial. *J Clin Psychopharmacol* 1992, **12**:251–261.

2. Boyer W: Serotonin uptake inhibitors are superior to imiprimine and alprazolam in alleviating panic attacks: a meta-analysis. *Int Clin Psychopharmacol* 1995, **10**:45–49.

3. Durham RC, Allan T: Psychological treatment of generalized anxiety disorder: a review of the clinical significance in outcome studies since 1980. *Br J Psychiatry* 1993, **163**:19–26.

Diagnosis

Symptoms

Tremor: in ~70% of patients; unilateral and usually noted in hand first; may be seen in jaw or leg. Most often unilateral at onset.

Poverty of movement, difficulty initiating movements and with repetitive movements: *e.g.*, shuffling gait, drooling, difficulty turning in bed, micrographia, softness of voice, constipation.

Rigidity: *e.g.*, poor balance, falls, muscle stiffness, pain.

Signs

Tremor: asymmetric, resting, "pill-rolling" at 3–5 Hz; usually disappears on intention; increased by anxiety; possibly postural tremor at 6–8 Hz.

Rigidity and bradykinesia: stooped, flexed posture; shuffling gait with poor swing of affected arm; cogwheel rigidity, may be enhanced by synkinesis; immobile facies, reduced blink and swallowing rates; rigidity usually noted first in axial muscles, *e.g.*, neck and shoulder.

Investigations

• No tests are available for Parkinson's disease; the diagnosis is based on clinical features alone.

• Investigation is indicated when the diagnosis is in doubt or presentation is atypical, especially in young-onset cases.

Testing of autonomic function: patients with multiple system atrophy may show abnormalities.

MRI: can show abnormal hypointensity in the putamen of patients with multiple system atrophy, can reveal strokes in some patients with parkinsonism.

Copper and ceruloplasmin measurement: in all patients with young-onset or atypical Parkinson's disease.

Complications

Depression, anxiety.

Postural imbalance: with falls and trauma.

Cognitive and psychiatric problems: frontal lobe dysfunction, bradyphrenia, fluctuating confusional state (dementia in 25% of patients); possible overlap with other syndromes, *e.g.*, diffuse Lewy body disease, senile dementia of Lewy body type.

Complications of L-dopa: dyskinesias, motor fluctuation.

Differential diagnosis

Drug-induced parkinsonism: *e.g.*, phenothiazines, butyrophenones; usually symmetrical and reversible.

Essential tremor: bilateral; absent at rest, exacerbated by intention, or maintaining posture; improved by alcohol; possible family history; should be treated with beta-blockers or primidone when necessary.

Multiple system atrophy or progressive supranuclear palsy: symptoms and signs usually symmetrical; tremor less usual; falls frequent; additional features, *e.g.*, pyramidal or cerebellar deficits, gaze palsies, or autonomic involvement including postural hypotension, and bladder dysfunction.

Wilson's disease: 40% present with neurological features, mainly parkinsonism and hypokinetic dysarthria; liver cirrhosis or psychiatric disease also occur; Kayser–Fleischer rings visible by slit lamp in most; low serum ceruloplasmin, high urinary copper; liver biopsy shows high copper and evidence of liver cell damage; should be treated with penicillamine.

Toxin-induced parkinsonism (*e.g.*, carbon monoxide).

Mitochondrial disorders; abnormal movements, usually dystonia or chorea.

Etiology [1]

• >80% dopamine depletion occurs in the striatum at presentation; neurons are lost in the substantia nigra (dopaminergic), locus caeruleus (noradrenergic), and substantia innominata (cholinergic). Intracytoplasmic inclusions, Lewy bodies, are found in surviving neurons.

• The cause of Parkinson's disease is not known, but environmental toxins and genetic susceptibility may play a role alone or in combination.

Epidemiology

• The incidence is ~20 in 100 000, with an overall prevalence of 150 in 100 000 (500 in 100 000 for those aged >50 years).

• The male : female ratio is equal.

• Younger-onset patients tend to develop more motor fluctuations, and older-onset patients have a much higher incidence of associated dementia.

Treatment

Diet and lifestyle

• Maintaining activity is important: a multidisciplinary approach, with physical therapy, occupational therapy, speech therapy, and social work contact is helpful; patients and caregivers may need support.

• Dietary protein should be reduced during the day; a main meal at night allows more predictable absorption of L-dopa.

Pharmacological treatment [2]

At diagnosis

• Most neurologists advocate selegiline.

Standard dosage	Selegiline (Eldepryl), 5 mg twice daily.
Contraindications	Possible interaction with tricyclic antidepressants or 5-HT reuptake inhibitors.
Special points	May delay requirement for L-dopa, although mechanism of action uncertain; some symptomatic benefit.
Main drug interactions	Concurrent L-dopa dose may need to be decreased 20%–50%; should not be administered with tricyclic antidepressants.
Main side effects	Gastrointestinal upset, hypotension, confusion.

At review

• Treatment is essentially symptomatic.

• L-Dopa is prescribed when clinical features interfere with life, or postural instability is noted on examination.

• Tremor and bradykinesia respond well, postural instability less well.

• The use of controlled-release L-dopa offers some improvement in patients with medium to advanced disease, especially in decreasing "off time"; transition to these drugs should be gradual because the bioavailability is different from that of the standard preparations; some neurologists use controlled-release preparations early to provide a more "physiological" prolonged drug exposure to dopaminergic neurons.

• Dopaminergic agonists may be used alone (early) or in combination with L-dopa.

Standard dosage	L-Dopa with a dopa decarboxylase inhibitor, initially at low dose and frequency, *e.g.*, 100 mg twice or 3 times daily, increased as necessary. Dopaminergic agonists, *e.g.*, bromocriptine or pergolide in low doses initially and built up gradually.
Contraindications	*L-Dopa:* closed angle glaucoma. *Dopaminergic agents:* hypotension, cardiac arrhythmias.
Special points	*L-Dopa:* generally, frequent small doses (up to every 2–3 hours) are better than infrequent large doses. *Dopaminergic agents:* may be used alone, but tolerance to these drugs develops quickly.
Main drug interactions	*Dopaminergic agents:* combination with L-dopa may improve control.
Main side effects	*L-Dopa:* gastrointestinal upset, postural hypotension, confusion, hallucination, dyskinesias and dystonia; neuropsychiatric side effects best treated by dose modification, but clozapine or olanzapine may be used (possible development of agranulocytosis). *Dopaminergic agents:* hypotension, hallucinations, confusion, gastrointestinal symptoms.

• Amantidine or anticholinergics may be useful adjunctive medications for tremor.

Treatment aims

To improve functional disability.

To avoid or minimize drug-related side effects.

To treat fluctuations when present.

Other treatments

• Posteroventral pallidotomy may be useful in selected patients to improve dyskinesias and motor fluctuations.

Prognosis

• Parkinson's disease progresses at variable rates.

• Patients with dementia have a significantly worse prognosis.

Follow-up and management

• The need for symptomatic treatment should be assessed.

• Correct use and titration of drugs should be monitored.

• Medical and support needs should be assessed.

Key references

1. Calne DB: Treatment of Parkinson's disease. *N Engl J Med* 1993, **329**:1021–1027.

2. Marsden CD: Parkinson's disease. *J Neurol Neurosurg Psychiatry* 1994, **57**:672–681.

Diagnosis

Symptoms

- Often no symptoms are manifest.

Mild feverish illness: in children.

Mild feverish illness with arthralgia or arthritis: in adults.

Symptoms of an aplastic crisis: in patients with hemolytic anemias or occasionally normal people; onset usually acute but self-limiting.

Symptoms of persistent severe anemia: in immunosuppressed patients.

Signs

- The illness, when accompanied by a rash, is known as erythema infectiosum, fifth disease, or slapped-cheek syndrome.

Rash: usually seen in children; appears on cheeks, giving slapped-cheek appearance; lasts 1 week; recurs for several months on exposure to sun or wind; variable but often reticular maculopapular rash may also develop on arms and legs but rarely affects palms or soles.

Lymph-node enlargement: in adults.

Arthralgia or arthritis: often involving wrists and knees in adults; can occur without rash; usually last 2–4 weeks, occasionally longer.

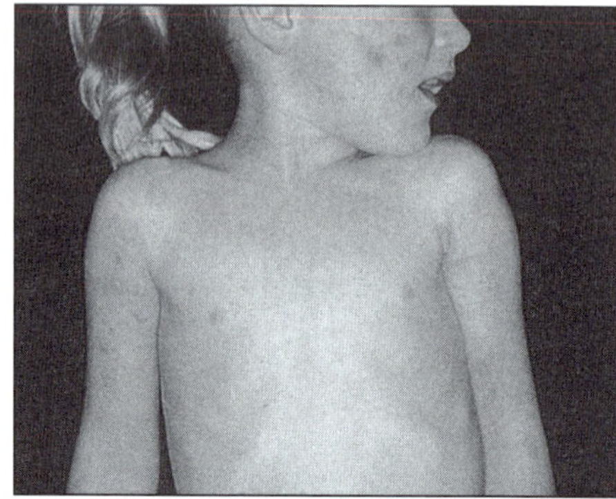

Slapped-cheek appearance of parvovirus B19 infection and reticular rash on arms. (*See* Color Plate.)

Investigations

Serology: IgM specific to parvovirus B19 manifest in early illness; parvovirus B19 IgG antibody develops early in illness and falls within 1–2 months.

Complications

Aplastic crisis.

Fetal anemia, hydrops fetalis, and death: especially during second trimester, although effect on pregnancy uncertain; about one-third of pregnant women with primary infection transmit it to fetus.

Treatment

Diet and lifestyle

• People known to be infected should avoid contact with pregnant women.

Pharmacological treatment

Analgesics, *e.g.*, acetaminophen.

NSAIDs for reactive arthralgia.

General references

Brown KE, Young NS: Parvovirus B19 in human disease. *Am Rev Med* 1997, **48**:59–67.

Gay NJ, *et al.*: Age specific antibody prevalence to parvovirus B19: how many women are infected in pregnancy? *Comm Dis Rep* 1994, **4**:R104–R107.

Levy R, Waissman A, Blomberg G, Hagay ZJ: Infection by parvovirus B19 during pregnancy: a review. *Obstet Gynecol Surv* 1997, **52**:254–259.

Pattison JR: Human parvovirus B19. *BMJ* 1994, **308**:149–150.

Diagnosis

Symptoms

Pericarditis

Mild to severe precordial pain: on inspiration or worse on inspiration; may radiate to neck and shoulders; worse on coughing, swallowing, or sneezing; improved by leaning forward.

Dyspnea, nausea.

Tamponade

Precordial discomfort: occasionally, due to large effusions.

Cough, hoarseness, tachypnea, dysphagia: due to pressure.

Malaise, cyanosis, dyspnea, sweating, anxiety, hypotension: rapidly developing.

Signs

Pericarditis

Fever.

Pericardial, often pleuropericardial, coarse rub: best heard at left sternal edge with patient leaning forward; may come and go over minutes to hours, may decrease with development of effusion.

Initially normal venous pressure.

Tamponade

Tachycardia: nearly always present.

Low blood and pulse pressures.

Pulsus paradoxus: pulse may disappear on inspiration; may also occur in asthma.

Raised venous pressure: with prominent "y" descent and no "x" descent; may increase on inspiration [1].

Investigations

• For any pericardial disease, the underlying cause must always be sought.

Pericarditis

Complete blood count, ESR and urine and electrolyte measurement.

Antistreptolysin O titer, antineutrophil factor, rheumatoid factor analysis.

Cardiac enzyme tests: enzymes may be normal or increase, but creatinine phosphokinase MB probably not significantly increased unless accompanying myocarditis.

Paired viral antibody screening: increase in neutralizing antibodies (up to 4 times) within 3-4 weeks of onset.

Mantoux test.

ECG: changes throughout all leads; raised ST segment, PR depression, inverted T waves only in some patients, pericardial effusion (low-voltage QRS and T wave in large effusions), electrical alternans (caused by heart swinging about).

Chest radiography: normal unless pericardial fluid >250 mL; cardiac contour may be globular, with no congestion in lungs.

Tamponade

Echocardiography: essential in any patient in whom pericardial fluid is suspected (*e.g.*, cardiomegaly on chest radiography with hypotension); right ventricular collapse characteristic of tamponade.

Complications

Relapsing or constrictive pericarditis, pericardial effusion and tamponade: complications of pericarditis.

Hypotension, renal failure: complications of tamponade.

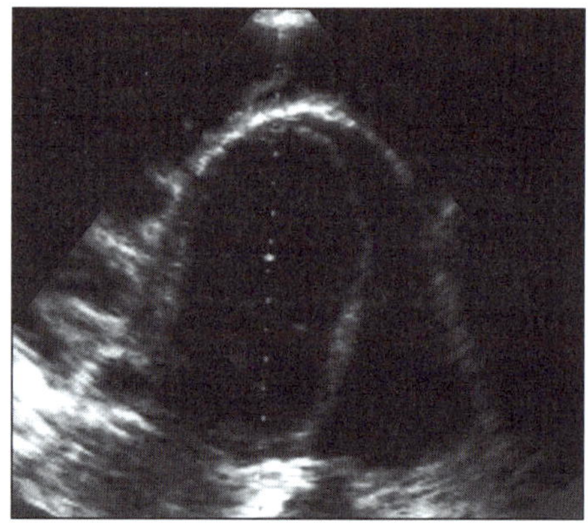

Pericardial space containing fluid (*top center*); bright pericardium (*mid center*); left ventricle (*lower center*); fibrinous strands in pericardial fluid (*lower left*).

Treatment

Diet and lifestyle

- No special dietary precautions are necessary.

- Overactivity is contraindicated until the symptoms have resolved.

Pharmacological treatment

- Drugs are used for pericarditis to decrease inflammation and treat the underlying cause.

- Aspirin usually settles both pain and fever; indomethacin is particularly useful in preventing recurrence; a short course of steroids may be needed.

- Specific treatment is needed for any related condition.

Standard dosage	Aspirin, 300–600 mg every 3–4 hours. Indomethacin, 50–200 mg in divided doses (adults). Prednisolone, 30 mg for 2–3 weeks, then reduced depending on symptoms.
Contraindications	*Aspirin:* peptic ulceration, hypersensitivity. *Indomethacin:* peptic ulceration. *Prednisolone:* osteoporosis, history of gastrointestinal symptoms, tuberculosis, pregnancy. Caution in renal or hepatic impairment.
Main drug interactions	*All:* warfarin. *Indomethacin:* aspirin, steroids. *Prednisolone:* aspirin.
Main side effects	*Aspirin:* dyspepsia. *Indomethacin:* gastrointestinal problems, including bleeding. *Prednisolone:* hypertension, peripheral edema, potassium loss, hyperglycemia.

Nonpharmacological treatment

- For tamponade, pericardial aspiration may be life-saving with large effusions.

- As much fluid as possible should be drained; blood-stained effusions usually signify malignancy, but all samples should be sent for cytology and bacteriology.

- Recurrent effusions may need balloon pericardotomy or surgical drainage.

- Chemotherapy can be started if malignant disease has been confirmed.

Treatment aims

To prevent adverse hemodynamic changes of tamponade.

To diagnose and treat underlying condition.

Prognosis

- Prognosis depends on the underlying condition: it is good for viral pericarditis but poor for malignant pericardial effusion [2,3].
- Patients with viral pericarditis usually recover completely in 1–2 weeks.

Follow-up and management

- Regular echocardiographic follow-up is necessary for pericardial effusions.

Key references

1. Fowler NO: Cardiac tamponade. A clinical or an echocardiographic diagnosis. *Circulation* 1993, **87**:1738–1741.

2. Friman G, Fohlman J: The epidemiology of viral heart disease. *Scand J Infect Dis* 1993, **88**:7–10.

3. Spodick DH: Pericarditis in systemic diseases. *Cardiol Clin* 1990, **8**:709–716.

Diagnosis

Definition [1]

• Personality disorders are dysfunctional patterns of thinking and behavior that reflect persistent ways of relating to self and others, which deviate markedly from the norm and are invariably accompanied by impairment of social role or major subjective distress.

•The specific personality disorders that appear in adolescence can be broadly categorized into three main areas:

Flamboyant: histrionic, emotionally unstable (borderline or impulsive), dissocial.

Eccentric: paranoid/schizoid.

Fearful: anancastic, anxious/avoidant, dependent.

• Others are acquired later in life and arise as a result of organic insult, psychiatric illness, or catastrophic stress.

Symptoms and signs

Suspicion, oversensitivity, querulousness, unforgiving: paranoid.

Emotional coldness, solitude, social insensitivity: schizoid.

Impulsiveness, emotional instability, poor self-control: emotionally unstable (impulsive or borderline).

Obsessions, perfectionism, rigidity, self-doubt: anancastic.

Social sensitivity, apprehension, feelings of social inferiority: anxious, avoidant.

Reliance on others, subordination of own needs, fear of abandonment: dependent.

Callousness, irresponsibility, blaming others, aggressiveness: dissocial.

Dramatics, suggestibility, seeking center stage, shallowness: histrionic.

Investigations

History: should be corroborated with other sources if possible (with patient's permission): personality characteristics of parents, early development, adverse life events and upbringing; school/social services (history of neglect, impoverishment, or abuse); legal sources (*e.g.*, probation office); spouse, cohabitee (partners may also have personality disorders); employer.

Standardized questionnaires: usually time-consuming but highly reliable; patients are asked tightly worded questions covering specific areas of personal and social function in order to avoid biased judgement on the part of the therapist; this is particularly important in the case of disorders with antisocial characteristics.

Munich Checklist for ICD-10: a good alternative [2].

EEG: finding may be abnormal in patients with dissocial disorder.

Complications

High suicide rate.

Self-harming behavior: may lead to frequent presentations in a wide variety of health care settings, *e.g.*, emergency departments, medical wards.

Alcohol addiction and drug abuse.

Harm to others: *e.g.*, violent assault or sexual abuse of children.

Differential diagnosis

Comorbidity with mental illness (AXIS I): cross-sectional studies show that ~40% of patients also manifest AXIS I disorders when they present in clinical settings.

Schizotypal disorder: frequently overlaps with borderline and schizoid disorders.

Prodromal or residual phase of schizophrenia.

Affective disorders: hypomania may mimic dissocial disorder; depression is frequent in patients suffering from borderline disorder.

Etiology

Genetic inheritance.

Abnormal developmental biology.

Failure to negotiate critical stages of emotional development.

Childhood trauma: sexual abuse is a more frequent feature in borderline disorders.

Social theories: abnormal parenting or lack of an appropriate role model.

Epidemiology

• Schizoid personality disorder appears to be rare because sufferers avoid society.

• The prevalence in the general population is 2%–6%; in primary care settings, 15%–34%; in psychiatric outpatients, 20%–40%; in psychiatric inpatients, 40%–60%; in forensic settings, 50%–90%.

Treatment

Diet and lifestyle

• No special precautions are necessary.

Pharmacological treatment [3]

• All drugs must be used with caution because of the dangers of overdose and abuse.

• Neuroleptics, *e.g.*, thioridazine or haloperidol in low doses, can alleviate symptoms, *e.g.*, hostility, anger, suspiciousness, and depressed mood, in borderline or dissocial conditions.

• Monoamine oxidase inhibitors may be useful in borderline conditions.

• Long-term use of benzodiazepines must be avoided because of the probability of addiction; they may cause paradoxical disinhibition.

• Mood stabilizers (lithium and carbamazepine) are most useful if there is evidence of mood swings or family history of affective disorder.

Nonpharmacological treatment

Psychotherapy
• Interpretative psychotherapies for flamboyant disorders are effective in mild to moderate conditions.

Behavior or cognitive therapy
• This is being developed but is not widely available; it is similar to therapies used in the treatment of depression and anxiety.

Supportive therapy
• This includes social support and is most useful for patients with severe disruptive personality disorders.

• Patients are encouraged to find practical solutions to present problems, *e.g.*, relationship difficulties, accommodation, other personal needs.

Group therapy
• Group therapy may help patients with some forms of personality disorders.

• It includes the use of therapeutic communities.

Treatment aims

To alleviate subjective distress and reduce impact of dysfunctional behavior.

Prognosis [4]

• Prognosis is usually poor in severely affected patients, but most improve with age (4th or 5th decade); improvement is more noticeable for the flamboyant group.

• The outcome is invariably worse when comorbid mental illness is present.

• Good prognostic features include intelligence and the presence of positive adaptive traits, *e.g.*, candor and introspectiveness.

Follow-up and management

• No treatment has universally proven effectiveness; the most useful approach is based on long-term supportive contact and crisis intervention when needed.

• Patients tend to arouse strong feelings in therapists; staff working in crisis situations particularly need regular support.

Danger

• Most patients with personality disorders are no more dangerous than unaffected people.

• A few people with severe disorders, especially those with paranoid or dissocial traits, can exhibit considerable aggression toward others; safety and surveillance is paramount in such circumstances.

• In community settings, the police should be involved to make the situation safe.

• Admission to secure units or forensic facilities may be needed.

Key references

1. Anonymous: *ICD-10 Classification of Mental and Behavioural Disorders. Clinical Descriptions and Diagnostic Guidelines.* Geneva: World Health Organization; 1992.

2. Bronisch T, *et al.*: The Munich diagnostic checklist for the assessment of DSM–III-R personality disorders for use in routine clinical care and research. *Eur Arch Psychiatry Clin Neurosci* 1992, **242**:77–81.

3. Stein G: Drug treatment of personality disorders. *Br J Psychiatry* 1992, **166**:67–84.

4. Stone M: Long term outcome in personality disorders. *Br J Psychiatry* 1993, **162**:299–313.

Diagnosis

Symptoms

Sore throat: with difficulty swallowing.
Concurrent coryza, laryngitis, productive cough: suggesting viral cause.
Malaise, fever, headache: common.

Signs

General

Injected mucous membranes of pharynx, tonsils, conjunctivae, and tympanic membranes.
Enlarged tonsils: sometimes with exudates.
Enlarged cervical lymph nodes.

Streptococcal infection

Grey exudates in tonsillar follicles.
Enlarged injected tonsillar and peritonsillar area.
Coated tongue with fetor.
Enlarged, tender cervical nodes.
Occasional meningismus.
Diffuse punctate erythema, flushed cheeks, circumoral pallor, reddened mucous membrane, white then red strawberry tongue: signs of scarlet fever.

Infectious mononucleosis

Prolonged fever: often for 10–14 days.
Nasal voice/"fish mouth" breathing.
Enlarged lymph nodes and splenomegaly.
Palatal petechiae and clean tongue.
Enlarged tonsils: sometimes almost meeting in middle, with confluent white exudates.
Faint maculopapular rash.

Coxsackie A virus

5–10 small aphthoid ulcers: scattered over oral cavity.
Firm vesicular lesions: along sides of fingers and on feet (usually few).
Papular lesions: especially on feet and lower legs, occasionally up to buttocks.

Diphtheria

Toxic, listless, tachycardia due to myocarditis: fever usually low-grade or nonexistent.
Adherent whitish membrane: spreading from tonsils to oropharynx or oral cavity.
Enlarged anterior cervical lymph nodes: with surrounding edema.

Investigations

Throat swab: to check for streptococcal infection and diphtheria; usually not needed for viral infections. Rapid streptococcal test.
Differential leukocyte count: elevated neutrophil leukocytosis indicates streptococcal infection; elevated, many atypical mononuclear cells indicate infectious mononucleosis.
Serology: for Epstein–Barr virus, mycoplasma.

Complications

Peritonsillar abscess, reactive phenomena (rheumatic fever, glomerulonephritis, erythema nodosum, Henoch–Schönlein purpura): with streptococcal infection.
Respiratory obstruction, hepatitis, splenic rupture: with infectious mononucleosis.
Nerve palsies, myocarditis: with diphtheria.
Erythema multiforme: with *Mycoplasma pneumoniae* infection.

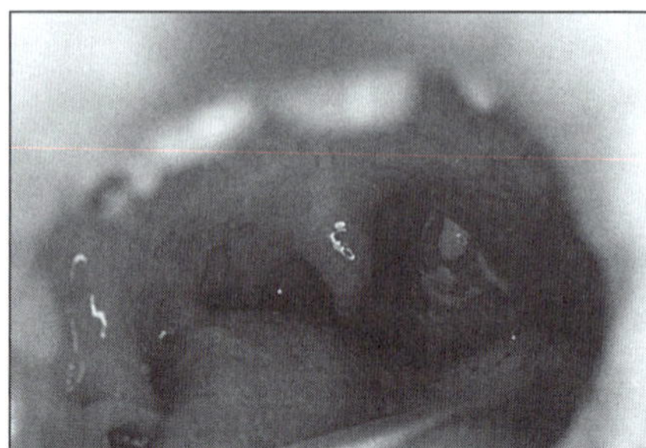
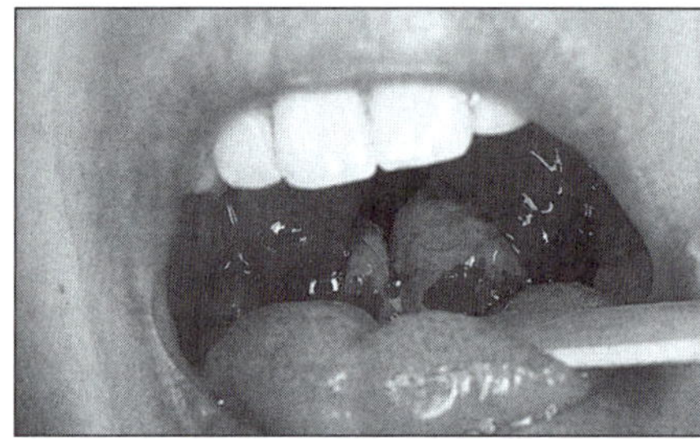

Streptococcal follicular tonsillar exudates (*top*) and confluent exudates (*bottom*) in infectious mononucleosis. (*See* Color Plates.)

Differential diagnosis

• Differential diagnosis depends on the underlying cause.

Etiology [1]

• Causes include the following:

Pharyngitis with nonspecific features
Viral infection, especially adenoviruses, enteroviruses, influenza or parainfluenza virus, Epstein–Barr virus, coronavirus. Beta-hemolytic *Streptococcus pyogenes* group A, C, or G.
M. pneumoniae, Corynebacterium diphtheriae, Neisseria gonorrhoeae.

Pharyngitis with clinically recognizable features
Streptococcus pyogenes infection: cause of follicular tonsillitis, scarlet fever.
Epstein–Barr virus infection: cause of infectious mononucleosis.
Coxsackievirus infection: cause of hand, foot, and mouth disease (A16), herpangina (A).
C. diphtheriae infection: cause of diphtheria.

Epidemiology

• Very common disease of adults and children.

• Adenoviral infection is the most common viral type identified in children with respiratory illnesses, which are more prevalent in crowded conditions.

• Enteroviral infection usually occurs in late summer or early autumn, with one or two types dominating (out of >70).

• Some influenza virus activity is usual each winter, with some larger outbreaks.

• Epstein–Barr virus circulates throughout childhood but is usually only manifest symptomatically in teenagers and young adults.

• Streptococcal infection occurs in late winter and early spring, especially in school children.

• Very few cases of diphtheria occur in the United States each year.

Treatment

Diet and lifestyle

• Infants should be breast-fed and subsequently provided with adequate nutrition throughout childhood.

• Respiratory secretions must be disposed of hygienically.

Pharmacological treatment [2]

• Immunization should be given as nationally recommended: *e.g.*, against diphtheria, influenza A.

• Symptomatic treatment is indicated for presumed viral infections: *e.g.*, throat lozenges, acetaminophen.

Antibiotics

• Penicillins are effective against streptococcal and diphtherial infections [3,4].

Standard dosage	Penicillin G, 1.2 MU i.m. Phenoxymethylpenicillin, 500 mg orally 6-hourly.
Contraindications	Hypersensitivity.
Special points	Erythromycin, 250 mg 6-hourly, or new macrolides are other options.
Main drug interactions	None.
Main side effects	Sensitivity reactions, diarrhea.

Antitoxin

• Antitoxin should be given immediately on clinical suspicion of diphtheria.

Standard dosage	Antitoxin 20 000–100 000 units i.v. (depending on disease severity).
Contraindications	Hypersensitivity (epinephrine should be available).
Special points	Test dose is needed before full dose because of equine origin of antitoxin.
Main drug interactions	None.
Main side effects	Sensitivity reactions, including serum sickness.

Treatment aims

To provide symptomatic relief.
To reduce infectivity.
To prevent rheumatic fever (in streptococcal infections).
To neutralize circulating toxins of diphtheria promptly.

Other treatments

Drainage of peritonsillar abscess, indicated by marked inferior and posterior displacement of tonsil.
Tracheostomy for respiratory obstruction.
Tonsillectomy in children with recurrent tonsillitis that disrupts schooling.

Prognosis

• Full rapid recovery is usual.
• Occasionally, patients suffer from post-viral fatigue, especially after influenza, Epstein–Barr, or enteroviral infections.
• Mortality from diphtheria is 5%–10%; survivors usually recover completely.

Follow-up and management

• Patients who have apparently recovered from streptococcal tonsillitis may continue to have enlarged and tender cervical nodes that subsequently spread infection as cellulitis or septicemia.
• Patients with diphtheria should be followed up after 2–6 weeks for late nerve palsies and myocarditis.

Notification

• Diphtheria and scarlet fever are legally notifiable diseases in the United States.

Key references

1. McIsaac WJ, Gael V, Slaughter PM, *et al.*: Reconsidering sore throats: problems with current clinical practice. *Can Fam Physician* 1997, **43**:485–493.

2. Carroll K, Reimer L: Microbiology and laboratory diagnosis of upper respiratory infections. *Clin Infect Dis* 1996, **23**:442–448.

3. Kline JA, Runge JW: Streptococcal pharyngitis: a review of pathophysiology, diagnosis, and management. *J Emerg Med* 1994, **12**:665–680.

4. Blumer JL, Goldfarb J: Meta-analysis in the evaluation of treatment for streptococcal pharyngitis: a review. *Clin Ther* 1994, **16**:604–620.

Diagnosis

Symptoms

Palpable swelling in the soft tissue overlying the sacrococcygeal junction.

Pain.

Drainage.

Fevers, symptoms of systemic infection: unusual.

Signs

Midline localized inflammation, most commonly in the region internatal or gluteal cleft.

Possible abscess formation.

Sinus tract: directed cephalad.

Absence of perianal inflammation or other signs of a perianal fistula.

Investigations

Careful digital rectal examination and if necessary anoscopy: to exclude perianal inflammation or communication with the anorectum.

Complications

Chronic abscess.

Persistent or recurrent cellulitis.

Sepsis and/or osteomyelitis: rare.

Squamous cell carcinoma: rare.

Differential diagnosis

Perianal fistula/abscess.

Hidradenitis suppurativa.

Carbuncle or furuncle.

Osteomyelitis.

Etiology

Acquired process from torsion on hair growing in the gluteal cleft resulting in folliculitis and sinus formation.

• Risk factors include family predisposition, prolonged sitting, obesity.

Epidemiology

• Incidence is 26 cases per 100 000.

• It is most common in the third decade and rarely occurs preadolescence.

• Male:female ratio is 3:1.

Treatment

Diet and lifestyle

• Patients with recurrent problems benefit from shaving the hairs in the sacrococcygeal region.

Pharmacological treatment

Cellulitis should be treated with a course of antibiotics that will cover *Staphylococcus* and *Bacteroides* spp. (*e.g.*, Augmentin).

Standard dosage	Augmentin, 500 mg every 8 hours for 10 days.
Contraindications	Penicillin allergy.
Main side effects	Antibiotic-related diarrhea.

Treatment aims

To relieve pain.

To control infection.

To prevent recurrence.

Other treatments

• Patients presenting with tender, localized nodules are best treated by surgical drainage rather than antibiotics.

• Definitive surgical management with resection of midline holes and pits that sustain abscesses is necessary in patients with recurrent disease.

• Sclerosing therapy is occasionally used to manage recurrent disease.

Prognosis

• 80% of patients are successfully treated long-term with simple drainage procedures.

Follow-up and management

• As noted earlier, removal of hair by shaving the sacrococcygeal region of the natal cleft probably reduces the recurrence of the disease.

General references

Armstrong JH, Barcia PJ: Pilonidal sinus disease: the conservative approach. *Arch Surg* 1994, **129**:914–918.

Barnett JL, Raper SE: Anorectal disease. In *Textbook of Gastroenterology*, edn 2. Edited by Yamada T. Philadelphia: JB Lippincott Co; 1995:2045–2049.

Sebastian MW: Pilonidal cysts and sinuses. In *Textbook of Surgery*, edn 15. Edited by Sabiston DC, Jr. Philadelphia: WB Saunders; 1996:1330–1334.

Diagnosis

Symptoms

• Platelet disorders may be manifest by bleeding or discovered incidentally in an otherwise asymptomatic patient.

Bruising.

Bleeding: usually mucosal, *e.g.*, gingival, nasal, gastrointestinal, menorrhagic; occasionally retinal (loss of vision) or intracranial (headache); after surgical procedures.

Deafness: in some familial disorders.

Signs

Petechiae, purpura, bruises.

Retinal hemorrhages.

Thrombosis and skin microinfarcts: in thrombotic thrombocytopenic purpura.

Capillary bleeding.

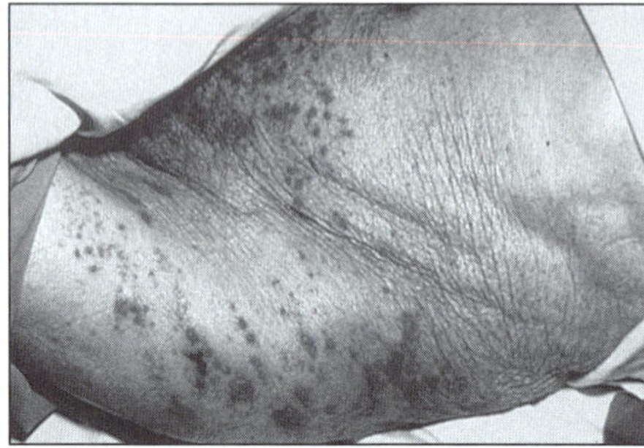

Purpura due to thrombocytopenia. (*See* Color Plate.)

Investigations

• Initial investigations are used to identify primary platelet disorder and to exclude von Willebrand's disease in patients with a strong family history and lifelong bleeding disorder.

Complete blood count: platelet count and mean platelet volume, to exclude other hematological disease and pseudothrombocytopenia due to clumping or EDTA (ethylene-diaminetetra-acetic acid)-induced aggregation.

Microscopic examination of film: for platelet morphology, to detect erythrocyte or leukocyte abnormality.

Coagulation screening: to exclude primary coagulopathy

Biochemistry profiles: to identify renal or hepatic disease.

Platelet function tests: bleeding time, if prolonged, suggests platelet function disorder or von Willebrand's disease (drugs that affect platelet function, *e.g.*, aspirin, should be avoided for 10 days before testing); spontaneous in vitro aggregation and response to ADP (adenosine diphosphate), collagen, and ristocetin should be recorded; if abnormal, response to other agonists (*e.g.*, epinephrine, thrombin, arachidonate) should be assessed; release reaction of radiolabeled 5-HT (5-hydroxytryptamine); measurement of platelet adenine nucleotides; hereditary and some acquired platelet disorders have characteristic aggregation responses.

Bone-marrow aspiration and biopsy: in most patients with thrombocytopenia, to assess number and structure of megakaryocytes and bone-marrow function.

Platelet serology: in posttransfusion purpura and in neonates with alloimmune thrombo-cytopenia, to identify specific antiplatelet antigen antibodies.

Platelet-associated immunoglobulin measurement: nonspecific, often increases in immune thrombocytopenias.

Flow cytometry: to quantify platelet membrane glycoproteins, using monoclonal antibodies to detect hereditary disorders.

Complications

Iron-deficiency anemia: caused by menorrhagia or recurrent epistaxis or gastrointestinal bleeding.

Neurological impairment or death: caused by intracranial bleeding.

Differential diagnosis

Bleeding disorders
Von Willebrand's disease.
Fibrinogen disorders.

Purpura
Vasculitis: *e.g.*, Schönlein-Henoch syndrome.
Amyloid.
Senile purpura.
Scurvy.
Steroid treatment.
Collagen disorders (*e.g.*, Ehlers–Danlos syndrome).
Hereditary hemorrhagic telangiectasia (does not cause purpura but can lead to low platelet count in extreme forms).

Etiology [1]

Decreased production
Bone-marrow failure: leukemia, metastatic tumor, idiopathic aplasia, infiltration, abnormal production, myelodysplasia, aplastic anemia, drugs (predictable, *e.g.*, cytotoxic drugs, or idiosyncratic reactions).

Increased consumption
Immune: autoimmune (idiopathic, post-viral, HIV, associated with other autoimmune disorders), alloimmune against platelet-specific antigens, *e.g.*, HPA-1.
Drugs: *e.g.*, quinine, heparin, sulfonamides, rifampin.
Coagulopathy: disseminated intravascular coagulation, thrombotic thrombocytopenic purpura.
Hypersplenism and splenomegaly.

Hereditary
Platelet membrane glycoprotein abnormal-ities, *e.g.*, Bernard–Soulier and Glanzmann's diseases.
Platelet storage pool abnormalities.
Other abnormalities, *e.g.*, May–Hegglin anomaly.

Acquired
Platelet storage pool defects: *e.g.*, aspirin, uremia, ethanol, cirrhosis, myeloprolifer-ative disorders.

Epidemiology

• Acquired disorders of platelet function are common and are associated with disorders such as chronic renal failure or the ingestion of aspirin.

• Chronic idiopathic thrombocytopenic purpura is relatively common (one group suggests that 0.18% of patients admitted to hospital in a 10-year period had the disease).

Treatment

Diet and lifestyle

- Patients should avoid trauma and contact sports.

Pharmacological treatment

For immune thrombocytopenia

- In children, the onset is usually acute and often follows a viral infection; spontaneous recovery is common, and treatment is given to those with severe or life-threatening bleeding to elevate the platelet count. In adults, the onset is more insidious, and it almost never remits spontaneously.

Standard dosage	*Children:* immunoglobulin, 0.4 g/kg i.v.daily (in 4–6 hours) for 5 days (sometimes 1.0 g/kg daily for 2 days); or prednisone 1 mg/kg. *Adults:* prednisone, 1 mg/kg daily initially until maximum response, then tapered off.
Contraindications	*Prednisone:* active infection, diabetes mellitus.
Main drug interactions	*See manufacturer's current prescribing information.*
Main side effects	*Immunoglobulin:* headache, hypertension, tachycardia. *Prednisone:* hypertension, diabetes mellitus, osteoporosis.

- Adults who do not respond or who relapse when steroids are reduced should be considered for splenectomy.

- Other treatments for adults failing steroids or splenectomy include i.v. immunoglobulin, azathioprine, vinca alkaloids, danazol, high-dose dexamethasone, or vitamin C.

For platelet functional defects [2]

- The bleeding tendency is often mild, and specific treatment (platelet transfusion, arginine vasopressin [DDAVP]) is needed for major hemorrhage or to cover surgical procedures. Antifibrinolytic agents may be helpful to control minor bleeding; antiovulatory treatment may be needed for menorrhagia.

Standard dosage	One single donor platelet pack/10 kg body weight or one platelet pheresis pack should raise the platelet count by $20{-}40 \times 10^9$/L. DDAVP, 0.4 µg/kg i.v. in 100 mL 0.9% saline solution in 15–20 minutes. Tranexamic acid, 0.5–1.0 g 3 times daily orally or i.v. Aminocaproic acid, 2–4 g 4 times daily orally.
Contraindications	*DDAVP:* coronary artery disease. *Tranexamic acid and aminocaproic acid:* history of thromboembolism and hematuria.
Special points	*DDAVP:* ineffective in Glanzmann's thrombasthenia.
Main drug interactions	*See manufacturer's current prescribing information.*
Main side effects	*Platelet transfusion:* allergic reactions, HLA or alloimmunization in multitransfused patients; hepatitis B (rare) or C transmission. *DDAVP:* nausea, tremor, vomiting, angina, myocardial infarction. *Tranexamic acid:* nausea, vomiting, diarrhea.

For bone-marrow disorders

- The risk of spontaneous hemorrhage increases when the platelet count is $<10 \times 10^9$/L. Prophylactic platelet transfusions are given to maintain the count above this level during the treatment of acute leukemia or aplastic anemia or during bone-marrow transplantation.

- In chronic thrombocytopenia due to bone-marrow failure, platelet transfusions are given for symptomatic bleeding.

For thrombotic thrombocytopenic purpura [3]

Supportive therapy of medical complications, *e.g.*, hemodialysis. Plasma exchange with fresh frozen plasma replacement (1.5 times plasma volume) for 7 days. Additional treatments include aspirin, dipyridamole, methylprednisone, and vincristine.

For alloimmune thrombocytopenia, neonatal and posttransfusion

Antigen-negative platelet transfusion, i.v. immunoglobulin, prednisone, or plasma exchange.

Treatment aims

To cure or alleviate symptoms, depending on underlying disease.

Other treatments

- Splenectomy is indicated for immune thrombocytopenia (not in children aged <6 years).
- Vaccination by Pneumovax and against *Haemophilus influenzae* type b and *Neisseria meningitidis* serogroups A and C should be given 1–2 weeks before surgery. Lifelong antipneumococcal prophylaxis (*e.g.*, penicillin V, 250 mg twice a day) is recommended for splenectomized patients.

Prognosis

- Up to 90% of children with idiopathic thrombocytopenic purpura remit spontaneously, with 50% recovering in 1 month.
- 80% of adults with idiopathic thrombocytopenic purpura remit after treatment by steroids alone or after splenectomy.
- The bleeding tendency in patients with hereditary platelet defects varies.
- In patients with acquired platelet function defects, the prognosis is related to the underlying disease.
- Mortality in patients with untreated thrombotic thrombocytopenic purpura is up to 90%; 60%–80% respond to treatment, reducing mortality to ~30%.
- Alloimmune thrombocytopenias are self-limiting but potentially fatal.

Follow-up and management

- The frequency of follow-up depends on the clinical severity and stability of the underlying disorder.

Key references

1. George JN, Shattil SJ: The clinical importance of acquired abnormalities of platelet function. *N Engl J Med* 1991, **324**:27–38.

2. Bolan CD, Alving BM: Pharmacologic agents in the management of bleeding disorders. *Transfusion* 1990, **30**:541–551.

3. Kwaan HC, Soff GA: Management of thrombotic thrombocytopenic purpura and hemolytic uremic syndrome. *Semin Hematol* 1997, **34**:159–166.

Diagnosis

Symptoms

• Patients are often asymptomatic if the effusion is small.

Breathlessness.

Chest pain: increased on deep inspiration or movement.

Positional discomfort or pain: with large effusions, causing mediastinal shift.

Symptoms of underlying disease.

Fever.

Signs

• Signs are clinically detectable only if the volume is ≥ 300 mL; loculated effusion may be very difficult to detect.

Decreased movement of chest wall on affected side.

Dullness to percussion.

Absent breath sounds in area of dullness.

Occasional bronchial breathing at upper margin of area of dullness.

Displaced trachea: large effusions only.

Decreased tactile tremitus.

Investigations [1,2]

Chest radiography: to assess extent of effusion and free-flowing character.

Ultrasonography: if doubt about nature of shadowing and to define loculated area for aspiration.

Aspiration: for cytology, Gram stain and Ziehl–Neelsen stain for acid-fast bacilli, culture, protein content, lactate dehydrogenase (LDH), cell count and differential, pH, glucose.

• Comparison of pleural protein content and LDH to plasma protein and LDH is essential to distinguish between transudative and exudative effusions [3].

Pleural biopsy: in experienced hands, much more reliable for diagnosis of tuberculosis and malignancy than simple aspiration.

Repeat radiography: after drainage of effusion, to visualize underlying lung.

Thoracoscopy: if doubt remains, to obtain better samples for histology.

CT: for visualizing loculated effusions and pleural and parenchymal disease.

Complications

Constrictive fibrosis of pleura and restricted lung function: caused by empyema and postpneumonic effusions.

Iatrogenic secondary infection.

Iatrogenic pneumothorax.

Unilateral pulmonary edema: after injudiciously rapid drainage (rare).

Hemorrhage: damage to intercostal vessels, especially after pleural biopsy.

Differential diagnosis

Infections: postpneumonic, tuberculosis.
Inflammation: pancreatitis, rheumatoid arthritis, SLE, polyarteritis nodosa.
Primary malignancy: mesothelioma.
Secondary malignancy: bronchogenic carcinoma, metastatic spread (especially breast, stomach, pancreas), lymphoma.
Infarction secondary to pulmonary embolism.

Etiology

Exudates

Unknown in ~20%, despite extensive investigation.
Infections: viral pleurisy, bacterial pneumonia, tuberculosis, empyema.
Secondary malignancy or secondary cancer (*e.g.*, lung, breast, stomach), leukemia or lymphoma.
Vascular: pulmonary infarction, pulmonary embolism.
Collagen disorders: rheumatoid arthritis.
Primary pleural malignancy (mesothelioma).
Uremia, chylothorax.

Transudates

Congestive heart failure, hypoalbuminemia (nephrotic syndrome and hepatic cirrhosis), constrictive pericarditis, pulmonary embolism.
Peritoneal dialysis.

Epidemiology

• Pleural effusion is frequently found with lung cancer and pneumonia.
• Tuberculosis is declining in importance but remains one of the most common causes of pleural effusion worldwide.
• Mesothelioma is rare. It is associated with asbestos exposure.

Treatment

Diet and lifestyle

• No special precautions are necessary.

Pharmacological treatment

Principles

• The principal aim is to treat any underlying cause and to treat the local problem by drainage.

• For transudates, the underlying disease must be treated.

• For infective causes (empyema, pneumonia), systemic antibiotics are indicated and intercostal drainage is essential; surgical drainage and decortication of pleura can be done if thick pleural rind develops.

• For tuberculosis, standard oral antituberculosis chemotherapy is indicated. The effusion should be aspirated to dryness. Tube drainage and surgery should be avoided if possible. *See* Tuberculosis, pulmonary *for details.*

• For malignant effusions, pleural effusion indicates inoperability; treatment is guided by symptoms. Intermittent aspiration is usually helpful. Tube drainage is the best method of preventing recurrence and achieving pleurodesis. In mesothelioma, tube drainage is best avoided if possible because of the risk of seeding tube tract [4,5].

• For noninfective nonmalignant causes, the effusion should be drained to dryness and followed with repeated chest radiographs.

• Pulmonary infarcts usually resolve without needing drainage, but formal anticoagulation with warfarin is usually appropriate (*see* Pulmonary embolism *for details*).

Chemical pleurodesis [5,6]

• Chemical pleurodesis is best done by specialists, who can consider the advantages and disadvantages in each individual case. It is usually reserved for malignant pleural effusions.

• Although many different agents ranging from antibiotics to antiseptics to antineoplastics to talc have been advocated, none is ideal.

• The agent most commonly used is talc. It may be insufflated via thoracoscopy or instilled as a slurry.

• Other approaches include the following:

Standard dosage	Doxycycline, 500 mg, or minocycline, 300 mg in 50 mL saline, after pleural fluid has been drained. A second dose may be given after 72 hours. Bleomycin, 60 U is an alternative for malignant effusions.
Contraindications	Transudate, bronchopleural fistulas, infection.
Main drug interactions	None.
Main side effects	Local pain, transient fever, hypersensitivity reaction.

Treatment aims

To achieve resolution of pleural effusion without residual fibrosis or functional deficit.

Prognosis

• Prognosis varies widely according to the underlying cause.

• If cleared by drainage, most bacterial effusions resolve, leaving some pleural scarring, which may need surgery if severe.

• Malignant effusions have poor prognosis, and treatment is mainly palliative, guided by symptoms.

Follow-up and management

• Serial chest radiographs should be taken, usually at 4–6-week intervals to assess recurrence.

• Lung function tests are needed to assess residual restrictive deficit if radiographic changes persist.

Key references

1. Collins TR, Sahn SA: Thoracentesis: complications, patient experience and diagnostic value. *Chest* 1987, **91**:817–819.

2. Bone R: The techniques of diagnostic and therapeutic thoracentesis. *J Crit Illness* 1990, **5**:371–379.

3. Light R, *et al.*: Pleural effusions: the diagnostic separation of transudates and exudates. *Ann Intern Med* 1972, **77**:507–513.

4. Keller SM: Current and future therapy for malignant pleural effusion. *Chest* 1993, **103(suppl)**:635–675.

5. Sahn S: Pleural effusion in lung cancer. *Clin Chest Med* 1993, **14**:189–200.

6. Light RW, Vargas FS: Pleural sclerosis for the treatment of pneumothorax and pleural effusion. *Lung* 1997, **175**:213–223.

Diagnosis

Symptoms

Fever, fatigue, weight loss: for weeks or months before respiratory symptoms develop.

Nonproductive cough, shortness of breath: initially on exertion, then at rest with disease progression.

• The absence of respiratory symptoms does not exclude *Pneumocystis carinii* pneumonia, especially in patients who are receiving prophylaxis or who have had previous episodes of infection.

Signs

Wasting, fever, diffuse lymphadenopathy, oral candidiasis, hairy leukoplakia, cutaneous Kaposi's sarcoma: general signs of immunosuppression secondary to HIV infection.

Tachypnea, rales without consolidation: revealed by auscultation, but often no pulmonary abnormalities.

Splenomegaly, fundal abnormalities: rare extrapulmonary signs of infection.

Investigations

• *P. carinii* pneumonia occurs in HIV-infected individuals who have a CD4 lymphocyte count $<200 \times 10^6$/L.

Complete blood count: to exclude anemia.

Plain chest radiography: may show diffuse interstitial infiltration; various other appearances, including lobar infiltrate cavity or pneumothorax occur. Chest radiograph may be normal.

Arterial oxygen tension measurement: hypoxia commonly occurs.

Exercise oximetry: a useful noninvasive test.

Sputum analysis: obviates need for routine bronchoscopy if laboratory is experienced; sputum induced by inhaled nebulized hypertonic saline solution; samples stained by Grocott or immunofluorescent stains.

Fiberoptic bronchoscopy: reserved for patients whose induced sputum test results are not diagnostic.

Complications

Pneumothorax.

Restrictive lung disease.

Extrapulmonic *P. carinii* infection.

Adult respiratory distress syndrome.

Differential diagnosis

Bacterial pneumonia.

Pulmonary Kaposi's sarcoma.

Pulmonary tuberculosis.

Toxoplasmosis.

Pulmonary lymphoma.

Asthma.

Cytomegalovirus pneumonitis.

Lipid interstitial pneumonitis.

Histoplasmosis.

Aspergillosis.

Etiology

• The pneumonia is caused by infection by *P. carinii* (possibly a fungus or protozoan).

• Acquisition may be common early in life (and controlled by the immune system) or occur shortly before the disease develops.

Epidemiology

• Most children have serological evidence of previous *P. carinii* infection by the age of 4 years; the disease was first recognized because of epidemics in orphanages after World War II.

• The disease is the most common AIDS opportunistic infection in people with HIV-induced immunosuppression, with no difference between genders or among races, although it occurs significantly less often in many developing countries.

Treatment

Diet and lifestyle

Not applicable.

Pharmacological treatment

Treatment of the disease

• Most treatment is based on inhibition of folic acid metabolism.

• The most effective agent is trimethoprim/sulfamethoxazole (TMP/SMX); in less severely ill patients, oral treatment may be used.

• Unfortunately, up to 40% of patients fail to complete a treatment course because of allergic or toxic side effects.

• Alternative treatment in bactrim-intolerant individuals with mild to moderate disease includes atovoquone, clindamycin and primaquine, or trimethoprim and dapsone. For patients with severe infection, the alternates to bactrim are pentamidine and trimethoprim.

• Corticosteroids have been shown to reduce mortality and the risk of respiratory failure in patients presenting with partial arterial oxygen pressure <8 kPa. The subsequent use of antiretrovirals has been shown to improve survival.

Standard dosage	TMP/SMX, 15 mg/kg i.v. every 6 hours.
Contraindications	Hypersensitivity.
Special points	Full blood count, U&E monitoring, and liver function tests must be done.
Main drug interactions	None.
Main side effects	Nausea and vomiting (antiemetic can be given), skin rash, leukopenia, thrombocytopenia, raised liver function tests.

Prophylaxis

• Primary prophylaxis is recommended in patients with clinical evidence of immuno-suppression (*e.g.*, buccal candidiasis) or other opportunistic infections or laboratory evidence (CD4 count $<200 \times 10^6$/L).

• Secondary prophylaxis should be offered to patients who have had previous episodes of *P. carinii* pneumonia.

Standard dosage	TMP/SMX, 1 tablet daily. Alternatively, dapsone, 100 mg daily, or pentamidine, 300 mg inhaled every month.
Contraindications	Allergy to sulfonamides or trimethoprim.
Special points	Cotrimoxazole may also reduce the incidence of subsequent toxoplasmosis and bacterial infection.
Main drug interactions	None.
Main side effects	Skin rash, nausea and vomiting, leukopenia, thrombocytopenia, raised liver function tests.

General references

Masur H: Prevention and treatment of Pneumocystis pneumonia. *N Engl J Med* 1992, **327**:1853–1860.

Moe AA, Hardy WD: *Pneumocystis carinii* infection in the HIV-seropositive patient. *Infect Dis Clin North Am* 1994, **8**:331–364.

Murray JF: Pulmonary complications of HIV infection. *Am Rev Med* 1996, **47**:117–126.

Santamauro JT, Stover DE: *Pneumocystis carinii* pneumonia. *Med Clin North Am* **81**:299–318.

Diagnosis

Symptoms

Common
• Onset may be abrupt or over days.

Cough: with sputum, which may be purulent, in two-thirds of patients.

Fever: possibly with rigors and diaphoresis.

Pleuritic chest pain: occasionally.

Dyspnea.

Less common
Hemoptysis, vomiting, diarrhea, myalgia.

Mental confusion: especially in patients with severe pneumonia and in elderly patients.

Signs

Fever.

Mental confusion, cyanosis, hypotension: suggesting severe illness.

Raised respiratory rate: suggesting severe illness.

Dullness on percussion.

Increased vocal fremitus.

Crackles.

Bronchial breathing: egobronchophony and whispering pectoriloquy; in one-third of patients.

Investigations [1]

To confirm diagnosis
Chest radiography: shows consolidation or infiltrates.

To assess severity
Arterial blood gas analysis: low partial oxygen pressure, raised partial carbon dioxide pressure, low pH.

Complete blood count: leukocytosis with left shift (leukocyte count <4 or >20 × 10^9/L indicates high risk).

To assess cause
Blood culture: for bacteremia.

Sputum Gram stain and culture: to exclude *Legionella* and *Pneumocystis* spp. and mycobacteria.

Pleural-fluid Gram stain and culture: if fluid present.

Serology: acute and convalescent sera for antibodies to viruses, chlamydia, mycoplasma, *Coxiella* spp., and legionella.

Bronchoscopy: often needed in immunocompromised patients but rarely in others.

Complications

Empyema, lung abscess, pulmonary embolus, adult respiratory distress syndrome.

Acute renal failure, hemolysis.

Sepsis.

Death: especially in the elderly, often despite appropriate therapy.

Differential diagnosis
Pulmonary edema.

Exacerbation of chronic bronchitis.

Pulmonary embolus.

Lung cancer.

Etiology [2–4]
• Pneumococcal infection is the cause of 50%–80% of community-acquired pneumonias.

• Gram-negative organisms (*e.g.*, *Escherichia coli* and *Pseudomonas* spp.) are the cause of 50% or more of nosocomial pneumonias.

• Anaerobic bacteria (*e.g.*, bacteroides) are important in aspiration pneumonia.

• Immunocompromised patients may be infected by a huge range of microorganisms, *e.g.*, unusual bacteria and fungi, many of which would not cause infection in immunocompetent patients.

Epidemiology [4]
• Pneumonia occurs at all ages but is most frequent in very young and very old patients.

• Primary care physicians see on average 10 cases annually.

• One patient in every five seen needs hospital admission.

• Most cases occur in the winter months.

• Mycoplasma infection affects mainly teenagers and young adults.

• Legionella infection may occur in epidemics related to water systems in buildings.

Classification
Community-acquired pneumonia.

Nosocomial pneumonia.

Aspiration pneumonia: caused by inhalation of oropharyngeal secretions, during vomiting, or when consciousness is depressed.

Immunocompromised pneumonia: *e.g.*, with HIV infection, organ transplantation, cytotoxic chemotherapy.

Treatment

Diet and lifestyle
• Smoking and smoking-related diseases are a major risk factor for pneumonia; smoking education is therefore important.

Pharmacological treatment [5,6]

General guidelines
Oxygen: to maintain partial oxygen pressure in arterial blood >60 mm Hg; may cause hypercapnia in patients with chronic obstructive pulmonary disease, so arterial blood gases should be monitored.

Oral or parenteral fluids: to correct dehydration.

Nonsedative analgesia: for pleuritic chest pain.

Physical therapy: especially if large sputum volumes are difficult to expectorate.

Intensive care, including assisted ventilation: valuable for patients in whom respiratory failure worsens despite treatment.

Antibiotics [7]
• Initial treatment must be empirical; this can be modified later if indicated by micro-biological results.

• Oral antibiotics are appropriate in mild infection, parenteral if infection is severe or accompanied by vomiting.

• Treatment should be for at least 7 days; severely ill patients need treatment for up to 3 weeks.

For mild community-acquired disease: azithromycin, penicillin, cephalosporin, or erythromycin.

For severe community-acquired disease: 2nd- or 3rd-generation cephalosporin (*e.g.*, cefuroxime), possibly with erythromycin.

For nosocomial infection: 2nd- or 3rd-generation cephalosporin, possibly with aminoglycoside; usually requires 2–3 weeks of therapy.

For aspiration: amoxicillin-clavulanate or clindamycin.

For immunocompromised disease: individually determined by causative pathogen.

Standard dosage	Amoxicillin, 500 mg 3 times daily. Erythromycin, 500 mg 4 times daily. Cefuroxime, 750 mg 3 times daily. Aminoglycoside guided by blood level. Clindamycin, 300 mg 3 times daily.
Contraindications	Hypersensitivity.
Main drug interactions	Warfarin.
Main side effects	Diarrhea.

Prophylaxis
Annual influenza vaccination: for patients >65 years of age or those with chronic heart or lung disease, renal failure, or diabetes mellitus and for immunosuppressed patients.

Pneumococcal vaccination: for patients who are >65 years of age; asplenic; or have sickle cell disease, chronic renal failure, or chronic lung, heart, or liver disease; and those with diabetes mellitus or who are immunocompromised.

Criteria for hospitalization: age >65 years, co-existing illnesses (*e.g.*, diabetes, chronic obstructive pulmonary disease), tachypnea, tachycardia, hypotension, signs of sepsis, leukopenia, or severe leukocytosis.

Treatment aims
To improve oxygenation.
To achieve rapid resolution of pneumonia and return to normal activities.
To prevent death or sepsis.
To relieve symptoms.

Prognosis
• Pyrexia usually settles within 48 hours of starting treatment.
• Lethargy after pneumonia often lasts weeks or months.
• Radiographic shadowing is slow to clear and lags behind clinical recovery.
• Death is unusual in patients managed at home.
• 5%–10% of patients admitted to hospital die.
• Up to 50% reaching intensive care die.
• The mortality in nosocomial pneumonia is up to 30% and may be higher in immuno-compromised patients.

Follow-up and management
• Patients should be seen 6 weeks after presentation, and chest radiography repeated to confirm recovery and exclude underlying lung disease, especially lung cancer.

Key references

1. Fine M, Smith D, Singer D: Hospitalization decision in patients with community-acquired pneumonia: a prospective study. *Am J Med* 1990, **89**:713–721.

2. Fang G, *et al.*: New and emerging etiologies for community-acquired pneumonia with implications for therapy. A prospective multicenter study of 359 cases. *Medicine* 1990, **69**:307–316.

3. Farr B, *et al.*: Prediction of microbial aetiology at admission to hospital for pneumonia from the presenting clinical features. *Thorax* 1989, **44**:1031–1035.

4. Mandell LA: Community-acquired pneumonia: etiology, epidemiology and treatment. *Chest* 1995, **108(suppl)**: 35S–42S.

5. Niederman MS, *et al.*: American Thoracic Society guidelines for the initial management of adults with community-acquired pneumonia: diagnosis, assessment of severity, and initial antimicrobial therapy. *Am Rev Respir Dis* 1993, **148**:1418–1426.

6. Fein A, *et al.*: When the pneumonia doesn't get better. *Clin Chest Med* 1987, **8**:529–541.

7. The choice of antibacterial drugs. *Med Lett Drugs Ther* 1996, **38**:25–34.

Diagnosis

Definition

• Autosomal-dominant polycystic kidney disease is a subset of renal cystic disorders in which cysts are distributed throughout the cortex and medulla of both kidneys, and the kidneys are enlarged.

Symptoms and signs

• Although the process is usually not clinically apparent until the third or fourth decade, it has been found in infants and aborted fetuses, and all carriers show evidence of disease by the eighth or ninth decade.

Abdominal pain.

Hematuria.

Polyuria or nocturia.

Hypertension.

Abdominal distension.

Nephromegaly.

Investigations

Palpation: very enlarged cystic kidneys are easily palpable.

CT: most sensitive; shows multiple cysts in kidneys and occasionally in liver, pancreas, and spleen.

Ultrasonography: only cysts >1 cm are detectable.

Radioisotope scanning: shows multiple cystic defects in isotope image.

Note: The presence of at least two renal cysts (unilateral or bilateral) in patients aged <30 years who are at risk is sufficient to establish the diagnosis of polycystic kidney disease 1.

APKD1/APKD2 **gene-linkage studies:** >95% predictive at any age if 3–4 affected family members can be tested.

Intravenous urography: shows stretched calyces.

Complications

Chronic renal failure.

Hypertension: in 50% of patients.

Cyst rupture: pain, hematuria, and intrarenal hemorrhage.

Nephrolithiasis and nephrocalcinosis: in 10%–18% of patients.

Infection: within renal cysts or above obstructed ureter (gallium scan useful).

Malignant tumors: occasional.

Obstruction: clot or stone (acute on chronic renal failure).

Polycythemia: occasionally.

Distal renal tubular acidosis.

Differential diagnosis

Autosomal-recessive polycystic kidney disease.

Tuberous sclerosis.

Cystic dysplasia of kidneys.

Benign noninherited cysts.

Acquired cystic disease of kidneys.

Etiology

Genetics

• The disease is autosomal dominant, with almost complete penetrance and variable expression.

• The spontaneous mutation rate is relatively high (20% no family history).

• 85% of cases are linked to abnormal gene on chromosome 16 (*APKD1* locus).

• Most of remaining cases link to *APKD2* gene.

Pathogenesis

• The disease probably begins *in utero*.

• Cysts are formed from proximal or distal tubules, only 1% of which are affected.

• Renal damage is caused by compression of normal kidney tissue.

Epidemiology

• The autosomal-dominant form is the most common polycystic kidney disease.

• Affects 1 in 1000 worldwide.

• The male : female ratio is equal.

• 10% of patients on dialysis suffer from the disease.

Associated extrarenal conditions

Aneurysms: berry, intracranial, abdominal aortic, dissecting thoracic, aortic root, and annulus aneurysms; 6% of patients with subarachnoid hemorrhage have autosomal dominant polycystic kidney disease; 10%–36% of patients with autosomal dominant polycystic kidney disease have intracranial aneurysms.

Liver cysts (in 20%–50% of patients): can cause obstructive jaundice and portal hypertension (rare); do not communicate with biliary tree; occasionally origin of cholangiocarcinoma.

Pancreatic cysts (in 5%–10%).

Cysts in other organs: ovary, uterus, spleen, thyroid, seminal vesicles, epididymis.

Valvular heart lesions: mitral incompetence, mitral valve prolapse (in 30%), tricuspid incompetence, pulmonary valve incompetence.

Diverticulosis (in 80%).

Hernia.

Treatment

Diet and lifestyle

• No special precautions are necessary in most patients; some are unusually susceptible to physical trauma.

• Genetic counseling should be offered.

• Low-protein diet may be of benefit.

Pharmacological treatment

• No specific treatment is available for the disorder, but the following can be considered:

Bed rest and analgesia for pain when bleeding occurs.

Overly aggressive blood pressure control may be detrimental.

Treatment of acidosis if present.

Treatment of renal failure when needed.

Prolonged antibiotic treatment for upper urinary tract infection.

Nonpharmacological treatment

• Hemodialysis and peritoneal dialysis are both suitable in patients with autosomal-dominant polycystic kidney disease.

• Polycythemia and repeated clotting of fistulas occasionally occurs in the hemodialysis group.

• Survival rate for these patients on dialysis is better than for patients with other renal diseases.

• Renal transplantation is the preferred method of treating end-stage renal disease due to polycystic kidney disease. No increased rate of mortality or morbidity is noted in these transplantation patients. The polycystic kidneys typically do not need to be removed.

See Renal transplantation *for details.*

Treatment aims

To treat complications as they arise.
To control blood pressure.
To prepare patient for renal replacement therapy.

Prognosis

• 50% of patients progress to end-stage renal failure by the age of 75 years.

Follow-up and management

• Annual monitoring of blood pressure and renal function is needed (more frequently in patients with impaired renal function) because when or whether renal failure will develop in an individual patient generally cannot be predicted.

• Opinion varies regarding the need to screen for intracranial aneurysms.

General references

Butler WE, Barker FG II, Crowell RM: Patients with polycystic kidney disease would benefit from routine magnetic resonance angiographic screening for intracerebral aneurysms: a decision analysis. *Neurosurgery* 1996, **38**:506–515 (discussion 515–516).

Elashry OM, *et al.*: Laparoscopy for adult polycystic kidney disease: a promising alternative. *Am J Kidney Dis* 1996, **27**:224–233.

Elles RG, *et al.*: Diagnosis of adult polycystic kidney disease by genetic markers and ultrasonographic imaging in a voluntary family register. *J Med Genet* 1994, **31**:115–120.

Fick GM, *et al.*: Causes of death in autosomal dominant polycystic kidney disease. *J Am Soc Nephrol* 1995, **5**:2048–2056.

Grantham JJ: The etiology, pathogenesis, and treatment of autosomal dominant polycystic kidney disease: recent advances. *Am J Kidney Dis* 1996, **28**:788–803.

Klahr S, *et al.*: Dietary protein restriction, blood pressure control, and the progression of polycystic kidney disease. Modification of Diet in Renal Disease Study Group. *J Am Soc Nephrol* 1995, **5**:2037–2047.

Ravine D, *et al.*: Evaluation of ultrasonographic diagnostic criteria for autosomal dominant polycystic kidney disease 1. *Lancet* 1994, **343**:824–827.

Diagnosis

Symptoms

Oligomenorrhea or amenorrhea with sometimes heavy menses: endometrium remains estrogenized, in contrast with other causes or anovulation.

Infertility: due to anovulation.

Mild androgenism: hirsutism, acne, seborrhea [1].

Severe virilization: alopecia, voice change, clitoromegaly (rare).

Signs

• The syndrome associated with polycystic ovaries is extremely variable; in most women with polycystic ovaries, the endocrine disturbance is subtle and the disorder has no outward signs.

Obesity.

Central adiposity.

Mild hypertension.

Hirsutism: documented by photography or Ferriman–Gallway score [1].

Acanthosis nigricans: feature of severe insulin resistance.

• Abdominal and pelvic examinations are rarely helpful but should be done to exclude ovarian masses.

Investigations [2,3]

• The aims are to make a positive diagnosis, to exclude other causes of anovulation, infertility, recurrent miscarriage and virilization as appropriate, and to screen for features of insulin resistance (syndrome X).

• Diagnosis of polycystic ovarian disease should incorporate both an endocrine and a morphological assessment.

For the disorder

Chronic anovulation, elevated androgen levels: diagnostic criteria.

• The presence or absence of ovarian cysts is an unreliable finding.

To rule out other causes of amenorrhea

Pelvic examination.

Ultrasonography: to examine endometrium, possibly with endometrial biopsy (menstrual disorder); to diagnose ovarian tumors (virilization).

Serum testosterone measurement: tumor more likely if concentrations are markedly elevated.

For cardiovascular risk factors

Blood pressure measurement.

Evidence of insulin resistance or frank diabetes.

Serum lipid measurements.

Complications

Endometrial cancer: despite anovulation, ovaries continue to secrete estradiol.

Diabetes mellitus, myocardial infarction, stroke: related to insulin resistance [4].

Recurrent miscarriages: probably due to elevated androgen levels.

Differential diagnosis

Classic polycystic ovarian syndrome.

Hypothyroidism.

Cushing's syndrome.

Acromegaly.

Androgen-secreting tumor.

Estrogenized amenorrhea.

Granulosa cell tumor.

Etiology [3]

• Excess androgen production is of unclear etiology, often combined with insulin resistance.

Epidemiology [3]

• 10%–20% of apparently normal women are found to have polycystic ovaries on ultrasonography.

• 1% of young women (aged 15–40 years) have clinically evident disease.

• Family studies show the prevalence of polycystic ovaries to be high among asymptomatic close relatives (80%).

• The disease is a factor in ~10% of couples with infertility.

Treatment

Diet and lifestyle

• In view of the increased risk of cardiovascular disease, advice should be given about diet, smoking, and exercise.

• A calorie-restricted diet may help by decreasing insulin resistance.

• Women with oligo- or amenorrhea not wishing to conceive should be warned of the small risk of conception.

Pharmacological treatment [3,5]

• Pregnancy must be ruled out before treatment begins.

• Polycystic ovarian syndrome is a diagnosis of exclusion, and other causes of amenorrhea must be investigated and ruled out.

For menstrual disorder

Combined oral contraceptive to improve regularity or reduce flow.

Cyclical progesterone or combined oral contraceptive to prevent endometrial neoplasia in women with oligo- or amenorrhea.

For anovulatory infertility

• Treatment should be carried out in conjunction with an appropriate specialist.

Antiestrogen treatment (clomiphene): acts through the hypothalamus.

Laparoscopic ovarian surgery.

Exogenous gonadotropin treatment: involves direct ovarian stimulation with human menopausal gonadotropin (hMG) or human follicle-stimulating hormone (hFSH), with human chorionic gonadotropin (hCG) to trigger ovulation.

Typical dosages	*Antiestrogen:* clomiphene, 100 mg orally daily on days 2–6 of cycle for up to 3 cycles. *Exogenous gonadotropin:* hMG or hFSH, 75 U daily.
Contraindications	Pregnancy, hormone-dependent tumors, undiagnosed abnormal menstruation.
Special points	*Antiestrogen:* near-normal conception rates expected; low risk of high-order multiple pregnancy (8% twin rate) and ovarian hyperstimulation; minimal monitoring needed (midluteal serum progesterone measurement). *Gonadotropin:* risk of multiple pregnancy and ovarian hyperstimulation; detailed monitoring mandatory (serial follicle scanning and estradiol measurement); no clear benefit of pure hFSH over hMG.
Main drug interactions	None.
Main side effects	*Antiestrogen:* hot flushes, mild abdominal discomfort, visual disturbance (rare). *Gonadotropin:* nausea, abdominal discomfort, allergy.

For virilization

Combined oral contraceptive: usual precautions for oral contraceptive use.

Flutamide or spironolactone: both are antiandrogens and may feminize a developing male fetus; therefore, contraception is of critical importance.

Special considerations

• The insulin-sensitizing agent troglitazone is currently being evaluated as a treatment for polycystic ovarian syndrome.

Key references

1. Fox R, *et al.*: Oestrogen and androgen states in oligo-amenorrhoeic women with polycystic ovaries. *Br J Obstet Gynaecol* 1991, **98**:294–299.

2. Fox R, *et al.*: Polycystic ovarian disease: diagnostic methods. *Contemp Rev Obstet Gynaecol* 1992, **4**:84–89.

3. Frank S: Polycystic ovary syndrome. *N Engl J Med* 1995, **333**:853–861.

4. Conway GS, *et al.*: Risk factors for coronary artery disease in lean and obese women with polycystic ovary syndrome. *Clin Endocrinol* 1992, **37**:119–125.

5. Jacobs HS: Polycystic ovary syndrome: aetiology and management. *Curr Opin Obstet Gynecol* 1995, **7**:203–208.

Diagnosis

Symptoms

Polymyalgia rheumatica

Pain and stiffness: bilateral and symmetrical, affecting neck, shoulder, and pelvic girdles; stiffness usually predominant, particularly severe after rest, and may prevent patient getting out of bed [1].

Giant-cell arteritis

Headache: in two-thirds or more of patients; severe pain, usually localized in the temple but may be occipital or be less defined and precipitated by brushing the hair [2,3].

Pain on chewing: due to claudication of muscles of mastication, in up to two-thirds of patients.

Visual disturbances: in 25%; visual loss evident in <10%.

Signs

Polymyalgia rheumatica

Unimpaired muscle strength: although pain makes interpretation of muscle testing difficult.

Tenderness of involved structures: with restriction of shoulder movement, if diagnosis delayed [1].

Peripheral synovitis: uncommon and transient.

Giant-cell arteritis

Scalp tenderness: particularly around temporal and occipital arteries; may disturb sleep [2].

Thickened, tender, and nodular arteries: with absent or reduced pulsation.

Partial or complete visual loss: due to anterior ischemic optic neuropathy [2,3].

Investigations

Baseline clinical investigations

• These are used to make the diagnosis and exclude other diagnoses.

ESR measurement: rate usually greatly raised, but can be normal [4].

Acute-phase protein (*e.g.*, CRP) measurement: concentration usually raised.

Complete blood count.

Biochemical profile.

Rheumatoid factor test.

Serum protein electrophoresis.

Thyroid function test.

Chest radiography.

Specific investigations

Temporal artery biopsy: for suspected giant-cell arteritis, not for polymyalgia rheumatica; findings can be focal, may be normal [2].

Complications

Visual loss: in up to 10% of patients, permanent blindness in giant-cell arteritis [5]; usually not reversible.

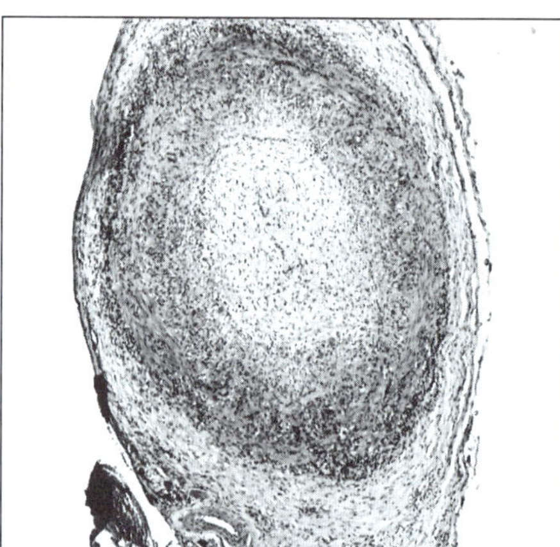

Occlusion of lumen due to intimal proliferation and inflammation of the media.

Treatment

Diet and lifestyle

• No special precautions are necessary.

Pharmacological treatment

• Patients with giant-cell arteritis should be referred as an emergency to a specialist to arrange a biopsy and to initiate treatment.

• Treatment by a systemic corticosteroid has long been recognized as mandatory in patients with giant-cell arteritis in order to prevent serious vascular complications, particularly blindness.

• Corticosteroids are usually also needed for patients with polymyalgia rheumatica.

• Many patients remain on treatment for years.

For polymyalgia rheumatica

Standard dosage	Prednisolone, 10–20 mg initially for 1 month, reduced by 2.5 mg every 2 weeks to 10 mg daily, then 1 mg daily every 2–4 weeks; maintenance dose 5–7 mg daily for 6–12 months; final reduction, 1 mg every 4 weeks [6].
Contraindications	Systemic infections; caution in pregnancy, hypertension, diabetes mellitus, osteoporosis, glaucoma, epilepsy, peptic ulceration.
Special points	In patients whose prednisolone dosage cannot be reduced because of recurring symptoms or who develop serious steroid-related side effects, azathioprine has been shown to have a modest steroid-sparing effect, and methotrexate may be more effective [7].
Main drug interactions	Rifampin and phenytoin reduce corticosteroid concentrations; anticoagulant dosage may need adjustment; reduced effect of NSAIDs.
Main side effects	Weight gain, edema, increased intraocular pressure, cataracts, glaucoma, gastrointestinal disturbances, peptic ulceration, diabetes, osteoporosis, skin atrophy [8].

For giant-cell arteritis without visual symptoms

Prednisolone, 40–60 mg daily initially for 8 weeks, reduced by 5 mg every 2 weeks to 10 mg daily; then as for polymyalgia rheumatica [9,10].

For giant-cell arteritis with possible or definite ocular involvement

Prednisolone, 60–80 mg daily initially for 8 weeks, reduced to 20 mg daily over next 4 weeks; then as for uncomplicated giant-cell arteritis [9,10].

Key references

1. Lestico MR, *et al.*: Polymyalgia rheumatica. *Clin Pharmacol* 1993, **12**:571–580.

2. Chmelewski WL, *et al.*: Presenting features and outcomes in patients undergoing temporal artery biopsy: a review of 98 patients. *Arch Intern Med* 1992, **152**:1690–1695.

3. Reech KA, *et al.*: Neurologic manifestations of giant cell arteritis. *Am J Med* 1990, **89**:67–72.

4. Kyle V, Cawston TE, Hazleman BL: Erythrocyte sedimentation rate and c reactive protein in the assessment of polymyalgia rheumatica/giant cell arteritis on presentation and during follow-up. *Ann Rheum Dis* 1989, **48**:667–671.

5. Wilke WS, Hoffman GS: Treatment of corticosteroid resistant giant cell arteritis. *Rheum Dis Clin North Am* 1995, **21**:59–71.

6. Kyle V, Hazleman BL: Treatment of polymyalgia rheumatica and giant cell arteritis. I. Steroid regimens in the first two months. *Ann Rheum Dis* 1989, **48**:658–661.

7. Krall PL, Mazanec DJ, Wilke WS: Methotrexate for corticosteroid-resistant polymyalgia rheumatica and giant-cell arteritis. *Cleve Clin J Med* 1989, **56**:253–277.

8. Kyle V, Hazleman BL: Treatment of polymyalgia rheumatica and giant cell arteritis. II. Relation between steroid dose and steroid associated side effects. *Ann Rheum Dis* 1989, **48**:662–666.

9. Behn AR, Perera T, Myles AB: Polymyalgia rheumatica and corticosteroids: how much for how long? *Ann Rheum Dis* 1983, **42**:374–378.

10. Hunder GG: Giant cell arteritis and polymyalgia rheumatica. *Med Clin North Am* 1997, **81**:195–219.

Diagnosis

Symptoms

Weakness of proximal limb muscles: evolving over weeks or months, with difficulty in lifting, running, climbing stairs, getting up from a squatting position or low chair.

Dysphagia: due to weakness of pharyngeal muscles.

Muscle pain and tenderness, fleeting arthralgia, inability to raise head, Raynaud's phenomenon, dyspnea and cough.

Signs

Weakness of neck flexors and proximal limb muscles, with retained, or absent tendon reflexes: muscle wasting minimal or absent in early stages.

Investigations [1]

General

Complete blood count, autoantibody screen, thyroid function tests: to identify overlap myositis and autoimmune thyroid disease.

Chest radiography, pulmonary function tests, ventilation perfusion studies: in patients with respiratory-muscle involvement or interstitial lung disease.

Video barium swallow: can be useful in patients with dysphagia.

ECG: to identify cardiac conduction defects and arrhythmias.

Special

Analysis of autoantibodies to aminoacyl transfer RNA synthetases: *e.g.*, Jo-1 antibody in patients with interstitial lung disease (positive in 70%).

Estimation of muscle creatine kinase activity in serum: activity usually increased 3–30-fold; serum creatine kinase concentration tends to reflect disease activity and is useful in monitoring treatment.

Needle electromyography: increased insertional activity with fibrillation potentials, positive sharp waves, and repetitive discharges; short and long duration, low amplitude, polyphasic motor unit action potentials; characteristic firing pattern.

Muscle biopsy: essential to establish diagnosis; samples from mildly to moderately affected proximal limb muscle (biceps or triceps brachii, vastus lateralis) that has not been needled for electromyography.

Light microscopy (cryostat sections): endomysial collections of inflammatory cells (lymphocytes, plasma cells, histiocytes) surrounding necrotic and nonnecrotic muscle fibers; regenerating muscle fibers with basophilic cytoplasm and prominent nucleoli; variable increase in endomysial connective tissue; necrotic fibers may be invaded by macrophages and lymphocytes.

Complications

Aspiration.

Interstitial lung disease.

Respiratory failure.

Raynaud's phenomenon: more common in dermatomyositis.

Cardiac conduction defects and dysrhythmias: rare.

• Malignancy is more common in polymyositis, especially dermatomyositis.

Differential diagnosis

General

Dermatomyositis, paraneoplastic myositis. Eosinophilic polymyositis.

Inclusion body myositis, sarcoid myopathy, mixed connective tissue disease, SLE, rheumatoid arthritis, Sjögren's syndrome, systemic sclerosis.

Myositides from other causes

HIV, influenza A and B virus, coxsackie virus, echovirus, adenovirus.

Spirochetes: *Borrelia burgdorferi* (Lyme disease).

Protozoa: toxoplasma.

Helminths: *Trichinella* spp., cysticerci.

Genetic disorders

Limb girdle dystrophies, late-onset nemaline myopathy, late-onset acid maltase deficiency, spinal muscular atrophy, lipid storage myopathies.

Drug-induced myopathies

Corticosteroids, penicillamine, lovastatin, cholestyramine, zidovudine, procainamide, chloroquine, colchicine, pancuronium with corticosteroids.

Other

Lambert–Eaton myasthenic syndrome. Polymyalgia rheumatica.

Etiology

• The cause of idiopathic polymyositis is unknown; the increased incidence of HLA haplotype B8, DR3 suggests genetic susceptibility.

Epidemiology

• Idiopathic polymyositis affects all age groups but occurs most often in the 5th and 6th decades.

• The annual incidence is ~3 in one million population.

• It is slightly more common in women.

Pathogenesis

• Idiopathic polymyositis is a major histocompatibility complex class 1 restricted T-cell-mediated myotoxicity [2].

• CD8+ cytotoxic T-lymphocytes expressing common alpha-beta receptor invade and destroy initially nonnecrotic muscle fibers.

• In a rare polymyositis variant, nonnecrotic fibers are invaded by CD4–, CD8– T lymphocytes expressing the gamma-delta receptor, which interacts with heat-shock proteins.

Treatment

Diet and lifestyle

• Alcohol consumption should be restricted.

Pharmacological treatment

First line

Standard dosage	Prednisone, 30–60 mg orally single daily dose for 4–6 weeks initially, tapered by 2.5–5 mg every 2–4 weeks depending on response and serum creatine kinase concentration to maintenance dose 10–15 mg daily. Azathioprine, 25–50 mg orally daily initially, increased to 2.5–3 mg/kg daily over 4 weeks; maintenance 1–2 mg/kg daily.
Contraindications	*Prednisone:* caution in hypertension, peptic ulcer, diabetes mellitus, osteoporosis, glaucoma, psychosis, previous tuberculosis. *Azathioprine:* rare hypersensitivity, pregnancy and breast-feeding.
Special points	*Prednisone:* calcium and potassium supplements may be needed on long-term treatment. *Azathioprine:* full blood count, platelet count, liver and renal function monitoring weekly for first 2 months, monthly for next 6 months, at least 3-monthly thereafter.
Main drug interactions	*Prednisone:* phenytoin, phenobarbital, oral anticoagulants, NSAIDs. *Azathioprine:* allopurinol, neuromuscular blocking agents, cytostatics.
Main side effects	*Prednisone:* dyspepsia, peptic ulcer, weight gain, hypertension, cushingoid changes, potassium loss, glucose intolerance, cataract, osteoporosis, vertebral fractures, avascular osteonecrosis, euphoria, psychosis, muscle weakness. *Azathioprine:* nausea, vomiting, diarrhea, bone-marrow suppression, disturbed liver function.

Second line

Pulsed methylprednisone, 0.5–1 g i.v. daily for 5 days.

Human immunoglobulin, 0.4 g/kg i.v. daily for 5 days [2,3].

Third line

• The following agents are indicated in refractory cases, usually with maintenance dose of oral steroids:

Methotrexate, 7.5–30 mg orally or 0.4–0.8 mg/kg i.v. weekly (adults).

Cyclophosphamide, 1–4 mg/kg orally daily.

Cyclosporine, 2–6 mg/kg orally daily (adults).

• All are contraindicated in hypersensitivity, pregnancy, and lactation.

• Monitoring of full blood count, platelet count, liver and kidney function is needed.

• Side effects include nausea, vomiting, diarrhea, alopecia, bone-marrow suppression, and hepatic and renal toxicity.

Treatment aims

To halt progression of disease and improve muscle strength.

Prognosis

• Remission is usually achieved and maintained in 50%–60% of patients with first-line treatment.

• Second-, third-, and fourth-line treatments have provided encouraging results in small uncontrolled trials, but their respective merits in cases refractory to first-line drugs have not yet been clearly established.

• Death is rarely due to muscle weakness and usually results from cardiopulmonary complications.

Follow-up and management

• Most patients need maintenance treatment for at least 1–2 years after remission has been achieved.

• Consider routine malignancy screen with chest radiograph, Hemoccult test, and so forth, as indicated.

Key references

1. Dalakas MC: Clinical, immunopathologic, and therapeutic considerations of inflammatory myopathies. *Clin Neuropharmacol* 1992, **15**:327–351.

2. Cherin P, *et al.*: Efficacy of intravenous gammaglobulin therapy in chronic refractory polymyositis and dermatomyositis: an open study with 20 adult patients. *Am J Med* 1991, **91**:162–168.

3. Soueidan SA, Dalakas MC: Treatment of inclusion-body myositis with high-dose intravenous immunoglobulin. *Neurology* 1993, **43**:876–879.

General references

Mastaglia FL, Walton JN (eds.): Inflammatory myopathies. In *Skeletal Muscle Pathology*. Edinburgh: Churchill Livingstone; 1992:453–491.

Mastaglia FL, Phillips BA, Zilko P: Treatment of inflammatory myopathies. *Muscle Nerve* 1997, **20**:651–654.

Diagnosis

Definition

• Postpartum depression is defined as a new episode of depression in a woman who has been well for at least the previous 6 months, with onset in the first 90 days postpartum.

• The illness may be manifest later in the puerperium.

Symptoms and signs

Postpartum "blues" [1]

• It develops within first 2 weeks after delivery; peak symptoms occur between 3rd and 7th day after delivery.

Insomnia, anxiety, tearfulness, headaches, irritability, appetite changes, feeling overwhelmed and oversensitive.

• Patients do not meet criteria for major depressive disorder (*see* Depression).

Postpartum depression

• It can occur up to 6 months after delivery; severe cases present early (within the first 6 weeks).

• Patients meet criteria for major depressive disorder (*see* Depression), characterized by depressed mood and/or loss of interest in activities; disrupted sleep and early-morning wakening; psychomotor retardation; or overvalued ideas or delusion of unworthiness, incompetence, and guilt; suicidal thoughts.

• Frequent intrusive, obsessional thoughts of failure as a mother or harm coming to the child are common manifestations.

Postpartum psychosis (bipolar or manic-depressive psychosis)

• Onset is abrupt and occurs between days 3 and 16 in most women. Within a week, the picture settles to become clearly that of an acute severe affective psychosis.

Perplexity, agitation, confusion (first few days) followed by hallucinations, delusions, emotional and behavioral disturbances: one-third of patients manifest manic symptoms (overactivity, elation, pressure of speech, flight of ideas), two-thirds manifest depressive symptoms (*see* above).

Investigations

• No special clinical investigation is needed beyond the normal physical postpartum investigations, including history, physical examination, and hemoglobin and thyroid-stimulating hormone levels.

Complications

Delayed detection and treatment of severe depression, physical morbidity.

Suicide and infanticide: rare but tragic and often unavoidable.

Failure to establish relationship with child.

Removal of child by family or social services.

Lasting problems in child's social, emotional, and cognitive development and physical health.

Marital difficulties.

Differential diagnosis

Transient hypothyroidism or thyrotoxicosis, profound anemia (fatigue), pituitary or adrenal disorders.

Acute confusional state (delirium, organic brain syndrome): rare, caused by infection, eclampsia, or other neurological disorder.

Distress: caused by social, marital, or relationship problems.

Etiology [2]

• Both biological and psychological factors are important.

• No current evidence suggests that the hormonal profile of mentally ill mothers differs from that of normal women; the postpartum drop to low progesterone concentrations is probably responsible for the "blues."

• Manic-depressive illness in a first-degree relative indicates a 1 in 3 risk for postpartum psychosis.

• Previous postpartum depression indicates a 1 in 3 risk after subsequent deliveries; previous nonpostpartum depression indicates a 1 in 5 risk or higher.

• Infertility, assisted reproduction, previous obstetric loss, or traumatic delivery may contribute to severe depressive illness.

• Marital conflict, social adversity, lack of confidante, single status, low socioeconomic status all increase the risk of a mild depressive episode.

Epidemiology

• 85% of new mothers experience a depressed mood after birth.

• 5%–20% of women who deliver develop postpartum depression.

• Two in 1000 women who deliver are admitted to a psychiatric hospital suffering from a postpartum psychosis.

Treatment

Diet and lifestyle [1]

• Counseling expectant mothers and fathers during the prenatal period about the symptoms and prevalence of postpartum depression will better prepare them for their upcoming roles and occupational changes.

• Expectant mothers should be taught to avoid self-blame if they are unable to meet their expanded responsibilities.

• Stress reduction and family therapy may also help women cope with the emotional and physical demands of their families.

Pharmacological treatment

• Women suffering from severe depression, with active suicidal or infanticidal ideation, and with postpartum psychosis should be treated in an inpatient psychiatric unit.

• Most postpartum depressive illnesses can be managed at home if the patient is not suicidal or infanticidal.

Postpartum "blues"

• Brief in-office counseling and supportive therapy are usually sufficient. Women with complicated social situations (*e.g.*, marital relational problems, threats of domestic violence) will benefit from more intense counseling services from a trained therapist.

Postpartum depression

• Most women (~60%) respond satisfactorily to antidepressants, such as selective serotonin reuptake inhibitors (SSRIs) or tricyclic antidepressants (TCAs). Both classes of antidepressants are excreted in breast milk, although concentrations are small for SSRIs. Long-term effects on neonates are unknown. Breast-feeding should either be discontinued (especially TCAs) or timed to avoid peak concentrations (SSRIs).

• Excessive sedation should be avoided because of childcare responsibilities.

• Women should always be referred to a psychiatrist if they are severely distressed, in a state of hopeless despair, or suicidal. *See* Depression *for details.*

Postpartum psychosis

• The immediate priority is to sedate the patient with neuroleptics to a level that makes her safe, allows adequate nutrition, and reduces her agitation, confusion, and fear.

• Treatment often requires both antipsychotic and antidepressant medication.

Standard dosage	Haloperidol, 5–20 mg daily orally for acute psychosis; alternatively risperidone, 1–3 mg twice daily.
Contraindications	*Neuroleptics:* hypersensitivity; caution in cardiovascular disease, hepatic impairment, epilepsy.
Special points	If no response occurs within 7 days, electroconvulsive therapy or lithium carbonate can be tried. Postpartum women are very sensitive to the extrapyramidal side effects of neuroleptic agents; close monitoring is needed. SSRIs and TCAs take 10–14 days to take effect. No psychotropic drug is of proven safety in breast-feeding.
Main drug interactions	*Neuroleptics:* antagonize anticonvulsants.
Main side effects	*Neuroleptics:* sedation, extrapyramidal effects, acute dystonias, akasthesia, parkinsonism.

Treatment aims

To provide early detection and prompt treatment in the setting most appropriate for safe recovery.
To give priority to the needs of the baby.
To avoid unnecessary separation of mother and baby.
To provide social and psychological support.

Psychosocial treatment

Adjunctive psychotherapy and specific counseling for all patients.

• Nondirective or cognitive therapy (6 sessions at weekly intervals) is effective for mild depressive illness.

• Practical social support and addressing of concurrent problems is essential.

• Psychosocial treatment is as effective as antidepressants for mild depressive illness.

Prognosis

• With early intervention and effective treatment the prognosis is excellent; improvement begins within 2 weeks and recovery within 6–8 weeks.

• Without treatment the illness may be prolonged, although 60% of patients recover spontaneously within 6 months.

Follow-up and management

• Treatment should continue for at least 6 months after the patient has recovered, longer in the case of a relapse.

• Patients with previous manic-depressive episodes should take lithium.

• For serious mental illness, the risk follows every childbirth: 1 in 3–5 risk of recurrent postpartum depression.

Key references

1. Susman JL: Postpartum depressive disorders. *J Fam Pract* 1996, **43(suppl):**S17–S24.

2. O'Hara MW: Social support, life events and depression during pregnancy and the peurperium. *Arch Gen Psych* 1986, **43:**569–573.

Diagnosis [1]

Symptoms and signs

• Pressure ulcers should be assessed for location; stage (*see* table); size; presence of sinus tracts, undermining, tunneling, exudate, necrotic tissue, and granulation tissue or epithelialization.

• Characteristics should be thoroughly documented.

• Pain associated with pressure ulcers should be assessed and treated with analgesics while the ulcer is healing.

Pressure ulcer staging	
Stage I	Nonblanchable erythema of intact skin
Stage II	Partial-thickness skin loss involving epidermis and/or dermis; the ulcer is superficial and appears as an abrasion, blister, or shallow crater
Stage III	Full-thickness skin loss involving damage or necrosis of subcutaneous tissue superficial to fascia; appears as deep crater with or without undermining of adjacent tissue
Stage IV	Full-thickness skin loss with extensive destruction, tissue necrosis, or damage to muscle, bone, tendon, or joint capsule; undermining and sinus tracts may be present

Risk factors [1]

Bed- and chair-bound status: especially with impaired ability to reposition.

Incontinence: fecal incontinence greater risk than urinary incontinence.

Poor nutritional status: albumin <3.5 mg/dL, total lymphocyte count <1800, patient not eating, weight <80% of ideal body weight. Vitamin deficiencies are common among nursing home residents and may contribute to ulcer formation and persistence.

Chronically moist or dry skin.

Friction and shear forces: pressure lateral to surface of the skin, as when repositioning patients by sliding or when patients sit up in bed without foot support.

• Risk assessment should be carried out periodically among patients with one or more risk factors. Serial use of assessment scales such as the Norton Scale (*see* table) help to measure patients' degree of risk and identify changes in risk status over time.

Norton scale*				
Physical condition	**Mental condition**	**Activity**	**Mobility**	**Incontinent**
Good = 4	Alert = 4	Ambulant = 4	Full = 4	Not = 4
Fair = 3	Apathetic = 3	Walk with help = 3	Slightly limited = 3	Occasional = 3
Poor = 2	Confused = 2	Chair-bound = 2	Very limited = 2	Usually (urine) = 2
Very bad = 1	Stupor = 1	Bed-bound = 1	Immobile = 1	Doubly = 1

*Scores are the total of individual scales (range, 5–20).

Investigations

Swab cultures: reflect surface colonization and have no diagnostic value.

Needle aspiration or tissue biopsy: should be used when necessary to obtain cultures.

Plain radiograph of underlying bone and nuclear medicine bone scan: for nonhealing pressure ulcers under appropriate treatment, may help diagnose underlying osteomyelitis.

Complications

Osteomyelitis, bacteremia, advancing cellulitis: most common.

Amyloidosis, endocarditis, heterotopic bone formation, maggot infestation, meningitis, perineal-urethral fistula, squamous cell carcinoma in the ulcer, sinus tract, or abscess formation: less common.

Differential diagnosis

• Commonly overlooked causes of non-healing ulcers include underestimate of ulcer stage, underlying osteomyelitis, and other complications such as squamous cell carcinoma (*see* Complications).

Etiology

• Pressure ulcers occur as a result of inadequate blood flow to capillaries in soft-tissue beds, in part due to mechanical pressure over the involved area.

• Tissue-threatening compromise of microvessel blood flow is a function of both pressure and time, and can occur as a result of high pressures for brief periods (*e.g.,* sitting on ischial tuberosities), low pressure for prolonged periods (*e.g.,* heel pressure in bedbound patients), or both (*e.g.,* trochanteric pressure in bed-bound patient).

Epidemiology

• Pressure ulcers occur in 10% of hospitalized patients; 20%–25% of nursing home residents; 60% of hospitalized quadreplegic patients; 66% of elderly patients admitted to hospitals for femoral fracture.

• 25% of nonhealing pressure ulcers are associated with underlying osteomyelitis.

• Total annual national cost of pressure ulcer treatment is estimated at $1.3 billion.

Treatment

Diet and lifestyle

Prevention [1]

• Minimize risk factors through skin care, ensuring adequate dietary intake, maximizing mobility.

• Skin massage over bony prominences may lead to deep tissue trauma and thus should not be used.

• Reposition patients at risk at least every 2 hours, using a written schedule. Because of higher pressure loads, seated patients must be repositioned every hour, by returning to bed if necessary. Seated patients who are able should be taught to reposition themselves every 15 minutes.

• Pillows or foam wedges should be used to keep bony prominences (knees, ankles) from direct contact with one another.

• Patients who are completely immobile should have a care plan that includes the use of devices that totally relieve pressure on the heels (*e.g.*, by raising them off the bed).

• Static support surfaces (foam rubber, "egg-crate" cushions) are helpful in patients who can be periodically repositioned (or reposition themselves). Doughnut cushions should be avoided.

Debridement [2]

• Devitalized tissue should be removed. Sharp debridement is necessary with advancing cellulitis or sepsis. Debridement by a surgeon is indicated for large ulcers or if the primary physician in inexperienced. Mechanical (*e.g.*, wet-to-dry dressings, hydrotherapy, wound irrigation, and dextranomers) or enzymatic (*e.g.*, collagenase) debridement is effective for small wounds.

Wound cleansing [2]

• Normal saline should be used to cleanse most wounds, initially at each dressing change. Antiseptic agents and skin cleansers are cytotoxic to normal tissues and should generally be avoided. Wound should be irrigated under mild pressure (*e.g.*, syringe with 19-gauge needle), adequate to remove bacteria and debris. Whirlpool treatment may be necessary for thick exudate, slough, or necrotic tissue.

Wound dressing [2]

• After debridement and wound cleansing, moist dressings (*e.g.*, continuously moist saline gauze, film, hydrocolloid dressing) are preferable to dry dressings.

• Dynamic support surfaces (air-fluidized, low-air loss, and alternating air support devices) are expensive but should be considered in patients with stage III or IV pressure ulcers on multiple turning surfaces.

Pharmacological treatment

• Stage II, III, and IV pressure ulcers are uniformly colonized with bacteria. Colonization per se need not (and should not) be treated with antimicrobial agents. Minimizing bacterial colonization enhances healing, however, and is best achieved through wound debridement and cleansing (*see* Wound dressing).

• Wound infection (purulence, foul odor) is initially managed by increasing the frequency of wound cleansing.

• For infected ulcers that produce exudate after 2–4 weeks of aggressive wound cleansing, or appear clean but nonhealing, a 2-week trial of a topical antibiotic is appropriate. The antibiotic should be effective against gram-negative, gram-positive, and anaerobic organisms (*e.g.*, silver sulfadizine, triple antibiotic). If resistant staphylococcal organisms are prevalent in the nursing home, mupirocin ointment should be used and susceptibility demonstrated.

• Choice of topical antimicrobial agents can be guided by culture of material obtained through needle aspiration or biopsy of ulcer tissue. Swab cultures are not helpful in guiding therapy, because all open pressure ulcers are colonized with bacteria.

• Appropriate systemic antibiotic therapy should be given for patients with bacteremia, sepsis, advancing cellulitis, or osteomyelitis. Systemic antibiotics are not required for pressure ulcers with only clinical signs of local infection.

Treatment aims
To achieve complete healing.
To provide patient comfort (in terminal illness).

Other treatments
• Electrical stimulation therapy, using proper equipment and trained personnel, may be helpful for stage III and IV and recalcitrant stage II ulcers.

• Hyperbaric oxygen, infrared, ultraviolet, and low-energy laser irradiation, and ultrasound therapy have not been demonstrated to be of benefit.

• Various topical treatments (sugar, vitamins, hormones), growth factors, and skin equivalents have not been demonstrated to be of benefit.

• Operative repair (*e.g.*, skin grafts, skin flaps, musculocutaneous flaps) should be considered for clean stage III or stage IV pressure ulcers not responding to optimal care.

• Vitamin C and zinc nutritional supplements may aid healing in the presence of deficiencies.

Prognosis
• A clean pressure ulcer should show evidence of some healing within 2–4 weeks. If no progress can be demonstrated, re-evaluate the adequacy of the overall treatment plan as well as adherence to the plan, including risk factor modification.

Follow-up and management
Monitor at least weekly, with documentation of pressure ulcer characteristics and revision of management plan as appropriate.

Key references

1. *Pressure Ulcers in Adults: Prediction and Prevention.* Rockville: Agency for Health Care Policy and Research, Public Health Service, U.S. Department of Health and Human Services; 1992 [AHCPR Publication 92-0047.] (Available at U.S. National Library of Medicine's Health Services/Technology Assessment Text (HSTAT) web page: http://text.nlm.nih.gov/).

2. *Pressure Ulcers in Adults: Treatment.* Rockville: Agency for Health Care Policy and Research, Public Health Service, U.S. Department of Health and Human Services; 1994. [AHCPR Publication 94-0075.]

Diagnosis

Symptoms

Symptoms of venous or arterial thrombosis.

Signs

• Patients to investigate include those with the following:

Venous thromboembolism before the age of 40–45 years.

Recurrent venous thrombosis or thrombophlebitis.

Thrombosis in an unusual site: *e.g.*, mesenteric vein, cerebral vein.

Unexplained neonatal thrombosis.

Skin necrosis.

Arterial thrombosis before the age of 30 years.

Relatives with a specific defect.

Unexplained prolonged coagulation screening tests.

Recurrent fetal loss, idiopathic thrombocytopenic purpura, SLE.

Investigations

• Functional and immunological assays are needed for a precise diagnosis.

• Screening tests and functional assays should be performed on fresh citrated blood samples collected with minimal venous stasis on all patients being investigated for a prothrombotic state.

Complete blood count and film.

Measurement of prothrombin, activated partial thromboplastin, and thrombin time; fibrinogen.

Assays for antithrombin III, protein C, protein S, activated protein C resistance (factor V Leiden), plasminogen, heparin cofactor II, anticardiolipin antibodies, lupus anticoagulant, factor XII, dysfibrinogenemia, and homocystinuria.

Fibrinolytic tests: before and after stimulation (*i.e.*, venous occlusion or DDAVP).

Fibrin plate, tissue-type plasminogen activator, and PA1-1 assays.

Platelet activation markers analysis: *i.e.*, GMP-140 expression, plasma β-thromboglobulin.

Complications

Arterial and venous thrombosis and embolism.

Differential diagnosis

Hyperviscosity.

Etiology

Common acquired causes of thrombosis
Diabetes mellitus, hyperlipidemia, malignancy, myeloproliferative disorders, chronic liver disease, SLE, paraproteinemias, nephrotic syndrome, antiphospholipid syndrome.

• These disorders cause predisposition to thrombosis in a multifactorial way; specific homeostatic assays are generally unhelpful in the investigation and management of individual patients.

Inherited defects with increased tendency to thrombosis
Antithrombin III, protein C, protein S, factor V Leiden, plasminogen, heparin cofactor II, factor XII, dysfibrinogenemia, homocystinuria.

• Most of these disorders represent autosomal dominant traits with variable penetrance.

• Deficiency in the heterozygous state predisposes to thrombosis either spontaneously or in association with other high-risk factors.

Pathophysiology
• The balance of the hemostatic mechanism can be shifted in favor of thrombosis in the following circumstances:
Increased coagulation system activity.
Increased platelet activity.
Decreased fibrinolytic activity.
Damaged vascular endothelial activity.

Epidemiology

• Epidemiological studies have shown an increased incidence of thrombotic events associated with raised concentrations particularly of fibrinogen, factor VII, and factor VIII:C, with a frequency of 1 in 2000–5000.

High-risk factors for thrombosis

Surgical and nonsurgical trauma.
Age.
Immobilization.
Heart failure.
Prior venous thrombosis and varicose veins.
Paralysis of lower limbs.
Obesity.
Estrogen treatment.
Pregnancy and puerperium.
Smoking.
Raised blood viscosity.

Treatment

Diet and lifestyle

• No special precautions are necessary.

Pharmacological treatment

Prophylaxis for venous thromboembolism [1]

• The degree of risk must be assessed depending on the predisposing factors.

Low risk: early ambulation, graduated compression stocking.
Moderate risk: standard unfractionated heparin, 5000 U s.c. every 8-12 hours.
High risk: low molecular weight heparin, s.c. every 12-24 hours, dose depending on type of heparin.

• The degree of risk for surgical prophylaxis may be defined as follows:

Low risk: <40 years, minor surgery lasting <1 hour.
Moderate risk: >40 years, abdominal or thoracic surgery lasting >1 hour.
High risk: >40 years, knee and hip orthopedic surgery, obesity, and malignancy.

Heparin

Standard dosage	Unfractionated heparin, 5000 U i.v. bolus, followed by 1000-2000 U/h i.v. for 5-7 days. Low molecular weight heparin s.c. once daily [2].
Contraindications	Rare hypersensitivity, risk of bleeding complications.
Special points	Activated partial thromboplastin time must be monitored 6 hours after start of treatment, then at least every 24 hours, with dose adjustment to maintain ratio at 1.5-2.5 times control.
Main drug interactions	Drugs that interfere with platelet aggregation or coagulation.
Main side effects	Bleeding, thrombocytopenia, rebound thrombosis, osteoporosis (if treatment lasts >3 months), rare alopecia, skin rash.

• Heparinization can be reversed by administering protamine sulfate, 1 mg, which neutralizes ~100 U heparin; maximum dose, 40 mg i.v. in 10 minutes.

Warfarin [3]

Standard dosage	Warfarin, 10 mg orally on days 1 and 2; 5 mg orally on day 3; then adjusted daily according to prothrombin time, maintained at 1-20 mg daily.
Contraindications	Pregnancy.
Special points	Prothrombin time must be monitored, with results expressed as INR with therapeutic range of 2.0-4.5.
Main drug interactions	Many medications potentiate or antagonize effect; for any new medication, prothrombin time should be checked.
Main side effects	Bleeding, skin necrosis after first few days of treatment in the case of protein C or S deficiency.

• Anticoagulant effects can be reversed by an infusion of fresh frozen plasma or factor II, IX, and X concentrate if bleed is life-threatening; vitamin K_1, 1-2 mg i.v., takes 6-24 hours to reverse warfarin effect.

Antiplatelet agents

• These are indicated for prophylaxis and prevention of further arterial thrombotic events when platelet activation has been shown to be a primary pathological factor, particularly myocardial ischemia and cerebrovascular thrombotic strokes, including transient ischemic attack, for secondary thrombocytosis (>800 × 10^9/L), and for essential thrombocythemia.

Aspirin, 75 mg orally daily or 300 mg twice weekly, or dipyridamole, up to 100 mg orally 3 times daily (dipyridamole may cause severe headaches).

Key references

1. Lowe GDO: Risk of and prophylaxis for venous thromboembolism in hospital patients. *BMJ* 1992, **305**:567–574.

2. The Columbus Investigators: Low molecular weight heparin in the treatment of patients with venous thrombolembolism. *N Engl J Med* 1997, **337**:657–662.

3. Poller L: Oral anticoagulation. *J Clin Pathol* 1990, **43**:177–183.

General reference

Thomas DP, Roberts HR: Hypercoagulability in venous and arterial thrombosis. *Am Int Med* 1997, **126**:638–644.

Diagnosis

Symptoms

Pruritus: in 20% of patients.

Unpleasant odor: in severe cases.

Joint pain, tenderness, and morning stiffness: in cases with psoriatic arthritis.

Chills: secondary to loss of body heat in patients with generalized psoriasis.

Signs

Scalp
Scaling.

Skin
Psoriatic plaques: especially on extensor surfaces and areas of trauma; some patients have pustules (pustular psoriasis) [1].

Oral mucosa
Glossitis or geographic tongue: in 10% of patients.

Nails
• 50% of patients have nail involvement.

Pitting.

Subungual keratotic debris.

Onycholysis.

Discoloration: yellow-brown ("oil spots").

Musculoskeletal system
Sausage digits.

Periarticular swelling: especially small joints of fingers and toes.

Asymmetrical oligoarticular arthritis: most common.

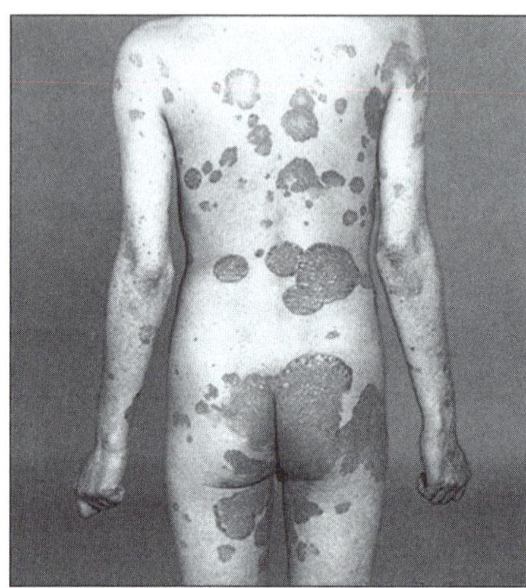

Chronic plaque psoriasis. (*See* Color Plate.)

Investigations

HIV test: if there is a history of sudden onset of severe psoriasis with no family history and no previous personal history [2].

Antistreptolysin O (ASO) titer: if guttate flare from recent streptococcal infection is suspected.

Complications

Exfoliative erythroderma.

Ankylosing spondylitis.

Psoriatic arthropathy.

Generalized pustular psoriasis: sheets of sterile pustules occurring in patients with psoriasis and associated fever, arthralgias, skin tenderness, and malaise.

Differential diagnosis

Lichen planus.

Tinea corporis.

Seborrheic dermatitis.

Reiter's disease.

Pityriasis rosea.

Secondary syphilis.

Subacute cutaneous lupus erythematosus.

Premycosis fungoides (parapsoriasis).

Drug reaction.

Atopic eczema: especially patients with advanced lichenification.

Etiology

• Psoriasis is a multifactorial disease with a definite genetic predisposition.

Positive family history in 30% of cases.

• Histocompatibility antigen HLA-Cw6 is strongly associated (relative risk of 24).

• The presence of HLA-B17 or B27 is associated with more severe disease or associated arthritis.

• Although immunological abnormalities of humoral and cell-mediated immunity have been described, no specific circulatory immune abnormalities have been identified.

• Epidermal transit time is rapidly increased (6–9-fold).

Precipitating factors

Streptococcal infections.

Trauma: Koebner's phenomenon.

Drugs: beta-blockers, antimalarials, lithium, oral corticosteroid withdrawal.

Stress.

Sunlight: a small subset of patients actually worsen with sun exposure especially sunburn.

Alcoholism: may be related to decreased compliance in alcoholic patients.

Epidemiology

• Incidence is 1%–3% of world population [3].

• It affects 2–8 million people in the United States.

• Peak onset is in the second decade of life, but it may appear at any age.

Treatment

Diet and lifestyle

• No specific precautions appear necessary.

Pharmacological treatment

• Cases of generalized pustular psoriasis of exfoliative erythroderma should be referred to a specialist immediately.

Topical treatment

Coal tar: safe and effective in plaque psoriasis; messy to apply (limiting compliance).

Steroids: effective and cosmetically acceptable; long-term use needs close supervision.

Vitamin D_3 analogues: calcipotriene appears safe and effective in mild to moderate psoriasis; may be irritating [4].

Phototherapy: ultraviolet B useful for chronic plaque and guttate psoriasis, alone or with other treatments such as topical applications.

Tazarotene (a recently developed receptor-selective retinoid): efficacious in mild to moderate plaque psoriasis. Once-daily application of a 0.1% or 0.05% gel affords rapid resolution of psoriasis lesions and some patients have a sustained therapeutic effect up to 12 weeks posttherapy.

Tazarotene is cosmetically acceptable and is minimally absorbed systemically with adverse events limited to local irritation [6].

Systemic therapy

• Treatment should be given under supervision of a specialist [5].

• Methotrexate is used in widespread plaque, acute generalized pustular psoriasis, and erythrodermic psoriatic arthropathy as short-term or maintenance treatment.

• Retinoids are effective particularly in acral or generalized pustular psoriasis.

• Cyclosporine is effective for severe refractory psoriasis and psoriatic arthropathy.

• Long-term photochemotherapy (oral or topical psoralens with UVA) is complicated by increased risk of cutaneous squamous cell carcinoma.

Standard dosage	This should be decided by a specialist who has experience with systemic therapy.
Contraindications	History of previous hypersensitivity to drug. *Methotrexate*: hepatic disease, alcohol abuse, malignancy [7]. *Retinoids*: hepatic and renal damage, pregnancy. *Cyclosporine*: renal disease, uncontrolled hypertension, infection, malignancy.
Special points	*Methotrexate*: pregnancy must be avoided. *Retinoids*: pregnancy must be avoided during treatment and for up to 2 years afterward. *Cyclosporine*: sudden withdrawal may lead to relapse within a few weeks but not to the severe rebound seen with systemic steroids; monitoring should include blood pressure, serum creatinine, and glomerular filtration rate.
Main drug interactions	*Methotrexate*: alcohol, salicylates, NSAIDs, probenecid, phenytoin, retinoids, pyrimethamine, furosemide. *Retinoids*: reduce effect of warfarin. *Cyclosporine*: NSAIDs may potentiate nephrotoxicity. The following drugs increase cyclosporine levels (inhibit P450): diltiazem, danazol, ketoconazole, nicardipine, bromocriptine, fluconazole, verapamil, metoclopramide, itraconazole.
Main side effects	*Methotrexate*: hepatic fibrosis (liver biopsy every 1.5 g cumulative dose), acute bone-marrow suppression. *Retinoids*: raised serum lipids, elevated liver enzymes (abnormalities return to normal on cessation of treatment), spinal changes after prolonged treatment (diffuse idiopathic skeletal hyperostosis). *Cyclosporine*: dose-related hypertension and nephrotoxicity (plasma creatinine should be monitored at baseline, then monthly).

Key references

1. Zelickson BD, Muller SA: Generalized pustular psoriasis: a review of 63 cases. *Arch Dermatol* 1991, **127**:1339–1345.

2. Zalla MJ, Sue WP, Franesway AF: Dermatologist manifestations of human immunodeficiency virus infection. *Mayo Clin Proc* 1992, **67**:1089–1108.

3. Farber EM, Nall ML: The natural history of psoriasis in 5600 patients. *Dermatologica* 1974, **148**:1–18.

4. Highton A, Quell J: Calcipotreine ointment 0.005% for psoriasis: a safety and efficacy study. Calcipotreine study group. *J Am Acad Dermatol* 1995, **32**:67–72.

5. Greaves MW, Weinstein GD: Treatment of psoriasis. *N Engl J Med* 1995, **332**:581–588.

6. Weinstein GD: Safety, efficacy and duration of therapeutic effect of tazarotene used in the treatment of plaque psoriasis. *Br J Dermatol* 1996, **135(suppl 49)**:32–36.

7. Petrazzuoli M, *et al.*: Monitoring patients taking methotrexate for hepatotoxicity: does the standard of care match published guidelines? *J Am Acad Dermatol* 1994, **31**:969–977.

Diagnosis

Symptoms

Precocious puberty
Pubertal development <8 years in girls, <9 years in boys.

Rapid growth.

Menstruation in girls.

Advanced skeletal maturation.

Behavioral disturbance.

Delayed puberty
Lack of pubertal development >14 years in girls, >15 years in boys.

Lack of pubertal growth spurt.

Small external genitalia in boys.

Possible anosmia.

Social difficulties.

Signs

Precocious puberty
Secondary isosexual sexual development.

Tall stature.

Short stature.

Cutaneous pigmentation: McCune–Albright syndrome.

Acne, clitoromegaly: indicating virilization in girls.

Delayed puberty
Lack of secondary sexual development.

Gynecomastia in boys.

Family history of delayed puberty.

Signs of Turner's syndrome in girls.

Chronic pediatric illness: *e.g.,* Crohn's disease, thalassemia.

Investigations [1,2]

Precocious puberty
Usually divided into gonadotropin-dependent (hypothalamic or pituitary) or gonadotropin-independent (*see* Etiology).

Hormone measurement: for gonadotropin and sex steroid concentrations.

MRI or CT of hypothalamic–pituitary region: to exclude structural lesion.

Ovarian ultrasonography: to assess ovarian development.

Adrenal CT: for precocious puberty secondary to adrenal tumors.

Delayed puberty
Hormone measurement: for gonadotropin and sex steroid concentrations.

Complete blood count, electrolytes analysis, liver function tests: to exclude chronic disease.

Karyotyping: in girls.

MRI or CT of hypothalamic–pituitary region: to exclude structural lesion.

Ovarian ultrasonography: to assess ovarian development.

Test of smell: to exclude Kallmann's syndrome.

Clomiphene test: in older patients, to exclude gonadotropin-releasing hormone deficiency.

Complications

Precocious puberty
Progression of pubertal development.

Early menstruation.

Premature completion of skeletal maturation.

Adult short stature.

Delayed puberty
No secondary sexual development.

Absence of pubertal growth spurt.

Emotional, physical immaturity.

Infertility.

Etiology [1,2]

True precocious puberty (gonadotropin-dependent)
Idiopathic (principally girls).
Structural lesions of hypothalamic region (tumors).
Postcranial irradiation.
Hydrocephalus.
Hypothyroidism.

Pseudoprecocious puberty (gonadotropin-independent)

McCune–Albright syndrome.
Familial male precocious puberty.
Adrenal tumors.
Congenital adrenal hyperplasia.
Gonadal tumors.
Human chorionic gonadotropin–secreting tumors.
Exogenous sex steroids.

Delayed puberty
Constitutional.
Chronic pediatric illness.
Malnutrition.
Hypopituitarism (idiopathic, tumors).
Isolated gonadotropin-releasing hormone deficiency and anosmia (Kallmann's syndrome).
Hyperprolactinemia.
Intensive exercise.
Turner's or Klinefelter's syndromes.
Radiotherapy, surgery, chemotherapy, autoimmunity.

Epidemiology

• No reliable estimates are available.

Treatment

Diet and lifestyle

• No special precautions are necessary.

Pharmacological treatment [1,2]

For central precocious puberty

• Primary CNS lesions, *e.g.*, tumors, must be treated.

Gonadotropin-releasing hormone analogue fixed dose s.c. injection monthly or cyproterone acetate, 50–100 mg daily; treatment continued until appropriate age for puberty to progress.

• Long-term cyproterone treatment may induce adrenal insufficiency.

For gonadotropin-independent precocious puberty

Treatment of underlying disease (*e.g.*, congenital adrenal hyperplasia).

Androgen antagonists (spironolactone).

Inhibitors of steroid synthesis (ketoconazole).

For delayed puberty

• The primary cause must be treated, *e.g.*, chronic illness, pituitary tumor, hyperprolactinemia.

For boys: testosterone, from 50 mg every 2 weeks to 300 mg every 3 weeks i.m. depending on age.

For girls: ethinyl estradiol, 2–10 µg daily, increasing to 30 µg daily with norethindrone or medroxyprogesterone acetate, 5 mg daily on days 1–14 of each calendar month.

Treatment aims

To replace hormones.

Prognosis

• Prognosis is good unless the disorder is caused by a tumor.

Follow-up and management

• Patients should be checked every 3–6 months to ensure that treatment is effective.

Key references

1. Bridges NA, Brook CDG: Premature sexual development. In *Clinical Endocrinology.* Edited by Grossman A. Oxford: Blackwell Scientific Publications; 1992:837–846.

2. Stanhope R, Albanese A, Shalet S: Delayed puberty. *BMJ* 1992, **305**:790.

Diagnosis

Symptoms

• Symptoms may be minimal.

Dyspnea, cough, sputum production, hemoptysis, chest pain, weight loss, fever.

• Hemoptysis with chest pain suggests Kaposi's sarcoma in those with AIDS but pneumonia in those with other forms of immunosuppression.

Signs

Tachypnea.

Cyanosis: indicating respiratory failure.

Consolidation: suggesting bacterial infection.

Collapse: suggesting infection or neoplasia.

Pleural effusion: suggesting mycobacterial infection or neoplasia.

Investigations

• The choice of investigation depends on the physical signs and symptoms and the degree of immunosuppression.

To assess degree of immunosuppression

Complete blood count, differential leukocyte count: in patients with acquired immunosuppression, *e.g.*, to assess neutropenia, after organ transplantation.

Immunoglobulin measurement, CD4 count: in patients with acquired immunosuppression; normal CD4 count in early stages of HIV infection, bacterial infection common; low CD4 count in late stages of HIV infection, opportunistic infection or neoplasia more likely.

To assess pulmonary complications of immunosuppression

Chest radiography: to identify focal or generalized abnormality.

CT: to assess pulmonary abnormalities in more detail (*e.g.*, intrathoracic lymph nodes).

Oximetry or arterial blood gas measurement: at rest or exercise, essential for early detection of respiratory failure.

Sputum for special stains and cytology: in patients with nonproductive coughs, sputum may be induced by inhalation of 3% nebulized saline solution.

Bronchoscopy, bronchoalveolar lavage, transbronchial biopsy, open lung biopsy: for tissue diagnosis.

Mediastinoscopy: if mediastinal lymph-node disease has been identified.

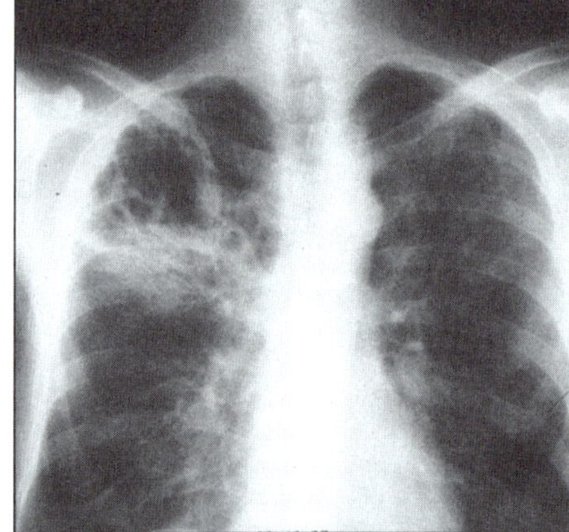

Chest radiograph showing cavitating aspergilloma.

Complications

Respiratory failure.

Disseminated infection.

Disseminated secondary malignancy.

Treatment

Diet and lifestyle

• Excessive alcohol consumption should be avoided.

• Cigarette smoking should be stopped because of the increased incidence of pulmonary complications in immunosuppressed patients who smoke.

Pharmacological treatment

• Treatment depends on diagnosis, which should be as accurate as possible.

• In deteriorating patients, treatment must be started empirically, depending on the most probable cause or agent; this is determined by the combination of symptoms, signs, degree of immunocompromise, stage of immunocompromise, and local pathogenic load.

Antibiotics

• If a specific organism is not detected and the patient is deteriorating, broad-spectrum cover should be used when there is purulence on the Gram stain.

Antituberculous drugs

• Four-drug treatment (ethambutol, rifampin, pyrazinamide, isoniazid) is recommended until sensitivity is available.

Antiviral agents

• Treatment should be initiated only if diagnosis is established.

For cytomegalovirus disease: Ganciclovir, 6 mg/kg twice daily initially, then maintenance dose depending on response.

Foscarnet, 90 mg/kg continuous infusion over 90 minutes twice daily depending on renal function.

• Renal function and leukocyte count must be monitored.

Antifungal agents

• Treatment should be initiated only if diagnosis is established.

Amphotericin B, 0.5 mg/kg daily i.v., increasing to 1 mg/kg daily, depending on renal function.

Itraconazole, 200 mg daily.

Antiparasitic agents

Trimethoprim, 15 mg/kg, may be used for *Pneumocystis* spp. infection.

Chemotherapy

• Chemotherapy may be used in certain patients with Kaposi's sarcoma or secondary B cell lymphoma or carcinoma.

• The choice of treatment is determined locally, and the use of chemotherapy combined with radiotherapy for symptomatic treatment must be considered.

Treatment aims

To eradicate infection and to prevent recurrence.

To relieve symptoms of secondary neoplasia or Kaposi's sarcoma.

Other treatments

Controlled oxygen therapy.

Continuous positive airways pressure.

Mechanical ventilation: needs careful consideration, ideally with the patient or a relative, before initiation.

Prognosis

• Prognosis depends on the cause of immunosuppression and the form of pulmonary complication.

• Mortality is 10%–20% in transiently neutropenic patients with bacterial infection.

• If the immunosuppression is reversible, recurrence is unlikely after the patient has recovered from an acute event.

Follow-up and management

• In continuing immunosuppression, follow-up and management depend on the specific diagnosis: for example, HIV-infected patients may need prolonged prophylactic treatment against recurrence of *P. carinii* infection.

General references

Dichter JR, Levine SJ, Shelhamer JH: Approach to the immunocompromised host with pulmonary symptoms. *Hematol Oncol Clin North Am* 1993, **7**:887–912.

Lartholory O, Dupont B: Antifungal prophylaxis during neutropenia and immunodeficiency. *Clin Microbiol Rev* 1997, **10**:477–504.

Verra F, *et al.*: Bronchoalveolar lavage in immunocompromised patients: clinical and functional consequences. *Chest* 1992, **101**:1215–1220.

Wade JC: Treatment of fungal and other opportunistic infections in immuno-compromised patients. *Leukemia* 1997, **11(suppl 4)**:S538–S539.

Diagnosis

Symptoms

Pleuritic chest pain, dyspnea, hemoptysis: indicating acute minor pulmonary embolism.

Acute-onset dyspnea, syncope, central chest pain: indicating acute massive pulmonary embolism.

Gradual-onset dyspnea, pleuritic chest pain, decreasing exercise tolerance: indicating subacute massive pulmonary embolism.

Increasing dyspnea, effort syncope: indicating chronic pulmonary embolism.

Signs

• Pulmonary embolism is manifest in several ways, depending on the extent of pulmonary vascular obstruction, the time during which the obstruction accumulates, and the presence or absence of pre-existing heart or lung disease [1].

Shortness of breath, pleural rub, signs associated with pleural effusion: indicating pulmonary infarction.

Tachypnea or hyperventilation, reduced cardiac output, right heart failure: indicating massive pulmonary embolism.

Pulmonary hypertension: indicating chronic pulmonary embolism.

Investigations

• The diagnosis of pulmonary embolism needs a high index of clinical suspicion, combined with the results of investigations that may confirm or refute these suspicions.

Pulmonary angiography: allows definitive diagnosis but is invasive and needs specialized facilities; emboli seen as filling defects within contrast-filled pulmonary arteries [2].

Chest radiography: helps to exclude other conditions; may show vascular markings or large pulmonary artery shadow in massive embolism; may also show linear basal atelectasis in pulmonary infarction; but this is a nonspecific sign.

ECG: the classic S_1, Q_3, T_3 pattern is nonspecific and unusual. Sinus tachycardia is usual, although atrial fibrillation or flutter may occur.

Ventilation perfusion scanning: easily performed, low-risk procedure; normal scan virtually excludes pulmonary embolus; nondiagnostic scans need investigation for presence of peripheral venous thrombosis to support diagnosis of pulmonary embolism (if negative, untreated patient has <3% chance of subsequent pulmonary embolism) or pulmonary angiography; high-probability scan usually diagnostic, with 98% specificity, 91% positive predictive value (74% in patients with previous pulmonary embolism), but low sensitivity (41%); investigation must not be delayed because 14% of high-probability scans and 45% of indeterminate scans become normal by day 7 of treatment [3].

Magnetic resonance angiography: shows promise as an alternative in "noninvasive" diagnosis of pulmonary embolism [4].

Echocardiography: primarily useful in differential diagnosis of dyspnea; thrombus seen within right heart or proximal pulmonary artery and high index of clinical suspicion may be considered diagnostic. Demonstration of right ventricular enlargement may lead to initial consideration of the diagnosis.

Doppler ultrasonography, phlebography, impedance phlethysmography: indirect investigations for proximal leg vein thrombosis; if positive, they may provide a useful alternative to pulmonary angiography in patients with suspected minor pulmonary embolism but indeterminate lung scan.

Complications

Death.

Pulmonary infarction, infection, cavitation, or hypertension.

Differential diagnosis

• Pulmonary embolism has a wide differential diagnosis and hence its reputation as "The Great Masquerader."

Acute minor pulmonary embolism
Pneumonia.

Acute massive pulmonary embolism
Septicemia.
Myocardial infarction.
Hypovolemia.
Pericardial tamponade.

Subacute massive pulmonary embolism
Pulmonary edema
Pneumonia
Hyperventilation.

Chronic pulmonary embolism
Primary pulmonary hypertension.

Etiology

• >90% of pulmonary emboli originate as deep venous thrombosis of the lower extremities.

• Common causes include the following:
Surgery within past 1 month.
Medical illness (*e.g.*, myocardial infarction or stroke).
Immobility, cancer, obesity, or oral contraception.
Pregnancy or estrogen therapy.
Indwelling central venous lines.
Hypercoagulable states, which may be acquired (*e.g.*, lupus anticoagulant, anticardiolipin antibodies) or inherited (*e.g.*, antithrombin III deficiency, protein C deficiency).

Epidemiology

• At necropsy, pulmonary embolism has been found in 9%–26% of all patients; it was suspected before death in only ~16%.

• Deaths are more common in women and increase with age.

Treatment

Diet and lifestyle

• Patients should avoid periods of sustained immobility, *e.g.*, during longhaul flights.

Pharmacological treatment

Anticoagulant treatment: heparin

• Heparin is used for acute treatment of hemodynamicallly stable patients; it prevents further fibrin deposition and thrombus extension.

• Treatment must be commenced immediately if clinical suspicion is high.

Standard dosage	Heparin bolus, 5000–8000 U, then i.v. infusion to maintain activated partial thromboplastin time at 1.5-2.5 times control.
Contraindications	Active bleeding, recent cerebral hemorrhage or brain, eye, or spinal-cord surgery, malignant hypertension.
Special points	High-dose s.c. heparin reduces need for i.v. infusion and increases patient mobility.
Main drug interactions	Oral anticoagulants or drugs that interfere with platelet function, *e.g.*, aspirin or dextran solutions.
Main side effects	Bleeding, heparin-induced thrombocytopenia.

Anticoagulant treatment: warfarin

• Warfarin has no role in immediate treatment but prevents recurrence; it impairs coagulation, thus reducing thrombus formation.

Standard dosage	Warfarin, 10 mg daily for 2 days (average-sized adult); maintenance dose adjusted to obtain INR 2.0-3.0
Contraindications	As for heparin; avoided in pregnancy.
Special points	Should be started at same time as heparin treatment.
Main drug interactions	Many drugs may enhance or reduce the activity of warfarin; manufacturer's prescribing information should be consulted.
Main side effects	Bleeding.

Thrombolytic treatment

• This is indicated for hemodynamically compromised patients with proven pulmonary embolism (*i.e.*, high clinical suspicion and high-probability lung scan or pulmonary artery thrombus seen on echocardiography or angiography).

• Treatment promotes the dissolution of recently formed thrombus. It produces a more rapid resolution of emboli and improvement in cardiopulmonary status than heparin therapy alone does. No reduction in mortality, however, has been shown.

Standard dosage	Streptokinase, 250 000 U for 30 minutes followed by 100 000 U/h for 24 hours. Urokinase, 4400 U/kg for 10 minutes followed by 4400 U/kg/h for 12-24 hours. Recombinant tissue plasminogen activator, 100 mg by continuous infusion for 2 hours.
Contraindications	Active bleeding, recent cerebrovascular accident, recent trauma, major surgery, or organ biopsy.
Special points	Local administration is no more effective and is not safer than peripheral administration, which is simpler. All thrombolytic agents appear equally effective. Should be followed by heparin treatment.
Main drug interactions	None.
Main side effects	Bleeding (the risk of major hemorrhage is twice that with heparin), allergic reactions to streptokinase.

Prophylactic treatment

• Most deaths from pulmonary emboli are sudden or occur in patients in whom the diagnosis was not suspected; therefore a significant reduction in mortality is only achieved by adequate prevention.

Physical measures: early mobilization, pneumatic calf compression, and graduated compression stockings.

Drugs: conventional heparin, 5000 U s.c. every 8-12 hours; low molecular weight heparin, 3500-5000 U once daily depending on type used, or low-dose warfarin.

• Percutaneous or surgical placement of inferior vena cava filter may prevent subsequent embolism in patients with recurrent pulmonary embolism despite effective anticoagulation [5].

Treatment aims

To reduce morbidity of acute episode.
To prevent recurrence of pulmonary embolism or chronic pulmonary hypertension.

Other treatments

Inferior vena cava filters: used when anticoagulation is contraindicated or fails.
Pulmonary embolectomy.

Prognosis

• One-third of acute or subacute pulmonary emboli result in sudden death or are undiagnosed during life.

• Patients with untreated clinically apparent pulmonary emboli have a 30% mortality from recurrent emboli; this is reduced to 8% with effective treatment.

• Survivors of the acute or subacute episode usually have no clinical sequelae.

• Chronic pulmonary embolism carries a grave prognosis and pharmacological treatment is generally ineffective; elective thromboendarterectomy may produce long-term improvement in some patients.

• Patients who have had pulmonary emboli are at increased risk of further thrombo-embolic episodes when exposed to situations in which thrombosis might occur.

Follow-up and management

• Oral anticoagulant treatment and monitoring are continued for at least 3–6 months but may be continued indefinitely if underlying risk factors cannot be controlled.

Key references

1. Goldhaber SZ, Morpurgo M, WHO/ISFC Task Force on Pulmonary Embolism: Diagnosis, treatment, and prevention of pulmonary embolism. *JAMA* 1992, **268**:1727–1733.

2. Stein PD, *et al.*: Complications and validity of pulmonary angiography in acute pulmonary embolism. *Circulation* 1992, **85**:462–468.

3. PIOPED Investigators: Value of the ventilation/perfusion scan in acute pulmonary embolism. *JAMA* 1990, **263**:2753–2759.

4. Meany JFM, *et al.*: Diagnosis of pulmonary embolism with magnetic resonance angiography. *N Engl J Med* 1997, 336:1422–1427.

5. Becker DM, Philbrick JT, Selby JB: Inferior vena cava filters indications, safety, effectiveness. *Arch Intern Med* 1992, **152**:1985–1994.

Diagnosis

Symptoms

• **Dyspnea:** Predominant symptom with primary pulmonary hypertension. The disease often has an insidious onset in an otherwise healthy person. The disease is typically diagnosed late in its course. Dyspnea on exertion is often the earliest presenting complaint.

Easy fatiguability, exertional chest pain, syncope, near syncope, cough, hemoptysis, hoarseness (due to compression of the left recurrent laryngeal nerve by a dilated pulmonary artery).

Angina: can occur from right ventricular ischemia.

Congenital heart disease, pulmonary embolism, pulmonary fibrosis, polycythemia vera, chronic obstructive pulmonary disease (COPD): with secondary pulmonary hypertension, symptoms of the underlying disease often predominate.

Signs

• Patients with mild and moderate disease may have no signs or may develop dyspnea with minimal exertion.

Increased P2 (pulmonic component to the second heart sound): physical examination may disclose this as the disease becomes moderate.

Diastolic murmur of pulmonic regurgitation: seen in severe disease.

Evidence of right ventricular dilatation with a peristernal heave, signs of right ventricular failure (increased jugular venous distention, hepatomegaly, ascites, and pedal edema): often present with severe disease.

Right ventricular S3: may be heard.

Reduced carotid pulse.

Investigations

Chest radiography: shows enlarged central pulmonary artery and clear lung fields in primary pulmonary hypertension.

Pulmonary function tests: often normal other than a reduced diffusing capacity for carbon monoxide; may show a mild restrictive pattern.

Arterial blood gases: show hypoxemia and hypocapnea in moderate and severe disease.

ECG: shows right ventricular hypertrophy often with acute right ventricular strain (S wave in lead I and Q wave and inverted T wave in lead III).

Echocardiography: may demonstrate enlargement of pulmonary arteries with right atrial dilatation. Enlargement of the right ventricle and parodoxical septal motion are often seen. Doppler echocardiography can estimate, often quite accurately, the level of pulmonary artery systolic and mean pressures.

Nuclear ventilation–perfusion scanning: helpful to rule out chronic pulmonary embolism as a secondary cause of pulmonary hypertension.

CT: can visualize the left and right ventricular size as well as the major pulmonary arteries. CT of the lungs is useful in ruling out underlying pulmonary causes of secondary pulmonary hypertension.

Cardiac catheterization: provides precise measurement of pulmonary arterial, capillary, and venous pressures. The severity of right ventricular failure can be quantified with cardiac output measurements and wall motion can be examined. Cardiac catheterization also can identify patients with congenital or acquired intracardiac shunts.

Pulmonary angiography: best method for identifying pulmonary embolism as a secondary reason for the development of pulmonary hypertension.

Complications

Severe right heart failure with cor pulmonale: occurs in severe disease.

Progressive right ventricular failure: leads to disability and death.

Sudden death: occurs more frequently in patients with primary pulmonary hypertension.

Differential diagnosis

Mitral stenosis.

Recurrent pulmonary emboli.

Congenital cardiac defects.

Sickle cell anemia.

Collagen vascular diseases.

• Most of these, when severe, can cause secondary pulmonary hypertension.

• Differentiating primary pulmonary hypertension from secondary pulmonary hypertension is necessary. Primary pulmonary hypertension classically presents as dyspnea that is not explained by other causes (intrinsic pulmonary disease, intrinsic cardiac disease, or severe anemia).

• Deconditioning with dyspnea can sometimes mimic early primary pulmonary hypertension.

Etiology and epidemiology

• Etiology of primary pulmonary hypertension is usually idiopathic. Women outnumber men in a ratio of ~4:1.

• Postulated causes for pulmonary hypertension include autoimmune disorders due to the high frequency of antinuclear antibodies seen in some cases of pulmonary hypertension.

• Appetite suppression medication has been implicated as a possible mechanism. One of these agents (Aminorex) was used in Europe in the late 1960s and was linked to an increase in unexplained hypertension.

• 7% of cases of pulmonary hypertension are familial, with an autosomal dominant method of transmission with variable expression.

• Secondary pulmonary hypertension is due to the underlying disease. Major causes of secondary pulmonary hypertension include massive acute pulmonary embolism or chronic recurrent embolization, COPD, living at high altitude with hypoxia, congenital heart disease, severe pulmonary vascular or parenchymal disease (including interstitial lung diseases, parasitic lung diseases, collagen vascular diseases, granulomatous lung diseases, and i.v. drug use), severe left ventricular failure, sickle cell anemia, chronic liver disease, and mitral stenosis.

Treatment

Diet and lifestyle

• Because of the link to appetite suppressant drugs, which are amphetamine-like in nature, caution is appropriate in the use of these agents for managing obesity. It is likely that there is some unknown susceptibility factor for this association. It should be stressed that this association is suspected but not proven.

Pharmacological treatment

• Pharmacological treatment for secondary pulmonary hypertension should be directed at the underlying cause.

• No satisfactory treatment exists for primary pulmonary hypertension. Logically, treatment that would decrease the pulmonary artery pressure or reduce pulmonary vascular resistance directly would be of benefit. However, most agents that achieve this also decrease cardiac output and systemic blood pressure. If pulmonary artery pressures are reduced in proportion to the decrease in cardiac output, there is little net benefit.

• General therapeutic measures include supplementing oxygen as needed to increase the arterial oxygen saturation above 85%. This permits adequate tissue oxygenation, thereby preserving functional ability and patient activity. Oxygen usually ameliorates patient dyspnea. Because hypoxia is a potent pulmonary vasoconstrictor, oxygen therapy often can result in some decrease in pulmonary artery pressures.

• Vasodilating agents have not uniformly been successful. Calcium channel blockers in high doses, *e.g.*, diltiazam, 120 mg 3 times daily, may be helpful. Unfortunately, only a minority of patients with primary pulmonary hypertension exhibit pulmonary vasoconstriction and benefit from medications that dilate pulmonary vessels. Most recently, prostacyclin has been tried and has been successful in some patients. Some preliminary studies suggest that prostacyclin may decrease pulmonary pressures. Vasodilator treatment for primary pulmonary hypertension should be started with a pulmonary artery catheter in place. Initial pharmacological evaluation can then proceed under direct monitoring of systemic and pulmonary arterial pressures, and cardiac output. The treatment of primary pulmonary hypertension remains unsatisfactory. Virtually every class of vasodilator drug has been investigated for treatment of primary pulmonary hypertension.

• Diuretic therapy may relieve dyspnea and peripheral edema but must be used cautiously so as to not markedly decrease cardiac output.

• Oral anticoagulant therapy has been advocated by some, suggesting that in situ thrombosis may occur. Some have suggested that anticoagulants increase survival; however, they do not reverse the disease.

• Heart/lung transplantation should be considered in patients with primary pulmonary hypertension. Patients who have <1 year predicted survival because of their disease are the best candidates. Recurrence of the disease has not been reported in transplantation patients.

Treatment aims

To reduce pulmonary artery pressure and minimize hypoxemia.

Prognosis

• Prognosis for primary pulmonary hypertension is poor. Mean survival of 2–3 years from time of diagnosis is the rule. Only rare patients survive >10 years. Sudden death is not uncommon.

Follow-up and management

• Routine monitoring of arterial oxygen levels is necessary.

• Patients should be monitored for disease progression.

General references

Abenhaim L, Moride Y, Brenot F, *et al.*: Appetite-suppressant drugs and the risk of primary pulmonary hypertension: International Primary Pulmonary Hypertension Study Group. *N Engl J Med* 1996, **335**:609–616.

D'Alonzo GE, Barst RJ, Ayres SM, *et al.*: Survival in patients with primary pulmonary hypertension: results from a National Prospective Registry. *Ann Intern Med* 1991, **115**:343.

Olschewski H, Walmrath D, Schermuly R, *et al.*: Aerosolized prostacyclin and iloprost in severe pulmonary hypertension. *Ann Intern Med* 1996, **124**:820–824.

Rich S, Brundage BH: High-dose calcium blocking therapy for primary pulmonary hypertension: evidence for long-term reduction in pulmonary arterial pressure and regression of right ventricular hypertrophy. *Circulation* 1987, **76**:135.

Rubin LJ: Primary pulmonary hypertension. *N Engl J Med* 1997, **336**:111–117.

Diagnosis

Symptoms

Symptoms of hypertension.

Symptoms of associated coronary, cerebral, and peripheral vascular disease: in atherosclerotic disease.

Acute dyspnea: in "flash" pulmonary edema.

Signs

Hypertension: typically severe, requiring >2–3 antihypertensive medications.

Epigastric or renal angle bruits.

Femoral bruits and absent leg pulses: in atherosclerotic disease.

Investigations

Plasma creatinine measurement.

24-hour urinary protein excretion measurement: non-nephrotic range or occasionally nephrotic range proteinuria can be seen with renal artery stenosis.

Plasma renin activity: elevated levels (>10) in patients in normal sodium balance is indicative of renal artery stenosis.

Renal ultrasonography: to measure kidney size (kidneys <8 cm long seldom worth revascularization); renal size asymmetry consistent with renal artery stenosis.

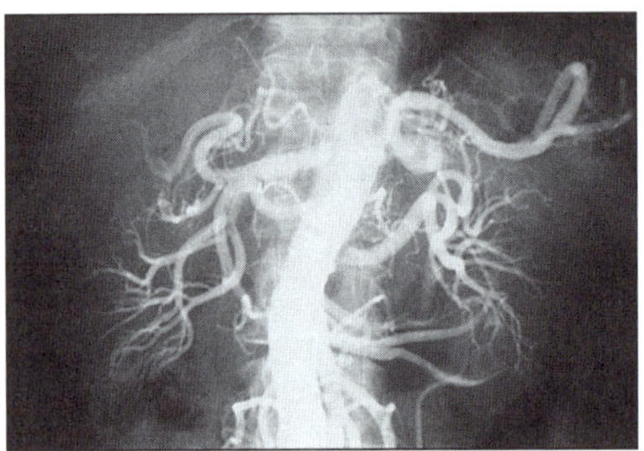

Widespread atherosclerotic disease in presence of renovascular disease, shown on angiography.

Nuclear medicine scanning: paired pre- and postcaptopril scans may increase sensitivity and specificity.

Renal angiography: use limited in patients with chronic renal insufficiency and severe aortosclerosis.

• Other examinations are those for atherosclerotic disease elsewhere.

Magnetic resonance angiography: no nephrotoxic contrast; expensive.

Spiral or helical CT scan: may well replace angiography and magnetic resonance angiography.

Complications

Malignant hypertension.

Chronic renal insufficiency.

End-stage renal disease: some patients may not need chronic dialysis if renal artery stenosis is diagnosed and treated.

Differential diagnosis

Other causes of hypertension.

Other causes of renal failure.

Left ventricular dysfunction.

Etiology

Fibromuscular disease: medial muscular hyperplasia.

Atherosclerotic disease: as for atherosclerosis elsewhere.

Large-vessel vasculitis, *e.g.*, Takayasu's arteritis.

Epidemiology

• Fibromuscular disease is rare (more common in younger female patients).

• Atherosclerotic disease occurs in 30% of patients with abnormal coronary angiograms and 42% with abnormal peripheral angiograms.

Treatment

Diet and lifestyle

• Patients should take measures to alleviate risk factors for atherosclerotic disease, *e.g.*, stopping smoking, losing weight, and reducing lipids.

Pharmacological treatment

• Hypertension is treated by the usual agents (*see* Hypertension *for details*), except in the following cases:

Fibromuscular dysplasia or bilateral renal artery stenosis: angiotensin-converting enzyme (ACE) inhibitors should be avoided because they may reduce renal function in kidneys with renal artery stenosis.

Atherosclerotic disease: beta-blockers should be avoided because most patients have peripheral vascular disease; ACE inhibitors may reduce renal function.

Angiographic treatment

• Newer experience with angioplasty and stenting is promising, especially for complicated medical cases.

• Risk of procedure-related atheroembolism is substantial in atherosclerotic individuals.

Note: the use of stenting even allows angioplasty management of ostial lesions.

Surgical treatment

Remains the gold standard for cases that appear amenable to reconstruction and have well-defined humoral hypertension and/or renal vascular–related renal failure.

Treatment aims

To control hypertension.

To preserve renal function.

To prevent "flash" pulmonary edema.

Prognosis

• The 5-year survival rate is 92% for fibromuscular disease and 67% for atherosclerotic disease; age is a major factor.

• Renal artery stenosis may recur, especially after angioplasty.

Follow-up and management

• Blood pressure and plasma creatinine measurement and imaging studies should be repeated, with re-angiography, if restenosis is possible.

General references

Dean RH, Benjamin ME, Hansen KJ: Surgical management of renovascular hypertension. *Curr Probl Surg* 1997, **34**:209–308.

Greco BA, Breyer JA: The natural history of renal artery stenosis: who should be evaluated for suspected ischemic nephropathy? *Semin Nephrol* 1996, **16**:2–11.

Kothari SS: ACE inhibitors and unilateral renal artery stenosis: what price? *Int J Cardiol* 1996, **53**:199–201.

Novick AC: Options for therapy of ischemic nephropathy: role of angioplasty and surgery. *Semin Nephrol* 1996, **16**:53–60.

Rubin GD: Spiral (helical) CT of the renal vasculature. *Semin Ultrasound CT MR* 1996, **17**:374–397.

Salvetti A, *et al.*: Renal artery stenosis in the nineties: screening dilemmas. *Contrib Nephrol* 1996, **119**:45–53.

Diagnosis

Symptoms

• The clinical features are usually dominated by those of the primary condition.

Nausea, vomiting, pruritus, malaise, lethargy, myoclonus: features of uremia develop if diagnosis unduly delayed.

Seizures and coma: in severe cases.

Signs

Oliguria: <400 mL urine daily; classic but not universal sign.
Edema.
Pericardial rub.
Asterixes.
Myoclonus.
Jugular venous distension.
Gallop rhythm.

Investigations

• Priorities are the detection and documentation of possibly life-threatening complications, exclusion of prerenal and postrenal factors, diagnosis of intrinsic renal disease, distinction of acute from chronic renal failure, and monitoring of response to treatment.

Blood electrolytes/chemistries: assess for hyperkalemia, acidosis, hyponatremia, hyperphosphatemia, hypo/hypercalcemia, degree of chemical uremia.

Central venous pressure monitoring and pulmonary capillary wedge pressure measurement: using Swan–Ganz catheter, if in any doubt about prerenal factors.

Chest radiography: assess for hypervolemia.

ECG, echocardiography: to exclude prerenal factors or pericardial changes, hyperkalemia.

Ultrasonography, plain abdominal radiography: to exclude postrenal factors.

Urine sodium and osmolality: can identify prerenal acute renal failure.

Urinalysis: proteinuria, dysmorphic erythrocytes, erythrocyte casts, other features of intrinsic renal disease.

Serology: for glomerulonephritis and vasculitis (anti–nuclear antibody, complement, anti–neutrophil cytoplasmic antibody, anti–glomerular basement membrane).

Creatine kinase and hydroxybutyrate dehydrogenase measurement: for rhabdomyolysis and hemolysis.

Blood film: for schistocytes and platelet count, to detect microangiopathic hemolytic anemia.

Blood cultures: for sepsis.

Coagulation tests, fibrinogen and fibrin degradation products analysis: for disseminated intravascular coagulation.

Liver function tests: for hepatorenal syndrome.

Renal biopsy: possibly indicated in patients with acute renal failure when intrinsic renal disease is suspected and may require specific therapy.

Ultrasonography, alkaline phosphatase measurement, bone radiography: for kidney size, evidence of metabolic bone disease, and anemia, respectively, to distinguish acute from chronic renal failure.

Immunoglobulin and protein electrophoresis: for myeloma in elderly patients.

Complications

Sepsis, adult respiratory distress syndrome (noncardiogenic pulmonary edema): usually seen in patients with multiple organ failure.

Gastrointestinal hemorrhage: caused by gastric stress ulceration.

Bleeding: uremic platelet-endothelial dysfunction and sepsis lead to a bleeding diathesis.

Opportunistic infections, poor wound healing, muscle wasting: due to hypercatabolic state associated with uremia and infection.

Hypertension: often related to fluid overload, sometimes to primary renal disease.

Hypotension: often related to sepsis, occasionally to occult myocardial ischemia.

Hyperkalemia: especially in presence of acidosis and tissue breakdown.

Treatment

Diet and lifestyle

• Acute renal failure is a medical emergency, usually occurring in hospital; diet is modified to supply sufficient energy while minimizing accumulation of toxins (protein 40–60 g, sodium 40–60 mEq, potassium 40–60 mEq daily).

• In the maintenance support of acute renal failure, more rigorous protein (>1.0 g/kg/day) and calorie (>25 kcal/kg/day) nutrition is recommended, with appropriate control for fluid balance.

• Acute renal failure does not occur in a vacuum and generally occurs in the setting of other acute illnesses.

Pharmacological treatment

For acute tubular necrosis
Diuretics only after restoration of euvolemia and maximization of cardiac output: escalating doses of a loop diuretic (bumetanide, 2–5 mg i.v. every 4–6 hours depending on urine flow rate) and dopamine (2.5–5 µg/kg/min) may restore urine flow; contraindicated in presence of obstruction, before hypovolemia is corrected, or if risk of cardiac arrhythmia.

For focal necrotizing and crescentic glomerulonephritis
Steroids, cyclophosphamide, and possibly plasma exchange only after biopsy confirmation if possible.

For acute interstitial nephritis
Withdrawal of offending drugs, possibly steroid therapy.

For infection
High-dose prolonged course of appropriate antibiotic (at least 4–6 weeks).

For hemolytic uremic syndrome and thrombotic thrombocytopenic purpura
Plasma exchange with fresh frozen plasma (*see* Hemolytic uremic syndrome *for details*).

For pigment nephropathy, myeloma kidney
Forced alkaline diuresis: 0.9% saline, 500 mL alternating with 1.26% sodium bicarbonate solution, 500 mL every 4 hours; bumetanide, 1–5 mg i.v. 8-hourly to maintain urine flow rate ≥100 mL/h; contraindicated in oliguria unresponsive to volume repletion and diuretics.

Nonpharmacological treatment

Optimization of vascular and extracellular fluid volume.

Maximization of perfusion of vital organs and exclusion of urinary obstruction.

Control of acidosis and hyperkalemia.

Enteral feeding, total parenteral nutrition if necessary; fluid balance must be controlled before feeding.

Hematological support: hemoglobin should be kept at ~10 g/dL, and albumin may be considered to support plasma oncotic pressure.

H2 blockers to prevent gastric stress ulceration.

Renal replacement therapy (dialysis or hemofiltration)
Indicated emergently for any combination of volume overload and congestive heart failure, hyperkalemia, severe acidosis, or symptomatic uremia in an oliguric patient.

Indicated semi-electively to support acute multisystem organ failure, nutritional administration, and fluid requirements in patients with moderate or severe renal failure who cannot be managed with diuretic therapy alone.

Uremic bleeding: consider i.v. vasopressin (0.3–0.6 mg/kg) × 1 dose, then conjugated estrogens (0.6 mg/kg/day) × 5 days.

General references

Alkhunaizi AM, Schrier RW: Management of acute renal failure: new perspectives. *Am J Kidney Dis* 1996, **28**:315–328.

Bellomo R, Ronco C: Acute renal failure in the intensive care unit: adequacy of dialysis and the case for continuous therapies. *Nephrol Dial Transplant* 1996, **11**:424–428.

Brady HR, Singer GG: Acute renal failure. *Lancet* 1995, **346**:1533–1540.

Conger JD: Interventions in clinical acute renal failure: what are the data? *Am J Kidney Dis* 1995, **26**:565–576.

Denton MD, Chertow GM, Brady HR: "Renal-dose" dopamine for the treatment of acute renal failure: scientific rationale, experimental studies and clinical trials. *Kidney Int* 1996, **50**:4–14.

Thadhani R, Pascual M, Bonventre JV: Acute renal failure. *N Engl J Med* 1996, **334**:1448–1460.

Diagnosis

Definition

• Irreversible renal impairment is most often recognized by persistently high urea (blood urea nitrogen [BUN]) and creatinine concentrations; it often progresses to end-stage renal failure.

Mild: glomerular filtration rate (GFR) 20–50 mL/min; creatinine 1.5–3.0 mg/dL.

Moderate: GFR 10–20 mL/min; creatinine 3.0–7.0 mg/dL.

Severe: GFR <10 mL/min; creatinine >7.0 mg/dL.

Symptoms

Constitutional symptoms, fatigue, reduced stamina, dyspnea on exertion.

Pruritus, malaise, anorexia, sleep disorders.

Drowsiness, twitching, blunting of intellect, diarrhea: late seizures and coma.

Symptoms of underlying disease.

Signs

Anemia.

Hypertension.

Pallor and pigmentation.

Pruritus, scratch marks, bruising.

Red eyes: high calcium–phosphate product, uremia.

Edema.

Peripheral neuropathy: sensory common, motor only in severe uremia.

Proximal myopathy: severe metabolic bone disease, nutritional deficiency.

Kussmaul's respiration: when acidosis is severe.

Pericarditis: causing tamponade when renal failure severe.

Investigations

Serum electrolytes, urea (BUN), creatinine, creatinine clearance, 24-hour urinary protein, calcium and phosphate measurement.

Plain radiography of abdomen: to detect calculi and nephrocalcinosis.

Ultrasonography of kidneys: to measure size and exclude obstruction.

Kidney biopsy: for changes specific to underlying disease; contraindicated for small kidneys or very late chronic disease.

Immunoglobulin electrophoresis, Bence–Jones protein measurement: to diagnose multiple myeloma in elderly patients.

Renal artery imaging: consider spiral CT or magnetic resonance angiography if renal artery stenosis suspected.

Complications

Anemia.

Renal osteodystrophy.

Hypertension.

Bleeding (platelet dysfunction).

Peripheral neuropathy.

Pericarditis.

Acute or chronic renal failure: aggravated by hypovolemia, hypertension, infection, toxic agents, overzealous control of blood pressure.

Accelerated atherosclerosis: increased risk of stroke, heart attack, and peripheral vascular disease.

Differential diagnosis

Acute renal failure: short history, examination shows features of underlying disease, normal hemoglobin, no evidence of renal osteodystrophy, normal or enlarged kidneys.

Etiology

• The cause varies depending on the patient's age; the following may have a role:

Chronic glomerulonephritis in 20%–30% of patients.

Diabetes mellitus in 20%–30%.

Hypertension in 20%–30%.

Chronic interstitial disease in 10%–20%.

Polycystic kidney disease in 10%.

Renovascular disease in ~10%.

Drugs in 2.5%.

Hypertension in 20%–30%.

Hereditary nephritis in affected families.

In elderly patients: multiple myeloma, atherosclerotic renal artery stenosis, obstruction, and amyloid.

In children: congenital absence or dysplasia, obstruction: posterior urethral valves, juvenile nephronophthisis (cystic disease).

Family or previous history of renal disease (*e.g.*, childhood urinary tract infection).

Epidemiology

• The annual incidence of chronic renal failure progressively to end-stage renal disease is 100–500/million depending on race and location.

Progression

• Although chronic renal failure often progresses to end-stage renal failure, function may not deteriorate quickly and, in some patients, remains stable, although significantly impaired, for several years.

• Measurement of serum creatinine is the most useful clinical test in assessing progression (serum creatinine is related to muscle mass and renal function).

• Serum creatinine rises exponentially with deteriorating renal function.

• A mild increase in serum creatinine may signal serious early loss of function.

• Plotting reciprocal serum creatinine values against time is a useful indicator of progression of renal failure.

Treatment

Diet and lifestyle

• Patients should eat a high-energy diet, with potassium restriction and protein intake restricted to 0.5–0.75 g/kg body weight daily; in later stages of chronic renal failure, decreased protein intake can help to control symptoms of nausea, vomiting, and anorexia.

• Phosphate intake should be restricted, and absorption reduced by phosphate binders (calcium carbonate in preference to aluminium hydroxide).

• Vitamin D supplementation is sometimes needed, using newer synthetic preparations.

Pharmacological treatment

• Specific treatment is directed at the underlying cause.

• Nephrotoxic drugs and NSAIDs must be avoided, and doses of other drugs must be adjusted for the degree of renal failure.

• Angiotensin-converting enzyme (ACE) inhibitors may help to control blood pressure, particularly in diabetic patients; diastolic pressure should be <90 mm Hg. Care is needed with these agents when renal artery stenosis is suspected or when serum creatinine is chronically elevated to levels >3.0 mg/dL.

• Erythropoietin can be used to treat anemia and improve well-being.

• Progression to end-stage chronic renal failure can be slowed by some or all of the following:

Aggressive control of systemic hypertension (120–130/70–80 mm Hg).

Reduction of glomerular blood pressure, using ACE inhibitors or calcium channel blockers.

Low-protein diets (in some patients).

Addressing the risk factors for accelerated atherosclerosis.

Nonpharmacological treatment

• Hemodialysis or peritoneal dialysis can be used to treat uremia, the prognosis depending on age, underlying renal diagnosis, and adequacy of the treatment regimen.

• Transplantation provides best long-term prognosis and quality of life, and all efforts should be made at the earliest reasonable time to evaluate patients with progressive chronic renal failure for transplant.

Treatment aims

To delay progression to end-stage renal failure.

To prevent renal bone disease.

To control hypertension.

To prevent acute or chronic renal failure (*e.g.*, by avoiding urinary tract infection, correcting obstruction).

Prognosis

• Timely dialysis or transplantation prolongs life.

• Comorbidity of multisystem diseases may limit survival.

Follow-up and management

• After chronic renal failure has been diagnosed, progress must be monitored at regular intervals; important parameters include the following:

Weight (for nutrition and fluid status).

Blood pressure (control may retard progression).

Urea/BUN (may alter with increased catabolism or protein intake).

Creatinine.

Hemoglobin.

Serum calcium (iatrogenic hypercalcemia must be avoided: calcium is nephrotoxic).

Serum phosphate.

Serum alkaline phosphatase.

Albumin (particularly helpful in assessing nutrition).

General references

Bushinsky DA: Bone disease in moderate renal failure: cause, nature and prevention. *Annu Rev Med* 1997, **48**:167–176.

Dunn CJ, Markham A: Epoetin beta: a review of its pharmacological properties and clinical use in the management of anaemia associated with chronic renal failure. *Drugs* 1996, **51**:299–318.

Holm EA, Solling K: Dietary protein restriction and the progression of chronic renal insufficiency: a review of the literature. *J Intern Med* 1996, **239**:99–104.

Hood VL, Gennari FJ: End-stage renal disease: measures to prevent it or slow its progression. *Postgrad Med* 1996, **100**:163–166, 171–176.

Lundin AP, Port FK: Adequacy of treatment for end-stage renal disease in the United States. *Adv Intern Med* 1996, **41**:323–363.

Steinman TI: Kidney protection: how to prevent or delay chronic renal failure. *Geriatrics* 1996, **51**:28–35.

Diagnosis

Symptoms

• History of previous renal stone disease and/or hematuria is common.

• Severe, intermittent, colicky abdominal pain, typically flank with possible radiation to groin, with no position of comfort.

Nausea, vomiting, diaphoresis, frequency, dysuria.
Chills and fever: if complicated by obstruction and infection.

Signs

Extreme restlessness, diaphoresis.
Hematuria: typically microscopic, may be gross.
Frequency of urination, tachycardia.
Flank tenderness on affected side, possible mild abdominal tenderness with deep palpation without peritoneal signs.
Fever: if associated with urinary tract infection.

Investigations

Acute evaluation

Plain radiograph of abdomen: is generally useful in rapidly demonstrating the presence and size of calcium-containing stones (radiopaque), but does not yield functional data.

Intravenous pyelogram (IVP): excellent in assessing all aspects of stone imaging and is readily available; however, is limited by need for i.v. contrast dye exposure.

Renal ultrasound: also yields comprehensive stone imaging data; however, it will not detect midureteral stones and is somewhat operator dependent.

Spiral or helical CT without contrast: probably the best imaging option and yields comprehensive data on all stone types and locations; however, this technology is not widely available.

Collect and strain all urine: to capture and save stone when it passes.

Serum chemistries: electrolytes, creatinine, complete blood count, urine culture.

• Must quickly rule out urinary tract infection proximal to an obstructing stone, *i.e.*, obstructive pyelonephritis. This could be potentially life-threatening due to urosepsis.

Basic evaluation

• This evaluation should be considered in uncomplicated, first-time renal stone patients.

Detailed history: to assess medical, lifestyle, dietary risk factors for renal stone disease.

Submit stone for radiographical diffraction crystallography evaluation, screen urine for cystine using nitroprusside test.

Screening blood tests: electrolytes, calcium, phosphorus, uric acid, creatinine.

Complete evaluation

• This evaluation should be done in patients with recurrent stone disease or who are in unusual demographic risk groups (*e.g.*, black females, children). It includes all the features of the basic evaluation in addition to the following:

Collect 24-hour urine on at least two occasions for the following values (includes optimal values):

Volume: >2–2.5 L	**Citrate:** >320 mg
Calcium: <300 mg in men, <250 mg in women	**Sodium:** <200 mEq
Oxalate: <40 mg	**Phosphorus:** <1100 mg
Uric acid: <800 mg in men, <750 mg in women	**pH:** >5.5 and <7.0

• Consider IVP, if not already done, to rule out medullary sponge kidney.

Complications

Chronic renal failure, pyelonephritis, perinephritic abscess, urosepsis.

Acute renal failure: if obstruction of single functioning kidney or if bilateral obstucting stone.

Recurrent stone formation, ureteral scarring.

Treatment

Diet and lifestyle

Increased fluid intake: approximately 3 L water intake per day, evenly spaced over the 24-hour period.

• Avoid dehydration and natural diuretics such as coffee or tea.

• Avoid high-salt and/or high-protein diet; both may increase calcium and uric acid excretion and decrease citrate excretion.

• Dietary recommendations may vary depending on stone work-up; general guidelines include the following:

Start a low-oxalate diet if hyperoxaluria.

Consider decreased purine diet for hyperuricosuria.

Cystine stone disease requires very aggressive water intake because it is necessary to achieve a urine output of 3–3.5 L/day; urine flow should be as high at night as during day; maintain cystine concentration below 250 mg/L in the urine.

Pharmacological treatment

Acute management

Prophylactic antibiotic: if more than 5 leukocytes/high-power field.

Narcotic pain medication.

Admit and initiate i.v. antibiotics: if obstructive pyelonephritis is possible.

Chronic management

• The following measures are dependent on data obtained from stone analysis and 24-hour urine studies.

Calcium stones:

Idiopathic hypercalciuria: hydrochlorothaizide, 25 mg daily; potassium citrate: 25–30 mEq twice daily.

Hyperuricosuria: allopurinol, 100 mg twice daily.

Hyperoxaluria: calcium carbonate, 1 g 3 times daily after meals.

Hypocitraturia: potassium citrate, 25–30 mEq twice daily.

Uric acid stones: sodium bicarbonate, 650 mg 4 times daily (to achieve urine pH >7.0); allopurinol, 100 mg twice daily.

Struvite stones: consider chronic antibiotic suppression (trimethoprim/sulfa-methoxazole).

Cystine stones: sodium bicarbonate, 650 mg 4 times daily; aggressive water intake (*see* Diet and lifestyle).

Nonpharmacological treatment

Expectant management with hydration, 2.5–3 L/day (drinking at time of all voidings).

Treatment is dependent on stone size:

<6 mm: Will pass spontaneously in 90%–95% (80% within 4 weeks).

6–10 mm: Decreased likelihood of passing; consider urologic consult.

≥10 mm: Urologic intervention.

With obstructing or large stones (≥0.6 cm) that are not passing:

Extract cystoscopically if located in the lower ureter.

If the stone is located in the upper ureter or renal pelvis, consider extracorporeal shock-wave lithotripsy (ESWL), percutaneous nephrolithotomy, endourologic procedures, or open surgery.

Most patients will not require admission if stone is <6 mm.

Treatment aims

To preserve native renal function.
To reduce or eliminate episodes of recurrent stone formation.

Prognosis

• Recurrent stone disease may result in chronic renal insufficiency, however, end-stage kidney disease is uncommon.

• Recurrent struvite stone is associated with the highest rate of progressive renal deterioration (28% over 7-year period).

• ESWL has made a revolutionary improvement in morbidity due to stone disease.

Follow-up and management

• During acute period of stone passage, follow on an every-day to every-week interval in order to monitor progress of stone movement.

• If stone is in a fixed position for 4 weeks, surgical intervention will likely be required.

• Formal evaluation of renal stone disease is typically initiated 1 month after stone passage.

• After stone passage, plan a 2-year period of therapy with regular checks.

General references

Begun FP, Foley WD, Peterson A, White B: Urolithiasis: patient evaluation, laboratory and imaging studies. *Urol Clin North Am* 1997, **24**:97–116.

Coe FL, *et al.* (eds.): *Kidney Stones: Medical and Surgical Management.* Philadelphia: Lippincott-Raven; 1996.

Hesse A, Tiselius H-G, Janen A: *Urinary Stones: Diagnosis, Treatment, and Prevention of Recurrance.* Basel, New York: Karger; 1997.

Monk RD: Clinical approach to adults with nephrolithiasis. *Semin Nephrol* 1996, **16**:375–388.

Pak CY: Southwestern Internal Medicine Conference: Medical management of nephrolithiasis: a new, simplified approach for general practice. *Am J Med Sci* 1997, **313**:215–219.

Teichman JM, Long RD, Hulbert JC: Long-term fate and prognosis after staghorn calculus management. *J Urol* 1995, **153**:1403–1407.

Selection

Patient criteria

• Factors to check for include the following:

Age: biological age more important than chronological age, upper limit is usually 65–75 years.

Cancer: must be excluded or at least 5 years free of recurrance.

Infection: *i.e.*, Staghorn calculi, tuberculosis, bronchiectasis, HIV must be excluded.

Cardiovascular status: angina detected by stress test (stress, thallium, dobutamine echocardiography) or coronary angiography; intermittent claudication detected by duplex Doppler or digital vascular imaging; myocardial infarction remains the most common cause of death after transplantation; presence of peripheral vascular disease may compromise leg perfusion after transplantation.

Bladder function: positive urological history obtained by flow rate and residual bladder ultrasonography or video cystometrography, possibly with cystoscopy; bladder outflow tract obstruction may compromise graft function.

Donor criteria

• The criteria have been relaxed over the past 10 years because of a shortage of donors. Sepsis is no longer a contraindication if the organism is cultured. Diabetic donors may be considered, but frozen section of the kidney is needed before transplantation.

Age 2–75 years.

Absence of chronic renal disease.

Hepatitis B virus, HIV, and hepatitis C virus negative.

No malignancies: except primary brain tumors.

• Live-related donors should always be sought: parents can only be a haplotype match (50%), but siblings can be HLA-identical (100%), a haplotype match (50%), or a complete mismatch (0%). Live-unrelated donors are considered reasonable candidates if there is a clear emotional connection to patient.

Matching

Tissue typing

HLA on chromosome 6. Class I = A and B, class II = DR.

• 1A, 1B, 1DR antigen is inherited from each parent.

• For matching, the importance is as follows: DR > B > A; *i.e.*, 1A, 2B, 2DR match is better than 2A, 1B, 2DR match.

Direct cross-match

• If donor lymphocytes combined with the patient's serum cause lymphocyte death, a positive cross-match is implied, and the kidney is unsuitable.

• Highly sensitized patients have high levels of anti-HLA antibodies; this may be secondary to previous transplantation, blood transfusion, or pregnancies; the incidence of positive cross-matches is increased.

Epidemiology

• 50% of patients on renal failure programs are unsuitable for transplantation because of age or coexisting diseases (*i.e.*, severe cardiovascular disease, cancer).

• >35 000 patients are on waiting lists in the United States.

• >11 000 kidney transplantations are currently done each year in the United States.

• 30% of transplants are taken from living donors in the United States.

• The waiting time in many states is now 2–3 years on average.

Transplantation or dialysis?

Advantages of transplantation

Improved quality of life.

No dialysis.

Correction of anemia.

Normal diet and fluid allowance.

Improved bone metabolism (however, increased osteoporosis from steroids).

Increased ease of travel.

Women of child-bearing age able to have children.

Less expensive than dialysis in the long run.

Disadvantages of transplantation

Emotional stress.

Surgical and anesthetic donor risks, minimal.

Approximate costs

Hemodialysis: $35 000–$50 000/year.

Transplantation: $50 000 in the first year, $5000–$10 000 in subsequent years.

Advantages of living donors

Improved graft survival.

Planned operation.

Much shorter wait.

Lower incidence of postoperative acute tubular necrosis.

Lower rate of rejection.

Treatment

Acute rejection

Clinical findings
• Careful monitoring of serum creatinine is essential because typically there are no clinical findings of rejection; however, possible findings include:

Tenderness over graft.

Pyrexia.

Decreased urine output.

Fluid retention.

Hypertension.

Investigation of graft dysfunction
Renal biopsy: open or needle biopsy; the standard method to diagnose rejection.

Urine analysis: midstream urine, proteinuria, cytology.

Blood analysis: increased blood urea nitrogen, creatinine, potassium, leukocyte count, interleukin 2R, cyclosporine concentration, blood cultures.

Ultrasonography: to exclude obstruction, possibly to diagnose rejection.

Renal isotope scans: show decreased perfusion.

Differential diagnosis
Acute tubular necrosis: 20%–50% of grafts have primary nonfunction lasting 1-2 weeks.

Cyclosporine toxicity.

Graft pyelonephritis.

Ureteric obstruction.

Renal artery stenosis.

Cytomegalovirus.

Histological features
Acute cellular rejection: lymphocyte infiltrate, macrophages, natural killer cells.

Acute vascular rejection: as above, with fibrinoid necrosis and infiltration of vessel walls.

Chronic rejection: fibrosis, chronic vascular changes (intimal proliferation) leading to vascular occlusion.

Treatment
Hyperacute rejection: extremely rare, usually due to circulating preformed antibody.

Simple acute cellular rejection: pulse corticosteroid (solumedrol, 250–500 mg IVPB daily $\times$ 3-4 days).

Steroid-resistant cellular rejection and vascular rejection: antithymocyte globulin, anti-lymphocyte globulin, OKT3; consider tacrolimus or mycophenolate rescue.

Chronic rejection: no effective treatment, aggressive renal sparing therapy (low-protein diet, excellent blood pressure control).

Immunosuppression

Agents
Combinations of corticosteroid, azathioprine, cyclosporine, and monoclonal and polyclonal antibodies.

New immunosuppressive drugs: tacrolimus, mycophenolate mofetil, sirolimus, others.

Side effects
All immunosuppressants: increased incidence of tumors (skin, reticuloendothelial system) and infection (*e.g.*, opportunistic infections, cytomegalovirus).

Azathioprine: bone-marrow suppression (leukocytes, hemoglobin, platelets), hepatotoxicity.

Steroids: cushingoid facies, buffalo hump, central obesity, striae, thinning of skin, bruising, proximal myopathy, acne vulgaris, hirsuitism, osteoporosis, aseptic necrosis of the hips, diabetes, hyperlipidemia.

Cyclosporine: hirsuitism, tremor, gum hyperplasia, nephro-, neuro-, or hepatotoxicity.

Tacrolimus: kidney and liver toxicity; neurotoxicity, diabetes.

OKT3 (anti-T-cell monoclonal antibody): first-dose effect (acute pulmonary edema), increased incidence of lymphoproliferative disorders.

Mycophenolate mofetil: upper and lower gastrointestinal complaints, leukopenia.

Sirolimus: elevated triglycerides, thrombocytopenia.

Blood transfusion and transplantation
• Donor-specific transfusion increases potential for patient sensitization, but patients who have received transfusion may have better outcome if they do receive a living transplant.

• The beneficial effect on transplantation outcome is less clear since the introduction of cyclosporine.

Surgical complications

Early
Hemorrhage, renal vein and renal artery thrombosis, urinary leak.

Late
Renal artery stenosis, ureteric stenosis, ureteric reflux.

Prognosis
• 1-year kidney graft survival rates are 90% (live) and 80%–90% (cadaveric).

• Graft loss is highest in the first 3 months.

• After the first year, ~4% of grafts are lost annually (mainly due to chronic rejection).

Follow-up and management
• Regular monitoring of immunosuppression and renal function (monthly or bimonthly).

• Regular outpatient visits are needed (3 times weekly initially, decreasing to once every 2 weeks, and eventually once every 4 months).

• A 20% rise in creatinine is investigated initially with ultrasonography and biopsy.

General references

Bennett WM: Mechanisms of acute and chronic nephrotoxicity from immuno-suppressive drugs. *Ren Fail* 1996, **18**:453–460.

Colvin RB: The renal allograft biopsy. *Kidney Int* 1996, **50**:1069–1082.

Danovich G (ed.): *Handbook of Kidney Transplantation*. Boston: Little, Brown and Co.; 1996.

Morris RE: Mechanisms of action of new immunosuppressive drugs. *Kidney Int Suppl* 1996, **53**:S26–S38.

Terasaki PI, Cecka JM (ed.): *Clinical Transplants 1996*. Los Angeles: UCLA Tissue Typing Laboratory; 1996.

Terasaki PI: High survival rates of kidney transplants from spousal and living unrelated donors. *N Engl J Med* 1995, **333**:3333–3361.

Diagnosis

Definition

• Renal tubular acidosis is a disorder of renal hydrogen secretion or bicarbonate reabsorption.

• The following subtypes of renal tubular acidosis have been defined:

Type 1 (distal): defect in distal hydrogen secretion, probably related to defect in hydrogen ATPase.

Type 2 (proximal): decreased proximal bicarbonate reabsorption, probably a defect in brush border sodium–hydrogen exchanger.

Type 3: described in older textbooks but does not exist.

Type 4 (*e.g.*, hyporeninemic hypoaldosteronism): decreased distal acidification due to lack of aldosterone and decreased distal sodium reabsorption (most commonly seen due to its association with diabetes mellitus).

Symptoms

• Renal tubular acidosis has no specific symptoms.

Weakness, musculoskeletal pains, low back pain: in type 1 disease.

Failure to thrive: in children in type 2 disease; often associated with Fanconi's syndrome or other chronic renal disease and symptoms including bone pain from osteomalacia.

Symptoms of diabetes mellitus: in type 4 disease (frequent association).

Symptoms of renal stone disease: in type 1 disease.

Signs

• These are rare.

Weakness leading to paralysis: in type 1 and type 2 disease (due to hypokalemia).

Signs of diabetes mellitus: in type 4 disease.

Investigations

• The diagnosis of renal tubular acidosis is indicated by a hyperchloremic metabolic acidosis defined from blood–gas analysis with a normal plasma anion gap (*see box*), defined by $(Na^+ + K^+) - (Cl^- + HCO_3^-)$; this differentiates it from an increased anion gap acidosis such as in lactic acidosis.

Plasma potassium analysis: to detect hypokalemia in patients with type 1 or type 2 disease.

Short ammonium chloride loading test: if urine pH >6.0 to diagnose type 1 disease.

Sodium bicarbonate loading test: if urine pH <6.0 to diagnose type 2 disease.

Plain abdominal radiography: in type 1 disease, to look for nephrocalcinosis.

Parathyroid hormone measurement: to detect primary hyperparathyroidism (associated with type 2 disease).

Complications

• These may be renal related as in type 1 disease or may be due to general complications of the underlying disease as in type 4 disease.

Nephrocalcinosis and nephrolithiasis: type 1 disease.

Diabetes mellitus leading to renal failure from diabetic nephropathy: most common condition associated with type 4 disease.

Hypokalemia: type 1 and type 2 disease; may be severe, resulting in paralysis.

Hyperkalemia: type 4 disease.

Childhood growth retardation: type 1 and type 2 disease.

Osteitis fibrosa: children.

Osteopenia: adults.

Differential diagnosis

Type 1 with nephrocalcinosis
Medullary sponge kidney, idiopathic hypercalciuria, hyperparathyroidism.

• Purgative abuse or chronic diarrhea can lead to a hyperchloremic acidosis with an abnormal short ammonium chloride loading test; this can be differentiated by the urinary ammonium excretion, which is normal in patients with diarrhea but low in patients with type 1 disease.

Etiology

Causes of type 1 disease
Idiopathic, Sjögren's syndrome, SLE, primary biliary cirrhosis, amphotericin, lithium, multiple myeloma.

Causes of type 2 disease
Idiopathic, cystinosis, Fanconi's syndrome, Wilson's disease, primary hyperparathyroidism, acetazolamide.

Causes of type 4 disease
Diabetes mellitus (most important in clinical practice), urinary obstruction, sickle cell disease; mimicked by potassium-sparing diuretics.

Epidemiology

• Types 1 and 2 are typically diagnosed in childhood.

• Type 4 is many times related to adult disease.

• Types 1 and 2 are rare; type 4 occurs relatively frequently.

Causes of normal anion gap acidosis

Failure of renal acidification due to renal tubular acidosis or acetazolamide.

Gastrointestinal loss of bicarbonate due to diarrhea, purgative abuse, pancreatic fistula, ureteric diversion (*e.g.*, ureterosigmoidostomy).

Ingestion of acid (*e.g.*, hydrochloric).

Parenteral nutrition.

Treatment

Diet and lifestyle

• No special precautions are necessary.

Pharmacological treatment

For types 1 and 2 disease

• Patients should be given oral sodium bicarbonate up to 1–2 mEq/kg (type 1) or 3–5 mEq/kg (type 2) daily, titrated to improve acidosis.

• Potassium and, in type 2 disease, vitamin D supplements may also be needed.

• Acidosis can never be completely corrected by oral supplements.

For type 4 disease

• Fludrocortisone or diuretics (loop or thiazide) with sodium bicarbonate are indicated.

• Potassium-sparing diuretics, NSAIDs, or angiotensin-converting enzyme inhibitors, which worsen hyperkalemia, must be avoided.

Standard dosage	Fludrocortisone, 100–400 µg daily. Bumetanide, 1–5 mg, and sodium bicarbonate up to 4 g daily.
Contraindications	*Fludrocortisone*: volume overload. *Bumetanide*: volume depletion. *Sodium bicarbonate*: volume overload.
Main drug interactions	None.
Main side effects	Fluid overload if inadequate diuretic given with sodium bicarbonate.

Treatment aims

To prevent nephrocalcinosis and nephrolithiasis in type 1 disease.

To treat bone disease with vitamin D if deficiency present in type 2 disease.

To avoid life-threatening hyperkalemia caused by concomitant medication in type 4 disease.

Prognosis

• Type 1 disease can progress to renal failure (not usual).

• The prognosis for types 2 and 4 disease depends on the associated conditions.

Follow up and management

• Acidosis and, in type 1 disease, nephrocalcinosis and nephrolithiasis must be monitored.

General references

Battle D, Flores G: Underlying defects in distal renal tubular acidosis: new understandings. *Am J Kidney Dis* 1996, **27**:896–915.

Kamel KS, *et al.*: A new classification for renal defects in net acid excretion. *Am J Kidney Dis* 1997, **29**:136–146.

Petersen-Smith AM: Renal tubular acidosis: when kids won't grow. *J Pediatr Health Care* 1995, **9**:131–133.

Sharma AM: Renal tubular dysfunction and acidosis. *Nephrol Dial Transplant* 1995, **10**:1544–1545.

Smulders YM, *et al.*: Renal tubular acidosis: pathophysiology and diagnosis. *Arch Intern Med* 1996, **156**:1629–1636.

Uribarri J, Douyon H, Oh MS: A re-evaluation of the urinary parameters of acid production and excretion in patients with chronic renal acidosis. *Kidney Int* 1995, **47**:624–627.

Diagnosis

Symptoms

Dyspnea.

Fatigue.

Ankle or abdominal swelling.

Signs

Restrictive cardiomyopathy

Raised jugular venous pressure.

Inspiratory increase in jugular venous pressure: Kussmaul's sign.

Palpable apex beat.

Mild or moderate cardiomegaly.

Third or fourth heart sounds.

Peripheral edema.

Ascites.

Constrictive pericarditis

Raised jugular venous pressure, with rapid diastolic "y" descent.

Kussmaul's sign.

Diffuse or impalpable apex beat.

Intercostal indrawing of apex in systole: Broadbent's sign.

Early diastolic pericardial "knock."

Widened splitting of second heart sound.

Investigations

• The two conditions overlap considerably, and separating them on clinical findings and investigations may be impossible; thoracotomy may be needed to exclude or confirm the diagnosis.

Chest radiography: *restrictive cardiomyopathy,* shows mild or moderate cardiomegaly; *constrictive pericarditis,* shows normal heart size and pericardial calcification.

ECG: *restrictive cardiomyopathy,* shows T-wave changes or bundle branch block, and atrial arrhythmias; *constrictive pericarditis,* shows nonspecific T-wave flattening and atrial fibrillation; *both,* show low-voltage complexes.

Echocardiography: *restrictive cardiomyopathy,* shows myocardial thickening and characteristic "ground-glass" appearance (in amyloid); *constrictive pericarditis,* shows normal myocardial thickness and may reveal thickened pericardium; *both,* show normal ventricular dimensions with enlarged atria and good systolic and poor diastolic function.

CT or MRI: *restrictive cardiomyopathy,* shows myocardial thickening and normal pericardium; *constrictive pericarditis,* shows normal myocardial thickness and pericardial thickening and calcification.

Cardiac catheterization: *restrictive cardiomyopathy,* shows left ventricular filling pressure exceeding right ventricular filling pressure and pulmonary artery systolic pressure often >45 mm Hg, with myocardial biopsy possibly diagnostic; *constrictive pericarditis,* shows identical left and right ventricular filling pressures and pulmonary artery systolic pressure usually <45 mm Hg, with normal myocardial biopsy; *both,* show rapid "y" descent in atrial pressure and early dip in diastolic pressure, with pressure rise to plateau in mid or late diastole.

Complications

Symptomatic hypotension.

Atrial and ventricular arrhythmias.

Progressive "heart failure": in constrictive pericarditis, the "heart" itself is not failing, but the resulting clinical features are similar to those of restrictive cardiomyopathy.

Hepatic failure: resulting from chronic hepatic venous congestion.

Nephrotic syndrome.

Conduction abnormalities: in restrictive cardiomyopathy.

Treatment

Diet and lifestyle

• Patients' daily activities are restricted by fatigue, breathlessness, and fluid retention.

Pharmacological treatment

Restrictive cardiomyopathy

• Specific measures are generally unsatisfactory.

• Amyloid has no known pharmacological treatment; however, avoidance of digitalis and calcium channel blockers is recommended.

• Patients with hemochromatosis should be given iron-chelating agents, *e.g.*, desferrioxamine.

• Corticosteroids are only effective during the acute myocardial phase of eosinophilia.

Constrictive pericarditis

• The only satisfactory treatment is surgical.

• Patients with tuberculous pericarditis should be pretreated with antituberculous therapy; if the diagnosis is confirmed after pericardial resection, full antituberculous therapy should be continued for 6–12 months after resection. *See* Tuberculosis, extrapulmonary *for details.*

Nonpharmacological treatment

Restrictive cardiomyopathy

Permanent pacing for conduction abnormalities in amyloid.

Bimonthly phlebotomy often for 2–3 years to reduce iron storage in hemachromatosis.

Endocardial resection after fibrosis is established in eosinophilia.

Transplantation occasionally.

Constrictive pericarditis

Complete surgical resection of the pericardium (myocardial inflammation or fibrosis may delay symptomatic response).

Treatment aims

To relieve symptoms.

To remove underlying causes.

Prognosis

• Prognosis is good after resection for constrictive pericarditis.

• Restrictive cardiomyopathy has poor prognosis, particularly due to amyloidosis or malignancy.

Follow-up and management

• Management is purely palliative.

General references

Maisch B: Pericardial diseases, with a focus on etiology, pathogenesis, pathophysiology new diagnostic imaging methods, and treatment. *Curr Opin Cardiol* 1994, **9**:379–388.

Spyrou N, Foale R: Restrictive cardiomyopathies. *Curr Opin Cardiol* 1994, **9**:344–348.

Ward D: Pericardial and myocardial disease. *Practitioner* 1993, **237**:929–932.

Diagnosis

Symptoms

• Acute rheumatic fever is a multisystem disorder occurring 1–5 weeks after group A streptococcal infection.

• Its manifestation is variable, involving any of the following:

Joint pain (migratory polyarthropathy): ranging from simple pain to disabling arthritis; classically involves large joints in succession, with "overlapping" involvement.

Breathlessness and chest pain (pancarditis): cardiac failure with occasional clinical pericardial involvement.

Rapid purposeless involuntary movements (Sydenham's chorea): including slurred speech, jerky movements, facial tics and grimacing, emotional lability; manifest only during wakefulness; may occur as late isolated feature of disease.

Subcutaneous nodules: painless firm lesions (up to 2 cm diameter) over bony prominences and tendons; tend to appear late and last 1–2 weeks.

Erythema marginatum: red rash extending circumferentially on trunk and proximal limbs; changes rapidly over minutes.

Signs

Joint involvement: joints may be exquisitely tender, red, swollen; refusal to bear weight (especially in children).

Signs of cardiac failure, tachycardia, cardiomegaly, pericardial rub, mitral regurgitation, Carey–Coombs aortic regurgitation, first-, second-, or third-degree atrioventricular block.

Chorea: "bag of worms" tongue of chorea (fasciculation on protrusion), "Milkmaid's grip" (squeezing and relaxing motion on gripping the hand), pendular knee jerks.

Skin rash and nodules.

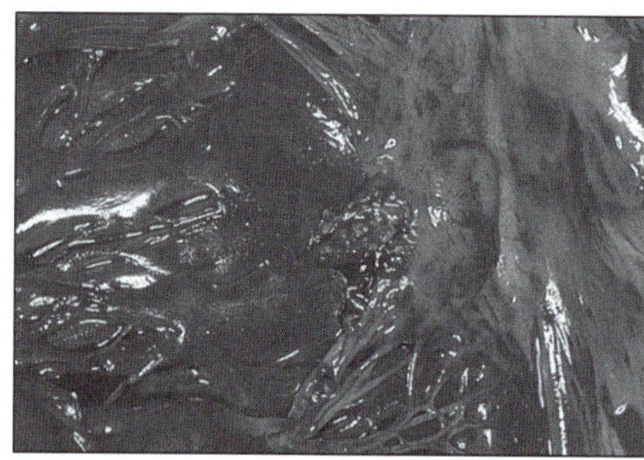

Vegetation on mitral valve, the major reason for continued prophylaxis after rheumatic heart disease. (*See* Color Plate.)

Investigations

• No single test is diagnostic; the diagnosis is simplified by application of the Duckett-Jones criteria.

• The most important laboratory contribution is evidence of antecedent streptococcal infection.

• No significant laboratory abnormality may be seen in pure chorea.

Throat swab: usually negative, but positive result indicates increased disease activity.

Antistreptolysin O, anti-DNAse B, antihyaluronidase titers: if all three done, 95% chance of positive result.

Complete blood count: leukocytosis common; moderate normochromic, normocytic anemia often seen.

ESR, CRP measurement: usually raised.

Liver function tests: aspartate transaminase possibly raised.

Urinalysis: sediment positive for leukocytes and erythrocytes (not pathognomonic of glomerulonephritis).

ECG: shows tachycardia and first-, second-, or, rarely, third-degree heart block.

Echocardiography: shows myocardial thickening and dysfunction, pericardial effusion, and valvular dysfunction.

Complications

Recurrent episodes: with continuing evidence of inflammatory activity.

Rheumatic heart disease: major long-term sequela.

Differential diagnosis

Other causes of polyarthropathy, fever, and cardiac involvement.

Viral arthritides, *e.g.*, rubella, hepatitis B.

Septic arthritis *e.g.*, *Neisseria* spp. infection.

Infective endocarditis.

Acute rheumatoid arthritis.

Stills' disease.

Serum sickness, *e.g.*, after penicillin.

SLE.

Prepurpuric phase Henoch–Schönlein purpura.

Lyme disease.

Etiology

• Acute rheumatic fever is an exudative, proliferative inflammation of connective tissues, especially heart, joints, and subcutaneous tissues.

• It only occurs after group A streptococcal infection of the upper respiratory tract.

• Particular serotypes, *e.g.*, types 5 and 18, are often implicated, whereas others, *e.g.*, type 12, are not.

Epidemiology

• The incidence of acute rheumatic fever mirrors that of acute streptococcal pharyngitis in a population.

• The peak incidence is at 5–15 years; it is rare in children aged <4 years but well described in adults.

• The overall male:female ratio is equal; women, however, are more likely to develop Sydenham's chorea and mitral stenosis.

Duckett-Jones criteria for diagnosing acute rheumatic fever

Modified by the American Heart Association.

• Acute rheumatic fever is indicated by two major or one major and two minor criteria if supported by evidence of preceding streptococcal infection.

Major manifestations

Carditis.
Polyarthritis.
Chorea.
Erythema marginatum.
Subcutaneous nodules.

Minor manifestations

Previous rheumatic fever or rheumatic heart disease.
Arthralgia.
Fever.
Raised ESR and CRP concentration, leukocytosis, prolonged PR interval.

Treatment

Diet and lifestyle

• Strict bed or chair rest is advised with mobilization according to clinical status.

Pharmacological treatment

Antibiotics

• Antibiotics do not modify an acute attack or influence the development of carditis.

• They are used to eradicate streptococci from the pharynx and tonsils to prevent recurrence and further valve damage, as prophylaxis for all rheumatic carditis patients, or to cover dental extractions and other surgical interventions (long-term penicillin G benzathine, i.m. 4-weekly).

Standard dosage	Penicillin V, 500 mg 4 times daily for 10 days (adults; *see manufacurer's current prescribing information for children*). Erythromycin, 250 mg 4 times daily for 10 days (adults; *see manufacurer's current prescribing information for children*).
Contraindications	Hypersensitivity.
Special points	Shorter courses may not eradicate streptococci from pharynx.
Main drug interactions	Oral anticoagulants, theophylline preparations (erythromycin).
Main side effects	Hypersensitivity and rash (penicillin), gastrointestinal intolerance.

Anti-inflammatory agents

• These do not cure or prevent subsequent development of rheumatic disease.

• Early indiscriminate use may obscure diagnosis in mild cases.

Standard dosage	Aspirin, 80–100 mg/kg daily (children), 6–8 g daily (adults); reduced after 2 weeks and continued for 6–8 weeks. *For more severe carditis or patients intolerant of high-dose salicylates:* prednisolone, 40–60 mg daily for 2 weeks, reduced over next 3–4 weeks, followed by aspirin.
Contraindications	*Aspirin:* breast-feeding, gastrointestinal ulceration, hemophilia. *Prednisolone:* current acute gastrointestinal blood loss.
Special points	*Aspirin:* one of the few indications for aspirin treatment in childhood. *Prednisolone:* possible adrenal suppression on sudden withdrawal.
Main drug interactions	*Aspirin:* anticoagulants. *Prednisolone:* danger of gastrointestinal hemorrhage if combined with NSAIDs.
Main side effects	*Aspirin:* hypersensitivity, gastrointestinal bleeding. *Prednisolone:* glucose intolerance, Cushing's syndrome, growth retardation.

Other options

Diuretics, possibly with angiotensin-converting enzyme inhibitors.

Digoxin.

Anticoagulants.

• Use is determined by the degree of carditis or cardiac failure and the stage of illness.

Prognosis

• Untreated acute rheumatic fever usually lasts up to 3 months.

• Severe carditis extends acute illness to 6 months.

• Most patients with valvular disease develop cardiological complications needing intervention by middle age.

• 6% of patients free of carditis during an acute attack have rheumatic heart disease at 10 years.

• 30% of patients with mild carditis and no pre-existing disease have murmurs at 10 years.

• 40% of patients with apical or basal murmurs in an acute attack have residual disease at 10 years.

• 70% of patients with cardiac failure or pericarditis in an acute attack have residual disease at 10 years.

• Exceptions are patients with "pure" chorea, who frequently develop rheumatic heart disease despite absence of signs of carditis at outset.

Follow-up and management

• Patients must be kept under strict supervision until signs of acute inflammation have subsided.

• Penicillin or alternative prophylaxis is needed at least until the age of 18 years (some clinicians advocate life-long prophylaxis).

• Adequate prophylaxis is needed for minor surgical interventions, *e.g.*, dental treatment.

General references

Homer C, *et al.*: Clinical aspects of acute rheumatic fever. *J Rheumatol* 1991, **18(suppl 29)**:2–12.

Simmons NA: Recommendations for endocarditis prophylaxis. *J Antimicrob Chemother* 1993, **31**:437–438.

Veasy LG, Hill HR: Immunologic and clinical correlations in rheumatic fever and rheumatic heart disease. *Pediatr Infect Dis J* 1997, **16**:400–407.

Diagnosis

Symptoms
• Symptoms are mostly trivial; patients are systemically well.

Mild fever.

Rash: in ~50% of infected patients.

Signs
Rash: fine, erythematous pink macules, almost confluent on trunk on second day, rarely lasts >3 days.

Reddened throat: sometimes with tonsillar exudates.

Enlarged lymph nodes: notably occipital, sometimes splenomegaly.

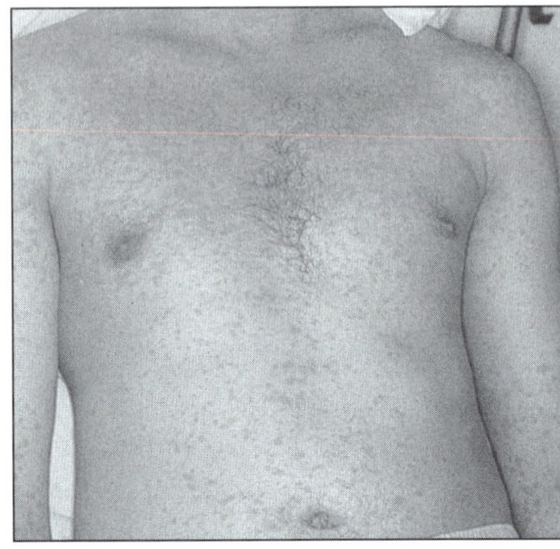

Fine nonblotchy rash of rubella. (*See* Color Plate.)

Investigations
• The diagnosis of rubella is established serologically.

• A patient's unconfirmed history of rubella should be discounted.

Serology: IgM detectable in serum within 1–2 days of rash; hemagglutination-inhibiting antibodies rise within 1–2 days of rash, peak in 6–12 days, and thereafter fade but remain detectable at lower levels.

Complications

General
Arthralgia or arthritis of fingers, wrists, and knees: usually in young women.

Encephalitis.

Thrombocytopenia.

Neuritis.

Congenital rubella
Cataract, retinopathy, microphthalmos, glaucoma.

Patent ductus arteriosus, ventricular septal defect, pulmonary stenosis.

Deafness.

Thrombocytopenic purpura, hepatosplenomegaly, hepatitis, CNS defects, bone lesions.

Differential diagnosis
• Patients with rubella are usually well and the rash is not blotchy.

Measles: marked prodrome, malaise, dusky-red maculopapular erythematous rash that travels down body over 3 days.

Adenovirus or enterovirus infections, mild scarlet fever, cytomegalovirus or Epstein–Barr virus infection, toxoplasmosis.

Etiology
• Infection is by rubella virus, an RNA virus.

• Transmission is by respiratory droplets.

• Fetal infection occurs secondary to maternal viremia; the incidence and type of defect are related to the age of the fetus at the time of infection.

• Significant defects are found with early infection.

Epidemiology
• Rubella occurs worldwide.

Infectivity
• ~16% of affected infants have major defects at birth after maternal rubella in the first trimester.

• Rubella is moderately infectious: patients are infectious during the rash and probably for ~7 days before and up to 5 days after illness, although the virus is detectable in throat secretions up to 10 days before and until 16 days after the rash.

• Babies with congenital rubella excrete the virus in throat and urine for prolonged periods.

Mean incubation period
~18 days.

Treatment

Diet and lifestyle

• No special diet is necessary.

• Affected patients should keep away from pregnant women.

Pharmacological treatment

Symptomatic

Analgesics, *e.g.*, acetaminophen.

Prophylactic

• Vaccination is by live attenuated virus: this may produce a mild rubella-like illness; women should not be pregnant or become so within 8–12 weeks of vaccination.

• It is routinely recommended in the second year of life as part of MMR, for girls aged 10–14 years at present, and any identified susceptible adult women of childbearing potential.

• Prompt serological testing of pregnant contacts of a patient with rubella is essential to assess susceptibility.

• The use of hyperimmune globulin should be considered if the risk is significant and if therapeutic abortion would not be considered should rubella develop later.

Treatment aims

To relieve symptoms.
To prevent congenital rubella.

Prognosis

• The prognosis in rubella is excellent.

• Deaths are rare and usually associated with encephalitis.

Follow-up and management

• Follow-up and management is not needed except in pregnancy, when risks and discussion of termination should be considered.

General references

Anonymous: *Immunization Against Infectious Diseases.* London: HMSO; 1992

Hall AJ, Peckham CS: Infections in childhood and pregnancy as a cause of adult disease: methods and examples. *Br Med Bull* 1997, **53**:10–23.

Miller E, *et al.*: Rubella surveillance to June 1994. *Comm Dis Rep* 1994, **4**:R146–R152.

Morgan-Capner P. Diagnosing rubella. *BMJ* 1989; **229**:338–339.

Diagnosis

Symptoms

• Patients may have no respiratory symptoms.

Dyspnea.

Cough: usually unproductive.

Chest discomfort: vague intermittent ache.

Fatigue, malaise, weight loss, fever, anorexia.

Symptoms of the complications of sarcoidosis.

Signs

Fine inspiratory crackles and wheezes: rarely.

Lymphadenopathy.

Uveitis, keratoconjunctivitis sicca, retinopathy.

Erythema nodosum, skin nodules, maculopapular rash, lupus pernio.

Hepatomegaly, splenomegaly, portal hypertension.

Bone cysts, polyarthralgia, myopathy.

Investigations [1]

Chest radiography: 90% of patients have abnormal radiographs, which show a wide variety of appearances (*see* Clinical staging).

Pulmonary function tests: may be entirely within normal limits, despite extensive radiographic shadows, or may show significant physiological dysfunction with clear radiographical lung fields. A restrictive defect is most common.

Skin test: anergy in two-thirds of patients.

Blood tests: leukocyte count may show lymphopenia; ESR may be raised; serum immunoglobulins and electrophoresis may show panhyperglobulinemia; serum angiotensin-converting enzyme increased in two-thirds of acute patients; hypercalcemia in ~18% of patients; liver function indices in a few may show intrahepatic cholestasis.

24-hour urine collection: hypercalciuria may be present despite normal serum calcium concentration.

ECG: arrhythmias, bundle branch block pattern in some patients.

Biopsy of lymph node, lung tissue, skin, liver, or other tissue: shows noncaseating epithelioid granulomata.

Fiberoptic bronchoscopy with transbronchial biopsy: the procedure of choice in patients with suspected pulmonary involvement.

Bronchoalveolar lavage: may be helpful adjunct to diagnosis; many patients with "active" sarcoidosis show increased percentage of lymphocytes and a high CD4/CD8 cell ratio.

• Ophthalmological assessment, including slit lamp examination and fluorescein angiography (needed in patients with associated occular symptoms).

Complications

Peripheral neuropathy, facial-nerve palsy, other cranial-nerve palsies, papilledema, meningitis, space-occupying lesions, epilepsy, cerebellar ataxia, hypopituitarism, diabetes insipidus.

Bundle branch block, arrhythmias, congestive cardiac failure, pericarditis, cardiomyopathy, cor pulmonale.

Disordered calcium metabolism, hypercalcemia, hypercalciuria, nephrocalcinosis.

Enlarged parotid and lacrimal glands.

Glaucoma, cataract: complication of chronic uveitis.

Differential diagnosis

Hilar lymphadenopathy
Tuberculosis, Hodgkin's lymphoma, infectious mononucleosis, metastases, enlarged pulmonary arteries.

Hilar lymphadenopathy with pulmonary infiltration
Tuberculosis, pneumoconiosis, lymphangitic carcinoma, idiopathic hemosiderosis, pulmonary eosinophilia, alveolar-cell carcinoma, histiocytosis X.

Diffuse pulmonary infiltration
The above and also chronic beryllium disease, honeycomb lung, rheumatoid lung, Sjögren's syndrome, interstitial lung disease, cystic fibrosis, hypersensitivity pneumonitis.

Noncaseating granulomata
Tuberculosis and other mycobacterial infections, fungal infections, leprosy, syphillis, cat-scratch disease, berylliosis, hypersensitivity pneumonitis, foreign-body reactions, lymphoma, carcinoma, biliary cirrhosis, Crohn's disease, hypogammaglobulinemia, granulomatous vasculitides, parasitic infection.

Etiology

• The cause is unknown, but alterations in the immune system is involved in its pathogenesis.

Epidemiology

• Sarcoidosis is usually manifest in the 20–40-year age group.

• It is more usual in temperate than in tropical climates.

• The prevalence rates are difficult to establish because the disease is often asymptomatic; in the United States, the incidence is 40 in 100 000 population.

• Sarcoidosis is more prevalent and tends to be more chronic in blacks, who have higher risk of nonrespiratory manifestations.

Clinical staging

Stage 0: normal chest (5%–10% of patients).

Stage I: bilateral hilar adenopathy (50%).

Stage II: bilateral hilar adenopathy and peripheral pulmonary infiltration; paratracheal nodes may also be enlarged (25%).

Stage III: parenchymal infiltration only (15%).

Treatment

Diet and lifestyle

• No special precautions are necessary.

Pharmacological treatment [2–4]

• Treatment is not needed in many patients because the disability is mild and remission is usual. Spontaneous total remissions occur in many. Constitutional symptoms or CNS involvement are some of the indications for systemic treatment.

Corticosteroids—drug of first choice

• These can suppress the manifestations of acute sarcoidosis, with rapid clearing of radiographic lesions; whether they alter the long-term outcome or prevent development of late fibrosis if started early remains unproven.

Standard dosage	Prednisone, 30–40 mg daily for 4–6 weeks; with rapid tapering to 15 mg daily for 3 months.
Contraindications	Uncontrolled hypertension, diabetes mellitus, infection, severe osteoporosis.
Special points	Relapses treated by increased dose; some patients with objective evidence of relapse on >3 occasions may need long-term low-dose maintenance prednisone.
Main drug interactions	Antihypertensive drugs.
Main side effects	Weight gain, edema, bruising, purple striae in skin (particularly abdomen), moon face, osteoporosis, collapse of vertebrae, diabetes mellitus, hypertension, myopathy (especially proximal girdle muscles), hirsutism, menstrual disturbances, psychotic reactions, cataracts, withdrawal phenomena.

Immunosuppressants

• Treatment should be given under specialist supervision.

• In resistant cases, immunosuppressants are sometimes partially effective (*e.g.*, methotrexate, azathioprine). Other agents rarely tried include cyclophosphamide, chlorambucil, and chloroquine.

Standard dosage	Methotrexate, 10 mg once weekly for 3 months; repeated courses every 6 months, possibly with oral steroids. Azathioprine, 100–200 mg daily.
Contraindications	Hepatic and renal impairment.
Main drug interactions	Alcohol, NSAIDs, antacids.
Main side effects	*Methotrexate:* hepatic fibrosis, acute bone-marrow suppression. *Azathioprine:* bone-marrow toxicity, gastrointestinal symptoms, rash, fever.

NSAIDs

• Anti-inflammatory agents are occasionally used in acute arthritic manifestations of sarcoidosis.

Standard dosage	Indomethacin, 50–200 mg daily in divided doses, with food.
Contraindications	Active peptic ulceration; severe renal, cardiac, and hepatic failure.
Main drug interactions	Angiotensin-converting enzyme inhibitors, anticoagulants, antidiabetics, antidepressants, 4-quinolones.
Main side effects	Gastrointestinal disturbances, ulceration, and bleeding, blood disorders (thrombocytopenia), headache, dizziness.

Treatment aims

To prevent development of irreversible pulmonary fibrosis.

Other treatments

• Lung transplantation or heart-lung transplantation has been done with end-stage disease.

Prognosis [2]

• 50% of patients remit spontaneously.

• Accompanying hilar adenopathy usually regresses within ~1 year.

• ~10% of patients develop parenchymal lesions, of which many resolve within 1 year.

• ~40% of patients resolve spontaneously within 1 year; the rest may progress with varying speed to irreversible fibrosis, which, in severely ill patients, may be complicated by upper-zone bullous disease and aspergillomas, with recurrent infection and haemoptysis.

Follow-up and management

• Regular clinical review is needed for patients being treated by steroids or immunosuppressants.

Key references

1. Winterbauer R, Belic N, Moores K: A clinical interpretation of bilateral hilar adenopathy. *Ann Intern Med* 1973, **78**:65–71.

2. Hunninghake G, *et al.*: Outcome of the treatment for sarcoidosis. *Am J Respir Crit Care Med* 1994, **149**:893–898.

3. Newman LS, Rose CS, Maier LA: Sarcoidosis. *N Engl J Med* 1997, **336**:1224–1234.

4. Lynch JP III: Pulmonary sarcoidosis: current concepts and controversies. *Compr Ther* 1997, **23**:197–210.

Diagnosis

Symptoms

• Symptoms of hypotensive shock are nonspecific; they include the following:

Restlessness.

Confusion or stupor.

Breathlessness.

Chest pain.

• Symptoms of the underlying cause may predominate.

Signs

Hypotension: a useful definition is systolic blood pressure <90 mm Hg.

Oliguria: <30 mL/h.

Cyanosis.

Confusion.

Peripheral vasoconstriction or vasodilatation: may indicate high or low systemic vascular resistance, respectively.

Tachycardia and third heart sound.

Investigations

Initial investigations
Complete blood count, hematocrit, urine and electrolytes, toxicology screen, and creatinine analysis.

Cardiac enzyme analysis: if myocardial injury suspected.

Blood culture: if any infective process known or suspected.

Arterial blood gas analysis: to assess hypoxemia and acidosis.

ECG and chest radiography: mandatory.

Circulatory assessment
• This should ideally be done in an intensive care unit.

Central venous cannulation: to measure central venous pressure.

Arterial cannulation: sphygmomanometry may be unreliable in shock.

Pulmonary artery catheterization: for pulmonary artery pressure, pulmonary capillary wedge pressure, and thermodilution cardiac output.

Echocardiography: for left ventricular function or if valve lesion, ventricular septal defect, or tamponade suspected.

Complications

Myocardial ischemia or infarction.

Acute renal failure.

Ischemic stroke.

Hepatic dysfunction.

Paralytic ileus.

Lactic acidosis: an indicator of severe tissue hypoxia.

Etiology

Low central venous pressure
Indicates hypovolemia.
Warm peripheries (low systemic vascular resistance): vasodilatation due to septicemia or drug overdose.
Cool peripheries (high systemic resistance): normal hemoglobin or hematocrit indicates hemorrhage; high hemoglobin indicates salt and water loss, *e.g.*, from peritonitis, pancreatitis, diabetic ketoacidosis, burns, polyuric phase of acute tubular necrosis.

Elevated central venous pressure
Indicates "pump failure."
Tension pneumothorax.
Pulmonary embolism.
Impaired myocardial contractility due to acute myocardial infarction or ischemia, sepsis, acidemia, electrolyte disturbance, negatively inotropic agents (*e.g.*, beta-antagonists, antiarrhythmic agents).
Arrhythmia.
Cardiac tamponade.
Ruptured interventricular septum.
Acute mitral or aortic valve regurgitation.
Aortic stenosis.

Epidemiology

Not applicable.

Septicemia and hypotensive shock

• The circulatory hallmark of sepsis is an unpredictable derangement of regional blood flow. Inappropriate vasodilatation of muscle and skin arterioles may coexist with profound vasoconstriction of the renal and splanchnic vascular beds.
• The hypotension has many causes, *e.g.*, a fall in systemic vascular resistance to <25% of normal, depression of myocardial contractility by hypoxemia and acidemia, dilatation of venous capacitance vessels resulting in low central venous pressure, and disruption of capillary function causing leakage of intravascular fluid and plasma proteins into alveoli, gastrointestinal tract, peritoneal cavity, and other tissues.
• The combination of myocardial impairment and damage to alveolar capillary basement membranes means that attempts to restore the blood pressure by rapid i.v. infusion of fluid will probably result in pulmonary edema.

Treatment

Diet and lifestyle
• No special precautions are necessary.

Pharmacological treatment
• Whenever possible, the underlying cause should be treated.

• Immediate measures include the following:

Provision of oxygen: hypoxemia contributes to lactic acid production.
Treatment of arrhythmias: cardioversion preferable to negatively inotropic antiarrhythmic drugs.
Plasma expander administration, if central venous pressure is reduced.
Correction of any electrolyte disturbance.
Broad-spectrum antibiotic treatment, if sepsis suspected.
Inotropic support for hypotension without hypovolemia, as follows:

For oliguria
• Dopamine is the first choice in oliguria; it enhances renal blood flow at a low dose, inotropic and vasoconstrictor at doses >5 µg/kg/min (beta$_1$-, alpha-agonism). It must be administered centrally.

Standard dosage	Dopamine, 3–5 µg/kg/min.
Contraindications	Pheochromocytoma.
Main drug interactions	Monoamine oxidase inhibitors.
Main side effects	Vomiting, tachycardia, angina, headache.

After myocardial infarction
• Dobutamine is the first choice after myocardial infarction; it is predominantly a beta$_1$-agonist; it improves myocardial oxygen supply:demand ratio and causes peripheral vasodilatation (hence its use if the systemic vascular resistance is high).

Standard dosage	Dobutamine, 5–20 µg/kg/min.
Contraindications	Outflow tract obstruction, proarrhythmic tendencies.
Main drug interactions	Hypotension with other vasodilators.
Main side effects	Tachycardia, local phlebitis, hypokalemia.

For severe hypotension
• Epinephrine is the most positively inotropic catecholamine; it acts as a beta-agonist at low dose, and an alpha-agonist at doses >10 µg/min and causes peripheral vasoconstriction (hence its use if systemic vascular resistance is low).

Standard dosage	Epinephrine, 2–40 µg/min.
Contraindications	Hypertension, tachyarrhythmias.
Main drug interactions	Inhalational anesthetics, tricyclic antidepressants.
Main side effects	Tachycardia, arrhythmias.

For bradycardia, atrioventricular block, and right heart failure
• Isoproterenol is used in bradycardia, atrioventricular block, and right heart failure; it causes pulmonary and systemic vasodilatation; it worsens myocardial supply:demand ratio and ventilation/perfusion mismatch.

Standard dosage	Isoproterenol, 1–10 µg/min.
Contraindications	Cardiac ischemia, hyperthyroidism.
Main drug interactions	Inhalational anesthetics, tricyclic antidepressants.
Main side effects	Atrial and ventricular tachyarrhythmias.

If systemic vascular resistance is profoundly low
• Norepinephrine is used if the systemic vascular resistance is profoundly low; its alpha agonism causes vasoconstriction; a rise in blood pressure occurs at the expense of a fall in cardiac output.

Standard dosage	Norepinephrine, 1–10 µg/min.
Contraindications	Myocardial dysfunction.
Main drug interactions	Tricyclic antidepressants.
Main side effects	Digit necrosis, myocardial ischemia.

Other treatments

Mechanical ventilation
• This allows effective correction of hypoxemia and eliminates the work of breathing (most useful in acute left ventricular failure).

Intra-aortic balloon pump
• This is a temporary measure (24–48 hours) while spontaneous improvement or definitive treatment (*e.g.*, valve or ventricular septal defect repair) is awaited.
• It is useful in cardiac surgery and refractory unstable angina.
• Complications, in 20% of patients, include leg ischemia, aortic dissection, hemolysis, thrombocytopenia, infection.

Surgery
• Surgery is indicated early in rupture of interventricular septum or papillary muscle, aortic dissection, and subacute myocardial rupture causing tamponade.

Prognosis
• The main determinant of outcome is the underlying disorder: for example, hypotension due to diabetic ketoacidosis in a young person has a favorable prognosis, whereas cardiogenic shock resulting from acute anterior myocardial infarction has a mortality of 80%–90%.

Follow-up and management
• No follow-up is needed.

Key reference

1. Colucci WS, Braunwald E: Pathophysiology of heart failure. In *Heart Disease*, edn 5. Edited by Braunwald E. Philadelphia: WB Saunders; 1997:394–415.

Diagnosis

Symptoms

Pain (supraspinatus tendinitis, deltoid, bicipital tendinitis, posterior, anterior, referred).

Functional impairment.

Sleep disturbance.

Diminished range of motion.

Weakness.

Signs

Atrophy.

Frozen shoulder.

Diminished range of motion.

Point tenderness.

Effusion.

Weakness.

Painful arc.

Yergason's drop-arm test.

Investigations

Radiography.

Electromylography.

Ultrasonography.

MRI.

Arthrography.

Arthroscopy.

• Sophisticated imaging studies are not generally required, unless there is failure of conservative initial management or compelling physical examination evidence or radiographical indication of rotator cuff tear.

Complications

Frozen shoulder.

Functional impairment.

Differential diagnosis

Periarticular disorders
Impingement syndromes.
Rotator cuff tendinitis.
Rotator cuff tears.
Adhesive capsulitis.
Cervical radiculopathy.
Reflex sympathetic dystrophy.
Fibromyalgia.
Diabetes mellitus.

Glenohumeral disorders
Osteoarthritis.
Osteonecrosis.
Septic arthritis.
Glenoid labral tears.
Adhesive capsulitis.

Regional disorders
Cervical radiculopathy.
Brachial neuritis.
Nerve entrapment syndrome.
Reflex sympathetic dystrophy.
Fibromyalgia.
Neoplasia.

Miscellaneous
Cholecystitis.
Splenic trauma.
Subphrenic abscess.
Myocardial infarction.
Diabetes mellitus.
Renal osteodystrophy.
Thyroid disease.
Hemarthrosis.

Etiology

Traumatic (acute injuries vs. chronic overuse).
Degenerative osteoarthritis.
Inflammatory.
Crystalline (hydroxyapatite).
Infectious.
Viscerogenic.
Hemorrhagic.
Infiltrative.
Neoplastic.

Epidemiology

• Shoulder disorders are among the most common presenting complaints in primary care.
• Duration of impairment may be 3–18 months.
• Risk factors include overhead work (*e.g.*, filing, reaching, painting), throwing sports, collision and contact sports.

Other information

• There is considerable overlap in the presentation and localizing symptoms and signs for many of the disorders listed above. An important concept to understand is the final common pathway of adhesive capsulitis (frozen shoulder).

Treatment

Diet and lifestyle

- Modification of work requirements may be necessary.
- Modification of exercise activities may be essential to recovery.

Pharmacological treatment

Acetaminophen.

NSAIDs.

Intra-articular corticosteroid administration.

- Intra-articular steroids are within the scope of the primary care physician.
- Standard procedure manuals outline the technique.

Nonpharmacological treatment

RICE—*R*est, *I*ce, *C*ompression, *E*xercise.

- Physical therapy modalities indicate the following:

Heat/cold.

Mobilization techniques.

Ultrasound.

Phonopheresis.

Iontophoresis.

- Other therapeutic options include arthroscopy, orthopedic surgery, and arthroplasty.
- Referral to musculoskeletal specialist may be needed early for surgical repair candidates (*i.e.*, return to work or to elite competition).

Treatment aims

- The goals of physical therapy are:
To relieve pain
To restore normal range of motion.
To restore strength.
To restore function.
To strengthen to prevent recurrence.

Prognosis

- With accurate, prompt diagnosis, most patients show improvement.
- Early institution of range-of-motion exercises prevents frozen shoulder.
- Long duration of symptoms must be met by support from physician and rehabilitation personnel, because encouragement enables patients to persist and ultimately improve.

Follow-up and management

- At the time of diagnosis, patients should be instructed on home exercises for the shoulder.
- Medications may be helpful adjunctive therapy.
- Physical therapy supervision may be necessary for refractory cases.
- Intra-articular steroids may be necessary for physical therapy failures or severely frozen shoulder.
- Patient expectations regarding the time course for improvement need to be reviewed at outset.

General references

Birrer RB (ed.): *Sports Medicine for the Primary Care Physician*, edn 2. Boca Raton, FL: CRC Press; 1994.

Garrick JG, Webb DR: *Sports Injuries: Diagnosis and Management.* Edited by Wickland E Jr. Philadelphia: WB Saunders; 1990.

Jahnke AH, *et al.*: A prospective comparison of computerized arthrotomography and magnetic resonance imaging of the glenohumeral joint. *Am J Sports Med* 1992, **20**:695–701.

Petri M, *et al.*: Randomized, double-blind, placebo-controlled study of the treatment of the painful shoulder. *Arthritis Rheum* 1987, **30**:1040–1046.

Warren RF: Shoulder pain. In *Manual of Rheumatology and Outpatient Orthopedic Disorders*, edn 2. Edited by Beary JF, *et al.* Boston: Little, Brown and Company; 1987:81–86.

Diagnosis

Symptoms

• Patients with SS and Sβ° thalassemia are generally more severely affected than those with SC, Sβ⁺ being the mildest disorder.

Acute painful vaso-occlusive crisis: causes >90% of hospital admissions affecting bones, joints, and muscles; initial presentation in one-third is the "hand foot" syndrome from age of 4 months; limb pain in older children, more central pain distribution in adolescents and adults.

Chronic pain: in hip or shoulders, caused by avascular necrosis.

Signs

• Often patients present with no signs in mild crisis.

Constitutional upset mimicking septicemia: in severe crisis (infection can precipitate crisis).

Localized swelling, tenderness, and redness of bone, joint, or muscle.

Abdominal pain mimicking more severe disease.

Limited range of hip or shoulder movement: with active avascular necrosis.

Investigations

For diagnosis

• Investigations should be made preferably when the patient is in a stable state.

Complete blood count: to establish degree of anemia.
Reticulocyte count: to establish degree of hemolysis.
Hemoglobin electrophoresis: to determine variant hemoglobins.
"Sickle test": to confirm presence of hemoglobin S.
Hemoglobin F estimation: high concentrations diminish severity.
Extended erythrocyte grouping: to ensure appropriate erythrocytes for transfusion.
Plasma blood urea nitrogen, creatinine, electrolytes analysis: to monitor renal function.
Liver function tests: to monitor hemolysis and exclude hepatitis.

In crisis

• The results should be compared with those from the stable state.

Complete blood count: hemoglobin raised with dehydration; falls in sequestration and aplasia.
Blood urea nitrogen, creatinine, electrolytes analysis: to detect dehydration.
Liver function tests: to measure dysfunction.
Cultures and viral screening: urine, blood, sputum, throat swab; to exclude infection (before antibiotic treatment); screening for parvovirus (not routine unless severely anemic).
Reticulocyte count.
Viral screen, chest radiography, blood gas and arterial oxygen saturation measurement: if patient has chest pain or signs.

Complications

Stroke: in 8% of patients, median age 7 years.
Sequestration syndromes: common cause of death; erythrocytes pooled in the organ, causing hemoglobin to fall by ≤2 g/dL, leading to dysfunction of the following organs: spleen (in infants; high risk of recurrence), liver (in children and adults), chest (a medical emergency, exchange transfusion if partial arterial oxygen pressure <60 mm Hg), splanchnic circulation (in adults, clinical picture of paralytic ileus that resolves spontaneously).
Infection: common and serious or life-threatening because of autosplenectomy, therefore susceptible to encapsulated bacteria, especially *Streptococcus pneumoniae* and *Salmonella* spp.; gram-negative infections, particularly *Escherichia coli*, account for 10% of deaths in adults; *Yersinia enterocolitica* infections in iron overloaded patients; aplastic crisis due to parvovirus B19.
Priapism, proliferative retinopathy, cholecystitis and cholelithiasis secondary to hemolysis.

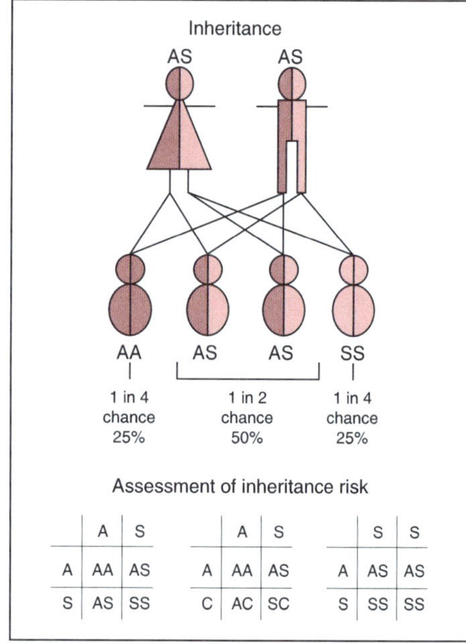

Assessment of inheritance risk. Among Jamaican and American sickle cell patients of African heritage, 50%–70% are Benin, 15%–30% are Bantu-CAR, and 5%–15% are Senegal haplotypes.

Treatment

Diet and lifestyle

• Patients should avoid factors that precipitate painful crisis, *e.g.*, infection, dehydration, exhaustion, cold, marked temperature changes, smoking, high altitude, and unpressurized aircraft; in some patients, stress is reported to be a precipitant.

Pharmacological treatment [1,2]

Analgesia

Standard dosage	*For mild to moderate pain*: acetaminophen, 12-15 mg/kg 8-hourly, codeine phosphate, 1-2 mg/kg 6-hourly (up to 3 mg/kg in 24 hours), or NSAIDs, all orally.
	For severe pain: morphine, 0.1 mg/kg i.v. loading dose, then 1-2 mg/kg i.v. infusion over 24 hours using patient-controlled analgesia system, or meperidine, 50-150 mg i.m. every 1-4 hours in adults.
Contraindications	*Oral drugs*: hepatic and renal impairment, peptic ulceration, asthma. *Parenteral drugs*: raised intracranial pressure.
Special points	*Meperidine*: respiratory rate must be monitored hourly, risk of seizures.
Main drug interactions	*Codeine and morphine:* alcohol, anxiolytics and hypnotics, dompetidone and metoclopramide, cimetidine. *Diclofenac:* caution with other analgesics, anticoagulants, antihypertensives, beta-blockers, and cardiac glycosides.
Main side effects	*Oral drugs*: rashes, blood dyscrasias, acute pancreatitis, constipation, respiratory depression. *Morphine*: respiratory depression, nausea, bronchospasm, severe pruritus. *Meperidine*: seizures.

Antibiotics

• Antibiotics are indicated for patients in severe crisis or when infection is suspected.

Standard dosage	Amoxicillin, 500 mg 3 times daily.
Contraindications	Penicillin allergy.
Special points	If pneumococcal infection is suspected, penicillin should be added.
Main drug interactions	Anticoagulants, antacids, oral contraceptives.
Main side effects	Nausea, diarrhea, rashes, pseudomembranous colitis.

Pharmacological augmentation of fetal hemoglobin production with hydroxyurea or 5-azacytidine [3,4]

• Reduces frequency of sickle cell crisis.

• Should not be administered without supervision of a hematologist.

Nonpharmacological treatment

Rehydration

Oral fluids increased in patients with mild pain; i.v. clear fluids in patients with severe pain at 80 mL/kg/24 h.

Oxygen treatment

60% oxygen if partial arterial oxygen pressure on air is <60 mm Hg; 35% if 60-70 mm Hg; 28% if 70-80 mm Hg.

Blood transfusion

See Transfusion medicine *for further details.*

Additive: when hemoglobin <5 g/dL and patient symptomatic from anemia; for aplastic crisis, sequestration, bleeding (*e.g.*, renal papillary necrosis).

Exchange: when hemoglobin >5 g/dL but improved oxygen transport needed.

Overall aim: hemoglobin S <20%, total hemoglobin 11-14.5 g/dL (possibly 3-4 procedures); for chest syndrome (if partial arterial oxygen pressure <60 mm Hg), priapism (if >4 hours), acute neurological deficit or splanchnic sequestration, severe or protracted crisis (occasionally), preoperatively in selected patients.

Long-term transfusion: to maintain hemoglobin at 11-14.5 g/dL, with hemoglobin S <25%; for neurological deficit, sickle chronic lung disease, prevention of pain (occasionally), pregnant women (selected).

Treatment aims

To provide early and effective relief of pain.

To treat infection.

To maintain hydration.

To maintain tissue oxygenation.

Prognosis

• All types of sickle cell disease are variable in clinical manifestations; no markers exist to predict severity for a particular patient.

• 87% of patients are alive at 20 years, 50% at 50 years.

• Deaths in childhood are most commonly due to infection.

• Deaths in adolescents and young adults are most commonly due to neurological and lung complications.

• Deaths in middle age are most commonly due to chronic organ failure.

• Successful outcome after bone-marrow transplantation has now been recorded and drugs that raise hemoglobin F levels look promising.

Follow-up and management

• Full education and counseling must be ensured, with family screening and genetic advice.

• Penicillin prophylaxis must be ensured for children, and antipneumococcal and hemophilus B vaccination should be considered.

• Children should be checked for upper airways obstruction.

Key references

1. Davies SC, Wonke B: The management of haemoglobinopathies. *Baillière's Clin Haematol* 1991, **4**:361–389.

2. Embury SH, *et al.*: *Sickle Cell Disease: Basic Principles and Clinical Practice.* New York: Raven Press; 1994.

3. Steinberg MH, Lu ZH, Barton FB, *et al.*: Fetal hemoglobin in sickle cell anemia: determinants of response to hydroxyurea. Multicenter study of hydroxyurea. *Blood* 1997, **89**:1078–1088.

4. Charache S, Barton FB, Morne KD, *et al.*: Hydroxyurea and sickle cell anemia: clinical utility of a myelosuppressive "switching" agent. *Medicine* 1996, **75**:300–326.

Diagnosis

Symptoms

Acute sinusitis

Headache or facial pain: involving either the maxillary, frontal, and ethmoid sinuses (pain directly over sinuses) or sphenoid sinuses (the great masquerader): pain may be retro-orbital, temporal, vertex, or occipital.

Purulent nasal discharge.

Maxillary toothache.

Poor response to decongestants.

Fever, malaise, cough, wheezing, postnasal drip, edema or erythema over sinuses.

Chronic sinusitis

Headache or facial pain: typically less severe than acute sinusitis, unless the infection involves frontal or sphenoid sinuses.

Purulent rhinorrhea: anteriorly and/or posteriorly (note: sphenoid sinusitis may present as only posterior rhinorrhea).

Nasal congestion.

Low-grade fever, malaise, halitosis, cough, wheezing edema, erythema over sinuses: less severe.

Signs

Purulent nasal secretions.

Nasal congestion and mucosal erythema.

Marked sinus tenderness on percussion or palpation: often nonspecific.

Abnormal translumination compared with contralateral side.

Facial edema or erythema.

Investigations

• Typically, diagnosis is made on clinical basis.

Indications for CT scan

To define extent of disease after "maximum medical treatment": in patients with chronic sinusitis who have been treated with 4 weeks of broad-spectrum antibiotics and topical steroid therapy.

Full CT scan: indicated in cases of suspected fungal disease, immunocompromised or diabetic patient with possible invasive fungal disease, suspected complication of sinusitis, suspected underlying mass.

Screening sinus CT: uncertainty of diagnosis.

Full or screening CT: indicated in cases of frequent acute sinusitis or failure to respond.

Other investigations based on clinical findings

Chest radiography: if suspected associated pneumonia or systemic illness such as Churg-Strauss syndrome, Wegener's disease, sarcoidosis.

ESR, urinalysis and sediment; antineutrophilic cytoplasmic antibody: to screen for Wegener's disease or (less commonly) Churg-Strauss syndrome or other systemic vasculitis.

Immunoglobulin levels (IgA, IgM, IgG, and IgG subclasses): for patients with unusually frequent bacterial respiratory infections.

Nasal smear: most commonly performed by allergist to identify bacteria as well as lymphocytes, neutrophils, or eosinophils as predominant cell type.

• Cultures (sinus tap vs. endoscopic middle meatus culture) are usually performed by an otolaryngologist.

Complications

Exacerbation of asthma, pneumonia, pharyngitis, otitis media, mucocele: general.

Periorbital or preseptal cellulitis (lid only); subperiosteal abscess; orbital cellulitis; orbital abscess; cavernous sinus thrombosis: ophthalmologic.

Subdural empyema; epidural empyema, cerebral abscess; meningitis: intracranial complications (higher risk with sphenoid and frontal sinusitis).

Invasive fungal disease: extension into orbit, brain, soft tissues of face, nasal cavity, and palate with tissue ischemia and necrosis.

Differential diagnosis

Allergic rhinitis with headache.

Nasal dryness and crusting (bacterial rhinitis).

Headache (migraine, tension, or ophthalmologic).

Temperomandibular joint or dental pain.

Gastroesophageal reflux laryngitis/pharyngitis (manifested as postnasal drip, hoarseness, cough).

Systemic diseases (Wegener's granulomatosis, sarcoidosis, Churg-Strauss syndrome).

Neuralgia and other neurological disorders.

Temporal arteritis.

Etiology and predisposing conditions

• The most common precipitating event is a bacterial or viral upper respiratory infection (URI).

• Common predisposing conditions include: Mucosal edema (rhinitis: allergic, vasomotor, bacterial, or viral).

Mechanical obstruction (polyps, septal deviation, trauma, tumor, foreign body).

Impaired ciliary motility or mucosal disease (Wegener's disease, sarcoidosis, cystic fibrosis, bacterial rhinitis/crusting).

Rapid change in altitude or pressure.

Dental infection.

Epidemiology

• Estimates are that 0.5%–5% of URIs in children will be associated with sinusitis.

• ~35 million adults in the United States suffer from "chronic sinusitis."

• Increasing incidence of bacterial resistance is expected.

Pathophysiology

URI.

Osteomeatal complex obstruction.

Sinus hypoxia, ciliary dysfunction, retained secretions, and cycle of infection.

Treatment

Diet and lifestyle

• Patients should avoid seasonal (pollens, grasses, trees) and perennial (dust, mold, danders) allergens.

• Patients should stop smoking.

• Saline sprays and/or saline bulb syringe irrigations are recommended.

Pharmacological treatment

Decongestants

Standard dosage
Oxymetazalone spray twice daily for 3–5 days (beware of rebound rhinitis medicamentosa if used >5 days).
Pseudoephedrine, short- or long-acting preparations (may elevate blood pressure or exacerbate urinary retention).

Antibiotics (acute sinusitis)

• Standard length of therapy is 10 days.

Standard dosage
First-line therapy: amoxicillin, 500 mg orally 3 times daily.
Bactrim DS, twice daily.
Alternative or second-line therapies (14–21 days' duration):
Clarithromycin, 500 mg twice daily.
Ceftin, 250–500 mg twice daily.
Augmentin, 875 mg twice daily or 500 mg every 8 hours (with food).
Ciprofloxacin, 500 mg twice daily.

Antibiotics (chronic sinusitis)

• Standard course of therapy is 3–6 weeks based on underlying comorbidities.

Standard dosage
Ceftin, 500 mg twice daily.
Augmentin, 500 mg every 8 hours (with food).
Biaxin, 500 mg twice daily.
Loracarbef, 400 mg twice daily.
Ciprofloxacin, 500 mg twice daily (± flagyl, 500 mg 3 times daily).

Special points
Prescription for antibiotics should avoid known allergies; consider compliance with dosing; and account for underlying comorbidities such as severe allergies or polyps, for which longer courses may be appropriate.
Patients with acute infections should be told to call their physician if symptoms, particularly pain and fever, are not responding to therapy after 48–72 hours.

For allergies

• Steroids sprays, antihistamine decongestants, immunotherapy are recommended.

When to refer for otolaryngologic evaluation and/or sinus surgery

Recurrent acute sinusitis 3–4 times a year documented by a screening CT.

Chronic sinusitis refractory to maximal medical treatment as evidenced by persistent obstruction of the sinuses or osteomeatal complex after 3–6 weeks of therapy.

Complication or impending complication of sinusitis.

Suspected fungal sinusitis (mycetoma, allergic fungal sinusitis, or invasive disease).

Immunocompromised patient not responding to therapy.

Bony erosive or destructive process on CT scan suggestive of more aggressive disease.

Nasal mass, tumor, or extension into other sinus.

Treatment aims

Treatment

To minimize symptoms of pain and rhinorrhea. To avoid development of complications.

Surgery

To widely open the osteomeatal complex, ethmoid, maxillary, and other sinuses to allow aeration of the cavity, restore mucociliary clearance of the sinuses, and thereby reduce the frequency and severity of infections.

Other treatments

Allergy testing and immunotherapy.

Skin testing appropriate for patients with allergic rhinitis refractory to avoidance, steroid sprays, antihistamines, and decongestants, or when allergens not readily identified; this may be followed by immunotherapy.

• Ideally, allergies should be maximally treated prior to sinus surgery (if required) to enhance mucosal healing.

Prognosis

• Majority of patients with sinusitis for several months will have such extensive irreversible mucosal disease that surgery may be necessary to establish drainage to allow resolution of the infection.

• 85%–90% of patients will be substantially improved by endoscopic sinus surgery.

Follow-up and management after surgery

Maintain or enhance mucociliary clearance with over-the-counter nasal saline sprays (*e.g.*, Ocean Spray) or salt water bulb syringe irrigations.

For patients with allergies and/or polyps: consider long-term daily steroid sprays.

Aggressive treatment of infections, especially in the first 3–6 months after surgery during which time mucociliary function is still compromised.

General references

Incauda GA, Wooding LG: Diagnosis and treatment of acute and subacute sinusitis in children and adults. In *Diseases of the Sinuses.* Edited by Gershwin ME. Totowa, NJ: Humana Press; 1995.
Kennedy DW, Gwaltney JM, Jones JG: Medical management of sinusitis: educational goals and management guidelines. *Ann Otol Rhinol Laryngol* 1995, **167**:22–30.

Diagnosis

Symptoms and signs

Impetigo
Isolated lesions or multiple small areas of golden yellow crusts, weeping areas, blisters: ruptured lesions leave raw areas.

Erysipelas
Inflammation substantially limited to skin and lymphatics, erythema with well-defined and palpable margins, swelling, local heat, mild superficial pain, fever and malaise; most common locations are face and lower extremities.

Deep infections
More swelling, deeper pain, less well–defined edges than in erysipelas, perhaps crepitus on palpation, and overlying skin necrosis: indicating cellulitis.

Boils or abscesses: focal areas of pus formation, often painful, abscesses may be enlarged and pointing.

Severe boil with central necrosis and multiple discharging sinuses: carbuncle.

Methicillin-resistant *Staphylococcus aureus* infections
• Patients are usually asymptomatic, *i.e.*, colonized, but some may have local or generalized life-threatening sepsis.

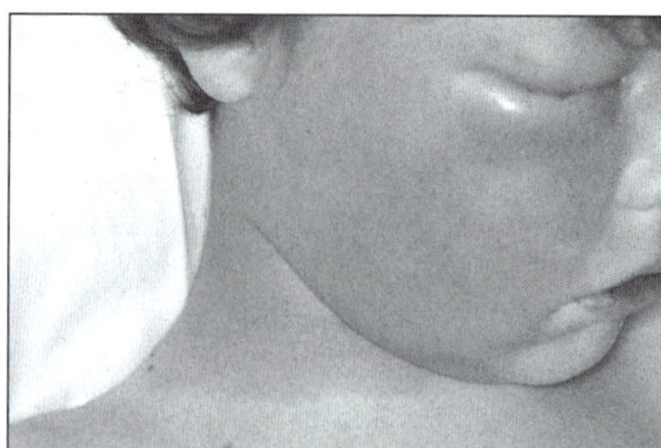

Erysipelas. (*See* Color Plate.)

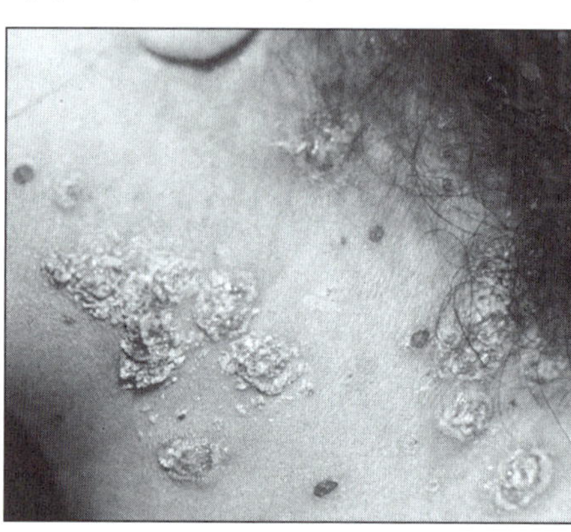

Impetigo. (*See* Color Plate.)

Investigations

Microbiology: areas of impetigo should be swabbed; methicillin-resistant *S. aureus* infection cannot be diagnosed clinically; swabs should be taken from nose, throat, perineum, eczematous areas, axillae, sputum, urine (if catheter present), any site of possible infection (including surgical wounds), i.v. access points; often not needed for classic erysipelas; if confirmation of causative organism of erysipelas or cellulitis desired, a few milliliters of saline solution can be injected into involved area and immediately aspirated (using same needle, which should not be withdrawn); site of entry of infection should be swabbed; abscess pus should be sent for microscopy and culture.

Blood culture: if skin is intact over areas of cellulitis.

Complications

Lymphangitis, scarlet fever, septicemia, poststreptococcal rheumatic fever: rare complications of erysipelas.

Spread of infection to contiguous tissue, septicemia: complications of cellulitis.

Rupture, septicemia: complications of boils.

Treatment

Diet and lifestyle

• No special precautions are necessary.

Pharmacological treatment

For erysipelas

• Erysipelas usually responds to penicillin parenterally if the illness is severe.

Standard dosage	Penicillin G, 300–600 mg i.v. 6-hourly Penicillin V, 500 mg orally 6-hourly.
Contraindications	Hypersensitivity.
Special points	Dicloxacillin or new macrolides are other options.
Main drug interactions	None.
Main side effects	Gastrointestinal disturbances, sensitivity reactions.

For cellulitis

• Usually dicloxacillin.

Standard dosage	Dicloxacillin, 500 mg 4 times daily.
Contraindications	Hypersensitivity.
Special points	Erythromycin is an alternative.
Main drug interactions	None.
Main side effects	Gastrointestinal disturbances, sensitivity reactions.

For boils and abscesses

• No antibiotics are needed in the case of free drainage, with no surrounding inflammation.

• Otherwise, floxacillin or erythromycin should be used.

For methicillin-resistant *S. aureus* (MRSA) infection

• If the patient is widely colonized, topical antiseptics can be tried (including tridosan, hexachlorophene, chlorhedixine, povidone-iodine), although success is uncertain.

• If the carriage is limited, particularly to the nose, topical mupirocin can be used.

• If the patient has an invasive infection or if eradication of MRSA is necessary to allow more appropriate treatment for underlying conditions, treatment with antibiotics under specialist supervision may be appropriate.

• MRSA strains are often sensitive to vancomycin or teicoplanin; fusidic acid, rifampin, or ciprofloxacin may also have a role.

Standard dosage	Hexachlorophene applied sparingly every 4–6 hours after washing. Mupirocin applied to nares 3 times daily for up to 10 days. Vancomycin, 1 g 2 times daily.
Contraindications	*Hexachlorophene*: damaged skin, pregnancy, breast-feeding, children <2 years of age. *Mupirocin, vancomycin*: hypersensitivity.
Main drug interactions	*Vancomycin*: cholestyramine, aminoglycosides, loop diuretics.
Main side effects	*Hexachlorophene*: redness (overgenerous application). *Mupirocin*: minor burning, stinging, itching. *Vancomycin*: hypotension, nephrotoxicity, ototoxicity, bone-marrow suppression, sensitivity reactions, phlebitis, muscle spasm.

• Clearance is accepted if weekly sets of screening swabs are negative over 3 weeks.

• Patients must initially be isolated on further admission, and continued carriage must be assessed.

Treatment aims

To eradicate infection.
To avoid spread of MRSA infection.

Other treatments

Surgical exploration to define the extent and nature of anaerobic cellulitis and to treat it.
Incision of abscesses.

Prognosis

• Further attacks of erysipelas are common at the same site; patients should report promptly for antibiotic treatment.

Follow-up and management

• All patients' feet should be regularly examined for the presence of athlete's foot, which is a common portal of entry for microorganisms that cause cellulitis of the lower extremity.

Prevention of spread of MRSA

• The patient must be isolated.
• The Infection Control Team must be contacted immediately.
• The source of the MRSA must be sought.
• The risk to other patients must be assessed.
• The patient's notes must be marked "MRSA infected."
• Infected staff must be identified and controlled.
• Hands must be washed after any patient contact.
• Gloves must be worn when infected tissue or dressings are being handled.
• Facemasks must be worn if exposure to infected aerosols is possible.
• "Infection Control" disposal of soiled material is vital.
• Rooms must be terminally disinfected.
• The patient can be discharged unless contacts are vulnerable; if discharge is not possible, infected individuals must be isolated (even if asymptomatic).
• Unnecessary staff–patient contact must be minimized (barrier nursing).
• The use of staff not familiar with the involved ward must be minimized.

General references

Duckworth DJ: Diagnosis and management of methicillin resistant *Staphylococcus aureus* infection. *BMJ* 1993, **307**:1049–1052.

Semel JD, Goldin H: Association of athlete's foot with cellulitis of the lower extremities: diagnostic value of bacterial cultures of ipsilateral interdigital space samples. *Clin Infect Dis* 1996, **23**:1162–1164.

Diagnosis

Definition

• Central sleep apnea is a clinical syndrome with a range of causes.

Neuromuscular weakness or chest-wall disease: the primary problem is inefficiency of the respiratory pump; patients may develop daytime ventilatory failure.

Periodic respiration (Cheyne–Stokes breathing): the primary problem is disordered respiratory feedback control; patients do not develop daytime ventilatory failure.

Pure central sleep apnea: characterized by hypoventilation despite normal airway, lungs, chest wall, and muscles; occurs in lesions of brainstem and with primary alveolar hypoventilation (Ondine's curse).

Symptoms

Daytime sleepiness, restless sleep, transient breathlessness: during the arousal and tachypnea that follow an apnea; symptoms of sleep disturbance.

Morning headache and nausea, poor exercise tolerance, ankle swelling, daytime breathlessness: only with neuromuscular or chest-wall disease; symptoms of respiratory failure.

Symptoms of primary causative disease.

Signs

Cyanosis, peripheral edema, raised venous pressure, signs of pulmonary hypertension or right ventricular hypertrophy: signs of ventilatory failure and cor pulmonale.

Raised venous pressure and edema: signs of heart failure.

Muscle fasciculation, weakness, loss of tendon reflex: signs of myopathy, dystrophy, motor neuron disease, postpoliomyelitis syndrome.

Supine breathlessness and paradoxical abdominal movement on sniffing: signs of diaphragm weakness due to bilateral phrenic palsy, acid maltase deficiency, or other muscular disease.

Upper motor neuron and brain stem signs: signs of stroke.

Chest-wall deformity: signs of scoliosis, thoracoplasty.

Investigations

Initial

Awake arterial oxygen saturation and blood gas analysis: for possible hypercapnia; alveolar–arterial oxygen gradient often normal.

Spirometry: to exclude chronic obstructive pulmonary disease and assess lung volume; daytime ventilatory failure with central sleep apnea rare if vital capacity >1.5 L standing; supine fall in forced vital capacity of >20% suggests marked diaphragm weakness.

Hemoglobin analysis: for polycythemia.

Nerve physiology, muscle biopsy, ECG, echocardiography: can also be considered.

Sleep studies [1]

• These are used to exclude obstructive sleep apnea, show characteristic apneas without continuing respiratory effort, show worsening hypoventilation during rapid eye movement sleep, and quantify the severity of the abnormality present.

• Complete study should include electroencephalography, electro-oculography, electromyography, oximetry, measurement of respiratory effort and airflow.

• Interpretation can be difficult because some patients with apnea due to pharyngeal collapse make little respiratory effort and some patients with a primary failure of respiratory drive have secondary airway collapse.

Complications

Ventilatory failure, cor pulmonale, pneumonia: in patients with neuromuscular or chest-wall disease.

Accidents: particularly motor vehicle accidents, due to poor daytime vigilance.

Differential diagnosis

Daytime sleepiness

Obstructive sleep apnea.

Narcolepsy.

Idiopathic hypersomnolence.

Periodic movements of legs during sleep.

Inadequate sleep.

Respiratory failure

Chronic obstructive lung disease.

Obstructive sleep apnea.

Etiology [2,3]

Neuromuscular or chest-wall disease

• Patients just able to sustain normal ventilation while awake hypoventilate as respiratory drive falls at onset of sleep.

• This worsens further with the muscle atonia of rapid eye movement sleep.

• How this contributes to the daytime ventilatory failure is not clear.

• The sleeping hypoxemia probably accelerates blunting of ventilatory drive, which allows further daytime ventilatory deterioration.

• Thoracic wall stiffness and respiratory muscle fatigue are probably also important.

Periodic respiration

• This develops when the feedback loop controlling respiration has an excessive feedback gain or delay.

• Contributing factors include excessive central drive levels (CNS disease), circulatory delay (heart failure), hypoxemia, hypocapnia, and arousal from sleep (high altitude).

Epidemiology [4]

• Neuromuscular causes of central sleep apnea are unusual.

• Sleeping periodic respiration affects >50% of patients with severe chronic heart failure and >20% of inpatients with neurological disease.

Treatment

Diet and lifestyle

- Changing diet and lifestyle do not alter central sleep apnea.

- Patients should not smoke: concurrent lung disease worsens respiratory failure.

Pharmacological treatment

- Patients with hypoventilation syndromes should be cautioned against the use of sedative medications, which may induce acute respiratory failure.

For neuromuscular or chest-wall disease [2]

- The mainstay of treatment for these conditions is nocturnal ventilatory support.

- Respiratory stimulants may be tried (*e.g.*, theophylline, acetazolamide, medroxyprogesterone), but their long-term efficacy has been disappointing..

For periodic respiration [3,4]

- Many patients with periodic respiration are asymptomatic and need no treatment; treatment of symptomatic periodic respiration remains experimental.

- Underlying heart failure or chronic obstructive pulmonary disease should be controlled.

- Oxygen, low-dose carbon dioxide, positive airway pressure, or acetazolamide may have a role.

Nonpharmacological treatment [3,5–7]

Nocturnal ventilatory support

- This is indicated for patients with central sleep apnea, daytime ventilatory failure and an otherwise good quality of life.

- It improves daytime symptoms, respiratory failure, and cor pulmonale, thereby improving prognosis.

- The first approach should be nasal continuous positive airway pressure. This allows for adequate ventilation in most patients.

- Older techniques include the rocking bed and tank and cuirass ventilators.

Advantages: corrects sleep disruption, daytime sleepiness, and respiratory failure.

Disadvantages: need for specialist care to acclimatize patient to ventilator and for follow-up.

Causes of treatment failure: ventilator or mask failure due to mechanical failure or air leaks, poor compliance due to mouth air leak, nasal obstruction, claustrophobia, inadequate patient education, or poor mask fit, upper airway collapse secondary to extrathoracic negative-pressure (tank or cuirass) ventilation, incorrect diagnosis (respiratory failure due to obstructive lung disease).

Oxygen

- Overnight oxygen (24%–28%) may improve symptoms of patients in whom ventilatory support is not appropriate; it has not been shown to improve prognosis in this group and may worsen daytime ventilatory failure.

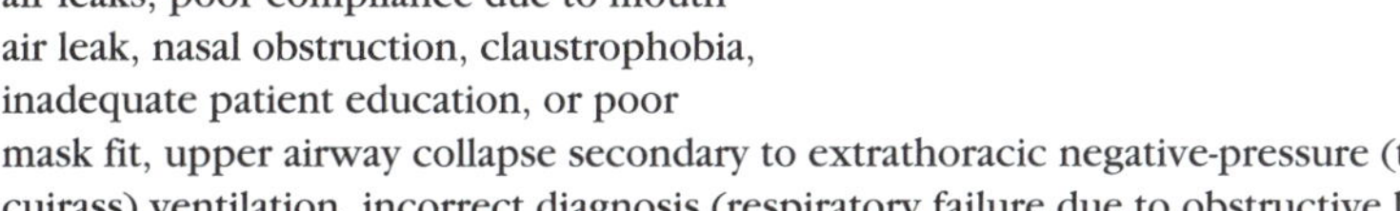

Improvements in awake arterial blood gases in seven patients with neuromuscular or chest wall disease and ventilatory failure after overnight support ventilation.

Key references

1. Bradley TD, Phillipson EA: Central sleep apnea. *Clin Chest Med* 1992, **13**:493–505.

2. Goldstein RS: Hypoventilation: neuromuscular and chest wall disorders. *Clin Chest Med* 1992, **13**:507–521.

3. De Backer WA: Central sleep apnoea, pathogenesis and treatment: an overview and perspective. *Eur Respir J* 1995, **8**:1372–1383.

4. Martin TJ, Sanders MH: Chronic alveolar hypoventilation: a review for the clinician. *Sleep* 1995, **18**:617–634.

5. Hill NS: Noninvasive ventilation. *Am Rev Respir Dis* 1993, **147**:1050–1055.

6. Meyer TJ, Hill NS: Noninvasive positive pressure ventilation to treat respiratory failure. *Ann Intern Med* 1994, **120**:760–770.

7. American Thoracic Society: Indications and standards for use of nasal continuous positive airway pressure (CPAP) in sleep apnea syndromes. *Am J Respir Crit Care Med* 1994, **150**:1738–1745.

Diagnosis

Definition

• Obstructive sleep apnea is a recurrent obstruction to breathing due to upper-airway narrowing or collapse during sleep.

• A mixed obstructive and central sleep apnea syndrome is often seen.

Symptoms [1]

• Symptoms are often manifest for several years before diagnosis.

Loud snoring, thrashing, restless sleep: usual adult presentation, often with history of witnessed apneas from partner.

Daytime somnolence, morning sluggishness, headaches, fatigue.

Nocturnal choking or panic attacks, irritability, nocturia, enuresis, impotence, cognitive dysfunction, memory loss, social disharmony, emotional disturbances: less common.

Behavioral disturbance, failure to thrive: nonspecific features in children, in addition to adult symptoms.

Signs

Obesity: particularly neck; characteristic but not invariable.

Small crowded pharynx with mucosal edema.

Retrognathia.

Tonsil hypertrophy: usual cause of obstructive sleep apnea in children.

Nasal obstruction.

Cyanosis.

Respiratory failure or cor pulmonale: in 10% of patients.

Features of hypothyroidism or acromegaly: rare.

Investigations

Initial

Awake arterial oxygen saturation or blood gas analysis, spirometry, hemoglobin analysis: for ventilatory failure (arterial oxygen and blood gases), obstructive pulmonary disease (spirometry), and polycythemia (hemoglobin).

Thyroid or growth hormone estimations: can be considered.

Sleep studies

• Sleep studies are needed to establish the diagnosis by showing upper-airway obstruction with continuing respiratory efforts; no ideal combination of physiological signals exists, but markers of respiratory effort, apnea, and sleep disturbances are needed.

Polysomnography: gold standard; includes EEG sleep staging, monitoring of ocular movements, oronasal airflow assessment, and measurement of thoracoabdominal movement or esophageal pressure; accurately identifies obstructive apneas but time-consuming and expensive and disturbs patient's sleep [2].

Complications

Respiratory failure, cor pulmonale: usually in patients with peripheral airways obstruction (often mild).

Accidents: particularly motor accidents, due to poor daytime vigilance.

Cardiovascular disease: increased vascular mortality (improves with effective treatment).

Treatment

Diet and lifestyle
• Weight loss can correct obstructive sleep apnea, but most patients also need other treatment.
• Reduced alcohol intake helps simple snoring and mild obstructive sleep apnea.
• Obstructive sleep apnea present only when patient is supine is improved by avoiding this posture.

Pharmacological treatment [3–5]
• Avoidance of alcohol and sedatives before bedtime is an important part of therapy.
• Drug treatment is secondary to continuous airways pressure.
• Hypothyroidism should be evaluated and treated.

Nasal steroids and decongestants
• These reduce simple snoring but have little effect on obstructive sleep apnea; they may be needed during continuous positive airway pressure therapy.

Standard dosage	Beclomethasone, 42–84 µg; or budesonide, 64 µg, twice daily in each nostril.
Contraindications	None.
Special points	Vasoconstrictor decongestants worsen nasal obstruction with sustained use and should be avoided.
Main drug interactions	None.
Main side effects	Nasal dryness.

Medroxyprogesterone
• Medroxyprogesterone has been useful in some patients with obstructive sleep apnea. Studies are conflicting, precluding overall endorsement.

Standard dosage	60–120 mg daily.
Special points	Obese females may be most appropriate candidates.
Main side effects	Impotence.

Tricyclic antidepressants
• Antidepressants have a minor role in mild obstructive sleep apnea by suppressing rapid eye movement sleep, when sleep apnea often worsens.

Standard dosage	Protriptyline, 10–20 mg orally at night.
Contraindications	Cardiac disease, epilepsy, mania, liver disease, glaucoma.
Main drug interactions	Alcohol, monoamine oxidase inhibitors, antihistamines, anticonvulsants.
Main side effects	Anticholinergic effects, arrhythmias, impotence, urinary retention.

Nonpharmacological treatment [4–6]
Nasal continuous positive airways pressure (CPAP) (usually 5–15 cm H_2O)
• This is the main treatment in most patients with substantial daytime sleepiness.
Advantages: dramatic correction of sleep disruption, daytime sleepiness, snoring, and apneas.
Disadvantages: unsightly, mask may be claustrophobic or cause nasal ulceration if badly fitted.
Causes of treatment failure: machine or mask failure; poor compliance due to nasal obstruction, claustrophobia, inadequate patient education, poor mask fit (air leaks or nasal ulceration), mouth air leak; incorrect diagnosis (central sleep apnea, narcolepsy, respiratory failure from another cause).

Surgery
• Surgery is indicated for patients with the following:
Structural nasal obstruction (*e.g.*, polyps, deviated septum).
Tonsil hypertrophy.
Facial maldevelopment.
Severe obstructive sleep apnea with continuous positive airways pressure failure.
• Tracheostomy is rarely indicated.
• Surgery (uvulopalatopharyngoplasty) should be attempted only in established centers.
• Soft-palette resection is not consistently curative.

Key references

1. Findley LJ, Weiss J, Jabour EP: Drivers with untreated sleep apnoea. *Arch Intern Med* 1991, **151**:1451–1452.

2. McNamara SG, Grunstein RR, Sullivan CE: Obstructive sleep apnoea. *Thorax* 1993, **48**:754–764.

3. Kryger MH: Management of obstructive sleep apnea. *Clin Chest Med* 1992, **13**:481–492.

4. American Thoracic Society: Indications and standards for use of nasal continuous positive airway pressure (CPAP) in sleep apnea syndromes. *Am J Respir Crit Care Med* 1994, **150**:1738–1745.

5. Strollo PJ Jr, Rogers RM: Obstructive sleep apnea. *N Engl J Med* 1996, **334**:99–104.

6. Hudgel DW: Treatment of obstructive sleep apnea. *Chest* 1996, **109**:1346–1358.

Diagnosis

Symptoms

Insomnia
Daytime fatigue, sleepiness.

Depression.

Obstructive sleep apnea [1]
Habitual snoring, witnessed apnea.

Breath holding.

Partial arousal.

Excessive daytime sleepiness.

Narcoleptic syndrome
Excessive daytime sleepiness.

Sudden weakness: with emotion or expectation of sudden event (cataplexy).

Short night sleep latency.

Excessive motor activity during sleep: leg kicking and sleep-walking.

Sleep paralysis (loss of muscle tone).

Hypnopompic or hyponagogic hallucinations.

Parasomnias
Somnambulism, confusional arousals, and night terrors: 60-90 minutes after sleep onset, during non–rapid eye movement (REM) sleep.

Acting out dream content (REM behavior disorder), cluster headache, nightmares: during REM sleep; accompanied by dreaming.

Other
Enuresis, sleep-talking, leg-kicking: common.

Bruxism, head-banging: less common.

Circadian sleep disorders
Sleep phase disturbance (lag or lead).

Signs
• No abnormal physical signs are manifest in most sleep disorders, although obstructive apneas are associated with retrognathia, micrognathia, macroglossia, or enlarged tonsils or soft palate.

Investigations
Polysomnography: necessary in most sleep–wake disorders, including the narcoleptic syndrome; allows detailed scientific sleep study and may occasionally clarify diagnosis of sleep disorder, particularly when combined with video monitoring [2].

Sleep oximetry: useful in evaluation of sleep apnea and review of treatment.

Multiple sleep latency test: in narcoleptic syndrome and other forms of daytime sleepiness; in narcolepsy, sleep latency is short and REM often begins within 15 minutes of sleep onset; ≥ 2 of 5 naps containing REM sleep is suggestive of narcolepsy.

Plasma and urinary screen: for hypnotic or CNS stimulant drugs, occasionally useful in suspected drug abuse or poor drug compliance.

Complications
• Sleep disorders may be as disabling as epilepsy.

Daytime sleepiness, depression, sleep "attacks."

Work and social problems: major cause of traffic accidents.

Differential diagnosis
Not applicable.

Etiology
• Insomnia is often multifactorial, with abnormal lifestyle, physical and psychological factors and sometimes hypnotic-stimulant drug or alcohol misuse.

• Familial insomnia is not uncommon.

• The narcoleptic syndrome has 99% association with HLA DR2 and DQw1; only 1 in 500 HLA DR2–positive patients, however, has the narcoleptic syndrome.

• Circadian sleep disorders are often due to shift work and/or psychological factors.

Epidemiology
• Chronic insomnia occurs in up to 20% of adults; it is more common in women than in men.

• Persistent excessive daytime sleepiness is usually caused by obstructive sleep apnea, the narcoleptic syndrome, or periodic leg movements with frequent arousals.

• Parasomnias including bed wetting and sleep walking are common, most frequently in childhood.

• Circadian sleep disorders caused by shift work occur in one-third of the workforce; shift work is tolerated better by younger people.

• The delayed sleep phase syndrome has an incidence of 1 in 10 000 people.

Treatment

Diet and lifestyle

• Good "sleep hygeine" with regular sleep and wake times, avoidance of books and TV while in bed, and finding another time for review of the day can improve insomnia. In some cases, initial sleep restriction is needed.

• In the narcoleptic syndrome, 2–3 planned short naps during the day may improve alertness.

• Sleep regularity with fixed stable bedtime and waketime is useful in the management of many parasomnias.

Pharmacological treatment

For insomnia

Standard dosage	Short-term (2–4 weeks) benzodiazepine or nonbenzodiazepine hypnotic, *e.g.*, temazepam, 2–3 times weekly, can be considered.
Contraindications	Pregnancy, psychiatric illness, sleep apnea.
Special points	Long-term nightly use to be avoided; can be combined with psychological support, although hypnotics not main-line treatment for most forms of chronic insomnia.
Main drug interactions	Enhanced sedative effect with many other drugs; metabolic interactions.
Main side effects	Waking sedation, tolerance.

For narcoleptic syndrome: daytime sleepiness [3]

Standard dosage	Methylphenidate, maximum 60 mg daily, pemoline, mazindol, dextroamphetamine; exact dose titration and timing essential.
Contraindications	Vascular disease, hypertension, pregnancy, prostatism, breast-feeding.
Special points	Stimulants ineffective for cataplexy. Regular monitoring of patients on long-term treatment needed.
Main drug interactions	Sympathomimetics, monoamine oxidase inhibitors.
Main side effects	Talkativeness, euphoria, gastrointestinal irritation, sweating, constipation.

For narcoleptic syndrome: cataplexy

Standard dosage	Clomipramine or imipramine, 10–50 mg once daily.
Contraindications	Recent myocardial infarction, heart block.
Special points	Cataplexy does not respond to stimulants, but these can be used in combination with clomipramine.
Main drug interactions	As for tricyclic antidepressants.
Main side effects	Appetite changes, sexual malfunction, or orthostasis.

Treatment aims

To restore normal waking alertness and mood.

To prevent sleep hypoxia, arousal, and cor pulmonale.

To alleviate symptoms of narcolepsy.

Other treatments

Continuous positive airways pressure: effective in patients with obstructive sleep apnea.

Consideration of surgery.

Prognosis

• The prognosis varies widely among the different sleep disorders.

• The narcoleptic syndrome does not remit.

• In many forms of insomnia, the prognosis is poor.

Follow-up and management

• Assessment of insomnia requires medical, psychiatric, and psychological review; a written treatment plan should be drawn up with the patient, aiming for sustained benefit in 3–6 months of treatment

• In patients with the narcoleptic syndrome, progress should be monitored using a sleep–wake diary; drug compliance can be ensured by monitoring plasma and urine concentrations.

Patient support

American Sleep Disorders Association, 1610 14th St NW, Suite 300, Rochester, MN 55901-2205; phone (507) 287-6006.

Driving regulations

• The general guideline is that driving ability with excessive daytime sleepiness depends on the success of and degree of compliance with treatment.

Key references

1. Hill NS: Noninvasive ventilation. *Am Rev Respir Dis* 1993, **147**:1050–1055.

2. Douglas NJ, Thomas S, Jan MA: Clinical value of polysomnography. *Lancet* 1992, **339**:347–350.

3. Thorpy MJ: *Handbook of Sleep Disorders*. New York: Marcel Dekker; 1990.

Diagnosis

Symptoms

• The neurological symptoms are progressive.

Localized back pain.

Radicular pain.

Numbness or paresthesia, weakness: below level of lesion; may be asymmetrical.

Loss of control of sphincters.

Signs

At level of lesion

Spinal tenderness or deformity: depending on the disease.

Weakness, wasting, reflex loss: root lesion.

Below level of lesion

• Signs may be asymmetrical, *e.g.*, Brown–Sequard's syndrome.

• With spinal cord lesions, sacral sensation may be relatively "spared," whereas perineal sensation is lost early in conus lesions.

Weakness.

Sensory loss.

Spasticity, clonus, hyperreflexia, extensor plantars: if above L1, *i.e.*, spinal cord.

Flaccidity, areflexia: if below L1, *i.e.*, cauda equina.

Investigations

• Laboratory investigations may indicate cause, suggest alternative diagnosis, or help in preparation for surgery.

Complete blood count and ESR measurement: may identify anemia or suggest infection.

Serum vitamin B_{12}, syphilis serology, serum acid phosphatase measurement, plasma protein electrophoresis: may be helpful in some patients.

Chest radiography: may show mass or infection.

Plain radiography of spine: may show loss of pedicle or vertebral collapse.

MRI, CT myelography: often needed urgently.

Plain CT: in some patients.

Spinal fluid: if a compressive lesion is not identified.

Complications

Irreversible neurological damage: due to infarction of cord or roots.

Urinary infection: due to neurogenic bladder.

Deep venous thrombosis and pressure sores: from immobility.

Differential diagnosis

Spastic paraparesis

Inflammatory myelopathies: acute transverse myelitis, multiple sclerosis, HIV infection, tropical spastic paraparesis, sarcoidosis (human T-cell leukemic virus I).

Vascular myelopathies: spinal stroke (anterior spinal artery distribution), vascular malformation.

Malformations: Arnold-Chiari (possible lower brain stem or cerebellar signs), syringomyelia (absent arm reflexes and suspended sensory loss).

Cerebral lesions: bilateral strokes, para-sagittal tumor.

Flaccid paraparesis

Flaccidity and absent reflexes (spinal shock) caused by acute spinal cord lesions; rare in compression.

Acute Guillain–Barré syndrome: symmetrical, distal sensory loss, areflexia.

Etiology

Extradural tumors: secondary carcinoma, lymphoma, myeloma [1].

Intradural–extramedullary tumors: meningioma, neurofibroma.

Intramedullary tumors: glioma, ependymoma, lipoma.

Disk protrusions: usually cervical or lumbar, usually spontaneous, often sudden onset.

Osteophytic ridges: may combine with narrow spinal canal, *i.e.*, cervical or lumbar canal stenosis.

Infection: pyogenic epidural abscess, tuberculosis.

Trauma: fractures or dislocations of vertebrae.

Hematomas: epidural and subdural (rare).

Epidemiology

Occurs in 5% of patients with systemic malignancy.

Treatment

Diet and lifestyle
• No special precautions are necessary.

Pharmacological treatment
Chemotherapy or radiotherapy: after decompression or biopsy of malignant lesion.

Steroids: before and after surgery to minimize spinal-cord edema (*e.g.*, dexamethasone, 24–100 mg daily in divided doses).

Nonpharmacological treatment
• If acute spinal cord compression is suspected, the patient must be referred to a neurosurgical unit immediately.

• Any delay may lessen the chance of recovery.

Decompression
• Lesions lying posterior to the spinal cord or within the dura mater should be removed from behind through a laminectomy.

• Lesions lying anterior to the dura mater, with the exception of lumbar disk protrusions, should be removed from the front.

Spinal stabilization
• Lesions that cause collapse of the vertebral bodies cause forward angulation; stabilization should be by insertion of a graft from the front or instrumental stabilization attached to laminae in extension, *e.g.*, Hartshill rectangle.

Radiotherapy
• Radiotherapy is useful alone or after surgery for metastatic lesions.

Treatment aims

To establish the diagnosis.

To reverse neurological deficit while preserving spinal stability, if lesion removable.

To prevent progression or recurrence, if lesion not removable.

Prognosis

• The prognosis depends on the underlying cause, the rate rather than degree of compression, and the delay in decompression.

• Patients with long-established myelopathy due to hard disk material or osteophytic bars have poor prognosis; those with soft disk protrusions do well.

• Myelopathies due to prostatic metastases have a relatively good prognosis.

• Metastases from breast or bronchus have a poor prognosis; direct invasion from bronchus has a very poor prognosis.

• Good recovery even from severe neurological deficit may follow successful surgical removal of benign tumors.

• Prognosis is good if decompression occurs before the onset of severe paraparesis.

Follow-up and management

• Patients need subsequent physical therapy, rehabilitation, surgical appliances (*e.g.*, walking aids, orthoses, wheelchair), occupational therapy, and home assessment.

• Patients should be referred to a spinal unit if the residual deficit is severe.

• Complications can be prevented by anti-embolism stockings, low-dose s.c. heparin, prevention of pressure sores, bladder care, and early treatment of intercurrent infection.

Key reference

1. Portenoy RK, *et al.*: Back pain in the cancer patient: an algorithm for evaluation and management. *Neurology* 1987, **37**:134–138.

Diagnosis

Definition

• Stroke is defined as rapidly developing (usually over minutes) clinical symptoms or signs of cerebral dysfunction lasting >24 hours, with no apparent cause other than that of vascular origin.

Symptoms

• Symptoms depend on the vascular territory involved.

Anterior (carotid) circulation

Combination of aphasia, unilateral, visuospatial, motor, or sensory loss: more common with cortical lesions.

Isolated contralateral sensory or motor loss: may indicate deeper hemispheric lesions.

• Extensive hemispheric involvement may eventually lead to altered consciousness due to cerebral edema.

Posterior circulation

Homonymous hemianopia or brain stem disturbance: *e.g.*, diplopia, vertigo, ataxia, gait imbalance, altered consciousness.

• Headache, loss of consciousness, and seizures are more common presenting features in subarachnoid or primary intracerebral hemorrhage than in cerebral infarction.

Signs

• Signs range from none or very subtle (*e.g.*, subjective sensory disturbance) to brain death.

Investigations

Serological

Prothrombin time/partial thromboplastin time, fibrinogen, platelet count, complete blood count, renal and hepatic function tests, sedimentation rates, cholesterol profile.

• In patients aged ≤50 years, add protein S & C, antithrombin III, anticardiolipin and antiphospholipid antibodies, homocystine levels, lactate/pyruvate, adrenoleukodystrophy and metachromatic leukodystrophy screen, where indicated.

Structural and etiological

CT or MRI of brain (MRI required for posterior circulation event).

MR angiography: for large- and medium-vessel disease.

Carotid ultrasonography.

ECG.

Transesophageal echocardiogram.

Angiography: for all patients with hemorrhage and needed for many without clear stroke etiology; often necessary to exclude vasculitis or dissection in young adults.

Temporary artery biopsy: if indicated.

Lumbar puncture: for hemorrhage or suspected vasculitis.

Complications

Infections (*e.g.*, aspiration pneumonia, urinary tract infection).

Venous thromboembolism.

Cardiac arrhythmias, cardiac failure, myocardial infarction.

Pressure sores.

Spasticity, contractures.

Mood disorders.

Seizures.

Falls, fractures.

Differential diagnosis

Intracranial tumor.

Subdural hematoma.

Etiology

Cerebral infarction

As for transient ischemic attacks (*see separate entry*).

Hypercoagulability.

Cerebral vasculitis.

Intracranial hemorrhage

Hypertension.

Aneurysm or arteriovenous malformation.

Epidemiology

• Stroke is the third most common cause of death in industrialized countries.

• It is the largest single cause of severe disability in people living at home.

Classification

• Stroke can be classified as follows:

Cerebral infarction: in 80% of patients.

Primary intracerebral hemorrhage: in 10%.

Subarachnoid hemorrhage: in 5%.

Uncertain: in 5%.

• Cerebral infarction may be further classified on clinical criteria, as follows:

Total anterior circulation infarction: hemiplegia, hemianopia, new cortical deficit.

Partial anterior circulation infarction: two of the above three, new cortical deficit alone, or motor or sensory deficit more restricted than lacunar infarction.

Lacunar infarction: pure motor or sensory stroke, sensorimotor stroke, or ataxic hemiparesis; thought to be caused by intrinsic disease of single perforating artery.

Posterior circulation infarction: evidence of brain stem lesion or homonymous hemianopia.

Treatment

Diet and lifestyle

• Attention to controlling hypertension, hyperlipidemia, and cessation of smoking are very important preventive measures.

Pharmacological treatment

• In acute stroke (≤180 minutes from initial symptoms), tissue plasminogen activator is recommended if patient meets inclusion criteria [1].

Standard dosage	0.9 mg/kg (up to 90 mg) given over 1 hour.
Inclusion criteria	No hemorrhage by CT, clearly defined onset.
Exclusion criteria	Improving or minor symptoms (2 weeks); blood pressure >185/110 (21 days); recent hemorrhage, surgery, head trauma (3 months); seizure; anticoagulant use.
Special points	Intensive care unit monitoring for BP and intracranial hemorrhage required.

Heparin: is currently indicated for posterior circulation ischemic stroke, cardiogenic emboli, and in many cases, for crescendo transient ischemic attacks and stroke in progression.

Aspirin: has been proved to be beneficial in reducing long-term risk after transient ischemic attacks in undifferentiated groups at risk.

Coumadin: is useful for most patients with embolic sources, atrial fibrillation, or nonoperable critical stenosis; broader use is under investigation.

Ticlopidine: 500 mg daily, is useful in some patients with small-vessel or posterior circulation disease but is associated with occasional neutropenia and requires close monitoring [2].

• The role of acute thrombolytic therapy is currently under investigation.

Nonpharmacological treatment

Surgery [3]

• Some patients with intracerebral hematomas may benefit from surgical drainage, although no universally acceptable selection criteria exist.

• Patients with subarachnoid hemorrhages should be managed in an intensive care unit and may require aneurysm repair.

• Carotid endarterectomy is indicated in symptomatic patients with stenosis >70% and in selected asymptomatic patients.

• Embolectomy is currently under investigation.

Rehabilitation

• Stroke units combining physical, occupational, and speech therapy save lives.

• Immobilized patients should wear antiembolism stockings.

• Support from the social services is an important but often neglected element in a patient's recovery.

• Physical, speech, and occupational therapy are vital to recovery.

Treatment aims

To prevent further cerebral damage or secondary complications.

To treat the cause of the stroke, where possible.

To enable survivors to achieve independence.

Prognosis

• For cerebral infarction, the overall 30-day case fatality is 10%.

• ~50% of survivors remain dependent.

• Important prognostic indicators include type and extent of stroke, age, and presenting level of consciousness.

• Intracranial hemorrhage carries a notably worse prognosis.

Follow-up and management

• The key aim is to identify and modify treatable risk factors (*e.g.*, hypertension, smoking).

• Lifelong antiplatelet treatment is indicated (aspirin, 75–150 mg daily) after cerebral infarction.

• Anticoagulation is effective as primary and secondary prophylaxis for cerebral infarction when atrial fibrillation is present.

• For patients who recover well from a limited carotid distribution stroke, endarterectomy may be indicated.

Key references

1. NINDS Stroke and PA Study Group: Tissue plasminogen activator for acute ischemic stroke. *N Engl J Med* 1995, **333**:1581–1587.

2. Hass WK, *et al.*: A randomized trial comparing ticlopidine with aspirin. *N Engl J Med* 1989, **321**:501–507.

3. ACAS Group: Endarterectomy for asymptomatic carotid artery stenosis. *JAMA* 1995, **273**:1421–1459.

General references

Baumlin KM, Richardson LD: Stroke syndromes. *Emerg Med Clin North Am* 1997, **15**:551–561.

Caplan LR: *Stroke: A Clinical Approach*, edn 2. Oxford: Butterworth Heinemann; 1993.

Diagnosis

Symptoms and signs

• Due to the low rate of suicide (11 per 100 000), predicting an individual suicide is very difficult; nonetheless, patients who attempt or commit suicide frequently consult their physician shortly before their attempt or death.

Risk factors [1]

Major depression (10-fold increased risk) or panic disorder (5-fold increased risk) within the previous year.

History of attempted suicide.

Current or recent alcohol or illicit substance abuse.

Lifetime history of any major psychiatric disorder.

Chronic debilitating medical illness.

Being separated or divorced.

Medical hospitalization within the past year.

Screening for suicidal behavior [1]

• Patients who have one or more risk factors for suicide should be asked: "Have you ever felt like hurting yourself or committing suicide?" or "Have you ever felt you wanted to die?"

• Answering "yes" to two or more questions on the Suicidal Ideation Screening Questionnaire may identify patients at high risk of suicide, but who may deny suicidal ideation on direct questioning [1].

Suicidal ideation screening questionnaire

1. Sleep disturbance: have your ever had a period of 2 weeks or more when you had trouble falling asleep, staying asleep, waking up too early, or sleeping too much?

2. Mood disturbance: have you ever had 2 weeks or more during which you felt sad, blue, depressed, or when you lost interest and pleasure in things that you usually cared about or enjoyed?

3. Guilt: has there ever been a period of 2 weeks or more when you felt worthless, sinful, or guilty?

4. Hopelessness: has there ever been a period of time when you felt that life was hopeless?

Investigations

• With patient's consent, further history should be obtained from available informants.

• Available databases should be checked for evidence of previous or present psychiatric care.

Complications

• Suicidal patients are at risk for social or occupational dysfunction, with resulting relational and/or financial stress on patient, spouse, and children.

• Unsuccessful suicide attempts can result in permanent injury (*e.g.*, vascular trauma) or functional impairment (*e.g.*, anoxic brain injury).

• Successful suicide creates tragic and long-lived consequences in the lives of family and relations.

Differential diagnosis

Threats or actual self-cutting or self-damage to relieve tension: often multiple superficial cuts on forearms.

Threats or actual self-mutilation in context of psychotic illness: especially schizophrenia.

Accidental ingestion of toxic substances: *e.g.*, tablets that look like sweets to children, weedkiller stored in a lemonade bottle.

Etiology

• Suicide has been conceptualized as a continuum, from ideation, to contemplation, to threats, to attempts, to completion [2]. Predicting the movement of an individual patient along the continuum, however, is difficult.

• One "overlap" model postulates that factors from five domains—psychiatric, personality, psychosocial and environmental, genetic, and biochemical—all contribute to suicide risk [3]. Adequate evaluation and treatment require assessment of all domains.

Epidemiology

• Suicide is the third leading cause of death in youths aged 15–24 years, and fifth leading cause of death in adults aged 25–64 years.

• ~30 000 Americans commit suicide each year.

• ~2%–3% of adults who receive care in general medical settings have had suicidal thoughts within the previous year.

Treatment

Diet and lifestyle

• High alcohol intake, social isolation, and lack of employment are all strong risk factors for suicide attempts, so efforts should be made among high-risk patients to change the lifestyle of the patients through therapeutic interventions.

• Family members of high-risk patients should be instructed to remove all potentially lethal objects (*e.g.*, guns, knives, medications) from the house.

Pharmacological treatment

• Adequate and early therapy of depressive illness (*see* Depression) and panic disorder (*see* Panic and generalized anxiety disorder) will reduce the likelihood of attempted or successful suicide.

• Antidepressants or other psychoactive medications should be prescribed in limited quantities (5–10 days) without refills to minimize risk of overdose and enhance follow-up.

• Except in emergencies, psychotropic drugs should be given only for treatment of specific mental illness, with psychiatric supervision when necessary.

• For the emergency management of violently mentally disturbed patients, a short-acting antipsychotic, *e.g.*, haloperidol in 5-mg increments i.m. every 15 minutes, should be used until symptoms are controlled, unless seizures are a risk. An antiparkinsonian drug, *e.g.*, procyclidine, 5–10 mg i.m., can be added to avoid dystonic reactions. Drugs should not be given i.v. when the cause of the mental disturbance is not known.

• When seizures are a risk, a benzodiazepine, *e.g.*, diazepam in 5-mg increments i.v. or lorazepam, 2–5 mg i.m., can be used. Benzodiazepines must be avoided in patients with severe respiratory impairment. Antipsychotic agents and benzodiazepines combined have an additive tranquilizing effect.

Nonpharmacological treatment [3]

Counseling

• Low-risk patients should be offered brief problem-oriented counseling, where available.

• Current or past high-risk patients should be asked about suicidal thoughts and plans at every visit.

• Patients with alcohol or substance abuse problems should be referred to the relevant specialist services.

• Relationship therapy should be offered to patients with relationship problems if both partners are agreeable.

• Open access or a telephone help-line may be offered, if available.

• Maintaining a strong therapeutic alliance is often an important "life line" for the patient.

Psychiatric referral

• Assessment and/or comanagement by a psychiatrist or experienced counselor is indicated when the primary physician needs assistance in suicide risk assessment, and for patients with recurrent or persistent suicidal ideation.

• Actively suicidal patients should be referred immediately for acute psychiatric intervention, usually on an inpatient basis. Compulsory inpatient admission must be considered in cases of psychiatric illness or serious suicide risk.

• Patients with major mental illness need urgent psychiatric treatment, usually on an inpatient basis.

• Emergency action in the patient's best interest is legally sanctioned in virtually every state; failure to act may be construed as negligence.

Treatment aims

To avoid attempted suicide by identifying and treating patients in earlier stages of the suicide continuum.

To treat any underlying mental disorder.

To help patient solve problems and to provide support through current crisis.

To strengthen the patient's future coping skills.

Prognosis

• Prognosis is largely determined by the underlying mental illness, substance abuse, or other risk factors.

• Repeat suicide attempts most often occur within the first 3 months of an episode.

• Among patients with a history of attempted suicide, long-term risk of completed suicide is ~1% at 1 year and 3% at 8 years.

• ~7% of patients with a history of attempted suicide make two or more attempts.

Follow-up and management

• Low-risk patients whose stressors and other risk factors have been addressed do not need special follow-up care.

• A telephone call should be placed to all currently or recently suicidal or high-risk patients who miss appointments.

• High-risk patients and those with mental illness need close monitoring.

Key references

1. Cooper-Patrick L, Crum RM, Ford DE: Identifying suicidal ideation in general medical patients. *JAMA* 1994, **272:**1757–1762.

2. Beck A, Kovacs M, Weissman M: Assessment of suicidal ideation: the scale for suicide ideation. *J Consult Clin Psychol* 1979, **46:**559–563.

3. Blumenthal SJ: A guide to risk factors, assessment, and treatment of suicidal patients. *Med Clin North Am* 1988, **72:**937–969.

Diagnosis

Definition
• Syncope is sudden, transient loss of consciousness and postural tone with subsequent spontaneous recovery.

Symptoms
• Symptoms are not always apparent; associations depend on the cause of syncope.

Presyncope.

Neurological (seizures, dizziness, vertigo, dysarthria, visual disturbance).

Postevent fatigue or confusion.

Chest pain.

Palpitations.

Dyspnea.

Emotional and/or physical stress.

Autonomic activation (*e.g.*, nausea, diaphoresis, pallor).

Generalized or focal weakness.

Signs
• Signs are not always apparent; findings vary depending on the cause of syncope.

Orthostatic hypotension.

Pulse deficit and asymmetric blood pressures in the arms: seen in aortic dissection.

Murmurs or physical findings consistent with cardiovascular abnormalities.

Focal neurological deficits.

Vascular bruits.

Investigations
• History and physical examination are critical in assessment.

• Sudden onset of symptoms without a prodrome may suggest arrhythmias, whereas protracted autonomic symptoms (pallor, diaphoresis, nausea) in association with a precipitating factor such as pain, extreme heat or emotion, or prolonged standing suggest vasovagal syncope. Exertional syncope suggests possible structural heart disease. Recovery from cardiac syncope is often brief (30 seconds); neurally mediated syncope (*e.g.*, vasovagal) is often accompanied by postevent fatigue or other symptoms of longer duration.

• Neurological syncope is suggested by brainstem findings (vertigo, dysarthria, ataxia, visual disturbances); postevent confusion is associated with seizures.

• Emphasis should be placed on the circumstances surrounding the syncopal event, associated symptoms, medication/drugs, family/psychiatric history, and presence of known cardiac disease. Observations from witnesses may be helpful.

• Routine nonselective neurological testing (CT, EEG, carotid Dopplers) and laboratory evaluations rarely provide useful diagnostic information. These tests and others (*e.g.*, nuclear scans, cardiac catheterization, cerebral angiography) should be selectively performed as directed by clinical data.

Carotid sinus massage: useful in elderly patients and those with features suggestive of carotid sinus syncope if not contraindicated.

12-lead ECG and rhythm strips: abnormalities can lead to the cause of syncope and/or direct additional testing; a normal ECG suggests a more favorable prognosis and makes arrhythmias less likely.

Ambulatory ECG monitoring (AEM): helpful when arrhythmia is detected and correlates with symptom reproduction; most helpful in patients with underlying heart disease.

Intermittent loop recorders: valuable in patients with frequent episodes not detected by AEM in which an arrhythmia is still suggested.

Head-up tilt testing: detects neurally mediated syncope, the most common cause of syncope in those without cardiac disease; the sensitivity, specificity, and reproducibility are variable.

Signal average ECG: possibly useful in patients with coronary artery disease and left ventricular dysfunction.

Electrophysiologic study: diagnostic value greatest in patients with abnormal ECG or AEM and structural heart disease.

Echocardiography: useful if cardiac disease is suspected or is manifest based on the history, physical examination, and ECG.

Exercise stress testing: consider if ischemic cause is suspected or with exertional syncope.

Psychiatric assessment: consider in syncope of unexplained cause with frequent recurrences and nonspecific complaints.

Complications
Sudden death.

Recurrent syncope.

Falls or accidents.

Differential diagnosis
Extensive, including common benign problems to life-threatening ones with potential for sudden death.

Need to exclude cardiogenic syncope in patients with structural heart disease, especially ischemic heart disease with left ventricular dysfunction.

Distinguish from patients with dizziness, seizures, drop attacks, or metabolic abnormalities such as hypoglycemia.

Etiology
• Syncope can be classified into four broad categories:

Neurally mediated syncope

Vasodepressor (vasovagal, neurocardiogenic), situational, carotid sinus syncope, psychiatric, and other causes.

Orthostatic hypotension

Drugs, autonomic insufficiency, volume depletion.

Cardiac syncope

Electrical (arrhythmic): tachyarrhythmias (ventricular tachycardia, supraventricular tachycardia, torsades de pointes, preexcitation) and bradyarrhythmias (sinus node dysfunction, atrioventricular block).

Mechanical/obstructive: valvular stenosis (aortic, mitral, pulmonic), prosthetic valve dysfunction/thrombosis, hypertrophic cardiomyopathy, aortic dissection, pulmonary embolism, pulmonary hypertension, myxoma, tamponade, subclavian steal, severe left ventricular dysfunction, myocardial infarction.

Neurological syncope

Transient ischemic attacks, seizures, vertebrobasilar syndromes.

• Syncope of unexplained etiology is a frequent finding.

Epidemiology
• Syncope is a common problem occurring in ≥3% of patients. It is a major reason for medical evaluation and hospitalization.

Treatment

Diet and lifestyle

• Avoidance of potential precipitating events is recommended, if possible, for example in neurally mediated syncope (*e.g.*, situational) or orthostatic hypotension (*e.g.*, volume depletion).

• In general, no special dietary precautions are required unless intake potentially aggravates the situation (*e.g*, caffeine and supraventricular arrhythmias).

• Increased salt intake is occasionally used in the treatment of orthostatic hypotension or neurocardiogenic syncope.

• Alcohol intake or lack of sleep may aggravate neurally mediated syncope.

Pharmacological treatment

• Treatment is individualized and directed toward the documented or presumed cause of syncope.

Neurocardiogenic syncope: difficult to make conclusive recommendations, but beta-blockers are effective and commonly used. Other options include a serotonin reuptake inhibitor, disopyramide, or transdermal scopolamine. Fludrocortisone has been used if expansion of central volume is a therapeutic goal.

Orthostatic hypotension: fludrocortisone combined with increased salt intake and nonpharmacological measures may be effective.

Cardiac syncope: antiarrhythmic therapy if clinically indicated for electrical cause.

Nonpharmacological treatment

• Implantable defibrillators should be considered in patients with cardiac syncope secondary to or at high risk for lethal ventricular dysrhythmias.

Dual-chamber cardiac pacing may be effective in the predominantly cardioinhibitory type of neurocardiogenic syncope. Cardiac pacing is effective for indicated bradyarrhythmias.

Compression garments/stockings have been used to help maintain central volume.

Treatment aims

To address the underlying cause of syncope and to prevent recurrent syncopal events.

• This is crucial for those with cardiac syncope because the major goal is to identify and treat the underlying heart disease.

• Treatment for neurally mediated syncope should be directed toward those with frequent, bothersome, or incapacitating symptoms.

• Consider that pharmacological drugs may be contributory to the cause of syncope and that withdrawal of a medication may alleviate the problem.

Prognosis

• Prognosis depends on the underlying cause of syncope.

• Cardiac syncope is associated with a high 1-year mortality (18%–33%) and an increased risk for sudden death. Noncardiac syncope and syncope of unexplained cause are associated with a better prognosis.

• The prognosis for neurally mediated syncope and for psychiatric patients with syncope is excellent. Recurrences, however, are common, especially in the psychiatric population.

Follow-up and management

• Management should be directed toward the identification and treatment of existing heart disease, if present. Otherwise, management should be individualized based on symptoms and the frequency of syncopal events.

• Patients with suspected or documented heart disease should be considered for referral to a cardiologist.

General references

Benditt DG, *et al.*: Syncope: causes, clinical evaluation, and current therapy. *Annu Rev Med* 1992, **43**:283–300.

Henderson MC, Prabhu SD: Syncope: current diagnosis and treatment. *Curr Probl Cardiol* 1997, **22**:237–296.

Kapoor WN: Workup and management of patients with syncope. *Med Clin North Am* 1995, **79**:1153–1170.

Kapoor WN, *et al.*: A prospective evaluation and follow-up of patients with syncope. *N Engl J Med* 1983, **309**:197–204.

Manolis AS, *et al.*: Syncope: current diagnostic evaluation and management. *Ann Intern Med* 1990, **112**:850–863.

Diagnosis

Symptoms

• Mild chronic hyponatremia (serum sodium concentration 125–135 mEq/L) may be asymptomatic.

• More profound hyponatremia (serum sodium concentration <120 mEq/L) can cause the following:*

Headache.	**Confusion.**	**Seizures.**
Malaise.	**Depression.**	**Coma.**
Nausea and vomiting.	**Cramps.**	**Death.**
Irritability.	**Drowsiness.**	

*The severity of the symptoms depends on the rate of fall of serum sodium as much as on the absolute value.

Signs [1]

• Mild chronic hyponatremia usually has no specific signs.

• Severe hyponatremia may cause the following:

Diminished reflexes.

Extensor plantar responses.

Cardinal features

Dilutional hyponatremia: plasma osmolality appropriately low for serum sodium.

Urine osmolality greater than plasma osmolality.

Persistent renal sodium excretion.

Absence of hypotension, hypovolemia, or edema-forming states.

Normal thyroid, renal, and adrenal function.

Investigations [1]

• Laboratory tests are not specific for the diagnosis but help to exclude other causes of hyponatremia and to identify underlying causes.

Chest radiography: to rule out a pulmonary process.

Serum sodium measurement: low concentration.

Plasma osmolality measurement: <270 mOsm/kg.

Blood glucose measurement: to exclude spurious hyponatremia in hyperglycemia.

Serum protein and lipoprotein measurement: to exclude pseudohyponatremia.

Serum uric acid measurement: low concentration.

Urine osmolality measurement: usually >300 mOsm/kg.

Renal function tests: creatinine clearance rate or serum creatinine concentration.

Thyroid function tests: free thyroxine, thyroid-stimulating hormone; to exclude hypothyroidism.

Adrenocortical tests: short cosyntropin test; to exclude cortisol deficiency.

Plasma vasopressin measurement: rarely checked.

Pituitary function tests: to exclude corticotropic hormone deficiency.

Complications

Permanent neurological deficit, high neurological morbidity and mortality: caused by prolonged profound hyponatremia or aggressive treatment leading to rapid rise in serum sodium concentration.

Differential diagnosis [2]

Hyponatremia associated with hypervolemia

Cardiac failure.

Cirrhosis.

Nephrotic syndrome.

Renal failure.

Hyponatremia associated with hypovolemia

Gastrointestinal fluid loss.

Severe burns.

Mineralocorticoid deficiency (*i.e.*, Addison's disease).

Salt-losing nephritis.

Etiology [2–4]

Neoplastic disease: *e.g.*, lung cancer, pancreatic cancer, lymphoma.

Chest disorders: *e.g.*, pneumonia, tuberculosis, abscess.

Neurological disorders: *e.g.*, head injury, infections, hemorrhage.

Drugs: *e.g.*, thiazides, cytotoxic agents, carbamazepine.

Epidemiology

• Hyponatremia is the most common electrolyte disturbance seen in hospitals (~10% of patients have serum sodium concentrations of <130 mEq/L).

• ~50% of all hyponatremia is due to the syndrome of inappropriate antidiuresis.

Treatment

Diet and lifestyle

- Fluid should be restricted to 0.5–1.0 L daily.
- Patients must eat a well-balanced diet.

Pharmacological treatment [1,5]

- The underlying cause of the syndrome should be treated (*e.g.*, cancer of the bronchus).
- Fluid restriction is the mainstay of therapy.
- Specific V_2-receptor antagonists to block the antidiuretic effect of vasopressin have been tested in humans.
- Treatment of severe hyponatremia is covered elsewhere (*see* Hyponatremia and Hyponatremia).

Induction of partial nephrogenic diabetes insipidus

Standard dosage Demeclocycline, 1.2 g in divided doses. Lithium carbonate 0.4–1.2 g daily.

Contraindications *Demeclocycline*: renal failure, pregnancy, children. *Lithium carbonate*: renal and cardiac disease.

Special points *Demeclocycline*: full effect may need up to 3 weeks of treatment. *Lithium carbonate*: narrow therapeutic level; plasma concentrations must be measured.

Main drug interactions *Demeclocycline*: warfarin. *Lithium carbonate*: diuretics, antibiotics, antihypertensives, sumatriptan.

Main side effects *Demeclocycline*: nausea, diarrhea, photosensitivity. *Lithium carbonate*: gastrointestinal disturbances, goiter, CNS dysfunction.

Inhibition of neurohypophysial vasopressin secretion

Standard dosage Phenytoin, 300 mg daily.

Contraindications Renal and hepatic dysfunction, porphyria.

Main drug interactions Antibacterials, anxiolytics, hypnotics, calcium antagonists.

Main side effects Drowsiness, ataxia.

Induction of diuresis and natriuresis

Standard dosage Furosemide, 40–80 mg daily, and sodium chloride, 3 g orally daily.

Contraindications Decompensated liver cirrhosis; caution in prostatism.

Main drug interactions Antifungals, potassium-losing drugs.

Main side effects Hypokalemia, gastrointestinal disturbances.

Treatment aims

To relieve symptoms of hyponatremia.
To increase serum sodium concentration to 125–140 mEq/L.

Prognosis

- Prognosis depends on the underlying cause.
- Patients with serum sodium concentrations <110 mEq/L have high morbidity and mortality (~50%).
- Development of osmotic demyelination syndrome indicates poor prognosis (~50% mortality).

Follow-up and management [1]

- Depending on the underlying condition, fluid restriction or drug treatment may be needed indefinitely.
- Serum sodium concentrations must be checked regularly.

Osmotic demyelination syndrome [6]

- This occurs after rapid correction of chronic severe hyponatremia, irrespective of the means of increasing serum sodium concentrations.
- It is found in central pontine and intracerebral structures.
- It is clinically evident 2–4 days after correction of serum sodium concentrations.
- It occurs rarely and predominantly when serum sodium is rapidly connected (>1 mEq/L/hr).

Key references

1. Robertson GL: Syndrome of inappropriate antidiuresis. *N Engl J Med* 1989, **321**:538–539.
2. Ayus JC, Arieff AI: Pathogenesis and prevention of hyponatremic encephalopathy. *Endocrinol Metab Clin North Am* 1993, **22**:425–446.
3. Baylis PH, Thompson CJ: Osmoregulation of vasopressin and thirst in health and disease. *Clin Endocrinol* 1988, **29**:549–576.
4. Berl T, *et al.*: Clinical disorders of water metabolism. *Kidney Int* 1976, **10**:117–132.
5. Arieff AI: Management of hyponatraemia. *BMJ* 1993, **307**:307–308.
6. Sterns RH, Riggs, J, Achochet SS: Osmotic demyelination syndrome following correction of hyponatremia. *N Engl J Med* 1986, **314**:1535–1542.

Diagnosis

Symptoms and signs

Tiredness: indicating anemia; one of the most difficult and resistant symptoms in systemic lupus erythematosus (SLE).

Polyarthralgias and nonerosive symmetric arthritis: involving predominantly small joints (rarely deforming) [1,2].

Rashes: photosensitive, discoid, and, less often, classic facial butterfly rash [1].

Vasculitic lesions of extremities: leading to gangrene of digits (rare).

Oral or pharyngeal ulcers.

Myalgia.

Pleuritic or pericardial pain: indicating serositis.

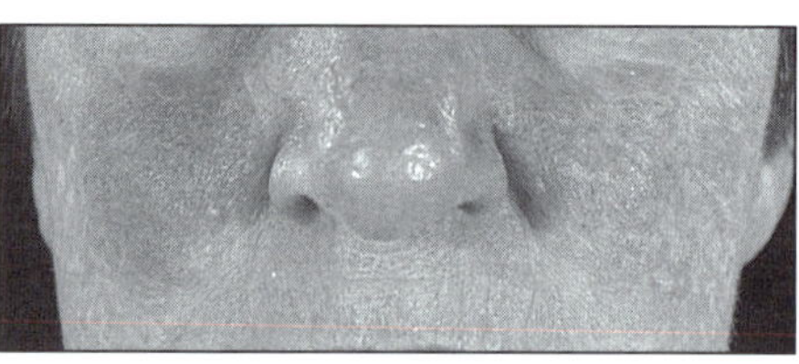

Classic butterfly rash. (*See* Color Plate.)

Epistaxis, bleeding gums, menorrhagia, purpura: symptoms of thrombocytopenia.

Visual and auditory hallucinations or epilepsy.

Edema or hypertension: *e.g.*, nephrotic syndrome or acute nephritic illness.

Alopecia [1].

Raynaud's phenomenon.

Lymphadenopathy.

Fever.

Livedo reticularis.

Investigations

Laboratory tests

• These are useful in the diagnosis of SLE, but no single diagnostic test is available [1].

Complete blood count: may reveal anemia, leukopenia, neutropenia, lymphopenia, or thrombocytopenia; raised ESR common in active disease; evidence of hemolytic anemia requires further investigation, *e.g.*, a Coombs' test [1].

Antinuclear antibody analysis: antibodies found in at least 95% of SLE patients but not disease-specific; antibodies to double-stranded DNA and Sm are relatively disease-specific but do not occur in all patients (~50% and ~5%, respectively); antibodies to Ro, La, and U1 ribonucleoprotein helpful in defining disease subsets and overlap syndromes; positive antiphospholipid antibodies and lupus anticoagulant define patients at risk from major arterial and venous thromboses [1].

For markers of disease activity or organ involvement

ESR measurement: raised ESR with normal CRP usual except when bacterial infection coexists [1,3].

Plasma-complement analysis: low C3, C4, and CH50 indicate activity.

Anti–double-stranded DNA antibody analysis: antibodies can rise with disease flares, especially those involving the kidney.

Dipstick testing of urine: for proteinuria and hematuria.

Microscopic examination: for red cell casts, leukocyte casts.

Measurements of renal function and 24-hour urine protein loss.

Complications

Severe renal involvement [3].

Cerebral involvement: infarcts or neuropsychiatric disease [3].

Infections secondary to immunosuppression.

Major thrombotic events: especially when high-titer antiphospholipid antibodies are present [4].

Differential diagnosis

Other connective tissue diseases: *e.g.*, rheumatoid arthritis, progressive systemic sclerosis.
Infection.
Malignancy.

Etiology

• Causes include the following:
Genetic factors and inherited defects of the early components of the classic complement pathway.
Environmental factors: *e.g.*, sunlight.
Drugs: *e.g.*, hydralazine, procainamide, phenytoin.

Epidemiology

• The prevalence of SLE in the United States is 45 in 100 000 women, 3.7 in 100 000 men [5].
• The highest incidence is in the 20–40 year age group.
• SLE is unusual in children.

Treatment

Diet and lifestyle

• Patients, especially those with photosensitivity, should avoid sunlight and should use high-factor sunscreen (ultraviolet A and B).

Pharmacological treatment

Indications

Discoid lupus erythematosus rashes: topical steroids.

Joint and skin involvement: hydroxychloroquine.

Systemic involvement: acute treatment by corticosteriods, introduction of cytotoxic agents, *e.g.*, azathioprine, chlorambucil, methotrexate.

Severe vasculitis (including cerebral and renal involvement): pulse cyclophosphamide and methylprednisolone [6,7].

Systemic treatment

Standard dosage	Hydroxychloroquine, 200 mg once or twice daily. Prednisone, 10–40 mg daily and azathioprine, 1–2.5 mg/kg daily to allow subsequent steroid reduction. Pulse methylprednisolone, 1 g i.v. daily for 3 days and pulse cyclophosphamide, 500–750 mg/m², adjusted downward for creatinine clearance <35 mL/min or myelosuppression. Cyclophosphamide is given i.v. monthly or 6 months, then i.v. every 3 months until clinical improvement or toxicity occurs. Cyclophosphamide dosing is complex and should be supervised by a specialist (*e.g.*, rheumatologist, nephrologist, pulmonologist).
Contraindications	Known hypersensitivity, systemic infections.
Special points	*Cyclophosphamide:* infusions must be preceded by a complete blood count to check for bone-marrow toxicity, in particular evidence of neutropenia.
Main drug interactions	*Cyclophosphamide:* concurrent allopurinol should be avoided because of enhanced toxicity.
Main side effects	*Hydroxychloroquine:* retinopathy, skin rashes. *Azathioprine:* bone-marrow suppression, gastrointestinal disturbances, liver toxicity. *Cyclophosphamide:* nausea and vomiting, hair loss, hemorrhagic cystitis, premature menopause [6]. *All cytotoxic agents:* teratogenicity (adequate contraception essential) [6,7].

Treatment aims

To alleviate disease flares.

Prognosis

• Renal and cerebral involvement and the complications of treatment, especially infection, are the major contributors to mortality.

• The survival rate has improved in the past 2 decades and is now ~95% at 5 years.

Follow-up and management

• Prompt treatment of lupus flares is mandatory.

• The use of oral cytotoxic drugs requires monthly blood counts to check for bone-marrow suppression and liver function tests with methotrexate.

Key references

1. Tan E, *et al.*: The 1982 revised criteria for the classification of systemic lupus erythematosus. *Arthritis Rheum* 1982, **25**:1271–1277.

2. Mills JA: Systemic lupus erythematosus. *N Engl J Med* 1994, **330**:1871–1879.

3. Boumpas DT, *et al.*: Systemic lupus erythematosus: emerging concepts. Part 1. Renal, neuropsychiatric, cardiovascular, pulmonary and hematologic disease. *Ann Intern Med* 1995, **122**:940–950.

4. Petri M: Systemic lupus erythematosus and pregnancy. *Rheum Dis Clin North Am* 1994, **20**:87–118.

5. Rothfield NF: Clinical features of SLE. In *Textbook of Rheumatology.* Edited by Kelley NN, *et al.* Philadelphia: WB Saunders; 1988.

6. Fox DA, McCune WJ: Immunosuppressive drug therapy of systemic lupus erythematosus. *Rheum Dis Clin North Am* 1994, **20**:265–291.

7. Pisetsky DS, Gilkeson G, St. Clair EW: Systemic lupus erythematosus: diagnosis and treatment. *Med Clin North Am* 1997, **81**:113–128.

Diagnosis

Symptoms

• Scleroderma is unlikely in the absence of Raynaud's phenomenon.

• It has two major subgroups of prognostic and therapeutic importance, as follows:

Limited cutaneous disease

• This occurs in 60% of patients.
• It was previously called CREST syndrome [1].
Swollen painful fingers: ulcers possible.
Thick skin on hands.
Calcium deposits.
Swallowing difficulty.

Diffuse cutaneous disease

• This occurs in 40% of patients.
Puffy hands, feet, arms, legs, tight skin.
Weight loss, fatigue.
Muscle and joint pain.
Breathlessness, dry cough, palpitations.
Indigestion, bloating, diarrhea [2,3].

Signs

Limited cutaneous disease

Early (<10 years)
• Distribution is limited to hands, feet, and face.
Sclerodactyly, swollen fingers, microstomia.
Pitting scars, pulp atrophy.
Digital ulcers.
Telangiectasia.
Calcinosis.

Late (>10 years)
Loud pulmonary second sound.
Right heart failure.
Abdominal bloating.
Wasting and other signs of malabsorption.

Diffuse cutaneous disease

Early (<5 years)
Diffusely puffy or sclerosed skin, including truncal changes.
Friction rubs.
Joint contractures.
Muscle weakness.
Digital pits and ulcers.
Basal crepitations, pericardial rub, arrhythmia.

Late (>5 years)
Dry, shiny skin.
Ulcers: atrophic, on fingers or elbows.
Muscle wasting.
Joint contractures.
Cardiac or respiratory failure.

Investigations

Complete blood count: to detect anemia of chronic disease.

Creatinine clearance measurement: to assess renal function.

Autoantibody tests: antinuclear antibodies are positive in 90% of patients; full screen useful to mark subsets of systemic sclerosis or overlap with other disorders.

Nailfold capillary tests (ophthalmoscope or microscopic): useful in "prescleroderma" and early disease; abnormal pattern of vessel drop-out and distortion.

Esophageal scintiscanning: to detect dysmotility (other "gut" tests as indicated).

ECG, echocardiography, Doppler ultrasonography: to detect cardiac involvement and to estimate pulmonary artery pressure.

Chest radiography, pulmonary function tests, high-resolution CT: to detect lung involvement; CT best test for presence and extent of early fibrosis.

Electromyography, biopsy: to diagnose inflammatory muscle disease in overlap disorders.

Joint radiography: to detect acro-osteolysis, calcinosis.

Skin biopsy: usually not needed in established disease, best used in early puffy stage for diagnosis or to differentiate systemic sclerosis from fasciitis.

Complications

Hypertensive renal crisis: in diffuse cutaneous disease, usually within first 5 years of disease; in 7%–10% of patients.

Pseudo-obstruction: late complication often of limited cutaneous disease; in <5%.

Carcinoma of lung: associated with pulmonary fibrosis.

Differential diagnosis

Eosinophilic fasciitis.

Mixed connective tissue disease.

Overlap syndromes.

Chronic graft-versus-host disease.

Eosinophilia-myalgia syndrome.

Vinyl chloride disease.

Toxic-oil syndrome.

Scleromyxedema.

Scleredema of Buschke.

Carcinoid syndrome.

Insulin-dependent diabetes mellitus skin changes.

Chronic reflex sympathetic dystrophy.

Idiopathic pulmonary fibrosis.

Primary pulmonary hypertension.

Cardiomyopathies.

Intestinal hypomotility syndromes.

Etiology

• In most cases, the cause is unknown, but the following may play a role:

Genetic: HLA classes II and III genes (weak association).

Environmental: organic chemicals (*e.g.*, vinyl chloride), epoxy resins, silica, rapeseed oil, drugs (*e.g.*, bleomycin).

Epidemiology

• Systemic sclerosis occurs worldwide.

• 12–20 in one million people are affected annually.

• The female:male ratio is 3:1 overall and 10:1 in people of child-bearing age.

• The disease is more severe in nonwhites.

• 30–60 years is the usual age of onset.

Treatment

Diet and lifestyle

• Patients should avoid cold and sudden drops in temperature.

• Patients should stop smoking.

• Skin care involves protection and moisturizers (cosmetic cover for telangiectasia).

• Patients should follow a daily exercise program to prevent, reduce, or delay contractures and to maintain strength and function.

Pharmacological treatment

For Raynaud's phenomenon and vascular insufficiency [4–7]

• Response can be variable, so more than one drug within a class is worth trying.

Standard dosage	Calcium antagonists: *e.g.*, nifedipine, 10–40 mg slow release twice daily. Angiotensin-converting enzyme (ACE) inhibitors: captopril, 6.25–18.75 mg daily; enalapril, 5–15 mg daily.
Contraindications	*Calcium antagonists:* pregnancy; caution in hepatic or renal disease. *ACE inhibitors:* pregnancy.
Special points	*ACE inhibitors:* may cause rapid fall in blood pressure.
Main drug interactions	*Calcium antagonists:* antiepileptics, antiarrhythmics. *ACE inhibitors:* must not be given with potassium-sparing diuretics.
Main side effects	*Calcium antagonists:* flushing, headache, edema. *ACE inhibitors:* dry cough, voice change, rashes.

For early diffuse disease

• No drug is of proven efficacy [5–7].

Standard dosage	D-Penicillamine, 750–1000 mg daily; methotrexate, 7.5–15 mg orally weekly; cyclosporine, 2.5–5 mg/kg orally daily; prednisolone, 20 mg on alternate days.
Contraindications	Pregnancy, existing liver and renal disease.
Main drug interactions	Cyclophosphamide with allopurinol, cyclosporine with ACE inhibitors.
Main side effects	Bone-marrow toxicity, renal and liver impairment, alopecia, rashes.

For esophageal involvement [5–7]

Standard dosage	Proton-pump inhibitor: omeprazole, 20 mg daily. Prokinetic drug: cisapride, 10 mg 3–4 times daily for 12 weeks, taken 30 minutes before meal or at bedtime.
Contraindications	Pregnancy, breast-feeding.
Special points	*Omeprazole:* can increase bowel colonization.
Main drug interactions	Oral anticoagulants, phenytoin, theophylline.
Main side effects	*Omeprazole:* constipation, headache, diarrhea. *Cisapride:* abdominal cramps, diarrhea.

For mid-gut involvement: bacterial overgrowth

• Rotation antibiotics can be used in various combinations, *e.g.*, metronidazole, 400–600 mg twice daily, tetracycline, 250 mg 3 times daily; erythromycin, 250 mg 4 times daily, or ciprofloxacin, 500 mg twice daily.

• These should be given for short periods, *e.g.*, 3–4 weeks, with "holidays" of 1–2 weeks.

Nonpharmacological treatment

Lumbar or digital sympathectomy for severe Raynaud's phenomenon with critical ischemia. Selective removal of calcinosis.

Key references

1. Medsger TA Jr: Systemic sclerosis (scleroderma), localized forms of scleroderma and calcinosis. *Arthritis and Allied Conditions* 1993, **2**:1253–1292.

2. Mitchell M, Bolster MB, LeRoy EC: Scleroderma and related conditions. *Med Clin North Am* 1997, **81**:129–149.

3. Penez M, Kohn SR: Systemic sclerosis. *J Am Acad Dermatol* 1993, **28**:525–547.

4. Kahaleh MB: Raynaud's phenomenon and vascular disease and scleroderma. *Curr Opin Rheumatol* 1994, **6**:621–627.

5. Medsger TA Jr: Treatment of systemic sclerosis. *Ann Rheum Dis* 1991, **50(suppl)**:877–886.

6. Van-den Hoogen FH, *et al.*: Treatment of systemic sclerosis. *Curr Opin Rheumatol* 1994, **6**:637–641.

7. Pope JE: Treatment of systemic sclerosis. *Rheum Dis Clin North Am* 1996, **22**:893–907.

Diagnosis

Definition

- Supraventricular tachycardias include the following:

Sinus tachycardia.

Atrial fibrillation.

Atrial flutter.

Atrial tachycardia.

Atrioventricular re-entrant tachycardia.

Atrioventricular nodal re-entrant tachycardia.

- Atrioventricular re-entrant and nodal re-entrant tachycardias, the two common supraventricular tachycardias arising from the atrioventricular junction, are discussed here.

Symptoms

Palpitation: paroxysms of regular palpitation at 140–240 beats/min, with sudden onset and offset [1].

Syncope: palpitation may be associated with syncope or presyncope at onset of attack, when blood pressure is probably at its lowest.

Chest pain: unusual but may occur during attacks, particularly in presence of ischemic heart disease.

Paroxysmal attacks: occasionally precipitated by postural changes or may be associated with particular times in menstrual cycle.

Signs

Fast, regular pulse.

Signs of left ventricular failure: unusual unless structural heart disease is coexistent.

- Atrioventricular dissociation is not evident (no cannon waves in neck).

- Blood pressure is usually well maintained after the first few seconds of an attack.

Investigations

ECG: regular rhythm present, usually with narrow QRS complexes; occasionally, preexisting or rate-related bundle branch block leads to broad QRS complexes [2].

Chest radiography: usually normal unless structural heart disease coexistent.

Electrophysiology: indicated if catheter ablation contemplated or for risk assessment in symptomatic patients with Wolff–Parkinson–White syndrome.

Complications

Left ventricular failure: caused by coexistent structural heart disease; supraventricular tachycardia may cause ventricular failure in the absence of pre-existing structural heart disease only if tachycardia is incessant and has continued uninterrupted for months or years.

Differential diagnosis

Atrial tachycardia or atrial flutter. Ventricular tachycardia: if atrioventricular re-entrant tachycardia is conducted with bundle branch block.

- When the history is being taken, establishing the presence or absence of structural heart disease, *e.g.*, cardiomyopathy or previous myocardial infarction, is important. A history or known diagnosis of either of these conditions makes a diagnosis of ventricular tachycardia much more probable than atrioventricular re-entrant or nodal re-entrant tachycardia. If the QRS complex is broad and has a pattern unlike that of classic left or right bundle branch block, then diagnosis is probably ventricular tachycardia.

Etiology

Atrioventricular re-entrant tachycardia

- The structural substrate is a congenital abnormality of the conducting system of the heart, whereby an extra electrical connection exists between the atria and the ventricles.

- Tachycardia arises when an electrical impulse passes from the atrium to the ventricle through the normal atrioventricular node but returns to the atria by the accessory pathway.

Atrioventricular nodal re-entrant tachycardia

- Patients have two functionally separate pathways within or close to the atrioventricular node.

- Tachycardia arises in a similar way to that arising in patients with atrioventricular re-entrant tachycardia.

Epidemiology

- These arrhythmias occur frequently and form most of the tachycardias in patients with structurally normal hearts.

- Men are more likely to have atrioventricular re-entrant tachycardia, and women atrioventricular nodal re-entrant tachycardia.

- Paroxysms of palpitation may start in infancy but more usually in teenage years or twenties.

Treatment

Diet and lifestyle

• If the tachycardias are initiated by atrial premature beats, abstinence from caffeine may help.

• Otherwise, no special precautions are necessary.

Pharmacological treatment

Acute treatment

Standard dosage Adenosine, i.v. bolus dose followed by saline flush, starting at 3 mg, with a second dose of 6 mg if tachycardia does not terminate after 60 seconds; a further dose of 12 mg is given if tachycardia does not terminate after another 60 seconds [3]. Verapamil, 5 mg i.v. slowly (30 seconds); if tachycardia has not terminated after 5 minutes, a second 5-mg dose may be given, if hypotension has not occurred.

Contraindications *Adenosine:* asthma.
Verapamil: poor ventricular function.

Special points *Adenosine:* although 12 mg is maximum adult dose recommended in product license, bolus doses of 18 mg may occasionally be need to terminate tachycardia; may exacerbate bronchoconstriction.
Verapamil: negatively inotropic and should not be given to patients with known abnormal ventricular function or with signs of cardiomegaly on chest radiography; best not given to patients with a broad complex tachycardia because it may cause cardiovascular collapse if erroneously given to patients with ventricular tachycardia; i.v. verapamil should not be given to patient taking oral beta-blockers because sinus arrest or dramatic hypotension may occur.

Main drug interactions *Adenosine:* increased effect with dipyridamole; decreased effect with theophylline.

Main side effects *Adenosine:* flushing and chest tightness (transient).

Prophylaxis

• Beta-blockade (*e.g.*, atenolol, 50–100 mg) is often effective in this role, particularly if the attacks are exercise-induced.

• Digoxin, 0.125 mg, and verapamil, 180–360 mg, may be effective but are contraindicated in the presence of a delta wave because they may increase the ventricular rate if atrial fibrillation complicates the Wolff-Parkinson-White syndrome.

Treatment aims

To terminate an acute paroxysm of tachycardia.
To suppress tachycardia.
To cure tachycardia.

Other treatments

Vagal maneuvers

• Deep breathing or the Valsalva maneuver (best done with patient lying down), with straining for at least 15 seconds, should terminate tachycardia a few seconds after strain release.

Radiofrequency catheter ablation [4]

• This is the treatment of choice for patients with recurrent symptomatic junctional tachycardias that do not respond to prophylactic drug treatment or as an alternative to chronic pharmacologic therapy. Ablation is also extremely effective in atrioventricular tachycardia owing to an accessory pathway. More recent advances include ablation of atrial flutter and modification techniques in atrial fibrillation.

Prognosis

• Prognosis is generally excellent, and life expectancy does not differ from that of the normal population.

• Symptomatic patients with the Wolff–Parkinson–White pattern on the ECG during sinus rhythm have a small risk of sudden death, associated with the development of atrial fibrillation. Symptomatic patients should undergo ablation.

Follow-up and management

• Oral aspirin is advisable for 6 weeks after catheter ablation because the damaged endothelium may provide a focus for thrombus formation.

• Patients should be assessed for recurrence of symptoms or re-emergence of the Wolff–Parkinson–White pattern on the ECG.

Key references

1. Bennett DH: *Cardiac Arrhythmias.* Oxford: Butterworth Heinemann; 1993.

2. Nathan AW: Cardiac arrhythmias. In *Essentials of Cardiology.* Edited by Timmis AD, Nathan AW. Oxford: Blackwell; 1993.

3. Camm AJ, Garratt CJ: Drug therapy: adenosine and supraventricular tachycardia. *N Engl J Med* 1991, **325**:1621–1629.

4. Jackman WM, *et al.*: Treatment of supraventricular tachycardia due to atrioventricular nodal reentry by radiofrequency catheter ablation of slow pathway conduction. *N Engl J Med* 1992, **327**:313–318.

Diagnosis

Symptoms

• Symptoms are not always manifest.

Palpitations.

Sudden shortness of breath.

Dizzy spells.

Blackouts.

Cardiac arrest.

Sudden death.

Signs

• Signs are not always manifest.

Tachycardia: 100–300 beats/min.

Hypotension and associated signs.

Cannon waves in jugular venous pressure, variable blood pressure, variation in intensity of first heart sound: signs of atrioventricular dissociation.

Investigations

12-lead ECG: initially, to confirm diagnosis, after treatment, for comparison of sinus rhythm; reveals tachycardia with QRS complexes 140 ms duration, evidence of atrioventricular dissociation (independent P waves, fusion beats, capture beats, second-degree ventriculo-atrial block), marked left or right axis deviation during tachycardia, absence of RS complexes in chest leads during tachycardia [1].

Adenosine test: initially, to distinguish from junctional or atrial tachycardia; if patient presents with stable tachycardia and if 12-lead ECG cannot be interpreted as showing ventricular tachycardia, incremental boluses of adenosine 0.05–0.20 mg/kg i.v. should be given, which terminates almost all junctional tachycardias, slows most atrial tachycardias, but affects almost no ventricular tachycardias except those arising in the right ventricular outflow tract.

Cardiac enzyme analysis: after treatment, if history suggests infarction.

Cardiac ultrasound: to determine whether there is underlying cardiomyopathic or valvular abnormality.

Exercise test: under supervision of arrhythmia specialist to look for coronary disease, to provoke arrhythmia, and to assess drug efficacy.

24-hour ambulatory ECG recording: to quantify frequency of ventricular arrhythmia and associated arrhythmias (*e.g.*, ventricular premature beat).

Echocardiography: to assess left and right ventricular function.

Left ventricular and coronary angiography.

Programmed electrophysiologic testing: to determine inducibility, morphology, and suppressibility of arrhythmia.

Complications

Cardiac arrest.

Sudden death.

Cardiogenic shock.

Pulmonary edema.

Differential diagnosis

Supraventricular tachycardia: either atrial or junctional, with either right or left bundle branch block.

• All wide-complex tachycardias should be considered ventricular in origin until proved otherwise.

Etiology

Acute ischemia: coronary obstruction by thrombus.

Large scar old infarction: previous surgery, dysplasias.

Microscopic scar infiltration: fibrosis.

No clinical disease: *e.g.*, right ventricular outflow tachycardia.

Right ventricular dysplasia.

Hypertrophic cardiomyopathy.

Viral myocarditis.

Functional disease: "fascicular" tachycardia.

Tumors, malformations, other causes (rare).

Epidemiology

• 2%–10% of patients suffering a myocardial infarction have a sustained ventricular tachycardia or cardiac arrest within 12 months.

Treatment

Diet and lifestyle

• Patients should avoid strenuous exercise and eat a normal diet unless they have evidence of coronary disease.

Pharmacological treatment

• The underlying disease process (*e.g.*, coronary artery disease) or associated cardiogenic fluid retention must be treated.

Emergency

Cardiopulmonary resuscitation if necessary.

Lidocaine, 50 mg i.v., in stable patients.

Direct-current cardioversion in unstable patients (synchronized) or if drug treatment fails.

• A succession of drugs is unwise, especially in patients with coronary disease and impaired ventricular function.

• Verapamil must not be given: it may cause profound collapse and even death.

Long-term

• Drug treatment should be supervised by a cardiologist with a special interest in arrhythmias.

• All antiarrhythmic drugs have proarrhythmic properties, especially when used in combination with other antiarrhythmic drugs [2].

• Whether long-term drug treatment improves prognosis is not known.

Standard dosage	Disopyramide, 250 mg slow release twice daily; alternatively, procainamide or quinidine. Flecainide, 100 mg twice daily; alternatively encainide or propafenone. Sotalol, 80 mg twice daily. Amiodarone, 200–400 mg daily.
Contraindications	*Disopyramide:* very poor left ventricular function. *Flecainide:* previous myocardial infarction; caution in patients with coronary disease [2]. *Sotalol:* as for beta-blockers generally.
Special points	*Flecainide:* increases pacing threshold [2]. *Sotalol:* prolongs action potential duration (unlike other beta-blockers). *Amiodarone:* in high doses may cause pulmonary fibrosis; long elimination half-life.
Main drug interactions	*Disopyramide:* antihistamines, antiepileptics. *Flecainide:* antidepressant, fluoxetine, antimalarial agents. *Sotalol:* as for beta-blockers generally. *Amiodarone:* digitalis, warfarin.
Main side effects	*Disopyramide:* vagolytic effects (dry mouth, slow stream). *Flecainide:* dizziness, arrhythmias. *Sotalol:* as for beta-blockers generally. *Amiodarone:* bradycardia, hypo- or hyperthyroidism, pulmonary fibrosis, blue skin deposits.

Treatment aims

To suppress recurrence of tachycardia (drug treatment).

To terminate recurrence of tachycardia (device treatment).

To destroy the arrhythmia "substrate," possibly offering a cure (ablation).

To correct mechanical heart disease and refractory arrhythmias (transplantation).

Other treatments

• Alternative long-term treatments include:

Implantation of automatic defibrillator device to terminate tachycardia: this also treats ventricular tachycardia by rapid pacing.

Ablation of localized focus or circuit causing tachycardia: radiofrequency energy and low-energy direct current are most popular sources.

Electrophysiologically guided surgery.

Transplantation in selected patients with severe ventricular impairment.

Prognosis

• Prognosis depends on the underlying disease process and presentation.

• 1-year mortality in patients resuscitated from cardiac arrest occurring out of hospital is up to 50%; defibrillator implantation probably reduces this significantly.

• Long-term prognosis is excellent for ventricular tachycardia associated with a normal heart.

Follow-up and management

• Patients should be referred to a center specializing in ventricular tachycardia to allow the correct treatment to be selected.

• Long-term drug treatment can be assessed by ambulatory monitoring (in patients with frequent ventricular premature contractions) or electrophysiological studies (in patients with inducible tachycardia).

• Ventricular tachycardia is not a curable disease and needs long-term follow-up.

Key references

1. Shenasa M, *et al.*: Ventricular tachycardia. *Lancet* 1993, **341**:1512–1518.

2. Echt DS, *et al.*: Mortality and morbidity of patients receiving encainide, flecainide, or placebo. *N Engl J Med* 1991, **324**:781–788.

Diagnosis

Symptoms

• β-Thalassemia is manifest during the first year of life in 90% of patients; a few present at 3–4 years (late-onset β-thalassemia major).

• 10% of patients with β-thalassemia major have a mild course (not dependent on transfusion).

• Patients may be asymptomatic; detection is from antenatal screening and diagnosis.

Poor weight gain.

Failure to thrive.

Fever.

Diarrhea.

Increasing pallor.

Distended abdomen.

Signs

Pallor.

Heart failure.

Splenomegaly.

Jaundice.

Investigations

Blood tests: low hemoglobin, mean corpuscular hemoglobin, mean cell volume; absent or reduced hemoglobin A (β° or β⁺ thalassemia), variable hemoglobin F and A_2 (using electrophoresis).

Genetic analysis: defines specific mutations, may help to predict disease severity and prognosis and facilitate first-trimester diagnosis.

Complications

Splenomegaly leading to hypersplenism (neutropenia, thrombocytopenia, anemia).

Anemia causing severe bone changes, short stature, and heart failure.

Differential diagnosis

Iron deficiency.

Etiology

• Thalassemia is caused by defective synthesis of the α- or β-globin chain (α- and β-thalassemia, respectively).

• The disorder is inherited (Mendelian recessive).

• It occurs in Mediterranean, Asian, Arabic, and Chinese groups because of a selective advantage against *Plasmodium falciparum*.

Epidemiology [1]

• Thalassemia is one of the most common inherited disorders throughout the world.

• Among blacks, approximately 30% of the population is either heterozygous or homozygous for the α-thalassemia-2 deletion.

• In southwest Europe, it is declining because of prevention programs; in consanguineous marriages, the birth rate of β-thalassemia increases by 30%.

Treatment

Diet and lifestyle

• Patients must avoid red meat and liver, and they should be encouraged to lead a normal active lifestyle.

Pharmacological treatment

Treatment of transfusional iron overload

• Desferrioxamine is infused s.c. over 8–12 hours from a portable syringe driver pump 5–6 nights/week.

• Chelation therapy is started when ferritin is 1000 µg/L (after 12–24 transfusions).

• Initial dose of 20 mg/kg desferrioxamine is diluted in 5–10 mL water for injection. Vitamin C, 100–200 mg orally (increases urinary iron excretion), is added when the patient is on desferrioxamine.

• In iron-overloaded patients, the desferrioxamine dose is 50 mg/kg daily.

• For cardiomyopathy, continuous desferrioxamine is given through an i.v. delivery device (Hickman Line, Port-a-Cath).

Complications of treatment

Alloimmunization to blood group antigens (in 25% of patients), febrile and urticarial transfusion reactions (in 75% of patients), cytomegalovirus infection and immunosuppression, transfusion-transmitted hepatitis B and C viruses: due to chronic transfusion (risk of HIV, 1 in 65 000).

Cardiomyopathy (most common cause of death), reduced growth, hypoparathyroidism, diabetes, failure of puberty: due to inadequate chelation.

Short stature, bone changes (pseudorickets), visual disturbances, hypersensitivity, hearing problems, pulmonary edema: due to desferrioxamine toxicity (overchelation).

Treatment aims

To provide good quality of life.

To provide a long life.

Other treatments

Bone-marrow transplantation: 94% success rate if patient compliant with desferrioxamine and has no liver fibrosis or enlargement; success rate affected by age and liver status.

Splenectomy for hypersplenism.

Prognosis

• Maintenance transfusion and regular iron chelation preserve excellent health, and the prognosis is now open-ended.

• Early death is generally the result of intractable heart failure secondary to iron overload and infections.

Follow-up and management [2–4]

• The patient's ferritin, liver function, and bone metabolism must be monitored 3 times yearly, with annual anti-hepatitis C virus, anti-HIV, and hepatitis B surface antigen checks.

• Oral glucose tolerance tests must be done yearly from the age of 10 years in patients with a family history of diabetes or from the age of 16 years in those without.

• Other endocrine and cardiac investigations should be made if clinically indicated.

• Patients should have yearly audiometry and twice-yearly eye tests.

• Splenectomized patients have higher risk of infection and may need vaccinations.

Key references

1. Davies SC, Modell B, Wonke B: *Access to Healthcare for People From Black and Ethnic Minorities.* London: Royal College of Physicians; 1993:147–168.

2. Piomelli S: The management of patients with Cooley's anemia: transfusions and splenectomy. *Semin Hematol* 1995, **32**:262–268.

3. Davies SC, Wonke B: The management of haemoglobinopathies. *Baillières Clin Haematol* 1991, **4**:361–389.

4. Kattamis CA, Kattamis AC: Management of thalassemias: growth and development, hormone substitution, vitamin supplementation and vaccination. *Semin Hematol* 1995, **32**:269–279.

Diagnosis

Symptoms

• Patients may be asymptomatic (thyroid swelling is noted by someone else).

Neck swelling: rapid increase in size raises level of concern.

Dysphagia, dyspnea, dysphonia: symptoms of local compression.

Pain in neck, radiating to jaw or ear.

Bone pain, hemoptysis, abdominal discomfort: may indicate metastases.

Symptoms of thyrotoxicosis: exceedingly rare.

Signs

Single nodule: most common presentation; often firm or hard.

Fixation of thyroid swelling to local structures.

Cervical lymphadenopathy.

Evidence of metastases (unusual): spinal cord compression, spastic paraparesis, hepatomegaly, bone swellings, tenderness.

Investigations

• No blood test of radiological study can distinguish benign from malignant thyroid lesions.

Fine-needle aspiration cytology: test of choice to diagnose malignancy in thyroid nodules.

Thyroid function tests: serum-free thyroxine and thyroid-stimulating hormone; used to diagnose hypothyroidism or hyperthyroidism.

Isotope scanning: hot nodules (suppressing surrounding thyroid tissue) are rarely malignant; nodules that are not hot should be evaluated by fine-needle aspiration.

Ultrasonography: best for accurately measuring size of nodules in patients who are being followed; can differentiate cystic vs. solid, but either may be malignant.

Serum calcitonin measurement: should be reserved for patients with known medullary thyroid cancer (MTC) and for screening members of families with inherited forms of MTC.

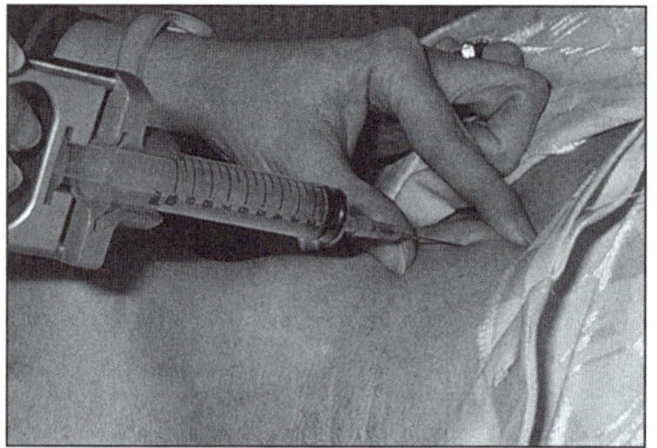

Fine-needle aspiration of a thyroid nodule, allowing rapid cytological examination of aspirated material. (*See* Color Plate.)

Thyroglobulin evaluation: minimal value in diagnosis of thyroid nodules; extremely useful for monitoring treated patients.

Antithyroid antibody tests: of little value in evaluating thyroid nodules.

Special considerations

• Hyperthyroid patients probably should have isotope scanning. If the nodule is hot (autonomously functioning thyroid nodule), malignancy is unlikely.

• A rapidly enlarging thyroid (diffuse or nodular) should raise the possibility of lymphoma.

Complications

Local infiltration of trachea, esophagus, nerves.

Metastases of bone, liver, lung.

Treatment

Diet and lifestyle

• No evidence indicates that environmental factors affect the prognosis of established thyroid cancer.

• An iodine-replete diet and avoidance of external irradiation to head and neck reduce the risk of developing thyroid cancer.

Pharmacological treatment [1–4]

• After surgery, patients can be considered for radioiodine treatment.

• No consensus has been reached on ^{131}I ablation of the thyroid in patients with small solitary papillary lesions.

• Routine ablation of thyroid remnant is indicated in patients with follicular thyroid cancer.

• Radioiodine has a clear role in the management of residual disease or established metastases.

• All patients with differentiated thyroid cancer need suppressive thyroxine treatment after definitive treatment; thyroxine is necessary in all patients rendered hypothyroid after treatment.

Nonpharmacological treatment

• The extent of surgery (simple lobectomy, near-total thyroidectomy, total thyroidectomy) depends on pathology and surgical preference.

• Surgery is the primary mode of treatment for papillary, follicular, and medullary thyroid cancers.

• Surgical removal of involved lymph nodes is indicated.

Treatment aims

To cure with minimal morbidity.

To minimize morbidity of diagnostic and therapeutic interventions.

Prognosis [1,2]

• Prolonged survival is usual.

• Patients with localized papillary or follicular thyroid cancers have an excellent prognosis, (10–20-year recurrence rates of 5%–10% and death rates of 2%–5%).

• Adverse prognostic factors include older age, greater degree of invasiveness, distant metastases, and abnormal chromosomal number within tumor tissue.

Follow-up and management [1–3]

• After radioablation of the thyroid, total-body radioiodine scans can detect recurrent or metastatic disease and may be performed at 12-monthly intervals.

• Following thyroidectomy, radioactive ablation, and suppressive doses of thyroid hormone, patients with differentiated thyroid cancer should have undetectable thyroglobulin levels. Measurable thyroglobulin levels suggest residual or recurrent tumor, and rising levels frequently represent tumor growth.

Key references

1. Kaplan MM, ed: Thyroid carcinoma. *Endocrinol Metab Clin North Am* 1990, 19:741–760.

2. DeGroot LJ, *et al.*: Natural history, treatment, and course of papillary thyroid carcinoma. *J Clin Endocrinol Metabol* 1990, **71**:414–424.

3. Utiger RD: Follow-up of patients with thyroid carcinoma. *N Engl J Med* 1997, **337**:928.

4. Samaan NA, *et al.*: The results of different modalities of treatment of well differentiated thyroid carcinoma: a retrospective review of 1599 patients. *J Clin Endocrinol Metab* 1992, **75**:714–720.

Diagnosis

Symptoms and signs

Daily use of cigarettes for at least several weeks.

Continued smoking of cigarettes despite knowledge of health risk.

Potential for nicotine withdrawal symptoms within 24 hours of abrupt cessation of smoking: dysphoria, insomnia, irritability, anxiety, restlessness, concentrating difficulty, increased appetite.

Impairment in social or occupational functioning: may occur due to withdrawal symptoms.

Investigations

ASK [1]: must have system in place to identify all tobacco users at every visit.

• Consider tobacco status as part of vital signs (*e.g.*, tobacco use status stickers on patient charts) or inclusion of "tobacco use disorder" on active problem list.

Fagerstrom Test for Nicotine Dependence [2]: assists in establishing level of physical dependence (*see* table). Correlation exists between high level of dependence (score >6) and severity of withdrawal symptoms, difficulty with abstinence, and relapse.

Fagerstrom test for nicotine dependence

Questions		Score
1. How soon after you wake up do you smoke your first cigarette?		
	<5 minutes	3
	6-30 minutes	2
	31-60 minutes	1
	>61 minutes	0
2. Do you find it difficult to refrain from smoking in places where it is forbidden, *e.g.*, church, library, movie theater?		
	YES	1
	NO	0
3. Which cigarette would you hate most to give up?		
	The first in the morning	1
	Any other	0
4. How many cigarettes per day do you smoke?		
	>31	3
	21-30	2
	11-20	1
	<10	0
5. Do you smoke more frequently during the first hours after waking than during the rest of the day?		
	YES	1
	NO	0
6. Do you smoke if you are so ill that you are in bed most of the day?		
	YES	1
	NO	0

Complications

Cancer: causally linked to lung cancer; strong associations with cancer of oral cavity, larynx, esophagus, bladder, kidney, pancreas, stomach, and cervix.

Chronic obstructive pulmonary disease: principal risk factor for chronic obstructive pulmonary disease; current smokers have lower forced expiratory volume in 1 second (FEV_1) and accelerated decline in FEV_1 than nonsmokers.

Coronary heart disease: 2–4-fold increased incidence of coronary heart disease and sudden death.

Cerebral vascular disease: nearly 2-fold increased risk of stroke.

Pregnancy: pregnant smokers with increased incidence of low birth weight babies, spontaneous abortion, placenta previa, and placental abruption.

Differential diagnosis

Not applicable.

Etiology

• Nicotine is the agent in cigarettes responsible for addictive properties.

• Dependence occurs via increased expression of brain nicotine receptors, changes in brain glucose metabolism, and release of catecholamines.

• Positive reinforcement occurs with delivery of nicotine via cigarettes and negative reinforcement occurs via withdrawal symptoms during quit attempts.

Epidemiology

• There are 1 billion smokers worldwide.

• 25% of American adults are smokers.

• 3000 teenagers start to smoke each day; most of those who become lifelong smokers start before high school graduation.

• 440 000 deaths per year in the United States are from diseases directly linked to smoking.

Treatment

Diet and lifestyle

• The major treatment for tobacco addiction is a lifestyle change: eliminating smoking activity from one's daily habits and social functions.

• Patients should 1) gather support of family, friends, and coworkers; 2) remove cigarettes from daily environment; 3) anticipate difficult situations and plan a nonsmoking coping mechanism.

Pharmacological treatment

• Nicotine replacement therapy should be offered to all patients smoking >10 cigarettes per day because it is proven to increase cessation success rates.

• Transdermal nicotine may allow for better compliance and may be more successful without formal counseling than nicotine gum; patient preference should be considered.

• Eight weeks of replacement therapy is just as successful as longer courses; weaning of patch dosage has not been proven to improve success rate, but may have psychological benefit.

Transdermal nicotine:

Standard dosage	If 5–10 cigarettes/day, use midrange dose (10–14 mg/24 h). If >10 cigarettes/day, use highest dose of given brand (precise patch dosages vary among manufacturers).
Contraindications	Pregnancy category D; unstable angina, myocardial infarction or revascularization procedure within prior 4 weeks, serious arrhythmia.
Special points	Choose hairless site and change site each day. Will require 2–3 days to achieve maximum systemic levels; may consider supplementation with gum during this time.
Main drug interactions	None with nicotine replacement; however, absence of other factors from smoke decreases metabolism of many drugs, including caffeine and theophylline, requiring dose reduction.
Main side effects	Skin reactions: pruritus, edema, rash; sleep disturbance.

Gum (polacrilex)

Standard dosage	<20 cigarettes/day or Fagerstrom score ≤6, use 2-mg stick. >20 cigarettes/day or Fagerstrom score >6, use 4-mg stick.
Contraindications	Pregnancy category C; cardiovascular contraindications as with transdermal nicotine.
Special points	~1 stick of gum/h; must chew and "park" between cheek and gums every 15–30 minutes; acidic beverages decrease absorption.
Main drug interactions	As with transdermal nicotine.
Main side effects	Jaw fatigue, hiccups, belching, nausea.

Nonpharmacological treatment

The "4 As" of smoking cessation counseling [1]:

Step 1: ASK: Identify all smokers at every visit.

Step 2: ADVISE: urge all smokers to quit with a personalized statement related to patients' health, social, or economic issues.

Step 3. ASSIST: once patient willing to make quit attempt, set a quit date; advise total abstinence; provide nicotine replacement therapy and supplemental materials.

Step 4. ARRANGE: schedule follow-up in person or by phone, ideally during first week. Congratulate successes and review potential reasons for failures.

Physician or counselor can use the "four Rs" [1] to motivate smokers to quit:
1. RELEVANCE: to patient's age, health, family or social situation, and so on.

2. RISKS: review health risks to both individual and family members.

3. REWARDS: have patient list rewards of quitting most relevant to self.

4. REPETITION: review above as needed.

Key references

1. The Smoking Cessation Clinical Practice Guideline Panel and Staff: The Agency for Health Care Policy and Research Smoking Cessation Practice Guideline. *JAMA* 1996, **275**:1270–1280.

2. Heatherton TF, Kozlowski LT, Frecker RC, Fagerstrom KO: The Fagerstrom test for nicotine dependence: a revision of the Fagerstrom Tolerance Questionnaire. *Br J Addict* 1991, **86**:1119–1127.

Diagnosis

Definition

• Definition criteria require fever, rash, hypotension, clinical or test evidence of involvement of three systems, negative results from blood (except in the case of *Staphylococcus aureus*), CSF, and throat culture, and exclusion of measles, leptospirosis, and Rocky Mountain spotted fever.

• Mild or near-miss toxic shock syndrome that does not reach the clinical severity of the full definition is almost certainly more prevalent and poorly recognized. It may resolve because of general antibiotic use or end of menstruation.

Symptoms

High temperature: often to 40°C.

Vomiting and diarrhea: usually watery.

Faintness: especially on standing.

Aching muscles.

Rash.

Signs

Hypotension: systolic blood pressure <90 mm Hg or postural drop of >15 mm Hg; below fifth percentile for age in children <16 years.

Rash: patchy erythema, likened to sunburn, especially on trunk, thighs, palms, soles.

Tender muscles.

Reddened mucosal surfaces: conjunctival, oral, vaginal.

"Red strawberry" tongue.

Confusion: without focal neurological signs.

Investigations

Hematology: thrombocytopenia usual.

Biochemistry: to assess renal function and liver inflammation; creatine kinase concentration often high.

Bacteriology: cultures of blood, stool, urine, vagina, cervix, wounds; *S. aureus* isolates to be forwarded for toxin production and phage typing.

Complications

Renal failure, coma, peripheral gangrene, adult respiratory distress: in varying combinations due to hypotension.

Marked desquamation: especially of palms, soles, and digits, 1–2 weeks after onset.

Hair loss, occasional nail loss: after 2–3 months.

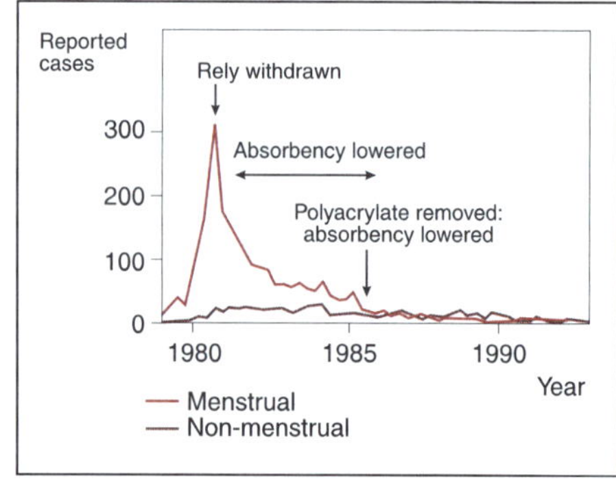

Incidence of toxic shock syndrome in the United States 1979–1993.

Treatment

Diet and lifestyle

• To reduce the likelihood of menstrually related toxic shock syndrome, women must wash hands before and after inserting tampons, use the lowest absorbency tampons that cope with their needs, change tampons regularly (at least every 4–6 hours), use pads overnight, remove and stop using tampons if acute symptoms develop during menstruation, and inform their physician of symptoms of current menstruation. Details of toxic shock syndrome are given on leaflets within tampon cartons, and a health warning is printed on the outside.

Pharmacological treatment

General resuscitation

• Severely ill patients need management and monitoring in intensive care units.

• Intravenous fluids should be used, initially with inotropic support.

• Other modalities, *e.g.*, dialysis, ventilation, should be used when indicated.

Antibiotics

• Although nafcillin does not improve case fatality rate, it reduces relapse rate.

Standard dosage	Nafcillin, 1 g i.v. every 4 hours ×10 days.
Contraindications	Hypersensitivity, porphyria.
Special points	Reduces recurrence rate in future menstrual periods. Third-generation cephalosporin can be used instead.
Main drug interactions	None.
Main side effects	Sensitivity reactions, jaundice.

Antitoxin

• The therapeutic usefulness of toxic shock syndrome toxin-1 antibodies (found in normal immunoglobulin or plasma) has not been determined.

Treatment aims

To limit hypoxic damage (prompt resuscitation).

To stop further toxin production and absorption (removal of tampons, drainage of pus, i.v. floxacillin).

To prevent subsequent relapses (floxacillin, advice on future tampon use).

Prognosis

• Mortality is 3%.

• Chronic morbidity varies and is related to acute ischemic damage to vital organs.

• The risk of recurrence during the next menstrual period is small, and symptoms tend to be milder.

• Recurrences may also follow nonmenstrual toxic shock syndrome, especially if anti-staphylococcal antibiotics are not used, and often follow subsequent skin or mucous membrane infection.

Follow-up and management

• Women should be advised against using tampons for the first few periods but can then reintroduce low-absorbency tampons, with frequent changing, and gradual return to advised standard routine thereafter.

• If further menstrual symptoms develop, tampon use must be stopped, and the patient should be given floxacillin and resuscitative measures in relation to symptoms.

General references

Kain KC, Schulzer M, Chow AW: Clinical spectrum of nonmenstrual toxic shock syndrome. *Clin Infect Dis* 1993, **16**:100–106.
Stevens DL: The toxic shock syndromes. *Infect Dis Clin North Am* 1996, **10**:727–746.

Diagnosis

Symptoms

Primary infection
Fever, neurological symptoms.

Secondary infection
Reactivation of tachyzoites: in cysts in any tissue, particularly brain, also eye, heart, and lung; symptoms are due to focal brain abscess, possibly with diffuse meningoencephalitis.

Focal symptoms
• Occur in 70% of patients.

• May be subacute in onset, evolving to persistent focal neurological deficits, including the following:

Hemiparesis, hemisensory loss, ataxia, visual field deficits, cranial nerve palsies, aphasia; cognitive changes may occur, depending on the intracranial location.

Focal and secondarily generalized seizures: in 38%.

Nonfocal symptoms
• These may predominate in up to 40% of patients; headache, fever.

Fever and malaise (variable), disorientation, psychosis, neck stiffness (in 5%), increasing confusion and coma.

Signs

• Focal signs, *e.g.*, cerebellar ataxia and hemiplegia may occur; they indicate multiple or focal CNS lesions.

• Signs of infection (fever, meningism) may be absent.

Investigations

Toxoplasma serology: IgG serology will be present in >95% of cases, representing reactivation of disease.

CT of brain with contrast: urgent; in 70%–80% of patients, shows single or multiple ring-enhancing lesions with edema (mainly in basal ganglia and bilaterally at corticomedullary junction).

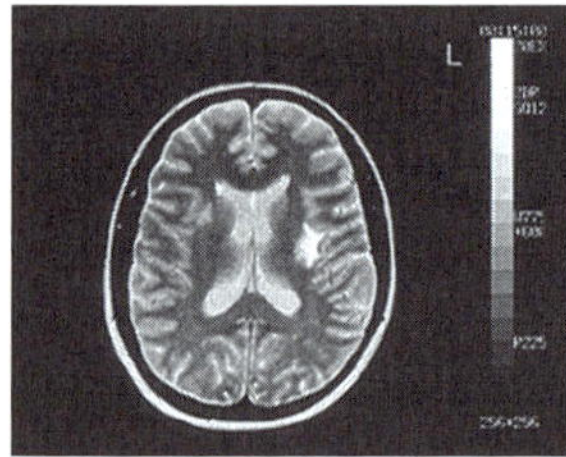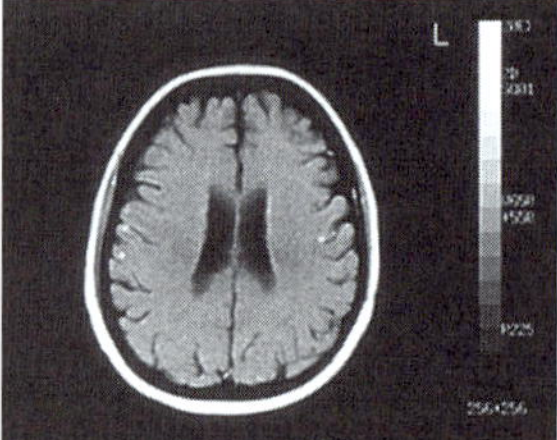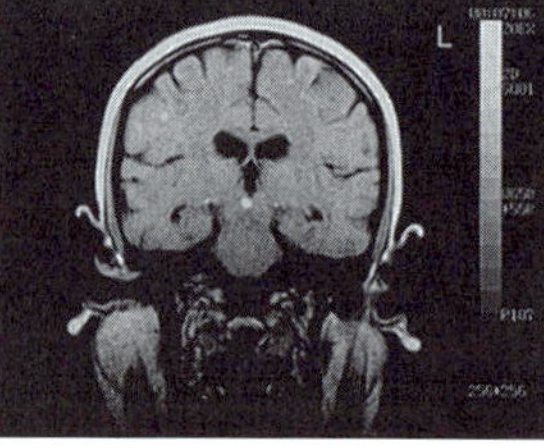

MRI of a patient with cerebral toxoplasmosis. Transverse section before (*left*) and after contrast (*middle*) shows multiple lesions; coronal section (*right*) shows several cortical lesions and one brain stem lesion.

MRI of brain: as alternative to CT scanning or for patients with single lesion on CT or lesions in cerebellum that do not appear on CT; demonstration of single lesion on MR strongly suggests cause other than toxoplasmosis.

Lumbar puncture: in absence of cerebral edema on brain scan; to detect intrathecal toxoplasma antibody production; CSF cellularity, protein, and glucose nonspecific in HIV.

Brain biopsy: indicated for single lesions on MRI or those patients who have negative serology to *Toxoplasma gondii*.

Complications

Seizures or hydrocephalus.

Panhypopituitarism, inappropriate antidiuretic hormone secretion, encephalopathy.

Differential diagnosis

Focal neurological dysfunction
Primary CNS lymphoma, metastatic non-Hodgkin's lymphoma, progressive multifocal leukodystrophy (common). Cytomegalovirus, herpes simplex virus, herpes zoster virus, cryptococcal meningitis, abcesses (*Tuberculosis, Nocardia, Candida* spp.), cerebrovascular disease (rare). Pyogenic abscesses.

Diffuse encephalitis
AIDS encephalitis, AIDS dementia syndrome, cytomegalovirus or herpes simplex encephalitis.

Etiology

• Toxoplasmosis is caused by infection with *Toxoplasma gondii*; spread is by the fecooral route.

• Silent chronic infection is characterized by tachyzoites in tissue cysts throughout the body.

• Acute reactivation involves cyst rupture, causing an encephalitis and a focal necrotizing vasculitic process.

Epidemiology

• Toxoplasmosis is ubiquitous in human populations.

• The incidence reflects the background seroprevalence in a given group: 10%–40% of adults in the United States are seropositive (90% in France).

• Up to 30% of HIV-infected people who are seropositive for *T. gondii* develop cerebral toxoplasmosis, usually with CD4 counts $<100 \times 10^6$/L.

• Overall, toxoplasma accounts for 40% of known CNS infection and 33% of intracerebral lesions in AIDS patients.

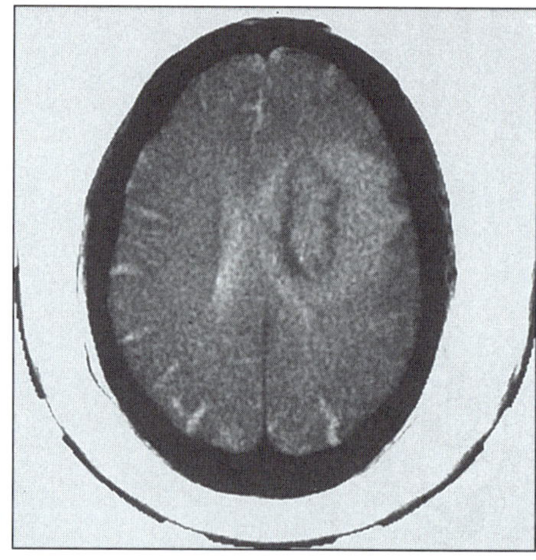

Contrast-enhanced CT of the same patient shows a single lesion in the left temporal lobe.

Treatment

Diet and lifestyle

• No special precautions are necessary.

Pharmacological treatment

• Treatment is begun empirically for a presumptive diagnosis of toxoplasma encephalitis based on clinical presentation and CT or MRI evidence (usually) of multifocal rung-enhancing lesions in a person who has positive serology to *T. gondii*.

• The main regimen is pyrimethamine and folinic acid with sulfadiazine. Clindamycin or atovaquone is used in sulfa-intolerant patients.

Standard dosage	Pyrimethamine, 75 mg to load (or 100–200 mg), then 50 mg orally daily. Folinic acid, 15 mg daily to prevent myelosuppression. Sulfadiazine, 4–6 g daily in divided doses. Clindamycin, 2400 mg daily in divided doses, if sulfa-intolerant. Atovaquone, 750 mg 4 times daily if cannot tolerate clindamycin.
Contraindications	*Pyrimethamine:* hepatic or renal impairment. *Sulfadiazine:* pregnancy, renal or hepatic failure, jaundice, porphyria. *Clindamycin:* diarrheal states.
Special points	Careful monitoring of neurological condition and repeat CT or MRI to check for improvement within 3 weeks. With clinical and radiographic improvement, treatment is normally continued for 4–6 weeks; if no improvement occurs in the first 14–21 days, stereotactic brain biopsy should be considered. *Pyrimethamine, sulfadiazine:* disrupt folic acid metabolism; blood count must be monitored weekly. *Clindamycin:* liver function and blood count must be monitored.
Main drug interactions	*Pyrimethamine:* increased antifolate effect with phenytoin and trimethoprim. *Sulfadiazine:* warfarin, phenytoin, pyrimethamine, cyclosporine. *Clindamycin:* neostigmine, tubocurarine.
Main side effects	*Pyrimethamine:* nausea, vomiting, myelosuppression (folate). *Folinic acid:* pyrexia. *Sulfadiazine:* nausea, vomiting, rashes, blood dyscrasias (treatment must be stopped immediately), nephrotoxicity, headache, hepatitis (rare); adverse reaction rate 40%. *Clindamycin:* nausea, vomiting, rash, diarrhea (rare but serious pseudomembranous colitis; treatment must be stopped immediately). *Atovaquone:* diarrhea, rash.

• In patients with significant mass effect or decreased consciousness level, steroids are indicated, *e.g.*, high-dose dexamethasone, 8 mg orally or i.v. 4 times daily.

• Steroids may complicate the interpretation of clinical improvement and CT or MRI resolution during empirical antitoxoplasma treatment.

• They should be reduced and withdrawn as soon as is reasonable and repeat scans performed to check for exacerbation.

General references

Minkoff H, Remington JS, Holman S, *et al.*: Vertical transmission of toxoplasma by human immunodeficiency virus–infected women. *Am J Obstet Gynecol* 1997, **176**:555–559.

Porter SB, Sande MA: Toxoplasmosis of the central nervous system in the acquired immune deficiency syndrome. *N Eng J Med* 1992, **327**:1643–1647.

Wong S, Israelski D, Remington J: AIDS-associated toxoplasmosis. In *The Medical Management of AIDS*. Edited by Sande M, Volberding P. Philadelphia: WB Saunders; 1995.

Indications

Erythrocytes

• A low hemoglobin level per se is not an indication for transfusion. Factors such as the patient's condition, the rate of fall of hemoglobin, and the cause of anemia must be considered to determine the correct treatment.

Whole blood
For acute massive blood loss.

For exchange transfusion of infants to avoid multiple donors.

Erythrocyte concentrates
For chronic blood loss or anemia.

For blood loss <1 blood volume in elective surgery (in additive solution).

Filtered blood
To prevent or delay nonhemolytic febrile transfusion reactions in patients who are erythrocyte dependent.

For newly diagnosed patients with aplastic anemia who are potential bone-marrow transplant recipients.

When cytomegalovirus-antibody–negative blood is indicated but not readily available.

For intrauterine transfusion.

Washed cells
For patients with proven hypersensitivity reactions to plasma proteins.

For neonates who have necrotizing enterocolitis.

Cryopreserved erythrocytes
For patients needing blood of rare phenotypes or blood compatible with multiple erythrocyte alloantibodies.

For patients with anti-IgA in the absence of IgA-negative blood.

Irradiated erythrocytes
For recipients at risk of graft-versus-host disease: in utero transfusion, after bone-marrow transplantation.

For rare cases of transfusions from relatives.

Platelets [1]

To prevent or treat bleeding in patients with thrombocytopenia and rarely to treat bleeding in patients with platelet function defects: the cause of thrombocytopenia and significance of hemorrhage influence the use of platelet transfusions.

For acute bone-marrow failure (e.g., due to aplasia, chemotherapy): if platelet count $10–50 \times 10^9$/L, serious spontaneous bleeding is unlikely, although minor bleeding (purpura, epistaxis) may occur; prophylactic platelet transfusions to maintain count $>10 \times 10^9$/L reduces risk of hemorrhage as effectively as keeping count higher and reduces morbidity but not mortality; patients with fever, infection, coagulopathy, or rapid fall in platelet count should be transfused to maintain platelets $>20 \times 10^9$/L.

For acute disseminated intravascular coagulation: when thrombocytopenia is associated with bleeding (not indicated in chronic disseminated intravascular coagulation without bleeding).

For massive blood loss: to maintain platelets $>50 \times 10^9$/L.

Prophylaxis for surgery: to maintain platelets $>50 \times 10^9$/L or $>100 \times 10^9$/L for surgery in a critical site, e.g., brain or eye (not routinely with cardiopulmonary bypass).

For autoimmune thrombocytopenia: platelet transfusions rarely used.

Fresh frozen plasma [2]

To replace single coagulation factor deficiencies when a specific or combined factor concentrate is unavailable.

For immediate reversal of warfarin effect.

For acute disseminated intravascular coagulation.

For thrombotic thrombocytopenic purpura.

For bleeding or disturbed coagulation associated with massive transfusion, liver disease, or cardiopulmonary bypass surgery.

Autologous transfusion [3,4]

Advantages

• The possibilities of alloimmunization, immunosuppression, and transfusion-transmitted infection are avoided.

Disadvantages

• Not all patients are eligible.

• Predeposited blood may be unused, e.g., if surgery is cancelled, or may be insufficient to meet the patient's needs.

• Collecting predeposited autologous blood is more expensive than using standard units.

Options

Autologous predeposit: up to 5 U of blood collected and stored during the weeks before surgery.

Acute normovolemic hemodilution: blood drawn from patient under anesthetic and replaced by crystalloid so that blood lost during surgery has a lower hematocrit; when blood loss starts or at end of procedure, patient's whole blood is returned.

Erythrocyte salvage: blood lost at operating site recovered and processed for transfusion.

Directed blood donations

• Blood donations from relatives or friends should be discouraged unless needed on medical grounds.

• Evidence suggests that "directed" donations are generally less safe than blood supplied by the American Red Cross.

Techniques

Erythrocytes

Whole blood: packed cell volume (PCV) 0.35–0.45, 1 U = 510 mL ± 10%; if blood loss and replacement exceed twice the blood volume, thrombocytopenia and abnormalities of hemostasis may develop.

Fresh blood (<24 hours): blood that has not been microbiologically tested must not be transfused.

Erythrocyte concentrates: PCV 0.55–0.75, 1 U = 220–340 mL.

Erythrocyte concentrates in additive solution: PCV 0.5–0.7, 1 U = 280–420 mL; not to be used for exchange or large-volume transfusion in neonates.

Filtered blood (leukodepleted $<5 \times 10^6$ leukocytes/U): PCV and quantity variable; rigorous validation of blood processing and component preparation needed [5].

Washed cells (residual protein <0.5 g/U): must be used within 24 hours of preparation.

Cryopreserved erythrocytes (thawed and washed): volume usually <200 mL; must be used within 24 hours of preparation.

Irradiated erythrocytes (minimum dose, 25 Gy): must be used within 1 day if for intrauterine transfusion because of increased potassium.

Platelets [6]

Administration

• Platelets for transfusion should preferably be of the recipient ABO and RhD group.

• If RhD-positive platelets are transfused to a RhD-negative woman potentially capable of childbearing, 250 IU anti-D immunoglobulin should be given subcutaneously with each dose of platelets.

Dose and response

• A standard dose of 300×10^9 may be issued as pooled or single platelet concentrates derived from individual donations or as a single apheresis donation, respectively, to raise the platelet count (adult) by $\sim 40 \times 10^9$/L.

• Patient factors, including sepsis, certain drugs, disseminated intravascular coagulation, splenomegaly, uremia, and platelet antibodies, can reduce the expected platelet increment.

• Patients who are repeatedly transfused with platelets may develop immunological refractoriness due to HLA alloimmunization and should receive platelets from HLA-matched donors.

• In some cases, platelet-specific alloantibodies develop, requiring type-specific platelet transfusions.

Fresh frozen plasma [2]

Administration

• Fresh frozen plasma (FFP) should be ABO and RhD compatible, although compatibility testing is not required.

• Group O FFP should be transfused only to Group O recipients.

• If an RhD-negative woman potentially capable of childbearing is transfused with RhD-positive FFP, 50 IU anti-D immunoglobulin should be given per unit of FFP transfused.

Dose

• A generally accepted starting dose is 12–15 mL/kg.

• The clinical and laboratory responses should be monitored to assess response and plan further management.

Key references

1. Murphy MF, *et al.*: Guidelines for platelet transfusion. *Transfusion Med* 1992, **2**:311–318.

2. Contreras M, *et al.*: Guidelines for the use of fresh frozen plasma. *Transfusion Med* 1992, **2**:57–63.

3. Contreras M: *ABC of Transfusion*, edn 2. London: British Medical Association; 1992.

4. Au Buchon JP: Blood transfusion options: improving outcomes and reducing costs. *Arch Pathol Lab Med* 1997, **121**:40–47.

5. Lumadue J, Ness PM: Current approaches to red blood cell transfusion. *Semin Hematol* 1996, **33**:277–289.

6. Mollision PL, Engelfriet CP, Contreras M: *Blood Transfusion in Clinical Medicine*, edn 9. Oxford: Blackwell Scientific Publications; 1993.

Diagnosis

Definition

• A transient ischemic attack is abrupt loss of focal cerebral or monocular function with symptoms lasting <24 hours, which, after adequate investigations, is presumed to be due to embolic or thrombotic vascular disease.

Symptoms

• Symptoms such as syncope, confusion, convulsions, incontinence, and isolated dizziness are not acceptable for transient ischemic attacks.

Carotid territory

• This is the site of 80% of transient ischemic attacks.

Unilateral paresis: weakness, heaviness, or clumsiness.

Unilateral sensory loss.

Aphasia.

Transient monocular visual loss: amaurosis fugax.

Vertebrobasilar territory

• This is the site of 20% of transient ischemic attacks.

Bilateral or alternating weakness or sensory symptoms.

Vertigo, diplopia, dysphagia, ataxia: patients must have two or more simultaneously.

Sudden bilateral blindness: in patients aged >40 years.

Uncertain arterial distribution

Hemianopia alone.

Dysarthria alone.

Investigations [1]

• Investigations are of little help in the recognition of transient ischemic attacks; they are directed at determining the cause of the attack.

Serological

Prothrombin time/partial thromboplastin time, fibrinogen, platelet count, renal and hepatic function tests, sedimentation rates, cholesterol profile.

• In patients aged ≤50 years, add protein S & C, antithrombin III, anticardiolipin and antiphospholipid antibodies, homocystine levels, lactate/pyruvate, adrenoleukodystrophy and metachromatic leukodystrophy screen, where indicated.

Structural and etiological

CT or MRI of brain (MRI required for posterior circulation event).

MR angiography: for large- and medium-vessel disease.

Carotid ultrasonography.

ECG.

Transesophageal echocardiogram.

Angiography: for all patients with hemorrhage and needed for many without clear stroke etiology; often necessary to exclude vasculitis or dissection in young adults.

Temporary artery biopsy: if indicated.

Lumbar puncture: for hemorrhage or suspected vasculitis.

Complications

None, by definition.

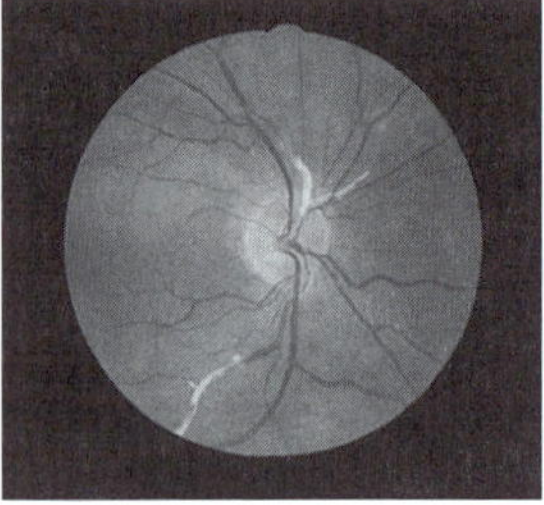

Cholesterol emboli seen on fundoscopy in a patient with amaurosis fugax. (*See* Color Plate.)

Treatment

Diet and lifestyle

• Treating raised blood pressure reduces the risk of stroke by 50%, even after only a few years; the effect on coronary events is less impressive. Targets should be a systolic and diastolic pressure of below about 180 mm Hg and 100 mm Hg, respectively.

• The effect of stopping smoking is most marked on reducing cardiac events, and all patients should be encouraged vigorously to stop.

• Reducing serum cholesterol leads to a reduced risk of cardiac events, but no reliable data for stroke are available. A diet low in saturated fats should be advised.

• Physical exercise should be encouraged and probably helps by facilitating weight, cholesterol, and blood pressure control.

Pharmacological treatment

Antiplatelet drugs

• Antiplatelet drugs have shown clear evidence of benefit in a meta-analysis of all trials: the risk of nonfatal myocardial infarction and stroke is reduced by one-third; the risk of all fatal vascular events is reduced by one-sixth.

• Aspirin is the most widely used agent.

Standard dosage	Aspirin, 75–325 mg.
Contraindications	Active peptic ulceration.
Main drug interactions	Increased risk of bleeding with warfarin.
Main side effects	Gastrointestinal hemorrhage.

• Ticlopidine is useful in patients with small-vessel or posterior circulation disease, and often is used if aspirin fails.

Standard dosage	Ticlopidine, 250 mg orally twice daily.
Contraindications	Bone-marrow disease.
Special points	Requires regular complete blood count analysis to exclude neutropenia.
Main side effects	Nausea/gastrointestinal upset, neutropenia.

Anticoagulants

• Anticoagulants are indicated when a definite cardiac source of emboli has been identified (*e.g.*, mitral valve disease with atrial fibrillation, prosthetic heart valve, recent myocardial infarction, dilated cardiomyopathy).

• In nonrheumatic atrial fibrillation, warfarin is superior to aspirin.

• Short-term warfarin may be used empirically for symptomatic treatment of frequent attacks resistant to aspirin. Warfarin may also be useful for intracranial stenosis and posterior circulation disease.

• Possible benefits of warfarin must always be weighed against definite side effects in individual patients.

Standard dosage	Warfarin sufficient to maintain INR at 2–4.
Contraindications	Bleeding diathesis, active peptic ulceration.
Special points	Requires regular blood monitoring.
Main drug interactions	Alcohol, NSAIDs, antiepileptics, antidepressants.
Main side effects	Hemorrhage.

Treatment aims

To prevent stroke or other serious vascular events (secondary prevention).

Other treatments

Carotid endarterectomy: for symptomatic carotid stenoses >70% only [3].

Prognosis

• The risk of stroke in the first year after a transient ischemic attack is 12%.

• Thereafter, the risk is 7% each year (seven times the risk in the normal population).

• The greatest risk occurs in the first month after the attack.

• Cardiac death occurs more often than stroke death after an attack.

• The combined risk of all serious vascular events (stroke, myocardial infarction, other vascular death) is ~9% annually.

Follow-up and management

• Risk factors (*e.g.*, hypertension) must be adequately controlled and antiplatelet therapy maintained.

Key references

1. Hankey GJ, Warlow CP: *Transient Ischaemic Attacks of the Brain and Eye*. London: WB Saunders; 1994. [Major Problems in Neurology 27.]

2. Dennis M, *et al.*: The prognosis of transient ischemic attacks in the Oxfordshire community stroke project. *Stroke* 1990, **21**:848–853.

3. European Carotid Surgery Trialist's Collaborative Group: MRC European Carotid Surgery Trial: interim results for symptomatic patients with severe (70–99%) or with mild (0–29%) carotid stenosis. *Lancet* 1991, **337**:1235–1243.

Diagnosis

Definition

• Tremor is an involuntary, rhythmic, smooth, sinusoidal oscillation of a body part. Faster tremors (6–12 Hz) are usually of fine amplitude; slower tremors (2–5 Hz) are coarse and of large amplitude. Tremors may be described according to the following:
Cause or underlying diagnosis.
Clinical circumstances of occurrence: rest (limb supported), postural (limb outstretched), kinetic (during voluntary movement), task-specific action (*e.g.*, during writing), intention (in terminal stages of movement).
Affected body part: *e.g.*, head, voice, hand, leg.
Frequency (cycles/s or Hz, considerable overlap).

Symptoms

Rhythmic shaking of hands, legs, trunk, or head: often resulting in clumsiness and loss of manual dexterity.
Slow voluntary movement (with rest tremor): suggesting Parkinson's disease.
Unsteadiness when standing (shaking legs), relieved by walking or sitting: suggesting primary orthostatic tremor.

Signs [1]

Parkinsonian
Rest ("pill-rolling"), possibly with postural tremor: 4–5 and 5–6 Hz, respectively; arms affected more than legs, which are affected more than jaws or lips.

Midbrain (rubral)
Rest, postural, intention tremor: 2–5 Hz; particularly affecting proximal arms.

Cerebellar
Postural, intention, kinetic tremor: 3–6 Hz; arms and trunk more than legs; titubation (head and truncal tremor).

Essential
Postural, kinetic tremor: 5–8 Hz; arms more than head more than legs; isolated.

Neuropathic
Postural, kinetic tremor: 4–6 Hz; arms more than legs.

Dystonic
Postural, kinetic tremor: 2–6 Hz; arms more than legs; exacerbated in certain postures.

Primary orthostatic
Tremor of legs and trunk when standing: 14–16 Hz.

Physiological
Postural tremor: 8–12 Hz; affecting arms; normal finding.

Exaggerated physiological
Postural tremor: 8–12 Hz; affecting arms; larger amplitude than physiological tremor.

Focal
Postural tremor: 4–8 Hz; affecting head, face, jaw, chin, tongue, voice, trunk (alone).

Task-specific action
Kinetic tremor during specific tasks: ~6 Hz; affecting arms, lips, and head.

Investigations

• Investigations are needed to exclude symptomatic tremor or identify the cause.
Serum ceruloplasmin, thyroid function, blood glucose measurement: for Wilson's disease, thyrotoxicosis, and hypoglycemia, respectively.
Nerve conduction studies, electromyography, serum immunoglobulin measurement: in patients with suspected neuropathy.
Brain imaging: if clinical suspicion of structural lesion, *e.g.*, hemitremor, focal neurological signs, midbrain or cerebellar tremor.

Complications

Clumsiness, loss of manual dexterity, difficulty writing, embarrassment.

Differential diagnosis

Repetitive myoclonus: brisk, abrupt jerks.

Chorea: flowing random variable movements.

Dystonia: intermittent fixed postures.

Etiology [2,3]

Hereditary
Essential tremor (50% of cases inherited autosomal-dominant).

Idiopathic
Physiological tremor.
Primary orthostatic tremor.
Task-specific action tremors.

Symptomatic
Parkinson's disease.
Akinetic rigid syndromes.
Dystonic tremor.
Thyrotoxicosis.
Cerebellar disease: multiple sclerosis, degenerative ataxias.
Midbrain lesions: multiple sclerosis, vascular.
Wilson's disease.
Peripheral neuropathy (especially demyelinating).
Exaggerated physiological tremor.
Drug-induced tremor.
Toxins.

Epidemiology

• Essential tremor occurs in 300 in 100 000 population.

• Parkinson's disease occurs in 200 in 100 000 population (increasing with age).

Diagnostic difficulties [4]

Drug-induced tremor
Beta-2 agonists, caffeine, theophylline, tricyclic antidepressants, 5-HT reuptake inhibitors, lithium, neuroleptics, amphetamines, valproate, steroids, thyroxine.

Toxin-induced tremor
MPTP (1-methyl-4-phenyl-1,2,3,6-tetrahydropyridine), mercury.

Drug-withdrawal tremor
Alcohol, barbiturates, benzodiazepines, opiates.

Exaggerated physiological tremor
Drugs (as above), drug withdrawal (as above), metabolic disease: thyrotoxicosis, hypoglycemia, pheochromocytoma, anxiety, fatigue.

Treatment

Diet and lifestyle

- Caffeine and fatigue may exacerbate tremor.
- Alcohol may help essential tremor, but addiction is a possibility.
- Aids for stability when standing (*e.g.*, shooting stick) help orthostatic tremor.

Pharmacological treatment

For essential tremor

Standard dosage	Propranolol, 60–180 mg long-acting preparation daily. Primidone, up to 50 mg 2 times daily.
Contraindications	*Propranolol:* obstructive airways disease, heart failure.
Main drug interactions	None.
Main side effects	*Propranolol:* hypotension, bradycardia, bronchospasm. *Primidone:* fatigue.

- Sometimes amantadine or anticholinergics are useful.

For parkinsonian tremor

L-Dopa, anticholinergics, amantadine, dopamine agonists in doses as for Parkinson's disease (*see* Parkinson's disease *for details*).

Treatment aims

To identify and remove causes of exaggerated physiological tremor.

To identify and treat causes of symptomatic tremor.

Other treatments

Thalamotomy or thalamic stimulation: in severe tremors refractory to drugs.

Prognosis

- The prognosis depends on the cause of the tremor.

Follow-up and management

- Follow-up depends on the cause of the tremor.

Key references

1. Weiner WJ, Land AE: *Movement Disorders*. New York: Futura Publishing Company; 1989:221–256.

2. Cleeves L, Findley LJ, Marsden CD: Odd tremors. In *Movement Disorders,* edn 3. Edited by Marsden CD, Fahn S. Oxford: Butterworth Heinemann; 1994:434–498.

3. Elble RJ: Central mechanisms of tremor. *J Clin Neurophysiol* 1996, **13**:133–144.

4. Findley LJ: Tremors: differential diagnosis and pharmacology. In *Parkinson's Disease and Movement Disorders*. Edited by Jankovic J, Tolosa E. Baltimore: Williams and Wilkins; 1993:293–313.

Diagnosis

Symptoms

• Disease may be focal, disseminated, or multifocal. Proportion by site: lymphatic ~35%; genitourinary, bone, joint ~15% each; disseminated, abdominal, cerebral <10% each; cutaneous, other sites <5% each.

• Systemic symptoms usually imply more widespread disease; focal disease may be acute or insidious (more usual).

Fever, malaise, fatigue, weight loss, night sweats.
Pain: in bone or joint, abdomen, gastrointestinal tract, or meninges.
Tissue swelling: in lymph node, joint, or peritoneum.
Frequency, dysuria, loin pain: in renal disease.
Cough, fever: in disseminated disease.
Headache, vomiting, confusion: in CNS disease.

Signs

Fever, wasting: due to tuberculous toxicity.
Erythema nodosum: a hypersensitivity reaction.
Choroidal tubercles: in miliary disease.
Nontender, fluctuant lymph node: perhaps discharging.
Hematuria.
Bone or joint deformity, cold abscess, spinal-cord signs.
Chest signs, pleural effusion, hepatosplenomegaly: in dissemination.
Ascites, abdominal distension, bowel obstruction.
Nuchal rigidity, obtundation, focal signs: indicating meningitis.

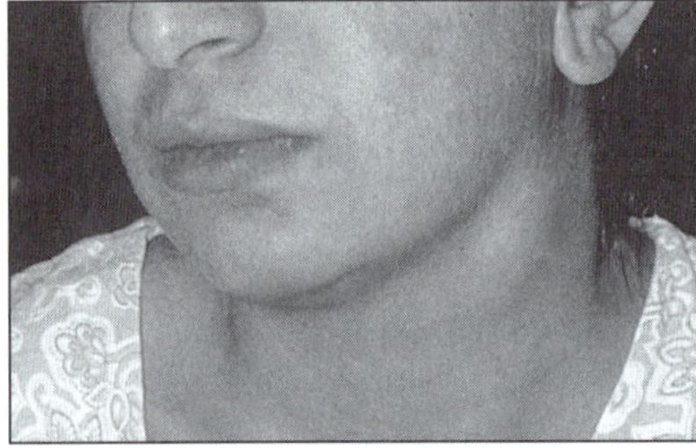
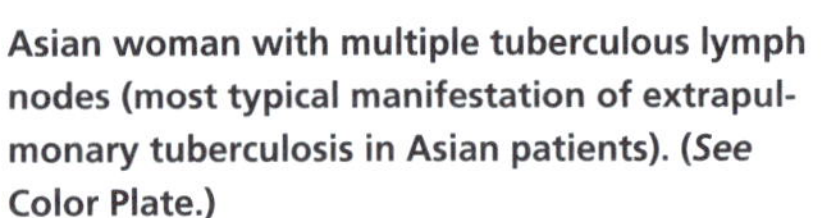

Asian woman with multiple tuberculous lymph nodes (most typical manifestation of extrapulmonary tuberculosis in Asian patients). (*See* Color Plate.)

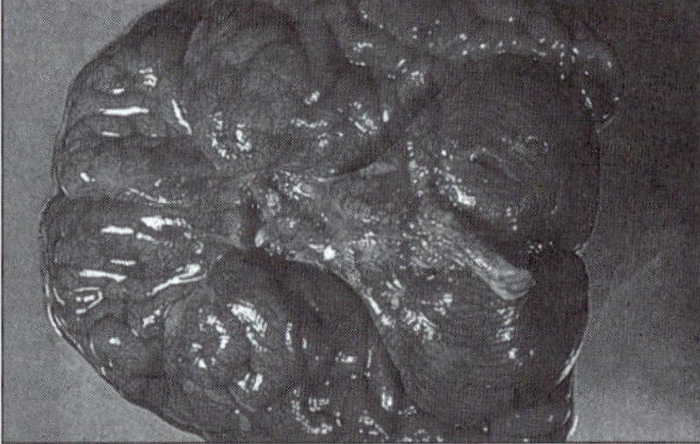

Massive cerebral edema typical of advanced tuberculous meningitis. (*See* Color Plate.)

Investigations

• Tests may suggest the diagnosis (ESR, skin test, radiography), identify the site (CT or specialized radiography, i.v. pyelography, isotope renography), or confirm the diagnosis (culture in ~50%, microscopy in ~35%, histology in ~35%).

Chest radiography: to check for apical or cavitary disease, pleural thickening.
Blood analysis: may show anemia, high ESR, pancytopenia, or leukemoid reaction.
Tuberculin skin test: possibly negative (especially in disseminated infection).
Sputum or urine culture.
Biopsy of bone marrow, liver, lymph node, joint, or bowel.

Complications

Cryptic disseminated tuberculosis, acute miliary disease, or meningitis: due to dissemination from a focal lesion.
Focal damage: from vasculitis, fibrosis, abscess, sinus formation, or caseation.
Hydrocephalus, spinal block, cerebral vasculitis.
Adult respiratory distress syndrome: in miliary disease.
Ureteric obstruction or renal destruction by caseation.
Spinal-cord involvement: in 20% of patients with vertebral disease.
Bone or joint deformity.
Gastrointestinal stenosis, adhesions, obstruction.

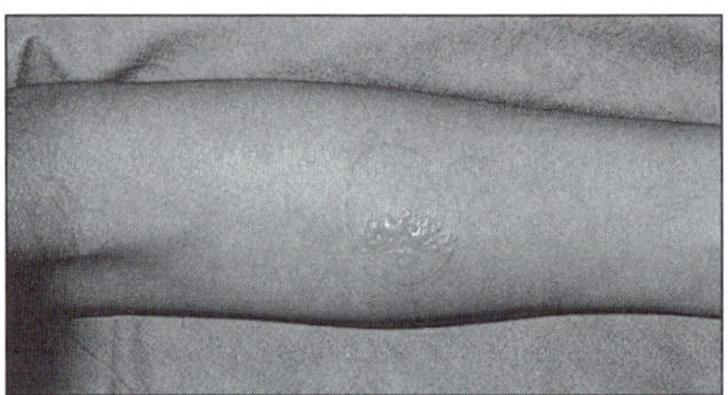

Strongly positive reaction to Mantoux test. (*See* Color Plate.)

Treatment

Diet and lifestyle

- Weight loss and malnutrition must be reversed.
- Alcohol or drug addiction should be treated.
- Social circumstances, *e.g.*, homelessness, should be improved.

Pharmacological treatment

- The advice of a tuberculosis specialist must be sought and the case reported to state authorities.
- In a seriously ill patient, empirical treatment is justified even when the diagnosis is unconfirmed; treatment is invariably instituted before sensitivities are available.
- Efforts should be made to establish diagnosis.
- Patients must comply with the drug regimen for the duration of treatment.

Standard chemotherapy

Standard dosage	*Initial phase (2 months):* 4 drugs, usually isoniazid, with pyridoxine, rifampin, pyrazinamide, and ethambutol. *Continuation phase (4–12 months):* two drugs, usually isoniazid and rifampin.
Contraindications	*Isoniazid:* drug-induced liver disease, porphyria. *Rifampin:* jaundice, porphyria. *Pyrazinamide:* liver damage, porphyria. *Ethambutol:* optic neuritis.
Special points	For suspected resistance: addition of ethambutol. For documented resistance: drugs as indicated by sensitivities. For cerebral, bone and joint, and drug-resistant infections: longer treatment (9 months). For unreliable compliance: intermittent, supervised treatment 2–3 times weekly.
Main drug interactions	*Rifampin:* oral contraceptive.
Main side effects	*Isoniazid:* neuropathy (pyridoxine prophylaxis), hepatitis, hypersensitivity reactions. *Rifampin:* hepatitis, gastrointestinal upset, influenza symptoms, purpura. *Pyrazinamide:* hepatitis, gastrointestinal upset.

Steroids

Patients with pericarditis or meningitis should receive steroids in order to prevent obstructive hydrocephalus.

Treatment aims

To secure survival (especially in disseminated and cerebral disease).
To preserve organ function and prevent deformity.
To relieve symptoms.
To prevent relapse by eradicating infection.
To prevent drug resistance by ensuring compliance.

Other treatments

- Surgery is often done both before and after the diagnosis is confirmed.
- It is indicated for the following forms of tuberculosis:
All: for biopsy diagnosis (>35% of patients), relief of obstruction due to inflammatory response, and correction of deformity.
Lymphatic: for chronic sinus and unresponsive or marked node enlargement.
Renal: ureteric obstruction or stricture, obstinate symptoms (*e.g.*, pain).
CNS: for hydrocephalus, cerebral edema.
Spinal: for cord pressure, bone graft.
Joint: to minimize deformity.
Gut: for obstruction, adhesions, strictures.
Pericardial: to relieve constriction.
Female genital: for stricture, infertility.

Prognosis

- Prognosis is related to the precariousness of the organ involved, the stage of disease progression, and the vulnerability of host.
- Mortality is significant in cerebral disease (10%–30%) and disseminated disease (10%–25%).
- Survival can be expected in other forms, although chronic sequelae may develop.
- The prognosis in lymph-node and dermatological tuberculosis is excellent.

Follow-up and management

- Drug toxicities that may affect compliance must be identified.
- The patient must be monitored for complications and long-term sequelae.

General references

Langdale LA, *et al.*: Tuberculosis and the surgeon. *Am J Surg* 1992, **163**:505–509.

Shafer RW, *et al.*: Extrapulmonary tuberculosis in patients with human immunodeficiency virus infection. *Medicine* 1991, **70**:384–397.

Diagnosis

Symptoms

Primary infection
• 90% of patients have no symptoms; the following are seen rarely:

Malaise, fever, erythema nodosum, phlyctenular conjunctivitis.

Postprimary infection (reactivation tuberculosis)
• Often no symptoms are seen.

Malaise, weight loss, fever, night sweats, anorexia, fatigue.

Cough, mucoid or mucopurulent sputum, hemoptysis, dyspnea, dull chest ache, pleuritic chest pain.

Malaise, weight loss, fever, meningism: symptoms of miliary tuberculosis; may be nonspecific, particularly in elderly patients.

Signs

• Physical examination is often unhelpful.

Evidence of weight loss, pyrexia, erythema nodosum: in primary infection.

Signs of pulmonary collapse, consolidation, or effusion, crackles (upper zones, increased after coughing), amphoric breath sounds over a large cavity.

Investigations

Chest radiography:
Primary: normal in 70% of patients; more often abnormal in children <5 years of age; typically shows unilateral hilar lymphadenopathy; bronchial compression can produce segmental or lobar collapse or hyperinflation, particularly in lower, lingula, and middle lobes; ulceration into bronchial tree, producing distal patchy consolidation, or into pleura, producing effusion.
Postprimary: classically shows bilateral upper-zone consolidation progressing to cavitation, fibrosis, and upper-lobe contraction; chronic tuberculosis lesions often calcified.

Tuberculin skin testing: positive test implies current or past infection or previous bacille Calmette–Guérin vaccination; positivity increases with age in United States; useful in identifying primary disease in younger patients. The larger the reaction, the greater likelihood exists that infection is present. A negative test does not rule out diagnosis.

Bacteriology: sputum samples stained (fluorescent auramine or Ziehl-Neelsen) and cultured (*e.g.*, in Löwenstein-Jensen medium); useful in establishing diagnosis in postprimary disease and in guiding management; sputum smear often positive in cavitating disease; examination of two good early-morning sputum samples allows identification of 90% of smear-positive cases; smear-positive sputum implies significant risk of infection; culture and sensitivity testing takes 4–8 weeks. DNA probes for *Mycobacterium tuberculosis* assist in the identification.

Complications

Lobar or segmental collapse or consolidation, pleural effusion, pericardial involvement, tuberculoma formation: in primary tuberculosis.

Postprimary or miliary tuberculosis, later infection at distant sites: caused by blood dissemination at time of primary infection.

Differential diagnosis

• Radiographical and some clinical features can be mimicked by the following:

Lung cancer.

Sarcoidosis.

Some bacterial pneumonias.

Allergic bronchopulmonary aspergillosis.

Pneumoconiosis.

Actinomycosis.

Etiology

General disease
Inhalation of *M. tuberculosis* from the cough of a patient with sputum-positive disease.

Postprimary disease
Reactivation of dormant *M. tuberculosis* disseminated at the time of primary infection; risk increased in patients with diseases causing depressed immunity (*e.g.*, malnutrition, alcoholism, diabetes, AIDS).

Epidemiology

• The estimated annual incidence in the United States is 4–20/100 000 people.

• The annual incidence in Indian, Pakistani, and Bangladeshi ethnic groups is ~170 in 100 000.

• Recently, the overall incidence has increased slightly.

• Persons infected with HIV are at increased risk of developing tuberculosis.

Atypical tuberculosis

• The frequency of atypical tuberculosis is increasing in elderly men with pre-existing lung disease.

• It is mostly caused by *Mycobacterium kansasii, malmoense, xenopi, avium,* or *avium-intracellulare* (*M. avium-intracellulare* particularly in later stages of AIDS).

• Presentation is similar to that of *M. tuberculosis* infection: 10%–40% of patients may be asymptomatic.

• Management is complicated, involving prolonged multidrug treatment: expert advice is needed.

Treatment

Diet and lifestyle

• Smoking must be stopped, and nutrition improved.

Pharmacological treatment

• Treatment must be supervised by a physician experienced in all aspects of tuberculosis management. Drug choice depends on susceptibility.

• Patients must be educated about the disease and the importance of prolonged treatment.

• Sputum-positive patients must be advised that they remain infectious for the first 2 weeks of treatment.

Standard 6-month unsupervised regimen

• A four-drug regimen consisting of isoniazid, rifampin, pyrazinamide, and ethambutol or streptomycin is recommended. The latter may be discontinued if the organism is susceptible to isoniazid and rifampin. Pyrazinamide is stopped after 8 weeks.

Standard dosage	Isoniazid, 300 mg daily (child, 5 mg/kg daily; maximum, 300 mg) for 6 months, rifampin, 450–600 mg daily (child, 10 mg/kg daily) for 6 months, pyrazinamide, 1.5–2 g daily (child, 15–30 mg/kg daily) for 2 months, and ethambutol, 15 mg/kg daily, or streptomycin, 15 mg/kg daily.
Contraindications	*All:* previous severe adverse event. *Isoniazid:* drug-induced liver disease, porphyria; caution in liver or renal disease. *Rifampin:* jaundice, porphyria; caution in liver disease. *Pyrazinamide:* liver disease, porphyria; caution in renal impairment, gout, or diabetes.
Special points	*Isoniazid:* isoniazid-resistant *M. tuberculosis* present in 4%–6% of patients. *Rifampin:* colors urine and tears orange; may stain soft contact lenses.
Main drug interactions	*Isoniazid:* binds to pyridoxine and may produce deficiency; inhibits phenytoin metabolism. *Rifampin:* hepatic enzyme induction increases metabolism and reduces effect of anticonvulsants, oral contraceptive pill, steroids, and digoxin. *Pyrazinamide:* interferes with renal testing for ketones; reduces renal excretion of uric acid. *Streptomycin:* may potentiate neuromuscular-blocking agents.
Main side effects	*Isoniazid:* gastrointestinal intolerance, exacerbation of acne, hepatotoxicity (in 1%–2% of patients; can be severe), peripheral neuropathy (in 2%; prevented by pyridoxine supplements 10 mg daily). *Rifampin:* nausea, abnormal liver function tests (usually mild and reversible), influenza-like reaction. *Pyrazinamide:* hepatotoxicity, arthralgia, precipitation of gout, urticaria. *Streptomycin:* 8th nerve damage, nephrotoxicity.

• Longer periods are needed for meningitis and with extensive disease.

• Pyridoxine, 10 mg daily, may be added when deficiency is a possibility.

• Supervised regimen and bi- or tri-weekly therapy are available options.

Other drugs

Corticosteroids: improve outcome in pericarditis and meningitis; of value in patients with severe infection, persistent pyrexia, or weight loss; higher doses needed if rifampin used.

Streptomycin, capreomycin, cycloserine, ethionamide for multiresistant or atypical infection: specialist advice must be sought.

Treatment aims

To achieve bacteriological and clinical cure.
To prevent resistance (with combination treatment).
To prevent or treat disease in contacts.

Prognosis

• ~6% of adults with pulmonary tuberculosis die of it before finishing chemotherapy.

• Only ~3% relapse if the full course of chemotherapy is taken; the rate is higher if compliance is poor.

Follow-up and management

• Close supervision is necessary throughout chemotherapy.

• Compliance must be checked; urine must be checked for rifampin.

• The patient must be checked for adverse effects.

• Response must be assessed: symptoms, weight gain, radiographic changes.

Prevention

• Notification of new cases to public health authorities for communicable disease control is a legal requirement.

• Care is needed in people with close contact with sputum-positive disease: 10% develop tuberculosis, mostly identified by initial tuberculin testing or chest radiography.

General references

American Thoracic Society: Diagnostic standards and classification of tuberculosis. *Am Rev Respir Dis* 1990, **142**:725–735.

Bass JB Jr, Farer LS, Hopewell PC, *et al.*: Treatment of tuberculosis and tuberculosis infection in adults and children. American Thoracic Society and The Centers for Disease Control and Prevention. *Am J Respir Crit Care Med* 1994, **149**:1359–1374.

Drugs for tuberculosis. *Med Lett Drugs Ther* 1995, **37**:67–70.

Stead WW: Management of health care workers after inadvertent exposure to tuberculosis: a guide for the use of preventive therapy. *Ann Intern Med* 1995, **122**:906–912.

Diagnosis

Symptoms

Persistent fever: developing after recent visit to endemic country.

Mounting fever, headache, malaise, anorexia, dry cough, constipation: abdominal pain in first week of illness.

Continuing fever, mental apathy: in second week.

Abdominal distension, "pea-soup" diarrhea: in third week.

Signs

Pyrexia: in first week.

Rose spots: 2–4-mm erythematous maculo-papules in crops on lower chest and upper abdomen in 30% of patients in second week.

Vagueness and withdrawal, splenomegaly, relative bradycardia: in second week.

Delirium or stupor, distended tender abdomen, dehydration, poor-volume rapid pulse, signs of complications: in third week.

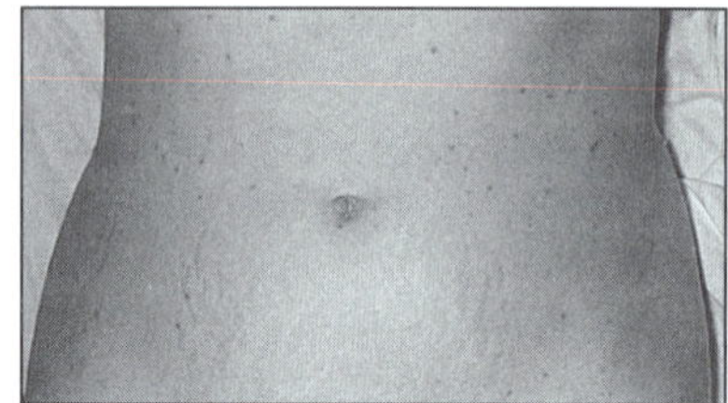

Rose spots in a patient with typhoid fever. (*See* Color Plate.)

Investigations

• Definitive diagnosis needs positive blood or bone-marrow culture.

Blood culture: highest positivity during first week (80%), declining thereafter; often negative if patient has already been given antibiotic.

Bone-marrow culture: often remains positive despite antibiotic administration.

Stool and urine culture: often positive from third week onwards; diagnostic only if clinical picture is compatible.

Widal's test: unreliable and difficult to interpret, so rarely performed.

Complete blood count: leukocyte count decreased, with relative lymphocytosis after first week.

Liver function tests: often mildly raised aspartate and alanine transaminase concentrations.

Complications

• Complications occur only in untreated patients after the second week.

Intestinal hemorrhage: indicated by sudden drop in temperature, rise in pulse rate, and rectal bleeding.

Intestinal perforation: signs of peritonitis may be difficult to detect in an already tender and distended abdomen; presence of gas under diaphragm and ascites may be the only signs.

Myocarditis: indicated by rapid, thready pulse and ECG abnormalities.

Jaundice: may be due to cholangitis, hepatitis, or hemolysis.

Typhoid abscesses: in different organs (rare).

Treatment

Diet and lifestyle

• Adequate nutrition and fluid replacement must be ensured.

• Chronic carriers, especially those handling foods, must practice strict hygiene because of the fecal–oral transmission of the disease; in such patients, attempts should be made to clear carriage.

Pharmacological treatment

General and supportive care

• Nutritional and fluid-electrolyte deficiencies should be corrected in patients presenting late.

Specific treatment

• 4-quinolones are currently the drug of choice in adults.

• Defervescence occurs in 3–5 days.

• Treatment failure, relapse, and chronic carriage are rare.

• Other drugs include third-generation cephalosporins and corticosteroids (in severe toxemia).

Standard dosage	Ciprofloxacin, 500 mg orally twice daily for 14 days (200 mg i.v. with vomiting or diarrhea). *In children (but see* Special points): 10 mg/kg orally or i.v. daily in 2 divided doses. Ceftriaxone, 3–4 g i.v. daily as single dose or 75–100 mg/kg i.v. daily in 2 divided doses for 7–10 days (shorter duration may be equally effective). Adjunctive dexamethasone, 3 mg/kg i.v. initially, then 1 mg/kg 6-hourly for 48 hours.
Contraindications	Hypersensitivity. *Dexamethasone:* caution in pregnancy, renal insufficiency, hypertension, and diabetes.
Special points	*Ciprofloxacin:* currently not recommended in pregnant women and children because of arthropathy in growing animals; this has not, however, been observed in children, and ciprofloxacin should not be withheld if benefits outweigh risks. *Ceftriaxone:* can be used in children and pregnant women but must be given intravenously.
Main drug interactions	*Ciprofloxacin:* NSAIDs, oral iron, anticoagulants. *Ceftriaxone:* probenecid. *Dexamethasone:* phenytoin, barbiturates, ephedrine or rifampin may increase the metabolic clearance of corticosteroids.
Main side effects	*Ciprofloxacin:* nausea, abdominal pain, diarrhea (all unusual). *Ceftriaxone:* headache, nausea, rash. *Dexamethasone:* fluid and electrolyte disturbances.

Treatment of chronic carriers

• Ciprofloxacin, 750 mg, or norfloxacin, 400 mg twice daily for 28 days, is highly effective.

Drug resistance

• Chloramphenicol, cotrimoxazole, and amoxicillin are highly effective if the infecting strains are sensitive to the above drugs.

Treatment aims

To achieve clinical cure.

To prevent complications and relapse.

To prevent chronic fecal carriage after recovery.

Other treatments

• Surgery is needed for intestinal perforation (hemorrhage managed conservatively).

• Cholecystectomy should be reserved for carriers with symptomatic gallbladder disease.

Prognosis

• Untreated, typhoid and paratyphoid fevers have a mortality of up to 20%, mostly from myocarditis and intestinal hemorrhage or perforation; these complications are rarely seen in the United States.

• Recovery begins in the fourth week in the absence of complications.

Follow-up and management

• ~10% of patients relapse, and 3% become chronic fecal carriers after treatment with chloramphenicol, cotrimoxazole, or amoxicillin but rarely after ciprofloxacin treatment.

• After clinical recovery, six consecutive negative stool and urine cultures should be obtained over 3 weeks.

General references

Lassere R, Sangalang RP, Santiago L: Three day treatment of typhoid fever with two different doses of ceftriaxone, compared to 14 day therapy with chloramphenicol: a randomised trial. *J Antimicrob Chemother* 1991, **28**:765–772.

Mandal BK: Modern treatment of typhoid fever. *J Infect* 1991, **22**:1–4.

Sack RB, Rahman M, Yunus M, Khan EN: Antimicrobial resistance in organisms causing diarrheal disease. *Clin Infect Dis* 1997, **24(suppl 1)**: S102–S105.

Diagnosis

Symptoms

Diarrhea: often bloody and with urgency.

Abdominal pain: tenesmus often a prominent feature and should not be confused with constipation.

Anorexia, fatigue.

Fevers, weight loss: in more severe disease.

Skin, joint, or eye symptoms in: <10%.

Signs

• Signs are typically absent in mild or moderate disease (*see* Clinical patterns).

Left lower quadrant abdominal tenderness: evidence of peritoneal signs or ileus requires prompt surgical consultation for perforation or toxic megacolon.

Hematochezia on digital rectal examination.

Fever, tachycardia: in severe disease.

Perianal disease (fissures, abscess, or fistulas): distinctly unusual.

Investigations

Stool culture: *Clostridium difficile*, *Entamoeba histolytica*, *Campylobacter* spp., and other bacterial infections should be excluded.

Complete blood count: to examine for anemia, leukocytosis.

Liver chemistry tests: to evaluate for hepatic inflammation.

Plain abdominal radiography: allows exclusion of dilatation and gives some indication of disease extent (bowel containing feces is probably not severely inflamed).

Colonoscopy with biopsies: allows accurate assessment of extent of disease and histological confirmation of inflammation or dysplasia. Inflammation almost always begins in the rectum extending proximally in a confluent pattern. Biopsies demonstrate crypt distortion, often with abscesses.

Barium enema: less frequently used because of inability to obtain histology.

• Colonoscopy and barium enema should be avoided in an acute attack because they may cause exacerbation; limited sigmoidoscopy with rectal biopsies can often be done in these settings to exclude or confirm the disease.

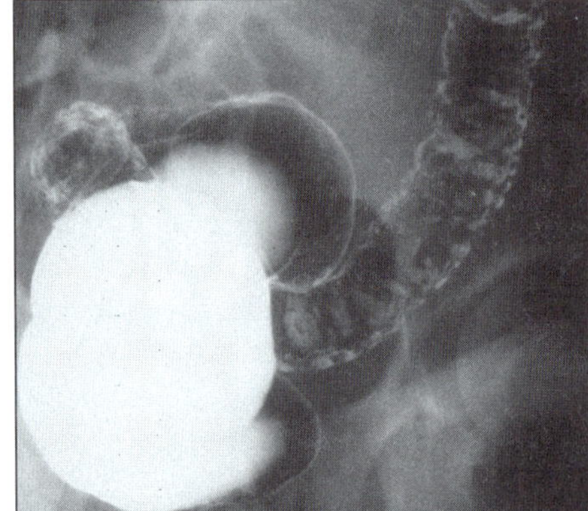

Double-contrast barium enema in severe ulcerative colitis, showing submucosal ulceration in sigmoid and descending colon.

Complications

Hemorrhage: chronic blood loss causing anemia common, life-threatening acute bleeding rare.

Perforation: in 5%, often a sequela of toxic megacolon; 50% mortality; avoidable with careful management and surgical referral.

Strictures: (unusual) colonoscopy and biopsy needed to exclude malignancy.

Colon cancer: risk is dependent on extent and duration of disease; increased risk observed after 10 years in patients with involvement of their entire colon.

Uveitis, episclera: 5%.

Erythema nodosum, pyoderma gangrenosum: 5%.

Arthropathy.

Sclerosis, cholangitis, cholangiocarcinoma: <5%.

Differential diagnosis [1]

Microscopic (lymphocytic) colitis.

Collagenous colitis.

Drug-associated disorders: oral contraceptives have been associated with a Crohn's-like colitis; NSAIDs and purgatives may cause microscopic colitis.

Diversion colitis.

Crohn's colitis.

Irradiation proctitis.

Ischemic colitis.

Bacterial or amebic infection (dysentery).

Irritable bowel syndrome: should not cause bleeding or nocturnal diarrhea.

Cytomegalovirus, herpes simplex, cryptosporidia in immunosuppressed patients.

Colon cancer.

Acute self-limited colitis

Etiology [2]

Cause is unknown but is probably related to an autoimmune process in genetically susceptible individuals; no specific infectious or dietary agents have been reliably identified to date. Overall risk in first-degree relatives is 5%–10%.

Epidemiology

• Patients present at any age; the highest prevalence is in the 2nd and 3rd decades, but a second peak in the 5th and 6th decades has been reported.

• The prevalence in northwestern Europe and the United States is 1 in 1500; it is rarely diagnosed in developing countries.

• An unexplained association with non-smoking exists (95% of sufferers are nonsmokers or exsmokers).

Clinical patterns

Mild disease: diarrhea ≤4 loose stools per day with at most scant amounts of blood.

Moderate disease: 4–6 loose stools per day with constitutional symptoms, abdominal symptoms, and no severe bleeding.

Severe disease: >6 bowel movements per day, persistent blood loss, abdominal tenderness, fevers, tachycardia, hypoalbuminemia.

• Symptoms correlate with length of colonic involvement. Proctitis (disease limited to the rectum) is the most common pattern, with more severe disease usually found in patents with pancolitis.

Treatment

Diet and lifestyle

- Smoking or nicotine patches often of benefit.
- No special precautions are necessary.

Pharmacological treatment [3–5]

For mild attacks

Standard dosage
Initially: sulfasalazine, 1 g 4–6 times daily; mesalamine, 1.2–3.6 g daily; or olsalazine, 1.5–3 g daily. Proctitis may be managed with rectal corticosteroid or 5-aminosalicylic acid preparations.
Maintenance: sulfasalazine, 1.5–4 g daily, mesalamine, 1.2–2.4 g daily, or olsalazine, 1.5–3 g daily; or 5-aminosalicylic acid enemas for disease limited to the distal colon [3].

Contraindications
All: salicylate intolerance, renal failure.
Sulfazalazine: sulfa allergy.

Special points
Regular complete blood counts and urea measurement advised. Increasing dose gradually and taking with food may reduce gastrointestinal side effects.

Main drug interactions
Sulfasalazine: warfarin, anticonvulsants.

Main side effects
Occasional nephrotoxicity.
Sulfasalazine: nausea, headaches, malaise, dyspepsia, reversible male infertility.
Mesalamine: occasional nausea, diarrhea, interstitial nephritis.
Olsalazine: diarrhea in 10%–20% of patients.

For moderate attacks

Standard dosage
Prednisone, 1 mg/kg (up to 60 mg) orally once daily, with oral 5-aminosalicylic acid preparation.

Contraindications
Systemic infections, hypersensitivity.

Special points
Weekly review essential; hospital admission if no improvement within 2 weeks.
Corticosteroids used in short courses; response should occur within 1–4 weeks then taper off drug over 6–8 weeks; if response poor, more severe attack should be assumed; corticosteroids of no value in maintaining remission.

Main drug interactions
None.

Main side effects
Occasional steroid-psychosis; hyperglycemia, asceptic necrosis; osteoporosis, hyperphagia, increased energy. Steroid-related side-effects uncommon if long-term treatment avoided.

For severe attacks

- Treatment includes admission to hospital for close observation, bed rest, high-dose i.v. corticosteroids (*e.g.*, solumedrol, 15 mg every 6 hours), total parenteral nutrition if patient is vomiting or malnourished, deep venous thrombosis prophylaxis. Cyclosporine 2–4 mg/kg/day is of benefit in patients who fail to respond to i.v. steroid therapy. However, complications of hypertension and renal insufficiency are common.
- The colonic diameter should be monitored by plain radiography daily.

For toxic dilatation

- Dilatation of the transverse colon to a diameter of >7 cm accompanied by signs of fever or tachycardia may be treated conservatively for up to 48 hours with nasogastric suction and avoidance of narcotics or other agents that reduce motility. Any clinical or radiographical deterioration during this period or failure to respond to treatment necessitates immediate surgery.

Treatment aims

To achieve and maintain remission.
To avoid life-threatening complications.

Other treatments

- 20% of patients need colectomy at some time; surgery is indicated for the following:
Failed full medical treatment for severe colitis (after 1–2 weeks of hospitalization on i.v. steroids or a trial of cyclosporine).
Toxic megacolon or perforation.
Persistent colitis, with poor quality of life.
Cancer or raised dysplastic lesion.

Prognosis

- Most patients have relapses interspersed with periods of prolonged remission; 90% are capable of full-time work.
- Life expectancy is normal.
- The risk of colon cancer is significantly increased beginning 10–15 years after onset of disease in patients with pancolitis.

Follow-up and management

- Patients should continue taking 5-aminosalicylic acid preparations for 1 year or, for severe or multiple attacks, until they have been free of disease for at least 5 years.
- Patients should be screened by colonoscopy for dysplasia or early colon cancer on a yearly basis if disease present >10 years.

Patient support

Crohn's and Colitis Foundation of America, 386 Park Ave S., New York, NY 10016-7374.

Key references

1. Hanauer SB: Inflammatory bowel disease. *N Engl J Med* 1996, **334:**841–848.

2. Kirsner JB, Short RG (eds.): *Inflammatory Bowel Disease*, edn 4. Baltimore: Williams & Wilkins; 1995.

3. Elton E, Hanauer SB: The medical management of Crohn's disease [review article]. *Aliment Pharmacol Ther* 1996, **10:**1–22.

4. Geier DL, *et al.*: New therapeutic agents in the treatment of inflammatory bowel disease. *Am J Med* 1992, **93:**1991–2008.

5. Reynolds PD, *et al.*: Pharmacotherapy of inflammatory bowel disease. *Dig Dis* 1993, **11:**334–342.

Diagnosis

Symptoms

Vomiting blood.

Passage of black, tarry stool: *i.e.*, melena.

Abdominal pain.

Syncope.

Weight loss.

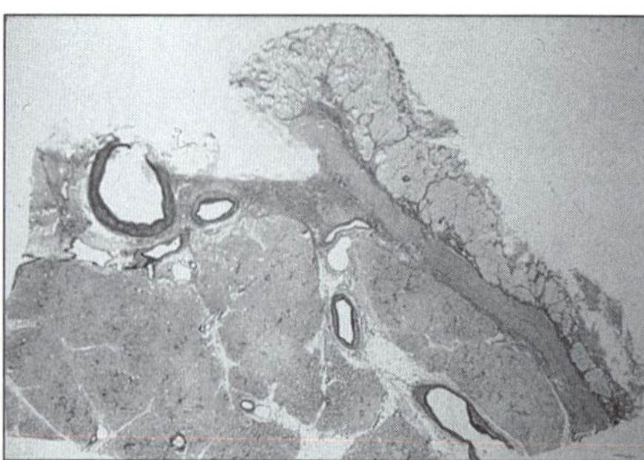

Large hole in an artery in the large duodenal ulcer in a patient who died.

Signs

Hematemesis.

Melena.

Tachycardia with orthostatic hypotension.

Abdominal tenderness: nonspecific.

Stigmata of chronic liver disease (*i.e.*, palmar erythema, spider angiomata, gynecomastia): should be assessed in all patients with upper gastrointestinal bleeding.

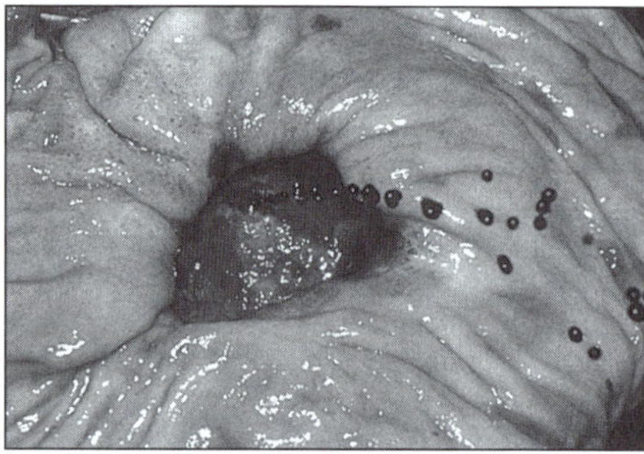

Bleeding gastric ulcer (*see* Color Plate).

Investigations

Complete blood count: evaluate anemia. Initial hemoglobin will not reflect severity of bleeding in acute presentations; presence of microcytosis (*i.e.*, mean corpuscular volume <80) suggests chronic blood loss; adequate platelets, prothrombin time, partial thromboplastin time, and iron stores should also be verified, particularly in patients with evidence of chronic liver disease. Blood urea nitrogen levels are often elevated with bleeding and may rise further in hypotensive patients.

Esophagogastroduodenoscopy: provides visualization of the proximal gastrointestinal tract to the level of the midduodenum. Allows prediction of rebleeding in patients with peptic ulcer disease (*i.e.*, rebleeding is more likely in patients with visible vessels), direct control of hemorrhage in patients with bleeding ulcers or varices, and biopsy of suspicious lesions.

Complications

Exanguination.

Perforation.

Cardiac or cerebrovascular ischemia.

Metabolic acidosis.

Prerenal insufficiency.

Aspiration.

Differential diagnosis

Epistaxis.

Swallowed blood from hemoptysis.

Ingestion of iron or bismuth-containing preparations creating the false impression of melena.

Etiology

Brisk or slow blood loss from the gastrointestinal tract proximal to the ligament of Treitz that most likely arises from one of the following conditions:

Esophageal varices.

Portal gastropathy.

Gastric ulcer.

Duodenal ulcer.

Erosive gastritis (from NSAIDs).

Hemorrhagic gastritis.

Esophagitis esophageal ulcer.

Mallory-Weis tear.

Gastric adenocarcinoma.

Lymphoma.

Hemobilia.

Aortoenteric fistula.

Epidemiology

• Estimated rate of hospitalization for upper gastrointestinal bleeding has been estimated at 150 patients per 100 000 members of the population.

• It is more common in patients with chronic liver disease, renal failure, diabetes mellitus, and individuals with coagulopathies.

• Elderly patients are particularly at risk in part due to limited compensatory reserve; the widespread use of NSAIDs in this population for management of arthritis is a major predisposing factor.

Treatment

Diet and lifestyle

• Patients with a history of peptic ulcer disease should refrain from the use of NSAID medications with the exception of acetaminophen, which does not significantly contribute to erosive disease or platelet dysfunction.

• Patients should not eat for 8 hours prior to endoscopy or surgery; at other times, no evidence suggests that allowing patients to eat will increase their tendency to bleed.

Pharmacological treatment

• *See* Esophagitis, Duodenal ulcer, Gastric ulcer, and Variceal bleeding *for specific treatment regimens*.

• Drug treatment has little if any role in the management of active upper gastrointestinal bleeding except in patients with bleeding from esophageal varices, in whom i.v. octreotide appears beneficial (*see* Variceal bleeding).

• Volume expansion should be rapidly achieved with i.v. crystalloid infusions via large-bore needles in patients with evidence of brisk bleeding or hemodynamic compromise; the patient's volume status and rate of bleeding should be used in conjunction with the hematocrit to determine the need for blood transfusion.

• Transfusion with packed red blood cells should be used judiciously to minimize the chances of iatrogenic infections and complications; avoid overtransfusion.

• In general, young healthy people who are euvolemic can tolerate a hematocrit as low as 20 without serious problems.

Nonpharmacological treatment

For peptic ulcer

Endoscopic treatment (laser, monopolar, bipolar, heater probe, and injection of adrenaline alone, adrenaline and a sclerosant, or alcohol): can reduce rebleeding rate, need for surgery, and mortality; repeat endoscopic treatment may be preferable to surgery in elderly patients [1–3].

Surgery: in patients with continued or recurrent bleeding in hospital; if surgery necessary, best done before repeated episodes of hypotension have impaired chances of recovery.

For bleeding varices

• *See* Variceal bleeding.

Endoscopic variceal injection sclerotherapy, using sclerosants such as monoethanolamine, alcohol, sodium tetradecyl sulfate, or sodium morrhuate: has been shown to reduce the incidence of further bleeding and to reduce mortality in patients with recent bleeding from esophageal varices, and it can stop bleeding from varices.

Endoscopic variceal band ligation: less invasive than surgery, has lower complication rate than endoscopic sclerotherapy.

Balloon tamponade: stops bleeding in 85% of patients, but bleeding recurs in 21%–60% and survival not improved; complications include esophageal rupture and aspiration pneumonia, with lethal complications of 10%.

Transjugular intrahepatic portacaval shunt: for patients who have recurrent variceal bleeding despite sclerotherapy or ligation therapy.

Surgery: for the few patients who do not respond to endoscopic treatment; options include portosystemic shunt, esophageal transection, devascularization, or hepatic transplantation [4].

• Patients with continued bleeding of 6–8 U over 24 hours despite endoscopic attempts at control require surgery.

Complications of treatment

After surgery: pneumonia, renal or cardiac failure, further bleeding.

After endoscopy for bleeding peptic ulcer: precipitation of acute bleeding, perforation, infarction of stomach or duodenum (with injection).

After endoscopy for bleeding varices: esophageal ulceration, perforation, septicemia, distant thrombosis, pleural effusion, aspiration.

Treatment aims

To halt bleeding.

To normalize the patient's volume status and erythrocyte mass.

To prevent further episodes of bleeding.

Prognosis

• For peptic ulcer bleeding, the risk of rebleeding in hospital is 15%–30%, of needing urgent surgery 15%–20%, and of death 5%–10%.

• The risk of death after admission with first variceal bleeding is 30%.

• 70% of patients with bleeding varices die within 1–4 years.

• Bleeding due to Mallory–Weiss tear, esophagitis, gastritis, and duodenitis has excellent prognosis.

• Most patients with bleeding upper gastrointestinal cancer die within 1 year.

Follow-up and management

• Ulcer patients with major bleeding should have follow-up endoscopy to check healing and eradication of *Helicobacter pylori*.

• Patients with a second major bleed should be considered for surgery.

• Patients with bleeding varices need re-peat endoscopy and sclerotherapy until varices are eradicated.

Key references

1. Consensus Development Panel, National Institutes of Health 1990: Consensus statement on therapeutic endoscopy and bleeding ulcers. *Gastrointest Endosc* 1990, **36**:S62–S63.

2. Cook DJ, *et al.*: Endoscopic therapy for acute nonvariceal upper gastrointestinal hemorrhage: a meta-analysis. *Gastroenterology* 1992, **102**:139–148.

3. Fleischer D: Endoscopic hemostasis in non-variceal bleeding. *Endoscopy* 1992, **24**:58–63.

4. Wheatley KE, Dykes PW: Upper gastrointestinal bleeding: when to operate. *Postgrad Med J* 1990, **45**:926–936.

General references

Laine L: Upper gastrointestinal bleeding. *Alimentary Pharmacol Ther* 1993, **7**:207–232.

Laine L, Peterson WL: Medical progress: bleeding peptic ulcer. *N Engl J Med* 1994, **331**:717–727.

Diagnosis [1]

Symptoms

• Many affected patients will not spontaneously mention urinary incontinence to their physician; routinely ask all patients >65 years of age (especially women): "Do you have trouble controlling your urine?"

• History should include detailed description of episodes, estimate of voided quantity (often inaccurate or unknown), onset, frequency, fluid intake patterns, change in bowel or sexual function, medications, menopausal status, mental status changes.

• 24-hour voiding record can be very useful in characterizing incontinence; should include time and amount of voids and associated symptoms (urgency, coughing, sense of complete evacuation).

Signs

• Physical examination should include assessment of intravascular fluid status (orthostatic BP), abdominal examination (distended bladder), genital, pelvic, and rectal examinations (cystocele, rectocele).

Classification

• To guide diagnostic evaluation and therapy, chronic urinary incontinence should be classified as being caused by detrusor muscle (cholinergic) under- or overactivity, and outlet (alpha-mediated smooth inner and somatic external sphincters), under- or overactivity, or a combination. The relationships of the traditional classification of urge, stress, and overflow incontinence to detrusor and outlet function are shown in the table.

Physiological causes of common types of chronic urinary incontinence

Detrusor underactivity (high PVR)	Detrusor overactivity	Outlet obstruction (high PVR)	Outlet insufficiency
DHIC (urge symptoms) Overflow	Urge	DSD (urge symptoms) Overflow	Stress

---

Investigations

Postvoid residual (PVR) measurement: indicated in virtually all patients; identifies detrusor underactivity and/or outlet obstruction. Normal PVR is <50 cc; borderline, 50–200 cc; abnormal >200 cc. PVR can be estimated via ultrasound if in-and-out catheterization is not feasible.

Urinalysis, serum creatinine, blood urea nitrogen, glucose, calcium.

Other investigations as indicated by initial workup: consider urinary cytology if hematuria and/or irritative voiding symptoms without urinary tract infection (UTI); i.v. pyelogram if hematuria.

Complications

Urinary retention, reflux, renal damage (detrusor underactivity, outlet obstruction).

Social impairment due to limitations in activities.

Treatment [1]

Diet and lifestyle

Bladder training: conscious delays in voiding; appropriate in detrusor instability (detrusor overactivity without UMN lesion) and stress incontinence.

Habit (timed) or prompted voiding: void on a regular basis, before urge is felt; timing parameters are based on incontinence record; most helpful for cognitively impaired patients with urge incontinence.

• Pelvic muscle ("Kegel") exercises improve stress incontinence among motivated women; they strengthen voluntary periurethral and pelvic muscles, exerting a closing force on the urethra. Exercise performed as 10-second flexion, 10-second relaxation. Target performing exercises 30–80 times a day for at least 6 weeks; can also be used in postsurgical incontinence due to outlet laxity.

Pharmacological treatment

Anticholinergic medications

Usual dosage	Oxybutynin, 2.5–5.0 mg 3–4 times daily.
	Tricyclic antidepressant (*e.g.*, amitriptyline, imipramine, doxepin), 10–25 mg 1–3 times daily.
	Probantheline, 7.5–30 mg 3–5 times daily.
Contraindications	Narrow-angle glaucoma.
Special points	Useful for low-PVR detrusor overactivity (urge) incontinence; PVR should be checked after obtaining therapeutic response or maximal tolerated dose, to rule out retention.
Main drug interactions	None.
Main side effects	Dry mouth, orthostasis, constipation, urinary retention.

Phenylpropanolamine

Usual dosage	50 mg twice daily (sustained release form).
Contraindications	Use with caution, if at all, in patients with hyperthyroidism, cardiovascular disorders, hypertension, diabetes, glaucoma, or prostatic hypertrophy.
Special points	Useful in mild stress incontinence; monitor blood pressure among hypertensive patients; some preparations contain tartrazine (yellow dye no. 5), a potent allergen in some patients.
Main drug interactions	Do not use with monoamine oxidase inhibitors; additive effects with other sympathomimetic agents.
Main side effects	Usually none or mild at therapeutic doses; can cause nervousness, restlessness, palpitations, elevations in blood pressure.

Treatment aims

To minimize or eliminate symptoms.
To maximize social function.

Other treatments

Refer to urologist or gynecologist for further diagnosis and treatment if:
High PVR.

Diagnosis uncertain and *either* no reasonable empiric plan *or* lack of consistent picture from symptoms and signs.

Failure to respond to empiric trial *and* candidate for further (usually surgical) therapy.

Hematuria without infection.

Other comorbidities that warrant investigation: suspected new systemic or local neurological condition, prostate nodule, severe symptoms of difficulty emptying bladder (suggests mass lesion), incontinence associated with recurrent UTIs (rule out structural defect), severe and symptomatic pelvic prolapse.

Prognosis

Urge incontinence: 90% of appropriately selected women will show improvement or cure with bladder training; up to 40% of women will be cured, and up to 80% improved, with pharmacological treatment (anticholinergic agents).

Stress incontinence: 15% cured and 60% improved with pelvic muscle or bladder training, 15% cured and up to 60% improved with pharmacological treatment (alpha-agonists), 80% cured with surgery.

Follow-up and management

As appropriate to condition and treatment, routine inquiry regarding recurrence of symptoms is indicated.

Key references

1. Urinary Incontinence Guideline Panel: *Urinary Incontinence in Adults: Clinical Practice Guideline.* Rockville: Agency for Health Care Policy and Research, Public Health Service, U.S. Department of Health and Human Services; 1992. [AHCPR publication 92-0038.] (800-358-9295 or http://text.nlm.nih.gov/).

2. Winograd CH, Resnick NM: Incontinence. In *Scientific American Medicine*, vol IX. Edited by Rubenstein E, Federman DD. New York: Scientific American Press; 1991.

Diagnosis

Symptoms and signs

Lower urinary tract infection

Cystitis: dysuria, frequency, and suprapubic tenderness.

Acute prostatitis: dysuria, frequency, fever, perineal pain, obstructive voiding dysfunction, tenderness.

Chronic prostatitis: relapsing infection, voiding dysfunction, abdominal or back pain.

Upper urinary tract infection

Acute pyelonephritis: fever, chills, prostration, back or flank pain and tenderness, dysuria, and frequency.

Renal abscesses: fever and chills, flank pain and tenderness, flank or abdominal mass, dysuria, and frequency.

Symptomatic bacteremia of urinary tract origin: clinical features of bacteremia often overshadow those relating to urinary tract.

Investigations

To establish presence of infection

Urine culture: $>10^2$ colony-forming units (CFU) coliforms/mL or $>10^5$ CFU noncoliforms/mL in symptomatic women, 10^3 CFU bacteria/mL in symptomatic men, $>10^5$ CFU bacteria/mL in asymptomatic patients on two consecutive specimens, $>10^2$ CFU bacteria/mL in catheterized patients, any growth of bacteria from a suprapubic aspirate in symptomatic patients.

Urine microscopy: pyuria (>10 leukocytes/mL unspun urine) supportive evidence of urinary tract infection but not specific; pus cells in "sterile" urine (sterile pyuria) may indicate fastidious organisms or previous antibiotic treatment; microscopic hematuria in 50% of patients.

Dipstick testing of urine: combined leukocyte esterase and nitrite test useful screening procedure, with negative predictive value of 96%-97% at level of 10^5 CFU/mL.

To establish site of infection

• Whether infection is confined to the lower tract or has ascended to the upper tract has important treatment implications; the distinction is usually made clinically.

Radiography

• Radiography is used to identify structural abnormalities of urinary tract, including reflux nephropathy, obstruction, calculi, congenital abnormalities, and, in children, vesicoureteric reflux.

• It is indicated in children and men in first infection and in women with recurrent infections, upper urinary tract infection, unusual infecting organism, fever persisting >48 hours after starting treatment, coexistent hypertension, or persistent microscopic hematuria.

Intravenous urography: investigation of choice in adults (usually delayed until after recovery); ultrasonography may be substituted or added in the case of renal impairment or when renal abscess or pelvic disease is suspected.

^{99m}Tc-DMSA scan and ultrasonography: with either voiding cystourethrography or radionuclide cystography; investigation of choice in children.

Complications

Reflux nephropathy: cortical scarring and clubbing of underlying calyces in infants with bacteriuria associated with vesicoureteric reflux.

Renal damage, perinephric abscess formation, septicemia: due to infection in presence of complicating factors (*e.g.*, obstruction, stones, vesicoureteric reflux).

Treatment

Diet and lifestyle

• A high fluid intake may help to alleviate dysuria during an acute episode; in the long term, it may be useful prophylactically.
• In women, postcoital voiding may be helpful; those using diaphragms and spermicides may benefit from changing to alternative contraceptive methods.

Pharmacological treatment

Indications

For lower urinary tract infections (uncomplicated): 3–5-day courses of trimethoprim, co-trimoxazole, nitrofurantoin, or co-amoxiclav; as effective as 7–14-day course; result in fewer relapses than single-dose treatment.

For lower urinary tract infections (complicated): antibiotic therapy as above continued for 7–14 days; short courses not suitable.
In pregnant women: 7–10-day course of amoxicillin, cephalexin, or nitrofurantoin; early screening and treatment of asymptomatic bacteriuria.
In men with prostatitis: trimethoprim, co-trimoxazole, or a quinolone for 4 weeks (longer for chronic prostatitis); nonbacterial prostatitis may respond to doxycycline or erythromycin.

For upper urinary tract infections (uncomplicated): severity of constitutional upset determines need for hospitalization.
In patients treated at home: oral trimethoprim, co-trimoxazole, co-amoxiclav, or quinolone for 14 days.
In hospitalized patients: initially, i.v. cefuroxime, cefotaxime, ciprofloxacin, co-amoxiclav, or co-trimoxazole; when fever subsides, oral treatment dictated by culture, continued for 14 days; relapses treated for 6 weeks.

For upper urinary tract infection (complicated):
In previously instrumented or catheterized patients: initially i.v. ceftazidime or amoxicillin with ciprofloxacin or gentamicin.
In patients with obstructed, infected upper tract: antibiotic therapy as above, with prompt drainage by percutaneous nephrostomy pending definitive surgery.
In patients with renal abscess: antibiotic therapy as above, with i.v. flucloxacillin, then 4–6-week courses of antibiotics based on cultures; percutaneous drainage usually needed.

Selected regimens

Amoxicillin, 500 mg orally 3 times daily.
Cefotaxime, 1 g i.v. 3 times daily.
Ceftazidime, 1–2 g i.v. twice daily.
Cefuroxime, 750 mg i.v. 3 times daily.
Cephalexin, 500 mg orally 4 times daily.
Ciprofloxacin, 500 mg orally or 200 mg i.v. twice daily.
Co-trimoxazole, 800 mg (sulfamethoxazole) and 160 mg (trimethoprim) orally twice daily.
Flucloxacillin, 500 mg i.v. 4 times daily.
Gentamicin, 80 mg i.v. 3 times daily, follow peak and trough levels.
Nitrofurantoin, 100 mg orally 4 times daily.
Ofloxacin, 200 mg orally twice daily.
Trimethoprim, 200 mg orally twice daily.

Antibiotics: contraindications and side effects

Chronic renal failure: nitrofurantoin ineffective, causes neuropathy; tetracyclines worsen uremia; aminoglycosides can be used but concentrations must be monitored to avoid nephrotoxicity and auditory/vestibular toxicity.

Pregnancy: tetracyclines cause bone or teeth dystrophy; trimethoprim possibly teratogenic; quinolones possibly cause arthropathy; aminoglycosides cause auditory/vestibular toxicity.

Infancy: tetracyclines cause bone or teeth dystrophy; sulfonamides cause hemolysis.

Prophylaxis

• Postcoital or nightly: trimethoprim, 100 mg, nitrofurantoin, 100 mg, or co-trimoxazole, 480 mg, reduces recurrence in women with normal urinary tracts.

• Prophylaxis is also useful after acute pyelonephritis in pregnancy.

Treatment aims
To relieve symptoms.
To prevent increase in prematurity and perinatal mortality.
To prevent and eradicate systemic sepsis.
To prevent progressive renal damage.

Prognosis
• Renal impairment in reflux nephropathy may progress without persisting infection and reflux.
• Adults with uncomplicated infection suffer minimal long-term sequelae if adequately treated.
• Complicated upper tract infections are potentially more damaging and may cause progressive renal scarring.

Follow-up and management
• Follow-up urine cultures are essential in pregnancy, after uncomplicated acute pyelonephritis, and after all complicated urinary tract infections.
• Any predisposing factors should be treated.
• Obstruction must be relieved by surgery or intermittent self-catheterization when indicated; calculi must be removed.

Recurrent infection
Relapse
• Relapse occurs soon after cessation of treatment.
• The same organism is involved.
• Relapse indicates inappropriate drug or duration of treatment, poor compliance, occult renal involvement, or underlying urinary tract abnormality.

Reinfection
• Reinfection occurs >6 weeks after cessation of treatment.
• A different organism is involved.
• Reinfection indicates failure of host defenses.

General references

Childs SJ, Egan RJ: Bacteriuria and urinary infections in the elderly. *Urol Clin North Am* 1996, **23**:43–54.
Funfstuck R, Smith JW, Tschape H, Stein G: Pathogenetic aspects of uncomplicated urinary tract infection: recent advances. *Clin Nephrol* 1997, **47**:13–18.
Rosenfeld DL, *et al.*: Current recommendations for children with urinary tract infections. *Clin Pediatr* 1995, **34**:261–264.

Diagnosis

Symptoms

Itching and swelling of skin.

Arthralgia: in severe urticaria or urticarial vasculitis.

Painful or burning sensation of the skin: in urticarial vasculitis.

Signs

Evanescent, red, elevated nonpitting papules or plaques: often with blanched centers or annular configurations.

Angioedema of the lips and periorbital regions: not uncommon.

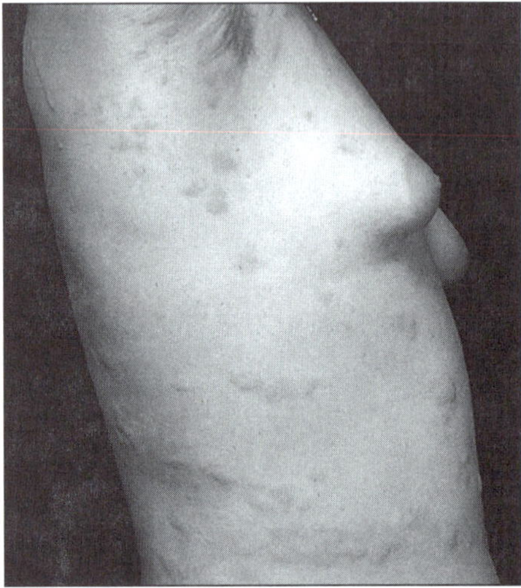

Scattered urticarial wheals on the trunk. (*See* Color Plate.)

Investigations

Acute urticaria (<6 weeks) [1,2]

• Usually an elaborate work-up is not warranted; a standard history is taken and a physical examination is performed with a special emphasis on food and drug ingestion.

Chronic urticaria (>6 weeks) [1,2]

• Very challenging and costly tests are rarely helpful.

• In the initial work-up, care should be taken to look for intolerance to aspirin and tartrazine (FDA yellow dye no. 5) and benzoic acid derivatives used as food preservatives. Low-grade chronic infections, especially *Helicobacter pylori* infection [3], should be ruled out.

• Chronic urticaria may be a presenting sign of underlying connective tissue disease or malignancy, especially in cases of urticarial vasculitis.

Complications

Underlying connective tissue disease or malignancy: can be missed in work-up of chronic urticaria [4].

Anaphylactic shock: in cases of IgE-mediated acute urticarial reactions.

Differential diagnosis

Urticarial vasculitis.

Urticarial component of bullous pemphigoid.

Erythema multiforme.

Herpes gestationis.

Erythema annulare centrifugum.

Erythema chronicum migrans.

Cutaneous larva migrans (creeping eruption).

Mycosis fungoides.

Erythema marginatum.

Erythema infectiosum (fifth disease).

Dermal contact dermatitis.

Cholinergic urticaria.

Solar urticaria.

Cold urticaria.

Pressure urticaria.

Hereditary angioedema: usually involves only mucous membranes with few urticarial skin lesions; life-threatening laryngeal spasm.

Etiology

• A cause is usually not identified except in cases of acute urticaria from food or drug ingestion.

• Chronic urticaria is most often idiopathic.

Epidemiology

• Urticaria affects 20% of population at some point in their lives.

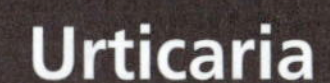

Treatment

Diet and lifestyle

• Known triggering agents such as food dyes and preservatives and aspirin must be identified and avoided.

Pharmacological treatment

• Topical steroids or antipruritic agents are often helpful.

H$_1$ and H$_2$ antagonists [5]

Standard dosage	Cetirizine HCl, 10 mg orally once daily.
	Terfenadine, 60 mg orally twice daily.
	Astemizole, 10 mg orally daily.
	Hydroxyzine hydrochloride, 25 mg orally every 6–8 hours.
	Doxepin, 10–50 mg orally 3 times daily.
	Cyproheptadine, 4 mg orally 3 times daily "used for cold urticaria."
	Loratadine, 10 mg orally 3 times daily.
Contraindications	Porphyrias.
Main drug interactions	*Terfenadine*, *astemizole* with concurrent erythromycin can cause fatal ventricular arrhythmias.
Main side effects	Drowsiness, anticholinergic effects, ventricular arrhythmias reported after concurrent use of terfenadine and astemizole with erythromycin.

Systemic corticosteroids

Often used in cases of acute urticaria.

Should be avoided as a first-line treatment in all but acute and severe cases of urticaria.

Standard dosage	Prednisone, 40–60 mg orally daily decreased over a 2- to 3-week period.
	Triamcinolone, i.m. 40–60 mg as a single dose.
Contraindications	History of peptic ulcer disease, tuberculosis, glaucoma, diabetes.
Main drug interactions	None.
Main side effects	Aseptic necrosis of bone, especially the femoral head; exacerbation of narrow-angle glaucoma; transient hyperglycemia.

Key references

1. Cooper KD: Urticaria and angioedema: diagnosis and evaluation. *J Am Acad Dermatol* 1991, **25**:166–174.

2. Huston DP, Bressler RB: Urticaria and angioedema. *Med Clin North Am* 1992, **76**:805–840.

3. Reborah A, Drago F, Parodi A: May *Helicobacter pylori* be important for dermatologists? *Dermatology* 1995, **191**:6–8.

4. Mehregan DR, *et al.*: Urticarial vasculitis: a histopathologic and clinical review of 72 cases. *J Am Acad Dermatol* 1992, **26**:441–448.

5. Ring J, Behrendt H: H$_1$ and H$_2$ antagonists in allergic and pseudoallergic diseases. *Clin Exp Allergy* 1990, **20**:43–49.

Diagnosis

Symptoms and signs

Major hematemesis or melena.

Chronic blood loss, with iron-deficiency anemia: indicating portal-hypertensive gastropathy.

• Sites of bleeding in patients with portal hypertension are esophageal (most frequent); fundal, lesser curve, antral, in hiatal hernia (gastric varices); ileostomy, colostomy, colonic, and rectal (ectopic varices). These may present with massive rectal bleeding [1].

Investigations

Esophagogastroduodenoscopy: to evaluate varices and gastric mucosa for portal gastropathy.

Doppler ultrasonography, angiography: to establish patency of portal vein.

Blood tests, CT, liver biopsy: to identify cause of underlying liver disease.

Measurement of portal venous, wedged hepatic venous, or intravariceal pressure: endoscopic needle, endoscopic pressure gauge; special investigations, mainly for research use in studies using pharmacologic agents.

Complications

Infection: in ~30% of patients during admission.

Renal failure: acute tubular necrosis, hepatorenal syndrome.

Delirium tremens, Wernicke–Korsakoff syndrome: related to alcohol withdrawal.

Ascites: precipitated by fluid overload.

Portal systemic encephalopathy: precipitated by blood in gut and liver hypoxia.

Aspiration pneumonia.

Spontaneous bacterial peritonitis.

Differential diagnosis

Bleeding caused by the following:
Peptic ulcer.
Mallory–Weiss tear.
Gastric erosions.
Gastric carcinoma.
Portal-hypertensive gastropathy.
Gastric vascular malformations.
Other sources of gastrointestinal bleeding.

Etiology

• Precipitants of variceal bleeding include the following:
Infection.
Drugs: *e.g.*, aspirin, NSAIDs.
Development of hepatocellular carcinoma or portal-vein thrombosis in cirrhotic patients.
Heavy alcohol binges in cirrhotic patients.

Epidemiology

• Varices develop in 90% of patients with cirrhosis; the risk of hemorrhage is highest in the first 2 years after identification.
• The risk of bleeding is highest in patients with large esophageal varices (>5 mm diameter), red signs on varices, and poor liver function.

Conditions complicated by variceal bleeding

Precirrhotic severe alcoholic hepatitis/fatty liver.
Cirrhosis.
Schistosomiasis.
Splenic-vein thrombosis: usually causes gastric fundal varices, with no esophageal varices.
Budd–Chiari syndrome.
Congenital hepatic fibrosis.
Idiopathic portal hypertension.
Nodular regenerative hyperplasia of liver.
Partial nodular transformation of liver.

Pugh's modified grading of the severity of liver disease

Points	1	2	3
Encephalopathy	None	Grade 1–2	Grade 3–4
Ascites	Absent	Slight	Moderate
Bilirubin (mg/dL)	<2.0	2.0–3.0	>3.0
Albumin (g/L)	>35	28–35	<28
Prothrombin (secs, prolonged)	1–3	4–10	>10

Pugh's grade A, 5–6; B, 7–9; C, 10–15 points.

Treatment

Diet and lifestyle

- Patients must avoid NSAIDs such as aspirin.

- Excessive amounts of acetaminophen (e.g, >4 g/day) should be avoided.

- Alcohol should be avoided if the liver disease is alcoholic cirrhosis.

- Patients should have ready access to aute care medical services.

Pharmacological treatment

Emergency drug treatment

- Octreotide is useful when emergency endoscopy is not available or is delayed; octreotide, 25–50 μg/h i.v. for 2–5 days [2].

Vasopressin: not as effective and associated with significant complications.

Prophylaxis: primary and secondary

- Propranolol reduces the risk of first hemorrhage; the resting pulse rate should be reduced to 60 beats/min or by 25% of the pretreatment rate. Treatment is recommended in cirrhotic patients with large varices and red signs. Beta-blockade also reduces bleeding from portal gastropathy and possibly reduces the risk of recurrent variceal bleeding.

- For prevention of recurrent hemorrhage, endoscopic banding or sclerotherapy should be repeated until varices are obliterated.

Nonpharmacological treatment

Resuscitation

Airway protection to prevent aspiration.

Insertion of large i.v. line (cross-matching of at least 6 units of blood).

Crystalloid and colloid infusion to maintain circulation while cross-matched blood is awaited.

Insertion of central venous line to guide further replacement therapy when systolic blood pressure >100 mm Hg.

Fresh frozen plasma to correct clotting abnormalities.

Platelet transfusion if thrombocytopenia exists.

Emergency treatment

Emergency endoscopy to confirm variceal bleeding.

Emergency endoscopic banding or sclerotherapy: treatment of choice; complications include fever, aspiration, esophageal perforation, and mediastinitis; gastric fundal varices respond poorly to sclerotherapy; complication rate of banding lower than that of sclerotherapy [3].

Balloon tamponade for temporary control of bleeding or bleeding refractory to sclerotherapy.

Other options

Transjugular intrahepatic portal-systemic stent shunt (TIPs): if emergency endoscopic treatment fails; also under evaluation for prevention of recurrent hemorrhages, but high rate of shunt occlusion (30% at 1 year) and encephalopathy (10%–20%) [4].

Emergency shunt surgery.

Emergency esophageal transection.

Liver transplantation: can be considered for prevention of recurrent hemorrhage in patients with liver failure.

Treatment aims

- The aims of treatment, in order of importance, are as follows:

To resuscitate the patient.

To control bleeding quickly.

To maintain liver function.

To identify and treat complications.

To prevent rebleeding.

Prognosis

- Esophageal band ligation or sclerotherapy has high success rates, with bleeding controlled in 90% of patients and variceal size reduced after 2–3 sessions.

- 70% of patients rebleed after balloon tamponade, so definitive treatment must be arranged.

- Mortality is 30%–40% with the first variceal bleed, 15%–20% with subsequent bleeds.

- Prognosis depends on the underlying liver function.

- ~ One-third of deaths in cirrhotic patients are related to bleeding.

Follow-up and management

- Patients should be followed-up every 3 months for the first year after the varices have been obliterated by band ligation or sclerotherapy.

- After TIPs placement, Doppler ultrasound should be performed every 6 months to evaluate shunt patency.

Key references

1. Burroughs A, Bosch J: Clinical manifestations and management of bleeding episodes in cirrhotics. In *Oxford Textbook of Clinical Hepatology*. Edited by McIntyre N, *et al.* Oxford: Oxford University Press; 1991:408–425.

2. Planas R: A prospective randomized trial comparing somatostatin and sclerotherapy in the treatment of acute variceal bleeding. *Hepatology* 1994, **20**:370–375.

3. Stiegman GV, *et al.*: Endoscopic sclerotherapy as compared with endoscopic ligation for bleeding oesophageal varices. *N Engl J Med* 1992, **326**:1527–1532.

4. Rossle M, *et al.*: The transjugular intrahepatic portosystemic stent-shunt procedure for variceal bleeding. *N Engl J Med* 1994, **330**:165–171.

Diagnosis

Symptoms

Crops of painful purple areas on skin.

Symptoms of the predisposing disease.

Signs

Painful, palpable purpura: the three "P's."

Crops of purple nodules: usually in dependent areas.

Lesions: tender; do not blanch; hemorrhagic blisters; black, necrotic, ulcerating in severe disease.

Finger pulp 2–3-mm lesions: indicating connective tissue disease, particularly rheumatoid arthritis.

Nail bed linear lesions: indicating trauma, connective tissue disease, or systemic infection.

Net-like pattern (livedo reticularis): indicating connective tissue disease, cryoglobulinemia, antiphospholipid syndrome, or polyarteritis nodosa.

Subcutaneous nodules along arteries: indicating polyarteritis nodosa.

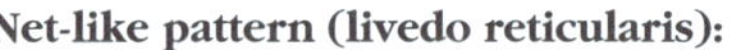

Cutaneous vasculitis on the legs, showing red/purple palpable painful lesions, some of which have overlying hemorrhagic blisters. (*See* Color Plate.)

Investigations

Urinalysis, urine microscopy, serum creatinine measurement: to identify renal involvement.

Blood culture, culture of possible sites of infection: to identify infective cause.

Measurement of rheumatoid factor, antinuclear antibodies, antineutrophil cytoplasmic antibodies, anticardiolipin antibodies: to identify connective tissue disorders.

Cryoglobulin measurement: collected after fasting and taken to laboratory at 37°C.

Skin biopsy: not indicated if clinical picture is typical, because histology often shows nonspecific leukocytoclastic vasculitis, but may help in patients with drug-induced, infective, or inflammatory vasculitis; may also be helpful in identifying infiltrating inflammatory cells, type and size of blood vessels involved, and whether granulomatous changes are present.

Complications

Ulceration: particularly on lower limbs; may follow skin biopsy.

Secondary infection.

Renal involvement: in 30%–60% of patients.

Joint, gastrointestinal tract, CNS, or lung involvement.

Differential diagnosis

Purpura.

Thrombocytopenia.

Platelet dysfunction.

Corticosteroid treatment.

Old age.

Scurvy.

Trauma.

Nonaccidental injury in children.

Hemangioma.

Kaposi's sarcoma.

Bacillary angiomatosis.

Etiology

Causes include the following:

Environmental factors
Gravitational stasis.
Cold exposure.

Infection
Acute: meningococcal meningitis (1–3 weeks after throat infection), gonorrhea.
Chronic: urinary infections, dental abscess, leprosy, hepatitis B and C.

Drugs
Antibiotics: *e.g.,* sulfonamides.
Warfarin (rarely causes hemorrhagic skin infarction).

Inflammation
Immune complexes: *e.g.,* connective tissue disorders.
Cryoglobulins: *e.g.,* in malignancy.
Autoantibodies: *e.g.,* antineutrophil cytoplasmic antibody in Wegener's granulomatosis (may be secondary phenomenon).

Epidemiology

- Vasculitis is a common condition.
- The male:female ratio is equal.
- It can affect people at any age.

Treatment

Diet and lifestyle

• Patients must avoid cold, gravitational effects (with bed rest during acute episodes), and tight garments.

Pharmacological treatment

• Drugs that are probable causes of vasculitis should be discontinued.

• Precipitating infections should be treated by antibiotics.

Prednisone

• Prednisolone may be ineffective, and side effects limit use to patients with severe progressive systemic disease.

Standard dosage	Prednisone, 60–80 mg daily initially.
Contraindications	Untreated infection; caution in pregnancy because causes neonatal adrenal suppression.
Main drug interactions	Antihypertensives, antidiabetics, diuretics, antiepileptics.
Main side effects	Diabetes, osteoporosis, mental disturbance, peptic ulceration, infections, suppressed growth in children, proximal myopathy, cataracts, hypertension, acute adrenal insufficiency.

Dapsone

• Dapsone is often effective against chronic vasculitis, although this is not mentioned on the manufacturer's prescribing information.

Standard dosage	Dapsone, 50–100 mg daily.
Contraindications	Porphyrias, severe anemia, glucose-6-phosphate dehydrogenase.
Special points	Folate supplements needed in pregnancy (causes neonatal hemolysis and methemoglobinemia). Regular blood checks necessary.
Main drug interactions	Probenecid.
Main side effects	Agranulocytosis, hemolytic anemia, headaches, nausea, neuropathy, exfoliative dermatitis, hepatitis.

Indomethacin

• Indomethacin is sometimes effective in urticarial vasculitis, although this is not mentioned on the manufacturer's prescribing information.

Standard dosage	Indomethacin, 50–150 mg daily.
Contraindications	Active peptic ulceration; caution in renal impairment, epilepsy, parkinsonism, salicylate hypersensitivity.
Special points	Excreted in breast milk.
Main drug interactions	Warfarin, angiotensin-converting enzyme inhibitors, haloperidol, digoxin, diuretics, lithium, probenecid.
Main side effects	Gastrointestinal discomfort, nausea, ulceration and bleeding, asthma, tinnitus, headache, vertigo, drowsiness, convulsions, fluid retention, renal failure, hypertension, corneal deposits, thrombocytopenia, angioedema.

Treatment aims

To alleviate discomfort.
To prevent skin ulceration.
To detect systemic involvement early.

Other treatments

• Plasmapheresis: has been used to remove immune complexes in patients with SLE; no evidence of benefit has been shown in controlled studies.

Prognosis

• Individual episodes may clear after 3–6 weeks.

• Relapse and chronic disease are common.

• Patients with infective or drug-induced vasculitis usually recover fully on removal of the cause, although chronic vasculitis or, rarely, fatal systemic necrotizing vasculitis occur.

• The prognosis of inflammatory vasculitis depends on the cause: up to 25% of patients with renal involvement develop chronic renal problems in Henoch–Schönlein purpura.

Follow-up and management

• Renal involvement must be detected by weekly urinalysis and microscopy during an episode and serum creatinine and blood pressure measurement every 2 weeks.

• Cutaneous complications must be treated.

• Patients must be monitored for side effects of treatment.

General references

Berlit P: The spectrum of vasculopathies in the differential diagnosis of vasculitis. *Semin Neurol* 1994, **14**:370–379.

Somer T, Finegold SM: Vasculidities associated with infections, immunization, and antimicrobial drugs. *Clin Infect Dis* 1995, **20**:1010–1036.

Watts RA, Scott DG: ABC of rheumatology, rashes, and vasculitis. *BMJ* 1995, **310(6987)**:1128–1132.

Diagnosis

Symptoms

• Symptoms depend on the size and site of the vessel involved. The following concentrates particularly on primary systemic vasculitis involving small- and medium-sized arteries.

Malaise, weight loss, fever, diffuse myalgia, arthralgia.
Symptoms of any underlying disease or secondary vasculitis: *e.g.*, rheumatoid arthritis, SLE.
Rash.
Epistaxis, nasal crusting, sinusitis: especially in Wegener's granulomatosis.
Chest pain, hemoptysis, dyspnea, cough, late-onset asthma (normally precedes Churg–Strauss syndrome).
Mouth ulcers, abdominal pain, diarrhea.
Numbness, weakness.

Signs

Pyrexia, lymphadenopathy, muscle wasting, weakness.
Microscopic hematuria or proteinuria, or both.
Skin purpura, ulcer, infarction.
Nasal crusting or collapse, septal perforation: especially in Wegener's granulomatosis.
Crackles, wheeze, cardiomyopathy, pericarditis: especially in Churg–Strauss vasculitis.
Mononeuritis or mononeuritis multiplex, peripheral neuropathy.
Arthritis: usually of large joints.

Investigations

Urinalysis: most urgent investigation because renal involvement influences prognosis.
Plasma urea and creatinine, 24-hour urinary protein and creatinine clearance measurement: to assess renal function.
Complete blood count: shows anemia, leukocytosis (leukocyte count normal or low in vasculitis secondary to rheumatoid arthritis or SLE), eosinophilia (especially in Churg–Strauss vasculitis), thrombocytosis.
ESR, CRP, and liver enzyme (*e.g.*, alkaline phosphatase) measurement: raised values.
Antineutrophil cytoplasmic autoantibody analysis: most useful for diagnosis; diffuse cytoplasmic staining (anti-proteinase III) in 80% of patients with systemic Wegener's granulomatosis, 50% limited Wegener's; perinuclear staining less specific (antimyeloperoxidase) but common in microscopic polyangiitis and idiopathic crescentic glomerulonephritis [1,2].
Other autoantibody tests: antinuclear antibody and rheumatoid factor nonspecific; may reflect underlying disease; C3 and C4 usually increased in primary vasculitis, low or normal in vasculitis associated with SLE and rheumatoid arthritis; high levels of cryoglobulins may indicate need for plasma exchange.
Von Willebrand's factor antigen test: measure of vascular damage; also increased in noninflammatory vascular injury (*e.g.*, thrombosis).
Viral studies: for hepatitis B, cytomegalovirus, Epstein–Barr virus.
Chest radiography: shows nodules, fibrosis, infiltrate.
Sinus radiography: shows sinusitis, bone destruction.
Angiography: shows microaneurysms in up to 70% of patients with polyarteritis nodosa; rarely with Wegener's granulomatosis and Churg–Strauss vasculitis.
Two-dimensional echocardiography: to exclude vegetations and atrial myxoma.
Biopsy: of kidney, skin, nose, muscle, sural nerve, rectum, or temporal artery.

Complications

Renal failure: acute, especially if diagnosis or treatment delayed, or chronic (<10% of patients dependent on dialysis).
Gangrene or infarction: can lead to amputation or chronic skin ulcer.
Neuropathy: possibly permanent (*e.g.*, footdrop), although 60% improve on treatment.
Subglottic stenosis: leading to tracheostomy.
Nasal collapse: permanent and may necessitate later plastic surgery.
Severe pulmonary hemorrhage: may cause breathlessness; and unexplained anemia.
Coronary arteritis: may cause myocardial infarction and heart failure.
Hypertension.

Treatment

Diet and lifestyle

• Because they are often immunosuppressed, patients should take precautions against possible infections.

Pharmacological treatment [3,4]

Steroids

• Steroids are only used alone in patients with small-vessel or large-artery disease (*see* Classification).

Standard dosage	*Continuous:* prednisolone, 15–60 mg orally depending on severity and type of vasculitis; usually reducing course. *Pulse:* methylprednisolone, 1 g i.v. or 100 mg orally for 3 days; dose and frequency varied according to response.
Contraindications	Infection (*e.g.*, subacute bacterial endocarditis).
Special points	Adrenal suppression may be a problem with long-term treatment.
Main drug interactions	Drugs that induce liver enzymes promote steroid metabolism; prednisolone antagonizes antihypertensive treatment.
Main side effects	Diabetes, hypertension, osteoporosis, mood change, cushingoid appearance.

Immunosuppressants

• Immunosuppressants are indicated for more severe vasculitis, particularly of small or medium artery.

Standard dosage	*Continuous:* cyclophosphamide, 2 mg/kg orally daily. *Pulse:* cyclophosphamide, 15 mg/kg i.v.; alternatively, 5 mg/kg orally daily for 3 days; dose and frequency vary according to response, renal function, and leukocyte count (measured at 7, 10, and 14 days).
Contraindications	Pregnancy (first trimester especially), uncontrolled infection.
Main drug interactions	None.
Main side effects	Bone-marrow suppression, hemorrhagic cystitis (rare with pulse treatment), nausea, alopecia, infertility.

Combination treatment

Pulse i.v. cyclophosphamide, 15 mg/kg, and methylprednisolone, 1 g 2-weekly for 6 courses (remission induction), then 3-weekly for 2 pulses, then monthly for 3 pulses (maintenance).

Pulse oral cyclophosphamide, 5 mg/kg daily, and prednisone, 100–200 mg daily for 3 consecutive days; interval between treatments as for pulse i.v. treatment.

Continuous oral cyclophosphamide, 2 mg/kg daily, and prednisone, 40–60 mg daily; prednisolone reduced to 20 mg daily by month 3, to 10 mg daily by month 6.

• Cyclophosphamide should be withdrawn at 9–12 months.

• Longer treatment or change to azathioprine, 2 mg/kg daily, is often needed in patients with Wegener's granulomatosis or rheumatoid vasculitis.

• Methotrexate may be an effective steroid-sparing agent.

Other drugs

Azathioprine: steroid-sparing and immunosuppressive.

Plasmapheresis: for pulmonary hemorrhage and severe renal disease.

Prognosis

• In patients with Wegener's granulomatosis or polyarteritis nodosa, 75% remit and 50% relapse with continuous oral treatment.

• The 2-year survival rate ranges from 10% with no treatment to 80% with cyclophosphamide treatment.

• For patients with small-vessel vasculitis, the prognosis is good.

Follow-up and management

• Long-term follow-up is essential, with regular clinical examination, complete blood count, renal function tests (especially urinalysis), and immunology.

• Daily steroids are more often used for large- and small-vessel vasculitis, with reduction in dose when the patient is in remission, aiming for alternate-day treatment.

• Early recognition of relapse is essential.

Key references

1. Gross WL, Schmitt WH, Caernok E: ANCA associated diseases: a rheumatologist's perspective. *Am J Kidney Dis* 1991, **2**:175–179.

2. Hoffman G: Wegener's granulomatosis: an analysis of 158 patients. *Ann Intern Med* 1992, **116**:488–498.

3. Chakravarty K, Scott DGI: Management of systemic vasculitis. *Rheumatol Rev* 1992, **1**:81–99.

4. Griffith ME, Gaskin G, Pusey CD: Classification, pathogenesis, and treatment of systemic vasculitis. *Ren Fail* 1996, **18**:785–802.

Diagnosis

Symptoms

• Most viral warts are asymptomatic, but occasionally they cause severe pain (especially plantar warts).

Signs

Common wart (verruca vulgaris)
Well-demarcated verrucous papule with "seeds" (*i.e.*, thrombosed capillaries).

Plantar wart (verruca plantaris)
Hyperkeratotic plaque: on the plantar surface of the feet, often painful to pressure.

Flat wart (verruca plana)
1–3-mm flat-topped papules: on face or legs (spread by shaving) or elsewhere.

Genital wart (condyloma acuminatum)
White moist cauliflower-like friable papules: occur anywhere on the anogenital skin or mucosa.

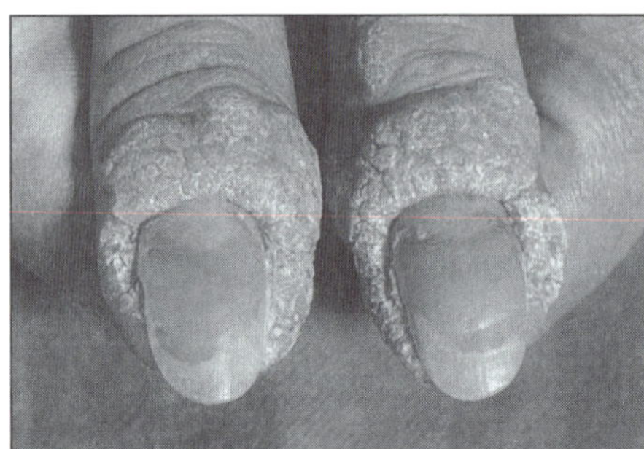

Periungual viral warts. (*See* Color Plate.)

Investigations

• A viral wart is a clinical diagnosis.

Rapid plasma reagin test: to rule out secondary syphilis in cases in which condyloma latum is considered.

Biopsy: in select cases to rule out verrucous carcinoma.

Colposcopy: in female patients with condyloma.

Proctoscopy and cytoscopy.

Complications

• Viral warts can have widespread involvement and spread in immunosuppressed patients (HIV-negative and HIV-positive).

Oncogenic potential: Bowen's disease (viral induced) on glans penis.

Urogenital dysplasia and carcinoma: associated with anogenital and laryngeal warts and cervical condylomata.

Squamous cell carcinomas in situ: secondary to human papillomavirus subtypes 6, 11, 16, 18, 31, 33.

Obstruction of urethral meatus: by urethral condyloma, making treatment extremely difficult.

Laryngeal condyloma: can develop in the birth canal in children born to mothers with condyloma acuminatum, causing respiratory difficulty in the infant; laryngeal condyloma can also occur in surgeons after treating condyloma with carbon dioxide laser [1].

Squamous cell carcinoma: from verruca vulgaris following irradiation [2].

Differential diagnosis

Molluscum contagiosum.

Stucco keratosis (form of seborrheic keratosis resembling verruca planae).

Flegel's disease.

Acrokeratosis verruciformis.

Epidermodysplasia verruciformis.

Pitted keratolysis.

Punctate keratoderma.

Arsenical keratosis.

Condyloma latum.

Acquired digital fibrokeratoma.

Recurrent infantile digital fibroma.

Acrochordon (skin tag).

Etiology

Cause
Human papillomavirus infections; sensitive DNA hybridization techniques have identified more than 60 types of viral DNA.

Spread
• Spread of viral warts is by contact (*i.e.*, skin to skin in verruca vulgaris; sexual contact with condyloma acuminatum; maternal genital tract for neonates).

Epidemiology

• Anogenital warts occur most often in young sexually active patients.

Treatment [3]

Diet and lifestyle

Condyloma acuminatum
• Close prenatal care and counseling is recommended for pregnant women.

• Education and the importance of examination and treatment of sexual partners should be emphasized.

• Condoms should be used.

Pharmacological treatment
• Treatment should be individualized, as treatment is difficult and no one method can be used in all patients with equal success.

For cutaneous warts

Standard dosage	Salicylic acid as ointments, plasters, gels (concentration from 10%–50%) applied nightly for 3–4 months. Combination of salicylic acid and lactic acid applied nightly for 3–4 months. Cantharidin is a blistering agent that is painless to apply and therefore a good treatment for children unable to tolerate cryotherapy. The solution is applied to a lesion, allowed to dry, and covered with a bandage for 24 hours. The dressing should then be removed and the medication washed off. A blister forms, and its roof dries and desquamates. Repeat biweekly or weekly for refractory lesions.
Contraindications	Local hypersensitivity.
Special points	The main objective is to cause inflammation but not infection or scarring.
Main drug interactions	None.
Main side effects	Skin irritation and pain.

Second-line treatment
Liquid nitrogen: either applied or sprayed onto the wart in order to cause a blister; repeated at 2–4-week intervals.

Electrodesiccation and curettage: often results in scarring.

CO_2 laser.

Pulsed dye laser.

Interferon injections for condyloma [4].

• Cimetidine therapy at a dose of 30–40 mg/kg/day has recently been discovered to be a useful adjuvant therapy for multiple viral warts in children. The mechanism of action is unknown but appears to up-regulate the immune system against the wart virus. Therapy should be continued for 3 months [5].

For anogenital warts

Standard dosage	Podophyllin or 5-fluorouracil applied sparingly to affected areas once daily, increased to twice daily as tolerated.
Contraindications	Widespread areas of involvement due to possible systemic absorption.
Special points	Treatment is individual with respect to severity of disease.
Main drug interactions	None.
Main side effects	Local irritation, burning, ulceration, pain, and blistering.

Other treatment
• Other treatment includes CO_2 laser.

Treatment aims
To clear clinical disease without causing scarring.

Other treatments
Hypnosis, particularly in children [6].
Contact sensitization.

Prognosis
• Warts spontaneously resolve in some patients.

Follow-up and management
• Routine cervical cytology in women with anogenital warts is warranted because of the oncogenic potential (colposcopy if indicated) [7].

Key references

1. Gloster HM Jr, Roenigk RK: Risk of acquiring human papillomavirus from the plume produced by the carbon dioxide laser in the treatment of warts. *J Am Acad Dermatol* 1995, **32**:436–441.

2. Kopelson PL, *et al.*: Verruca vulgaris and radiation exposure are associated with squamous cell carcinoma of the finger. *J Dermatol Surg Oncol* 1994, **20**:38–41.

3. Drake LA, *et al.*: Guidelines for care of warts: human papillomavirus. Committee on Guidelines of Care. *J Am Acad Dermatol* 1995, **32**:98–103.

4. Reichman RC, *et al.*: Treatment of condyloma acuminatum with three different interferon-alpha preparations administered parenterally: a double-blind placebo-controlled trial. *J Infect Dis* 1990, **162**:1270.

5. Bauman C, *et al.*: Cimetidine therapy for multiple viral warts in children. *J Am Acad Dermatol* 1996, **35**:271–272.

6. Ewin DM: Hypnotherapy for warts (verruca vulgaris): 41 consecutive cases with 33 cures. *Am J Clin Hypn* 1992, **35**:1–10.

7. Krays SJ, Stone KM: Management of genital infection caused by human papillomavirus. *Rev Infect Dis* 1990, **12**:S620–S632.

Diagnosis

Symptoms

Fatigue, weakness and weight loss: in >80% of patients.

Bleeding tendency: in 60%.

Sensorimotor peripheral neuropathy: in 15%.

Headache, dizziness, vertigo, confusion, stroke, drowsiness, breathlessness, dependent edema: features of hyperviscosity syndrome in 20%.

Epistaxis, gastrointestinal hemorrhage, dependent purpura.

Signs

Lymphadenopathy: in 40%.

Splenomegaly: in 30%.

Hepatomegaly: in 30%.

Peripheral neuropathy: in 15%.

Ataxia; nystagmus; hemiplegia; dementia; coma; signs of congestive cardiac failure; dependent purpura; hemorrhage; dilated, tortuous retinal veins with "sausage-like" segmentation; retinal hemorrhage; papilledema: signs of hyperviscosity syndrome.

Investigations

Complete blood count: shows normocytic, normochromic anemia in 80% of patients; rouleaux, sometimes spuriously raised mean cell volume, neutropenia, thrombocytopenia; lymphocytes may be increased but seldom >5 × 10⁹/L.

Cell marker analysis: surface immunoglobulin of single light chain class (κ or λ); CD19⁺, CD20⁺, CD37⁺, CD38⁺, CD5⁻, CD10⁻.

Bone-marrow aspiration: increase in small lymphocytes and plasmacytoid lymphocytes, sometimes in plasma cells.

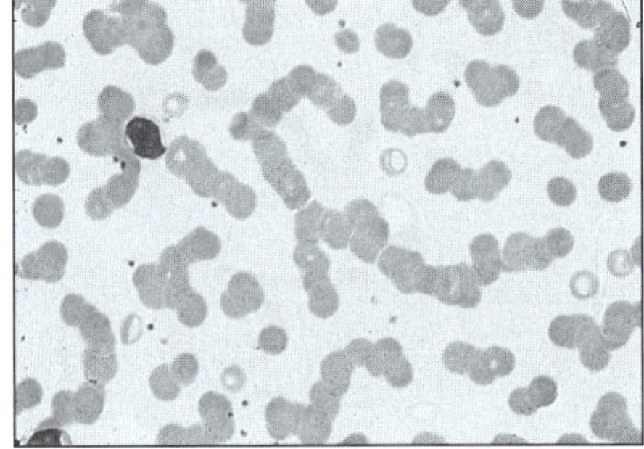

Rouleaux on Romanowsky-stained blood film. (*See* Color Plate.)

Serum electrophoresis: monoclonal spike in beta or gamma globulins; identifiable as IgM by immunoelectrophoresis; serum IgG and IgA often reduced.

Plasma viscosity measurement: raised; hyperviscosity syndrome only if relative serum viscosity >4 times water.

Cryoglobulin analysis: proteins that precipitate at 4°C found in 15% of patients.

Cold agglutinin analysis: erythrocyte autoantibodies (anti-I or anti-i) agglutinate erythrocytes in the cold; idiopathic acquired variety monoclonal IgM.

• Clotting studies may indicate a pseudo von Willebrand's state with prolonged activated partial thromboplastin time, bleeding time, and abnormal platelet function.

Complications

Amyloid: in <10%.

IgM monoclonal protein autoantibody activity: occasionally.

Peripheral neuropathy, cold agglutination syndrome, acquired hemophilia: due, respectively, to antimyelin, antierythrocyte, and anti–factor VIII antibodies.

Treatment

Diet and lifestyle

• The patient should be encouraged to live as normal a life as possible.

Pharmacological treatment

• Chlorambucil, given under specialist supervision, is the mainstay of treatment, but only ~50% of patients respond.

• Other alkylating agents give similar responses and probably could be used interchangeably.

• Recent reports have suggested that fludarabine and 2-chlorodeoxyadenasine [1,2] are useful drugs. Reports indicate that interferon-α may be of value [1].

Standard dosage	Chlorambucil orally daily for 2 weeks every 4 weeks.
Contraindications	No absolute contraindications.
Special points	Full blood count essential because chlorambucil may cause bone-marrow suppression.
Main drug interactions	No major interactions known.
Main side effects	Bone-marrow suppression, nausea and vomiting, diarrhea, oral ulcers, hypersensitivity rashes, occasionally myelodysplasia, acute leukemia.

Treatment aims

To relieve symptoms.

To prolong life.

Other treatments

• Plasma exchange should be instituted urgently for hyperviscosity syndrome; one plasma volume exchanged at regular intervals until relative viscosity <4 times that of water.

• Maintenance plasmapheresis alone may be sufficient to control the disease; viscosity need not be restored to normal.

Prognosis

• The disease is not curable.

• Median survival is 4 years in patients who respond to treatment, 2 years in non-responders; the peripheral neuropathy is frequently unresponsive.

Follow-up and management

• Patients should be followed up at regular intervals.

• Full blood count and IgM concentrations should be monitored.

• Plasma viscosity indicates whether plasmapheresis is indicated.

• No large controlled trials are available to guide the physician. By analogy with other low-grade lymphomas, it is reasonable to withhold treatment in asymptomatic patients.

Key references

1. Dimopoulos MA, O'Brien S, Kantarjian HM, *et al.*: Fludarabine therapy in Waldenström's macroglobulinemia. *Am J Med* 1993, **95**:49–52.

2. Dimopoulos MA, Kantarjian HM, Estey E, *et al.*: Treatment of Waldenström macroglobulinemia with 2-chlorodeoxyadenosine. *Ann Intern Med* 1993, **118**:195–198.

Diagnosis

Definition

• Myocardial activation from atrial to ventricular myocardium occurs over an accessory connection (accessory to the normal His-Purkinje system).
• If conduction occurs in sinus rhythm, pre-excitation is apparent on the ECG.
• The substrate for atrioventricular re-entry tachycardia is present; conduction in tachycardia from ventricle to atrium over the accessory connection is orthodromic (90%) or from atrium to ventricle is antidromic.

Symptoms

• Most patients who are found to have the Wolff–Parkinson–White syndrome are asymptomatic; the only feature is the presence of pre-excitation on the surface ECG.

Palpitation: most common symptom; caused by re-entry tachycardia (sudden onset and termination, regular, rapid—often >200 beats/min); may also be caused by paroxysmal atrial fibrillation (in ~5% of patients).

Chest pain: during tachycardia; pain or discomfort similar to angina; rarely indicates coronary artery disease.

Impaired consciousness: dizziness or faintness common; syncope less frequent (5%) and usually follows vasodilatation occurring as a secondary response to tachycardia.

Polyuria: accompanying sustained episodes of tachycardia.

Signs

• In sinus rhythm, no clinical signs indicate the presence of the condition; during tachycardia, clinical signs associated with the impaired circulation and abnormal cardiac action may be found, principally the following:

Rapid pulse.
Hypotension.
Alteration in the venous pulse wave form.

Investigations

Pre-excitation ECG: pre-excitation is the QRS configuration generated by fusion of ventricular activation wave fronts from normal His-Purkinje system and accessory atrio-ventricular connection; myocardium activated through accessory connection gives rise to delta wave (slurred initial QRS); precise delta wave pattern depends on location of accessory connection on atrioventricular ring, and QRS configuration may be subtly or dramatically changed from normal; pre-excitation ceases with temporary cessation of anterograde conduction through accessory connection, or pre-excitation changes may vary depending on balance of activation between normal conduction system and accessory connection, (both influenced by autonomic tone); PR interval shortening results from myocardial activation through the accessory connection, which lacks decremental conduction properties.

ECG during tachycardia: usually (90%) narrow complex tachycardia; retrograde atrial activation may be seen as P waves of altered configuration inscribed in ST segments; rate-related bundle branch block (aberrancy) or antidromic tachycardia results in broad QRS complex tachycardia.

Ambulatory monitoring: paroxysms of tachycardia may be seen on 24-hour or 48-hour monitoring; usually too infrequent for capture of tachycardia to be probable; self-activated recording devices (cardiac memo/wrist recorder) with transtelephonic transmission to a recording center may be more useful.

Electrophysiological study: cardiac extrastimulation techniques and recording of endo-cardial ECG allows diagnosis and characterization of the condition in almost all cases; complex studies rarely done for diagnosis alone but used as prelude to radiofrequency catheter ablation of accessory connection; single wire study determines ventricular response rate through accessory connection conduction during atrial fibrillation to assess risk of malignant arrhythmias secondary to rapid ventricular activation; this is an imprecise means of assessing the risk of sudden death.

Exercise stress testing: no role in defining connection conduction properties.

Complications

Atrial fibrillation.
Sudden cardiac death: rare.

Differential diagnosis

Atrioventricular nodal re-entry tachycardia: tachycardia due to dual atrioventricular node physiology allowing re-entry within the atrioventricular node; other types of supraventricular tachycardia (*e.g.*, atrial flutter, fibrillation, ectopic atrial tachy-cardia, Mahaim re-entry).

Ventricular tachycardia: broad QRS complexes (due to antidromic tachycardia or aberrant conduction) may be misdiagnosed as tachycardia arising from a ventricular focus; algorithms are available to aid ECG differentiation.

Etiology

• Wolff–Parkinson–White syndrome is not inherited.

• During early cardiac development, direct physical continuity exists between ventric-ular and atrial myocardium; in growth of atrioventricular sulcus, tissue at a later stage in cardiac development interrupts this, but defects may persist into neonatal and subsequently adult life.

• Term infants have frequently been found to have these connections, but they are presumed to be nonfunctional in most.

• Accessory connections appear microscop-ically to be normal myocardial muscle bundles bridging atrial and ventricular myo-cardium; they may have subepicardial or subendocardial locations; they are multiple in ~10% of patients with the condition.

• Ebstein's anomaly is associated with their presence, and multiple pathways are more common in these patients.

Epidemiology

• Early studies have suggested that ECG evidence of pre-excitation can be found in 0.3% of the population; probably only a few of such patients are symptomatic, but the evidence is conflicting.

• Depending on the nature of the popula-tion studies, documentation of tachycardia has varied from 5% to 90% of patients.

Treatment

Diet and lifestyle

• In patients with frequent symptoms, lifestyle is restricted by the occurrence of palpitations (often apparently related to stress or exertion) or by the side effects of drug treatment.

Pharmacological treatment

• Drugs are now considered second-line treatment for the Wolff–Parkinson–White syndrome.

• Asymptomatic patients need no drug treatment unless their occupation demands removal of all risk of tachycardia (*e.g.*, airline pilots, certain military, police, and fire-brigade personnel).

• Symptomatic patients who need treatment but who do not wish to have radiofrequency catheter ablation can be given antiarrhythmic drugs; these exert their effect by altering atrioventricular nodal conduction or accessory connection conduction, or both, so that re-entry tachycardia will less probably be sustained.

• Drugs that slow atrioventricular nodal conduction but enhance accessory pathway conduction (*e.g.*, digoxin) should not be used in isolation.

• Antiarrhythmic drugs often have unacceptable side effects, and some have been shown to have dangerous proarrhythmic effects.

• Drugs must be taken continuously, and not on an ad-hoc basis, to give optimal control of symptoms; even then, abolition of symptoms is rare.

• Adenosine can be used as an i.v. bolus to abort an episode of atrioventricular re-entry tachycardia.

Nonpharmacological treatment

Catheter ablation

• Catheter ablation is technically demanding but is associated with very low mortality and morbidity in skilled hands [1].

• Apposition of an ablation electrode to the endocardial location nearest the accessory connection results in cessation of accessory connection conduction on delivery of radiofrequency energy through the electrode.

• This is a low-voltage, high-frequency energy source, which results in heating of the electrode tip, in turn producing a small endocardial lesion (5–7 mm) that extends into the myocardium.

• Primary success is >90%.

• Failure to achieve complete abolition of accessory connection conduction leads to a small recurrence rate after apparently successful procedures.

• Radiofrequency catheter ablation is the treatment of choice because it is curative; other energy sources are available but are associated with various disadvantages.

Surgery

• Although curative, surgical division of accessory connections needs major cardiac surgery and so is associated with higher morbidity and mortality than catheter ablation.

• It should be reserved for patients in whom catheter ablation has been a repeated failure.

Treatment aims

To abolish accessory connection conduction and therefore risk of tachycardia and palpitation.

To remove risk of sudden cardiac death.

To assess risk in asymptomatic patients.

Prognosis

• The prognosis is probably that of the normal population after successful catheter ablation.

• Lesions induced by radiofrequency catheter ablation have not been associated with impairment of ventricular function or arrhythmogenic complications except in infant hearts, when lesions may grow with heart size.

• Untreated asymptomatic Wolff–Parkinson–White syndrome carries a good prognosis; the risk of sudden death in asymptomatic patients is probably very small.

Follow-up and management

• Recurrence of pre-excitation may occur early after a primarily successful catheter ablation (within 6 weeks) in as many as 10% of patients; occasionally, recurrence is not accompanied by symptom recurrence because of modification of the connection conduction properties.

• Late recurrence after successful catheter ablation (>3 months) is rare; patients usually experience short-lived episodes of palpitation or rhythm irregularity for some months after successful ablations, which may relate to a learning effect through which individuals have become sensitized to any short-lived change in heart rhythm (*e.g.*, ectopic activity) because, before treatment, these heralded onset of tachycardia; these symptoms resolve with time and reassurance.

• After surgical treatment, standard follow-up is needed.

• Follow-up of patients treated by anti-arrhythmic drugs is determined by their symptoms and drug side effects.

Key reference

1. Jackman WM, *et al.*: Catheter ablation of accessory atrioventricular pathways (Wolff–Parkinson–White syndrome) by radiofrequency current. *N Engl J Med* 1991, **324**:1605–1611.

Basis of recommendations

Beginning in the 1970s, three groups, the US Preventive Services Task Force (USPSTF) [1], the American College of Physicians (ACP)[2], and the Canadian Task Force on the Periodic Health Exam [CTF] [3], produced disease screening and prevention recommendations for a wide spectrum of diseases based on explicit criteria that measure and report the strength of scientific evidence to support each recommendation. Practitioners should monitor the recommendations of these evidence-based groups in determining optimal disease screening and prevention practices for their patients.

Recommended practices for asymptomatic, low-risk adults

The table summarizes the recommendations for disease screening and prevention developed at The University of Michigan's health maintenance organization (M-CARE) in 1996, based primarily on the recommendations of the CTF, USPSTF, and ACP.

Breast cancer

USPSTF: screening for breast cancer every 1–2 years (mammography ± clinical breast examination [CBE]) for women aged 50–69 years. Recommendations for or against routine mammography or CBE in women aged 40–49 years cannot be made based on current evidence.

ACP: mammography every 2 years for women aged 50–74 years.

CTF: annual CBE and mammography for women aged 50–69 years only.

Other: American Cancer Society, American College of Radiology, American Medical Association, and American College of Obstetrics and Gynecology recommend screening with annual CBE and biannual mammography beginning at age 40 years, and annual CBE and mammography beginning at age 50 years.

Hyperlipidemia

USPSTF: total cholesterol levels (nonfasting) should be measured in men aged 35–65 years and women aged 45–65 years.

ACP: total cholesterol levels (nonfasting) should be considered in men aged 35–65 years and women aged 45–65 years with fewer than two additional risk factors and without a strong family history of coronary artery disease [4].

CTF: total cholesterol measurement should be considered in men aged 30–59 years.

Other: National Cholesterol Education Program (NCEP) [5] advocates screening all adults for hyperlipidemia.

Cervical cancer

USPSTF: Papanicolaou (Pap) smears at least every 3 years beginning with onset of sexual activity; discontinue testing after age 65 years in women who have had regular previous screenings in which the smears have been consistently normal.

ACP: Pap smears every 3 years for women aged 20–65 years and every 2 years for women at high risk; screening is recommended for women aged 66–75 years every 3 years if they have not been screened from age 56–66 years.

CTF: annual Pap smears beginning at age 18 years or the onset of sexual activity. After two normal smears, screen every 3 years to age 69 years.

Other: American Cancer Society, National Cancer Institute, American Medical Association, and American College of Obstetrics and Gynecology recommend annual Pap smears for all women who are or have been sexually active or who have reached age 18 years.

Colorectal cancer

USPSTF: annual fecal occult blood testing (FOBT) or sigmoidoscopy (interval unspecified), or both, for all persons aged 50 years and older.

ACP: screening options for patients aged 50–70 years include flexible sigmoidoscopy, colonoscopy, or air-contrast barium enema, repeated at 10-year intervals; FOBT is recommended for patients who decline these screening tests.

CTF: there is insufficient evidence to support screening of asymptomatic individuals over age 40 years.

Other: American Cancer Society recommends annual digital rectal examination for all adults beginning at age 40 years, annual FOBT beginning at age 50 years, and sigmoidoscopy every 3–5 years beginning at age 50 years.

• The Agency for Health Care Policy and Research, in conjunction with several specialty societies, released a consensus statement in 1997 that included colonoscopy every 10 years (among other alternatives endorsed by other groups) as a recommended screening method [6].

Prostate cancer

USPSTF: routine screening for prostate cancer not recommended.

ACP: individualized screening based on patient and physician preferences.

ACP: the routine use of prostate-specific antigen (PSA) is not recommended. Qualified support for digital rectal examination (DRE) in men aged 50–70 years.

Other: American Cancer Society recommends an annual DRE for both prostate and colorectal cancer beginning at age 40 years; annual serum PSA determination for African-American men aged 40 years and older, other men aged 50 years and older; similar recommendations have been issued by the American Urological Association.

Key references

1. U.S. Preventive Services Task Force: *Guide to Clinical Preventive Services*, edn 2. Baltimore: Williams & Wilkins; 1996.

2. Sox HC: Preventive health services in adults. *N Engl J Med* 1994, **330**:1589–1595.

3. Canadian Task Force on the Periodic Health Examination: *Canadian Guide to Clinical Preventive Health Care*. Ottawa: Canada Communication Group; 1994.

4. Guidelines for using serum cholesterol, high-density lipoprotein cholesterol, and triglyceride levels as screening tests for preventing coronary heart disease in adults. *Ann Intern Med* 1996, **124**:515–517.

5. Summary of the second report of the National Cholesterol Education Program (NCEP) Expert Panel on Detection, Evaluation, and Treatment of High Blood Cholesterol in Adults (Adult Treatment Panel II). *JAMA* 1993, **269**:3015–3023.

6. Winawer SJ, Fletcher RH, Miller L, *et al.*: Colorectal cancer screening: clinical guidelines and rationale. *Gastroenterology* 1997, **112**:594–642.

M-CARE Preventive Care Guidelines, 1996 (minimum levels of preventive care for asymptomatic, low-risk adults)

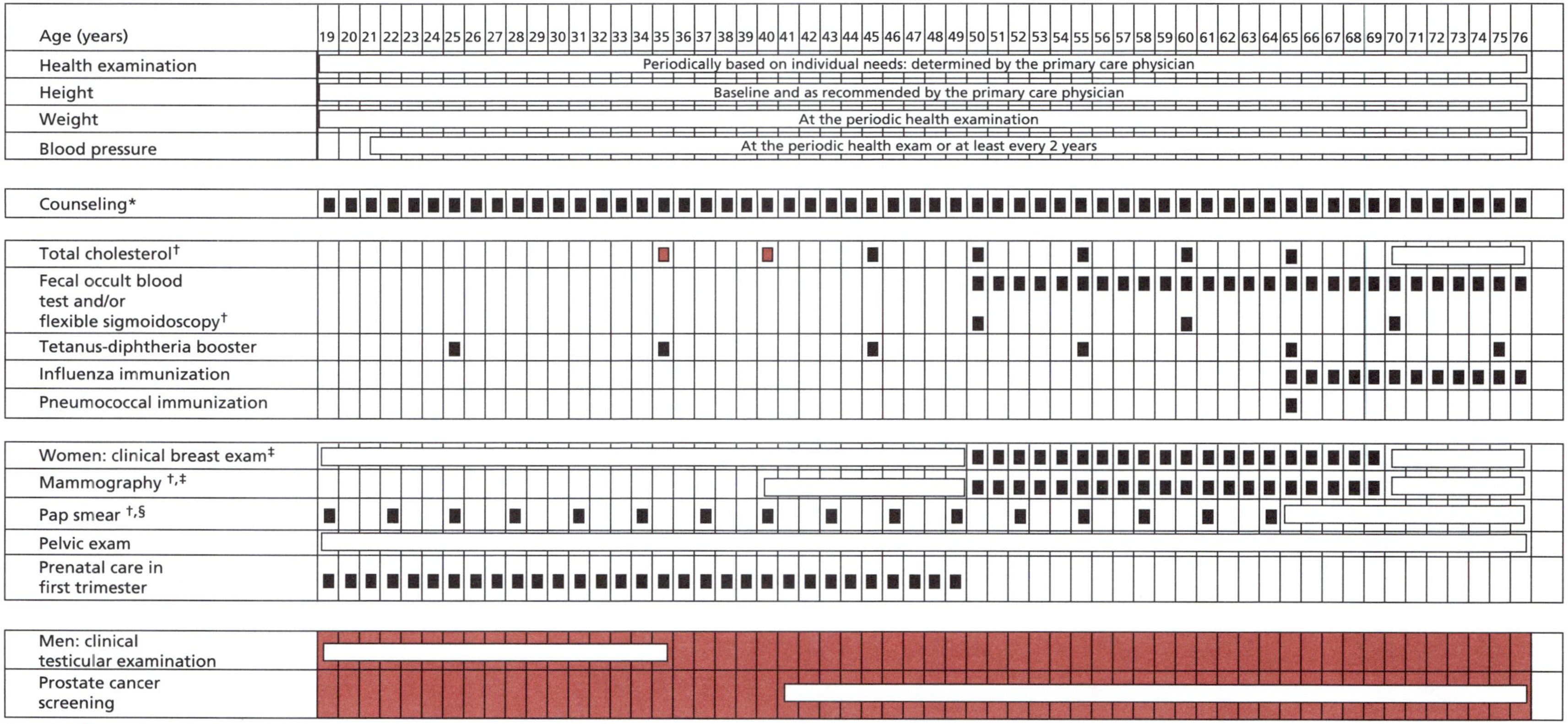

Age (years): 19–76

	Recommendation (ages 19–76)
Health examination	Periodically based on individual needs: determined by the primary care physician
Height	Baseline and as recommended by the primary care physician
Weight	At the periodic health examination
Blood pressure	At the periodic health exam or at least every 2 years

Key to the schedule grid below: ■ = recommended; □ = white box (as recommended by the primary care physician); ■r = red box (men only).

Ages 19–40

	19	20	21	22	23	24	25	26	27	28	29	30	31	32	33	34	35	36	37	38	39	40
Counseling*	■	■	■	■	■	■	■	■	■	■	■	■	■	■	■	■	■	■	■	■	■	■
Total cholesterol†																	■r					■r
Fecal occult blood test and/or																						
flexible sigmoidoscopy†																						
Tetanus-diphtheria booster							■										■					
Influenza immunization																						
Pneumococcal immunization																						
Women: clinical breast exam‡	□	□	□	□	□	□	□	□	□	□	□	□	□	□	□	□	□	□	□	□	□	□
Mammography†,‡																						□
Pap smear†,§	■			■			■			■			■			■			■			■
Pelvic exam	□	□	□	□	□	□	□	□	□	□	□	□	□	□	□	□	□	□	□	□	□	□
Prenatal care in first trimester	■	■	■	■	■	■	■	■	■	■	■	■	■	■	■	■	■	■	■	■	■	■
Men: clinical testicular examination	□	□	□	□	□	□	□	□	□	□	□	□	□	□	□	□	■r	■r	■r	■r	■r	■r
Prostate cancer screening	■r	■r	■r	■r	■r	■r	■r	■r	■r	■r	■r	■r	■r	■r	■r	■r	■r	■r	■r	■r	■r	■r

Ages 41–58

	41	42	43	44	45	46	47	48	49	50	51	52	53	54	55	56	57	58
Counseling*	■	■	■	■	■	■	■	■	■	■	■	■	■	■	■	■	■	■
Total cholesterol†					■					■					■			
Fecal occult blood test and/or										■	■	■	■	■	■	■	■	■
flexible sigmoidoscopy†										■								
Tetanus-diphtheria booster					■										■			
Influenza immunization																		
Pneumococcal immunization																		
Women: clinical breast exam‡	□	□	□	□	□	□	□	□	□	■	■	■	■	■	■	■	■	■
Mammography†,‡	□	□	□	□	□	□	□	□	□	■	■	■	■	■	■	■	■	■
Pap smear†,§			■			■			■			■			■			■
Pelvic exam	□	□	□	□	□	□	□	□	□	□	□	□	□	□	□	□	□	□
Prenatal care in first trimester	■	■	■	■	■	■	■	■	■									
Men: clinical testicular examination	■r	■r	■r	■r	■r	■r	■r	■r	■r	■r	■r	■r	■r	■r	■r	■r	■r	■r
Prostate cancer screening	■r	□	□	□	□	□	□	□	□	□	□	□	□	□	□	□	□	□

Ages 59–76

	59	60	61	62	63	64	65	66	67	68	69	70	71	72	73	74	75	76
Counseling*	■	■	■	■	■	■	■	■	■	■	■	■	■	■	■	■	■	■
Total cholesterol†		■					■					■	□	□	□	□	□	□
Fecal occult blood test and/or	■	■	■	■	■	■	■	■	■	■	■	■	■	■	■	■	■	■
flexible sigmoidoscopy†		■										■						
Tetanus-diphtheria booster							■										■	
Influenza immunization							■	■	■	■	■	■	■	■	■	■	■	■
Pneumococcal immunization							■											
Women: clinical breast exam‡	■	■	■	■	■	■	■	□	□	□	□	□	□	□	□	□	□	□
Mammography†,‡	■	■	■	■	■	■	■	■	■	■	■	□	□	□	□	□	□	□
Pap smear†,§			■			■	□	□	□	□	□	□	□	□	□	□	□	□
Pelvic exam	□	□	□	□	□	□	□	□	□	□	□	□	□	□	□	□	□	□
Prenatal care in first trimester																		
Men: clinical testicular examination	■r	■r	■r	■r	■r	■r	■r	■r	■r	■r	■r	■r	■r	■r	■r	■r	■r	■r
Prostate cancer screening	□	□	□	□	□	□	□	□	□	□	□	□	□	□	□	□	□	□

* Counseling topics include tobacco cessation, alcohol/drug use, diet (limit fat and cholesterol; maintain caloric balance; emphasize grains, fruits, vegetables; adequate calcium-rich foods for women; recommend breast-feeding, if appropriate), regular physical activity, injury prevention (lap/shoulder belts, apprpriate helmet use, smoke detector use, safe storage/removal of firearms, violence prevention, poison control, fall prevention), sexual behavior (sexually transmitted disease prevention, unintended pregnancy), dental health, multivitamin with folic acid for women of childbearing age, hormone prophylaxis in peri- and postmenopausal women, and skin cancer counseling if family history of skin cancer and fair skin, eyes, or hair.

† More frequently and/or at an earlier age, based on risk factors.

‡ Screen every 1 or 2 years with mammography alone or with mammography and clinical breast examination.

§ Regular screening may be discontinued after age 65 years in women who have had regular screenings that have been consistently normal.

■ Red boxes indicate men only; □ white boxes indicate as recommended by the primary care physician.

M-CARE— University of Michigan's health maintenance organization.

Indications for nutritional support

Malnourished patients unable to maintain adequate oral intake of nutrients (*e.g.*, surgical patients with prolonged ileus, medical patients with pancreatitis, or severe diabetic gastroparesis).

Well-nourished patients who will be NPO for >10–14 days.

Patients who are not able to maintain adequate oral intake when full nutrition is required (*e.g.*, burn patients, trauma patients, Crohn's disease patients.)

Nutritional therapy, such as providing branched-chain amino acids (BCAAs), to patients with portasystemic encephalopathy.

Nutritional requirements

Fluid

• ~35 mL/kg/day or 1 mL/kcal is required for patients without excess fluid loss; additional fluid is needed to replace losses from nasogastric suction, diarrhea, third-spaced fluid, and burns.

Caloric requirements

Maintenance requirements: 25 kcal/kg/day.

Trauma, febrile, pancreatitis: 30 kcal/kg/day.

Minor burns, sepsis: 35 kcal/kg/day; major burns: 40 kcal/kg/day.

Carbohydrate

• Glucose (8%–25% solution) is the main source of calories in parenteral formulas. Although glucose can provide all nonprotein calories, this requires large fluid volumes for delivery, resulting in edema, fluid overload, hyperglycemia, and fatty liver.

Protein

• A positive nitrogen balance is maintained by adequate protein intake (amino acid infusion) and sufficient nonprotein calories to prevent protein breakdown (gluconeogenesis). The recommended dietary protein intake is 0.8 g/kg/day but can be increased to 1.5 g/kg/day in stressed patients (*e.g.*, burn, trauma, postoperative patients).

Fat

• Lipids are emulsions of soybean or safflower oil and contain linoleic acid, an essential fatty acid. In standard formulas, lipids provide ~30% of nonprotein calories. Patients with respiratory failure can be given a higher percentage of lipid calories to decrease CO_2 production. Excessive use of lipid can result in hyperlipidemia and increased risk of infection via impairment of neutrophilic function.

Electrolytes

• Electrolyte replacement should be closely monitored, particularly in patients with renal disease, cirrhosis with ascites, congestive heart failure, diarrheal states, nasogastric suction, and third spacing of fluids. Potassium and phosphorus requirements may be high in malnourished patients beginning total parenteral nutrition (TPN).

Minerals and vitamins

• Commercial multivitamin products (*e.g.*, MVI-12), which typically do not include vitamin K, are required. Trace elements (*e.g.*, zinc, copper, and selenium) should also be added for patients who require prolonged nutritional support. Iron cannot be given with lipids and may need to be given separately. Patients with diarrhea may need extra zinc replacement.

Assessment of nutritional status

• Often the clinician's overall assessment of the patient's nutritional status is most accurate.

• Helpful indicators of poor nutrition include the following:

Patient is 15% below ideal body weight.

Signs of muscle wasting, decreased hand grip strength.

Serum albumin <3.0 g/dL.

Anthropomorphic measurements:
Triceps skin fold: female <15 mm; male <11.4 mm.
Midarm muscle circumference: female <25.8 mm; male <26.4 mm.

Central TPN

• Patients needing complete nutrition parenterally require central TPN. To provide total calories intravenously requires a large osmotic load that must be given through a large central vein where the mixture is quickly diluted. Solutions with up to 25% glucose can be used. In peripheral veins, osmolality must be kept <900 mOsmL with glucose concentration <10% to prevent unacceptable phlebitis.

Standard TPN solution/24 hours

Volume: 2600 cc.

Total calories: 2000.

Calorie to nitrogen ratio: 131:1.

Macronutrients

Glucose (15% solution): 350 g (60% of total calories).

Amino acids: 80 g (16% of total calories).

Lipid emulsion (20%): 240 mL (24% of total calories).

Electrolytes

Sodium: 120 mEq.

Potassium: 80 mEq.

Chloride: 140 mEq.

Acetate: 20 mEq.

Phosphorus: 30 mmol.

Calcium gluconate: 9.2 mEq (2 g).

Magnesium sulfate: 16.8 mEq (2 g).

Vitamins

MVI-12: daily.

Vitamin K: 5 mg/week (do not use in patients requiring anticoagulation with coumadin).

Peripheral parenteral nutrition (PPN)

• Patients who require additional calories to supplement oral intake or patients who are not malnourished and require short-term nutritional support may use PPN. Roughly 1000 kcal/day can be delivered via PPN. Isotonic fat emulsions have greatly increased the amount of calories that can be delivered peripherally, but exclusive reliance on these products would result in hyperlipidemia.

Laboratory monitoring

• Prior to starting parenteral nutrition, a complete blood count, electrolytes, blood urea nitrogen, creatinine, albumin, total protein, liver chemistries, triglycerides, weight, and 24- hour urine for urea and creatinine should be obtained. After initiating parenteral nutrition, electrolytes/creatinine/blood urea nitrogen and weight should be obtained daily to detect significant electrolyte shifts for the first 2 weeks. Glucose should be monitored closely including every-6-hour bedside monitoring until the serum glucose is <200 g/dL. Liver function tests, triglycerides, and renal function should be followed weekly. Stable patients on long-term parenteral nutrition are followed at less-frequent intervals.

Complications

Electrolyte abnormalities.	Gallstones.
Hyperglycemia.	Cholecystitis.
Hypoglycemia.	Sepsis.
Elevated transaminases.	Pneumothorax.
Fatty liver.	Air embolus.
Hyperlipidemia.	Broken catheter embolus.
Fluid overload.	Catheter/venous thrombosis.
Hyperosmotic coma.	Mineral deficiences.

Enteral nutrition

• If the patient's gastrointestinal tract is functional, this is the preferred method of nutritional support. Supplements include standard formulas with complex carbohydrates, intact protein, and fat such as vegetable oil. Some are modified- to high-calorie (2 kcal/mL), high-fiber, high-protein, low-protein, or volume-restricted formulations. Elemental dietary supplements are expensive preparations designed for patients with impaired digestion, short gut syndrome, or as a possible therapeutic modality in Crohn's disease.

Oral supplementation

• If patients are able to eat without aspiration but not taking an adequate amount of food, liquid supplements such as Ensure (1 kcal/mL) can raise caloric intake enough to maintain weight.

Nasogastric tube

• Nasogastric bolus tube feeding can be used in patients with normal gastric emptying. Patients should be placed in the upright position during administration and over the subsequent hour. Complications include aspiration, gastric ulcers, perforation, bleeding, and gastroesphageal reflux.

Small-bore nasoduodenal tube

• Small-bore nasoduodenal tubes are moderately well tolerated and can be used for long-term feeding. A pump is required to deliver a continuous infusion because the small bowel cannot tolerate bolus feeding. Complications include tube occlusion, accidental removal, difficulty replacing the tube, diarrhea, aspiration.

Percutaneous gastric tube

• Percutaneous gastric tubes have the advantage of using a large-bore tube that is not easily clogged and cannot be pulled out accidentally during sleep. Patients should have a normally functioning stomach. Care should be taken in patients with a history of aspiration pneumonia and significant gastroesophageal reflux. Complications include gastric ulcers, gastric bleeding, gastric outlet obstruction, wound infection, necrotizing fasciitis, and rapid closure of the fistula if the tube falls out.

Surgical jejunostomy tube

• In patients who have a nonfunctioning stomach, recurrent aspiration pneumonia, recent gastric surgery, or duodenal and gastric outlet obstruction, a surgical jejunostomy-tube may be necessary. A pump and continuous infusion is required. Complications include diarrhea, wound infection, small bowel obstruction, and jejunal ulcers.

General references

Stenson WF, Eisenberg P: Parenteral and enteral nutrition. In *Textbook of Internal Medicine*, edn 3. Philadelphia: Lippincott-Raven; 1997.

Alpers DH, Stenson WF, Bier D: *Manual of Nutrition Therapeutics*. edn 3. Boston: Little, Brown; 1995.

Indications for immunization

Hepatitis A virus (HAV)

• HAV vaccine is recommended for travelers to endemic areas. HAV vaccine should replace the use of immunoglobulin for foreign travelers. It is recommended for adults and children living in communities with high rates of HAV or periodic outbreaks of HAV, staff and clients of group homes for disabled persons, daycare centers, homosexual men, and i.v. drug users.

Serum immunoglobulin: for postexposure prophylaxis (*e.g.*, outbreaks in daycare centers or household contacts), the vaccine does not offer acceptable protection and immune globulin should be given. For short trips, immunoglobulin alone is still an acceptable alternative (vaccine is preferred), and for those who must depart on short notice, a combination of immunoglobulin and vaccine can be given.

• Patients who are already serum IgM HAV antibody–positive (indicating acute HAV infection) or serum IgG HAV antibody–positive (indicating past exposure to HAV) will not benefit from vaccination or serum immunoglobulin.

Hepatitis B virus (HBV)

• HBV vaccine is recommended for all children as part of childhood immunization series and previously unvaccinated adolescents. It is recommended for household contacts of HBV carriers, infants born to HBsAg-positive mothers, health care workers, homosexual men, i.v. drug users, people living or traveling in endemic areas; and people with postexposure prophylaxis.

• Patients who are serum HBsAg positive are chronic carriers (or acutely infected) and will not benefit from vaccination. Patients who are HBsAb positive have either been exposed to HBV in the past or have been vaccinated previously. In either instance vaccination is not needed. Patients who are HBsAb positive, HBsAg negative, and HBcAb positive have had past HBV infection and recovery. Serum HBsAb-positive, HBsAg-negative, HBcAb-negative results indicate past vaccination.

Hepatitis C virus (HCV)

• No vaccine is available. Serum immunoglobulin is not recommended for postexposure prophylaxsis.

Hepatitis D virus (HDV)

• Because HDV infection requires previous or simultaneous infection with HBV, vaccination against HBV effectively prevents infection with HDV.

Investigations

• Preimmunization testing to determine if recipient has already been exposed to HAV or HBV is not routinely recommended. Patients who are already HBsAg positive or HBsAb positive do not need to be vaccinated. Postimmunization testing is not recommended but may be indicated in patients who are immunocompromised, suspected of having a poor response to immunization, or in those patients considered to be at high risk for exposure (*e.g.*, a surgeon or phlebotomist).

Complications of immunization

HAV

Soreness, erythema at the sight of the injection: common.

Fever.

Anaphylactic reactions, Guillain-Barré syndrome: rare.

HCV

• Outbreaks of HCV infection from contaminated serum immunoglobulin and specialized immunoglobulins such as RhoD have been reported.

Immunization dosage and schedule

HAV
Standard dosage

Adults: 1440 ELISA U/1 mL (Havrix) or 50 U/0.5 mL (Vaqta) given at 0 and 6–12 months.

Children: 720 ELISA U/0.5 mL (Havrix) or 25 U/0.5 mL (Vaqta) given at 0 and 6–12 months.

Newborns: neither vaccine is approved for children <2 years of age.

Serum immunoglobulin: 0.02 mL/kg IM for postexposure prophylaxis or foreign travel lasting <3 months; for longer trips 0.06 mL/kg provides protection for up to 6 months.

HBV
Standard dosage

Adults: one 1-mL dose given at 0, 1–2, and 4–6 months for a total of three doses (Recombivax HB 10 µg/1.0 mL or Engerix-B 20 µg/1.0 mL).

Children: one dose given at 0, 1–2, and 4–6 months for a total of three doses (Recombivax HB 2.5 µg/0.5 mL for children aged 1–10 years, Recombivax HB 5.0 µg/0.5 mL for children aged 11–19 years; Engerix-B 10 µg/0.5 mL for children aged 1–19 years).

Newborns: one dose given at 0–2, 1–4, and 6–18 months for a total of three doses (Recombivax HB 2.5 µg/0.5 mL; Engerix-B 10 µg/0.5 mL).

For newborns of HBsAg-positive mothers: within 12 hours of birth give HBIG along with first dose of vaccine given at a separate site (Recombivax HB 5.0 µg/0.5 mL; Engerix-B 10 µg/0.5 mL).

Postexposure prophylaxis

For needle-stick injuries from a patient who is HBsAg positive, if the injured person has not been vaccinated previously, give hepatitis B immunoglobulin and first dose of vaccine at a separate site, then complete vaccine schedule. If the injured person has been vaccinated consider checking HBsAb level and give vaccine booster if undetectable.

Immunocompromised patients

One dose given at 0, 1, and 6 months (Recombivax HB 40 µg/1.0 mL; Engerix-B 40 µg/2.0 mL).

Causes of pharmacologic treatment failure

Gluteal injections associated with decreased response to HBV vaccination; immunocompromised patients such as renal transplant patients and AIDS patients; HBV mutants.

General references

Lemon SM, Thomas DL: Vaccines to prevent viral hepatitis. *N Engl J Med* 1997, **336**:196–204.

McDonnell WM, Askari FK: Immunizations. *JAMA* 1997, in press.

C

F

I

M

S

T

U

Index

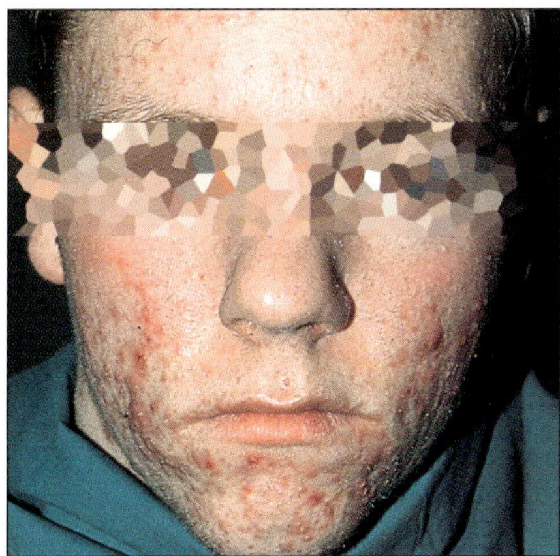

Acne, page 6.

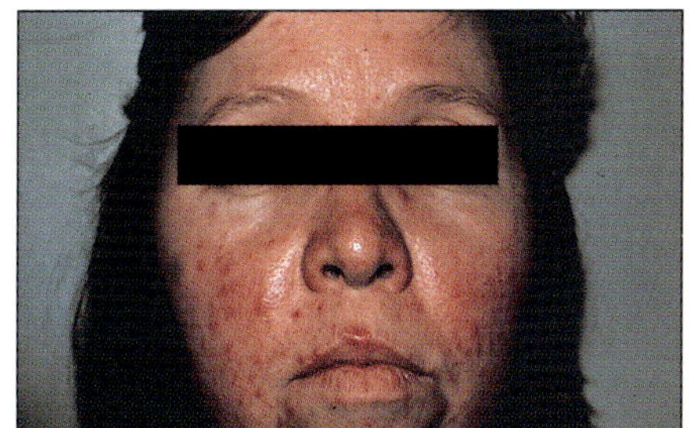

Acne rosacea, page 8.

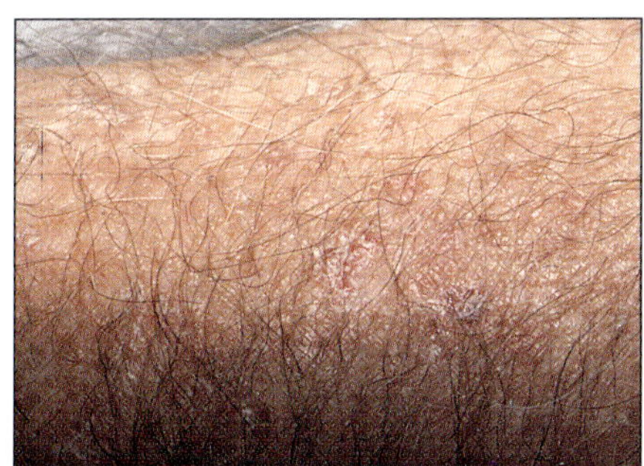

Actinic keratoses, page 10.

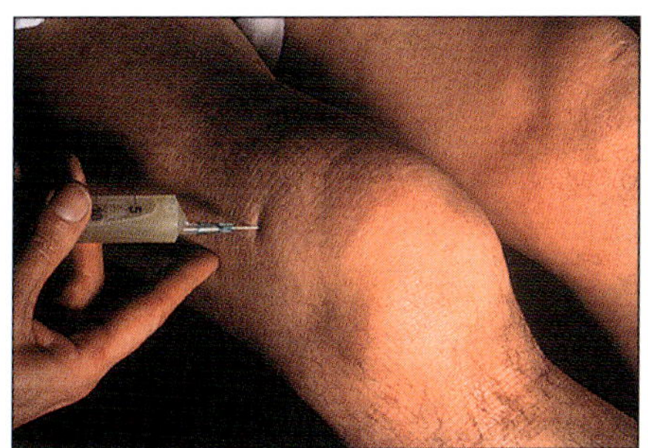

Acute crystal synovitis, page 12.

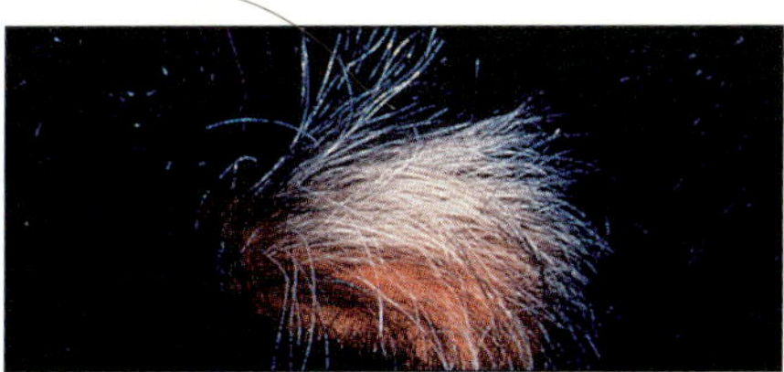

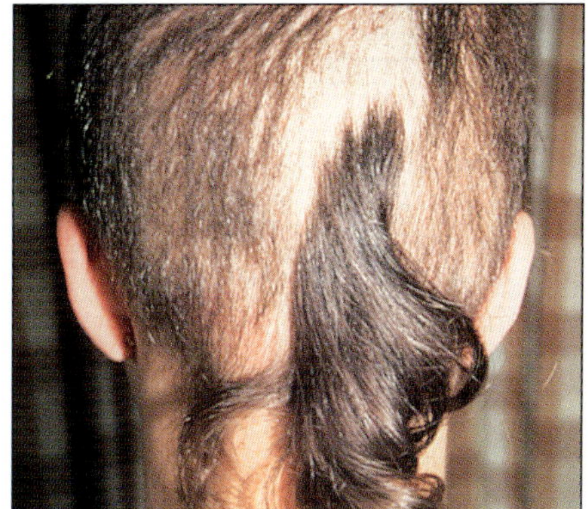

Alopecia, page 24.

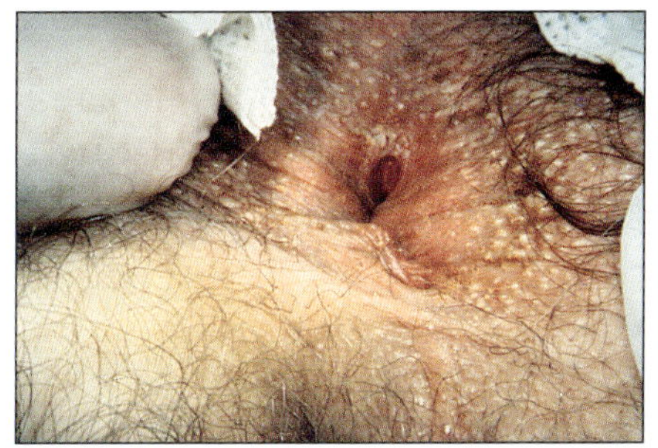

Anal fissure, page 26.

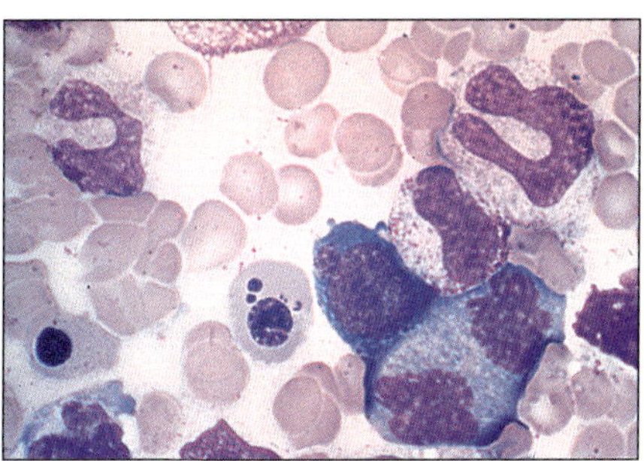

Anemia, megaloblastic; page 30.

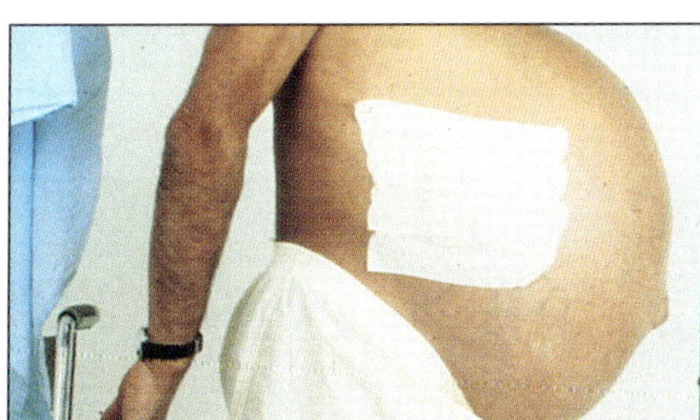

Ascites, page 54.

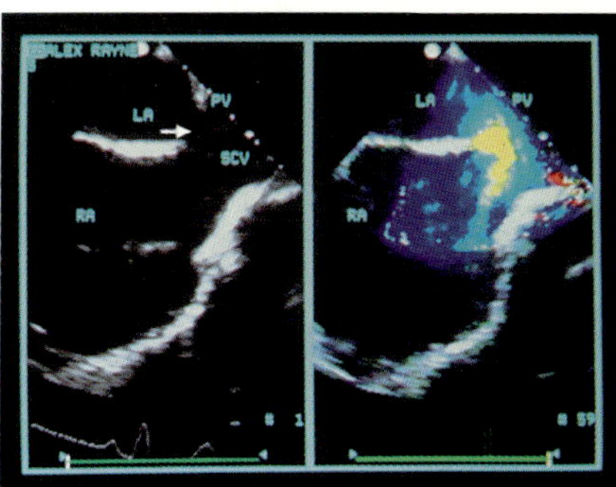

Atrial septal defect, page 62.

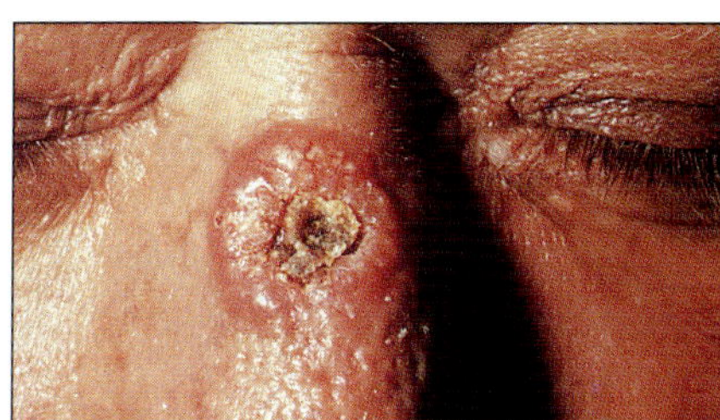

Basal cell carcinoma, page 66.

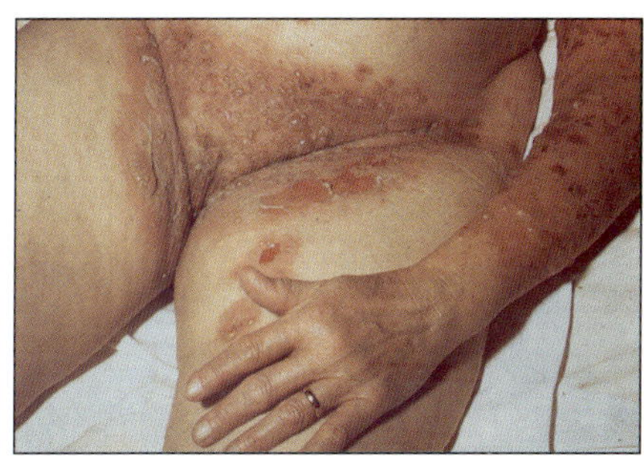

Bullous disorders, page 74.

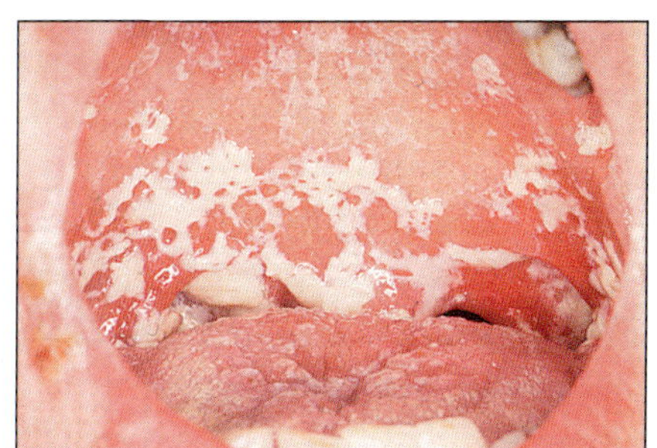

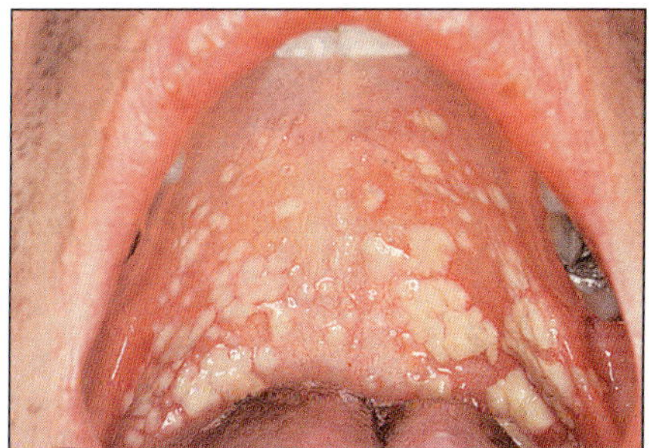

Candidiasis, buccal and esophageal in AIDS; page 76.

Color plates

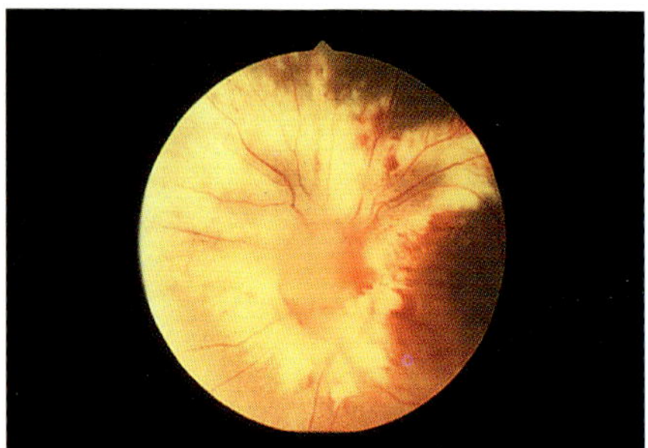

Cytomegalovirus infection in AIDS, page 110.

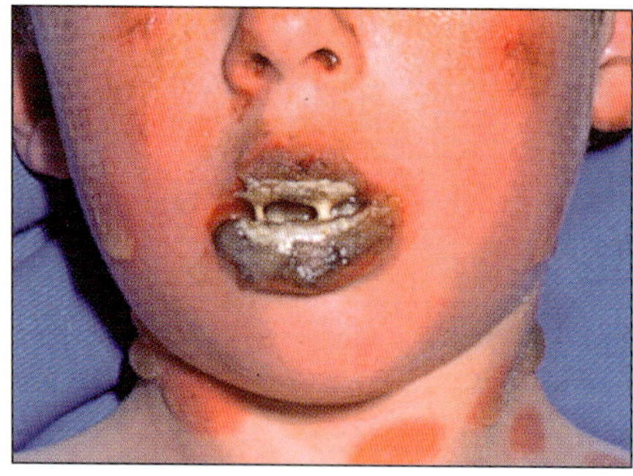

Erythema multiforme and Stevens–Johnson syndrome, page 148.

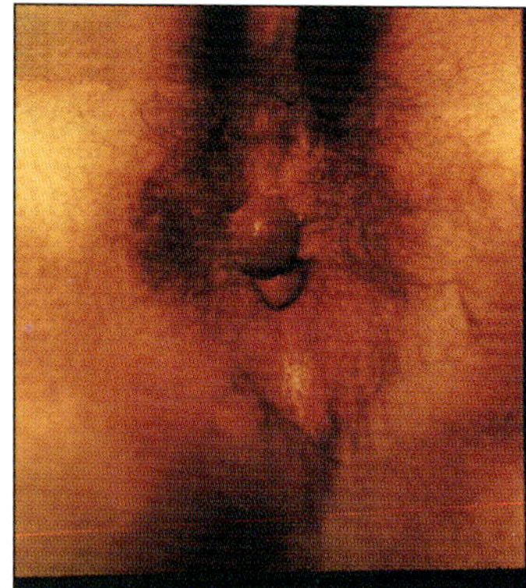

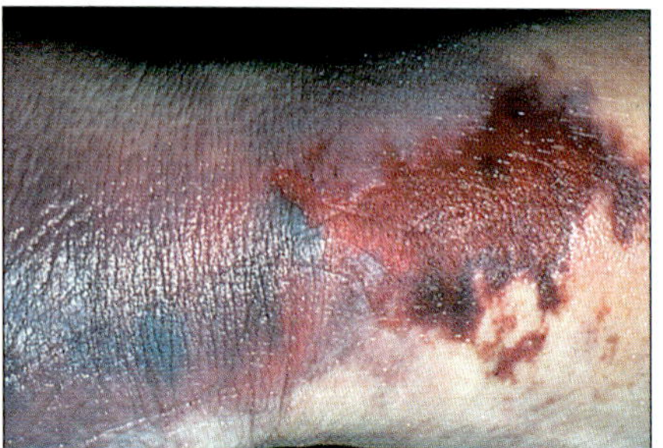

Disseminated intravascular coagulation, page 130.

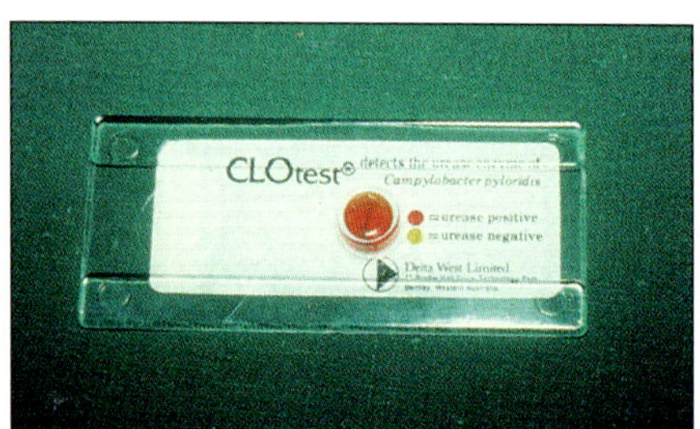

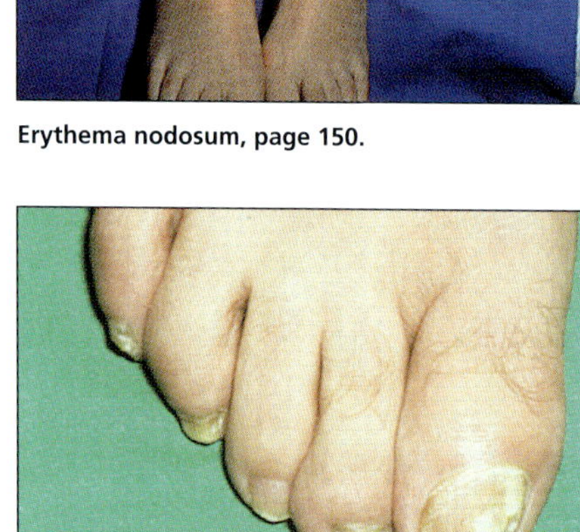

Erythema nodosum, page 150.

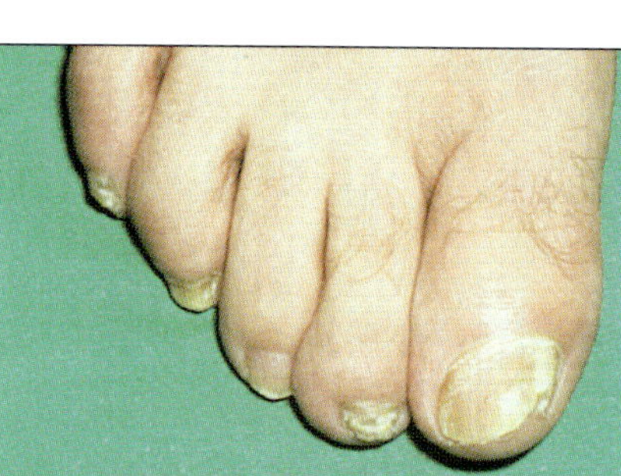

Duodenal ulcer, page 134.

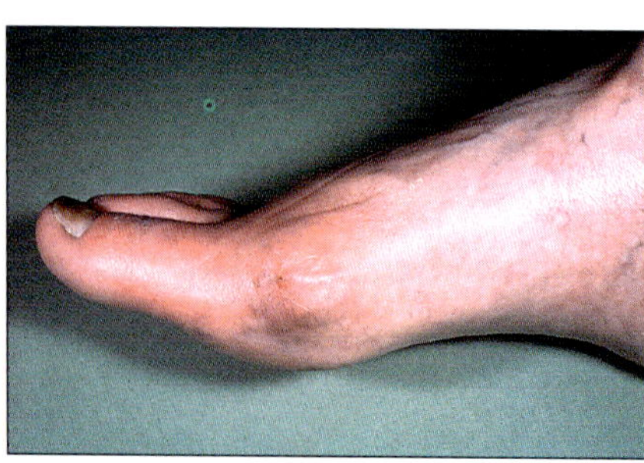

Fungal nail infection, page 160.

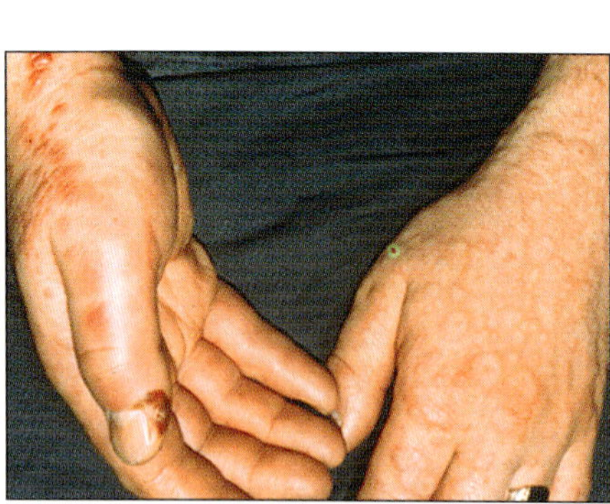

Erythema multiforme and Stevens–Johnson syndrome, page 148.

Gout, page 170.

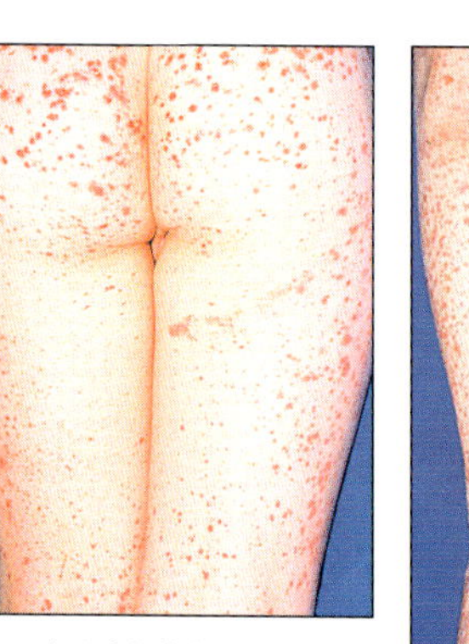

Hemorrhoidal disease, page 188.

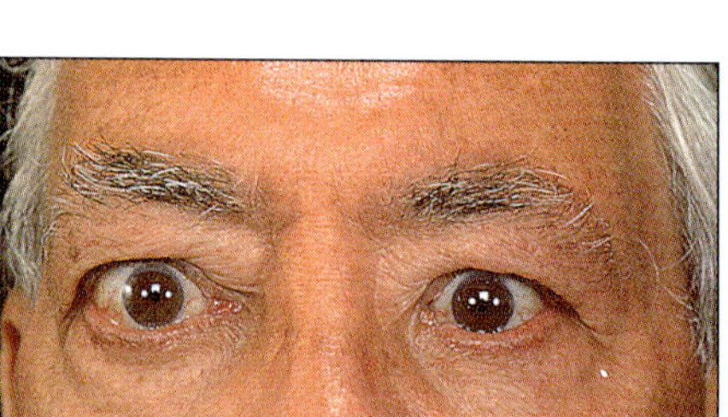

Henoch-Schönlein purpura, page 190.

Hyperthyroidism, page 218.

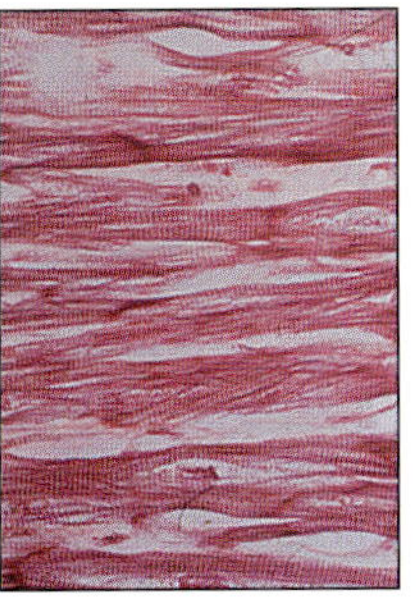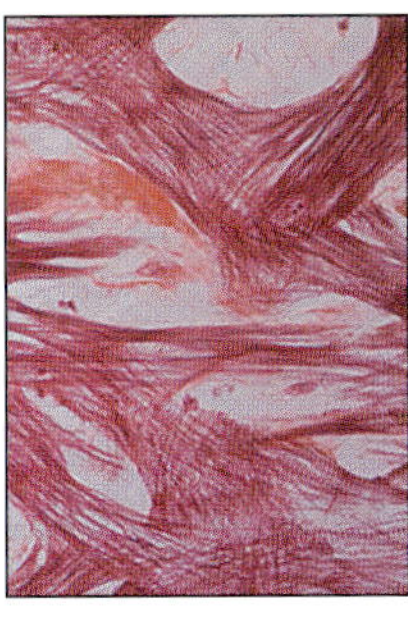

Hypertrophic cardiomyopathy, page 220.

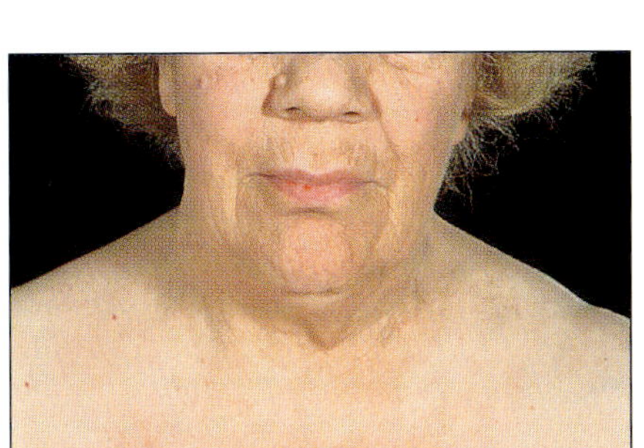

Hypothyroidism, page 228.

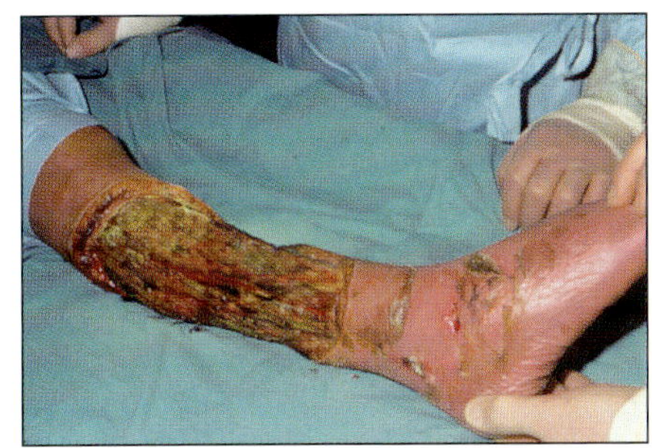

Infections in hematological malignancy, page 230.

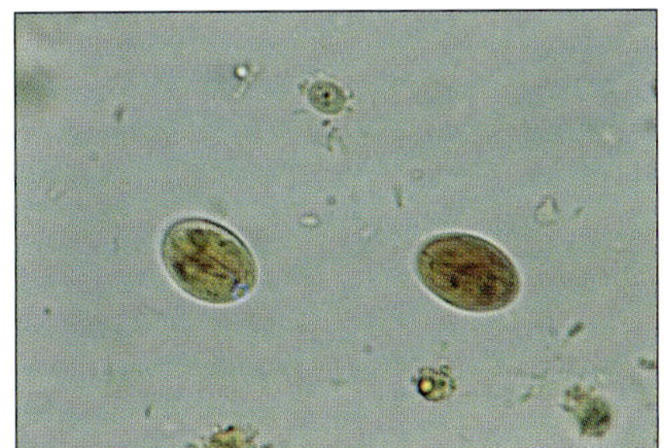

Infectious diarrhea, page 232.

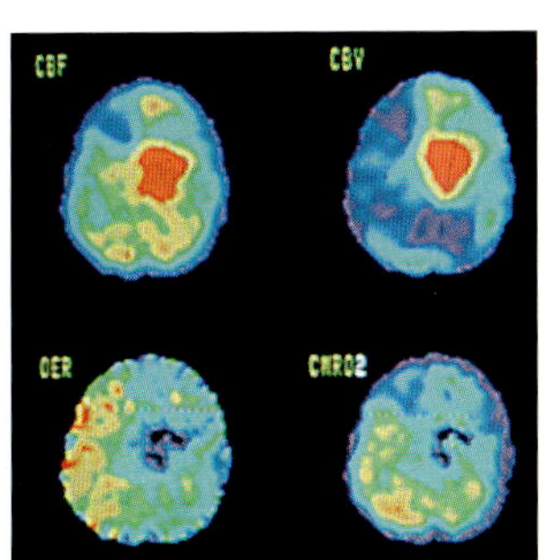

Intracerebral hemorrhage, page 236.

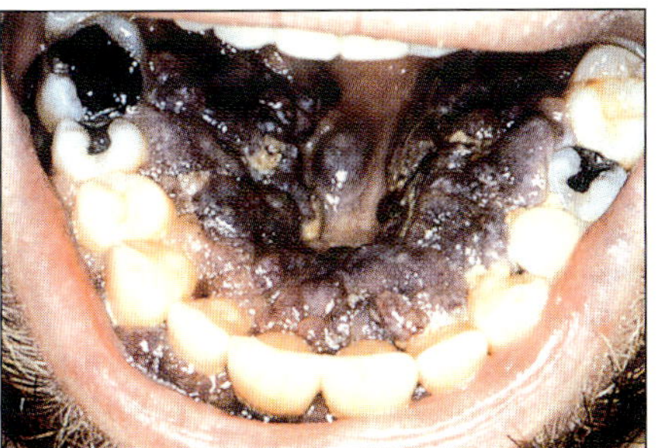

Kaposi's sarcoma in AIDS, page 240.

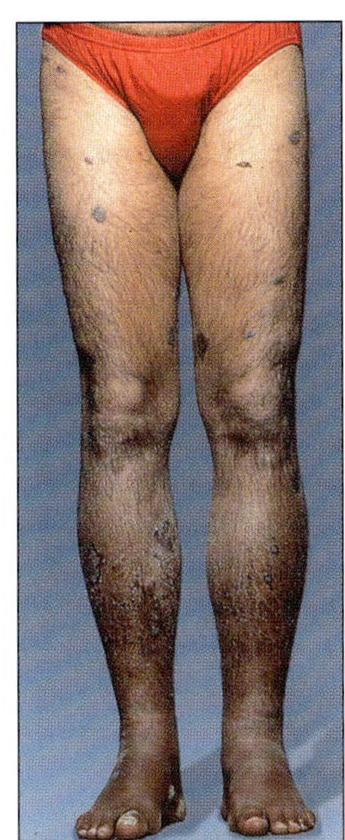

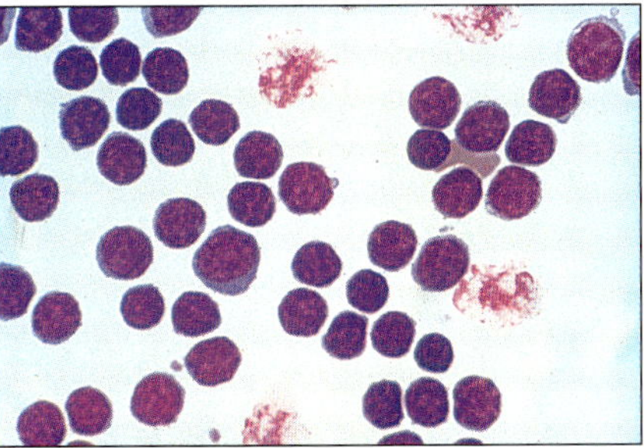

Leukemia, chronic lymphocytic; page 252.

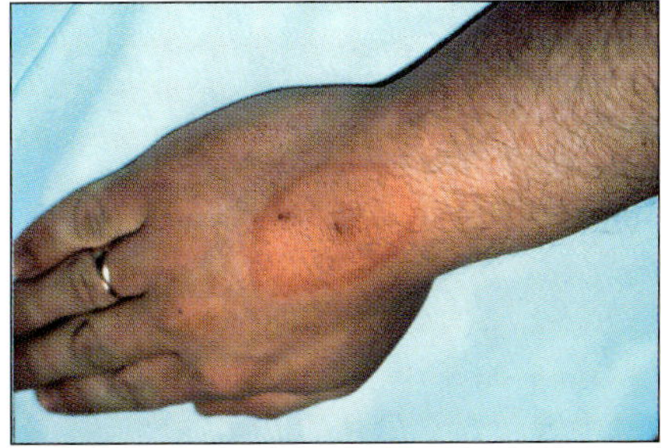

Lyme disease, page 264.

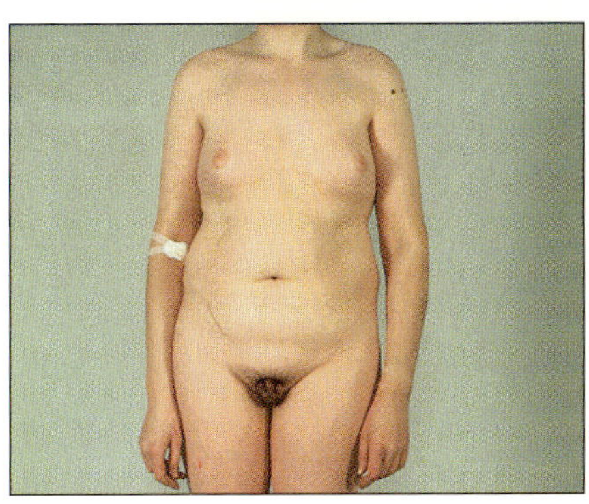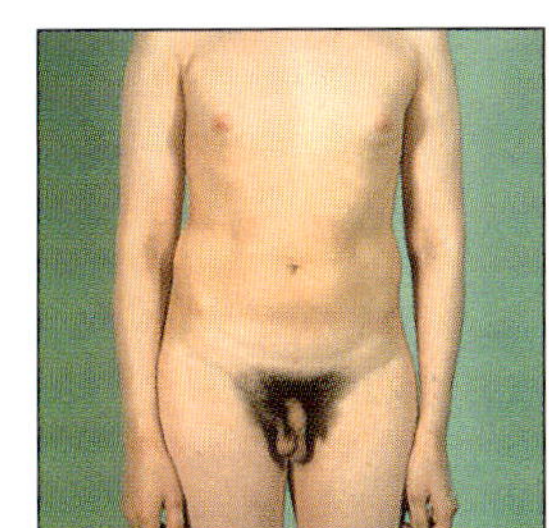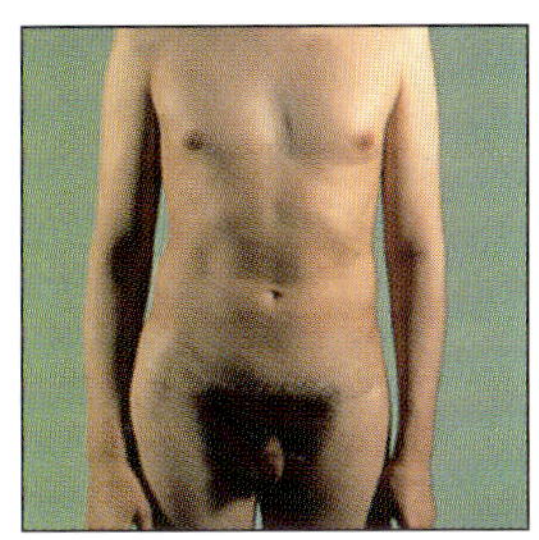

Male hypogonadism, pages 266–267.

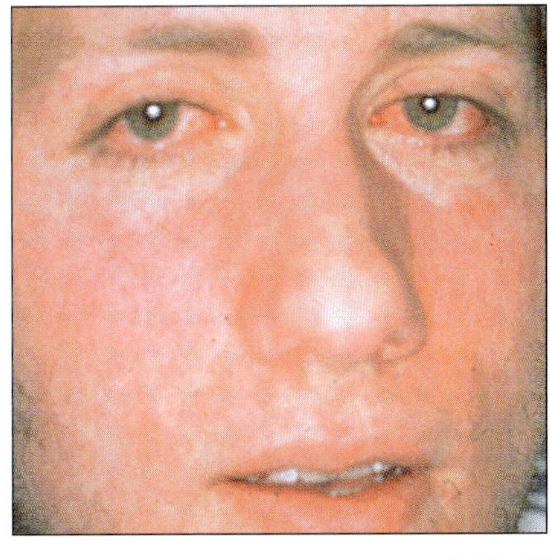

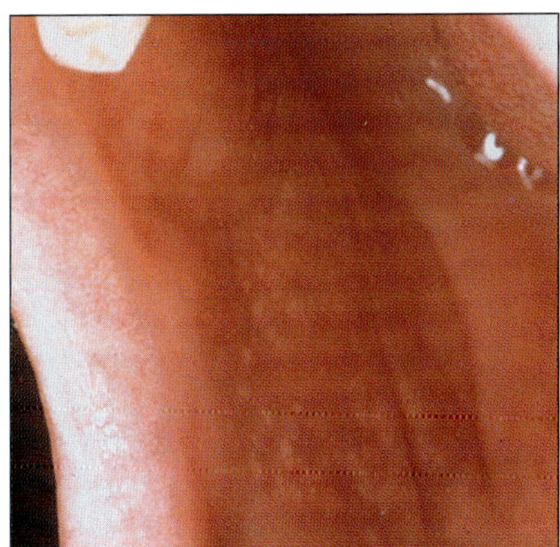

Measles, page 270.

Color plates

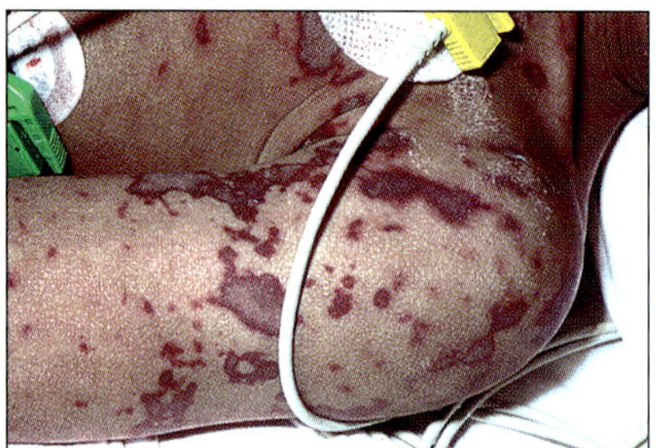

Meningitis, bacterial; page 272.

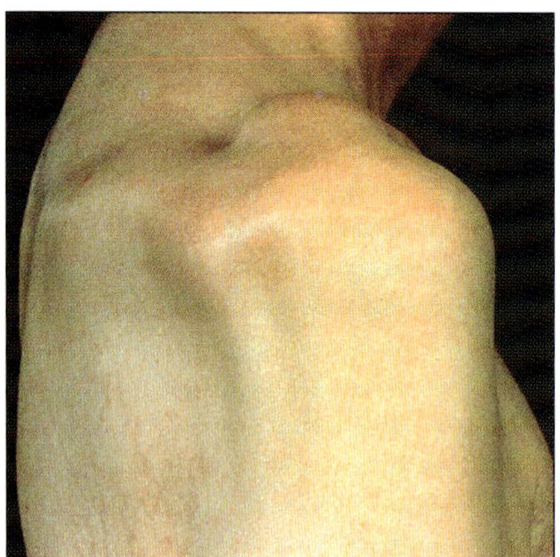

Motor neuron disease, page 284.

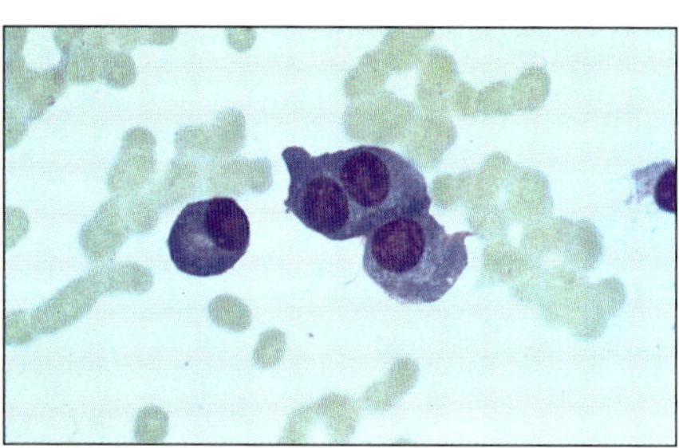

Multiple myeloma, page 286

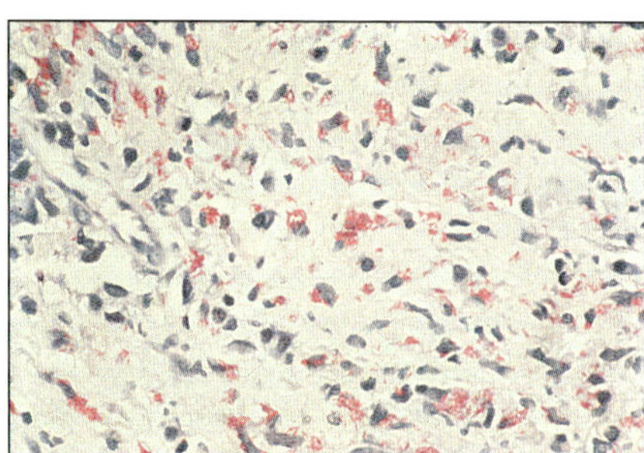

Mycobacterium avium complex infection in AIDS, page 292.

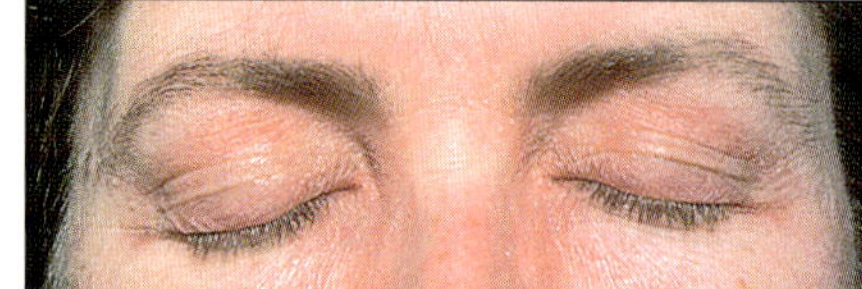

Myositis, inflammatory; page 298.

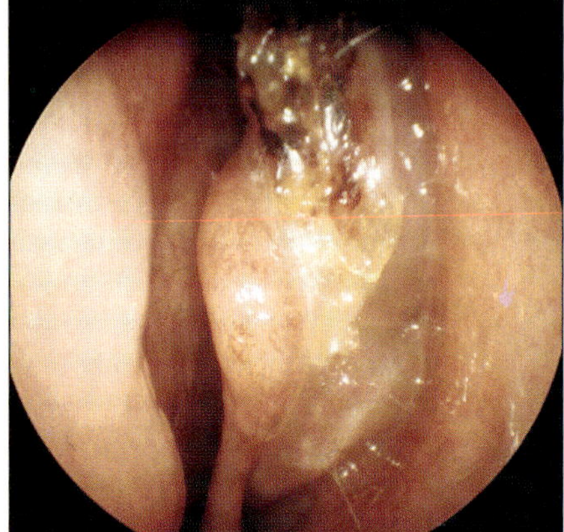

Nasal polyposis, page 300.

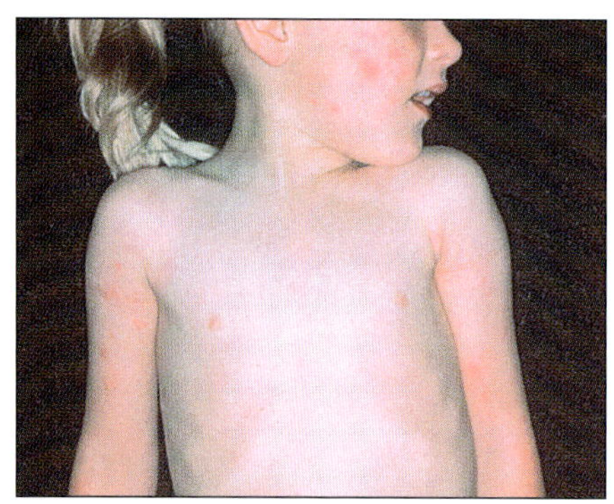

Parvovirus B19 infection, page 328.

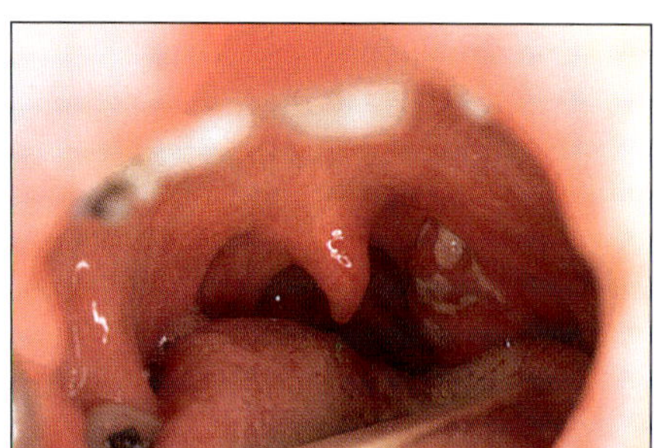

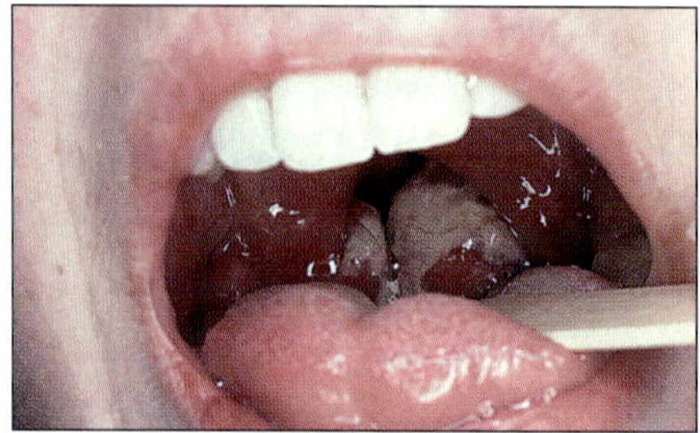

Pharyngitis, page 334.

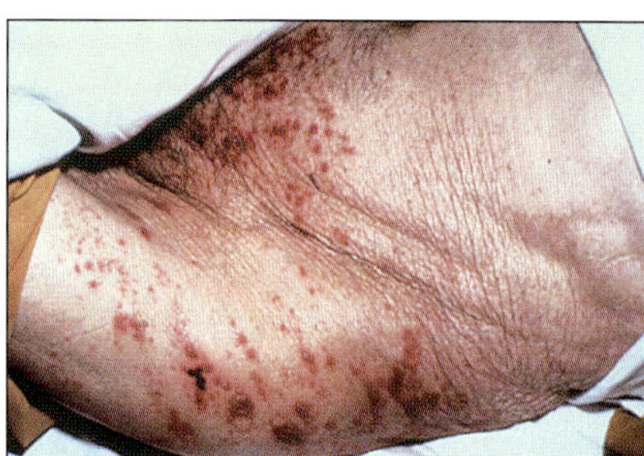

Platelet disorders, page 338.

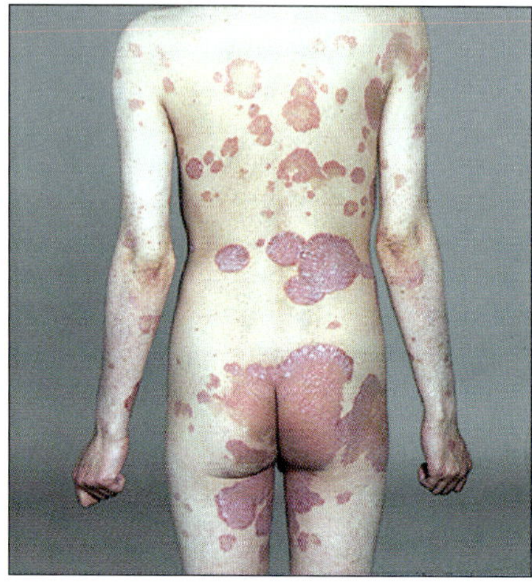

Psoriasis, page 360.

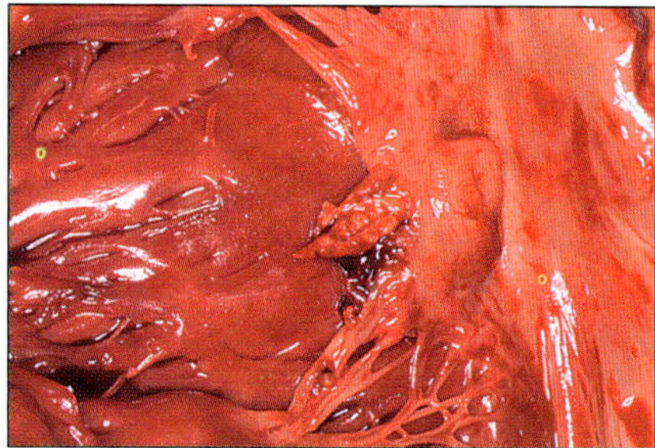

Rheumatic fever, acute; page 384.

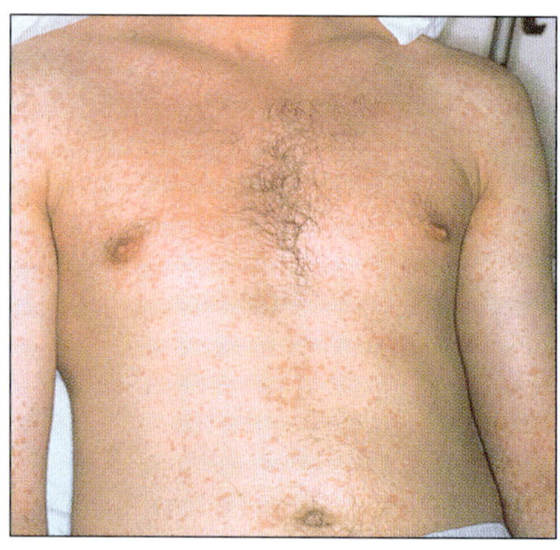

Rubella (German measles), page 386.

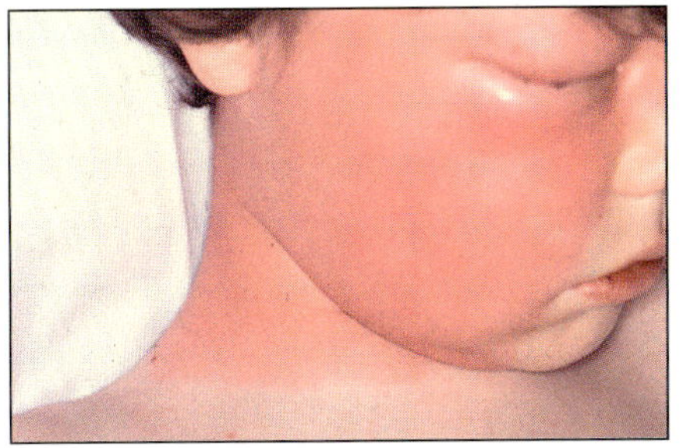

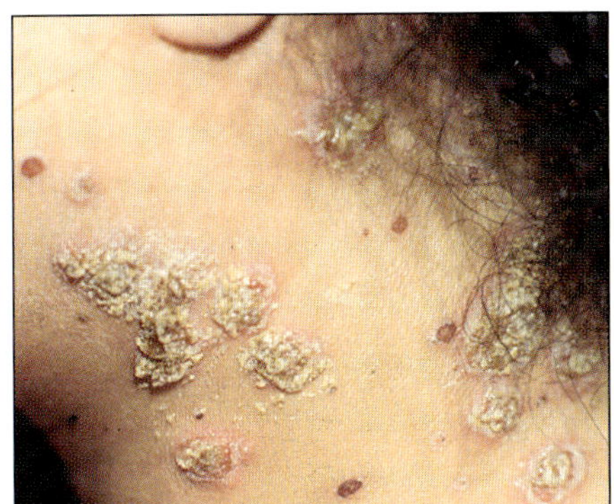

Skin infections, page 398.

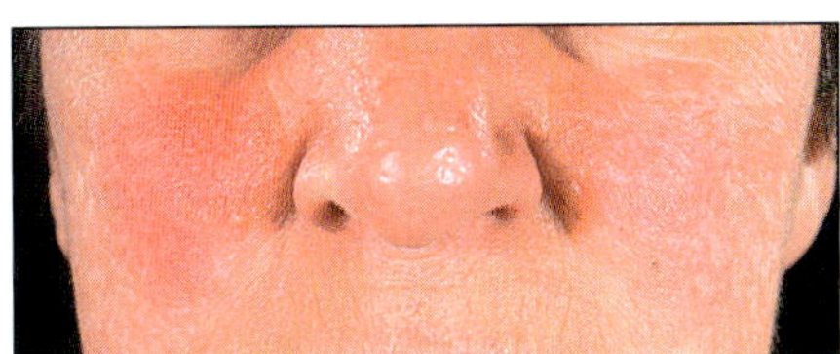

Systemic lupus erythematosus, page 416.

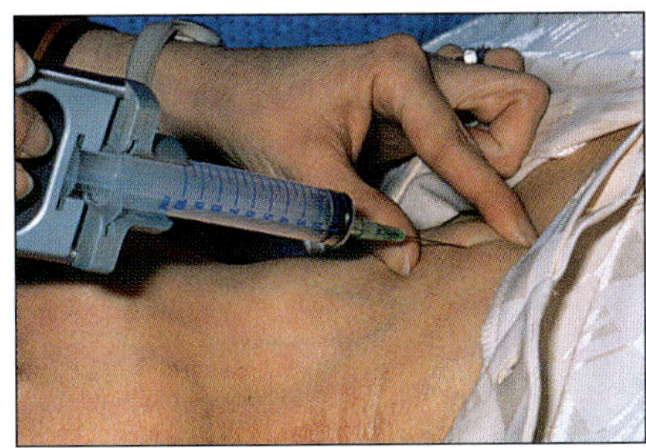

Thyroid carcinoma, page 426.

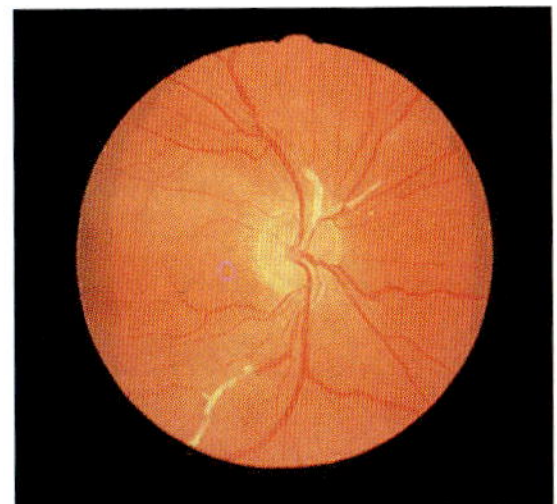

Transient ischemic attacks, page 436.

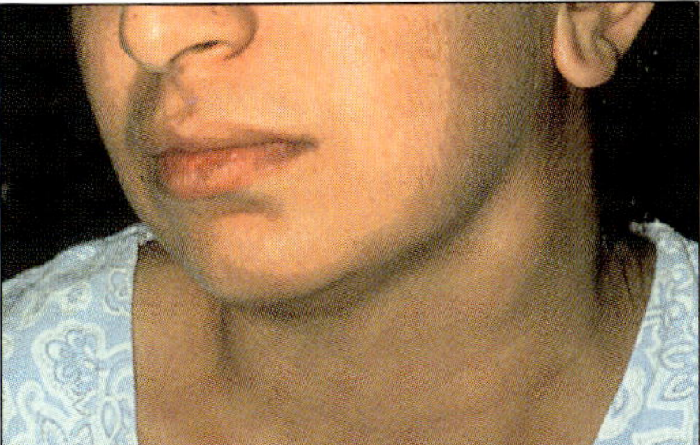

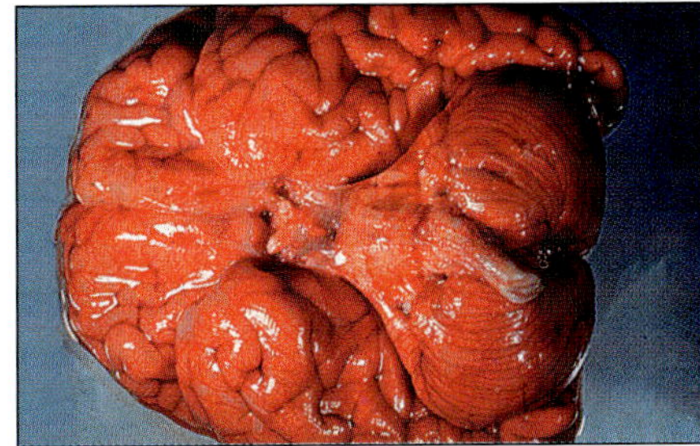

Tuberculosis, extrapulmonary; page 440.

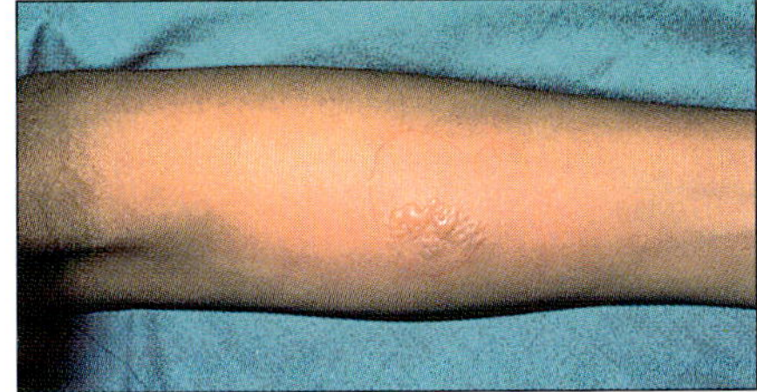

Typhoid and paratyphoid fevers, page 444.

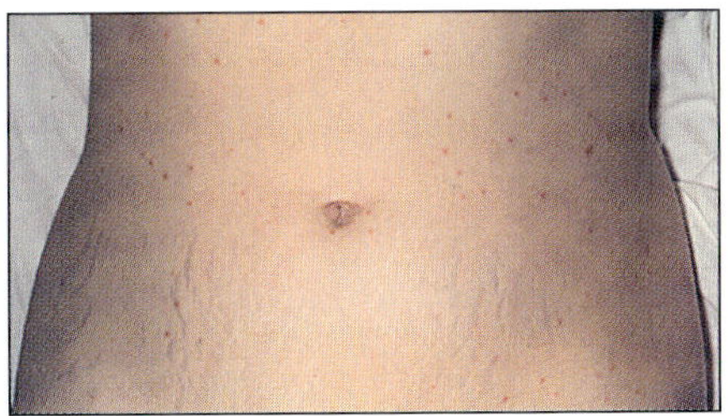

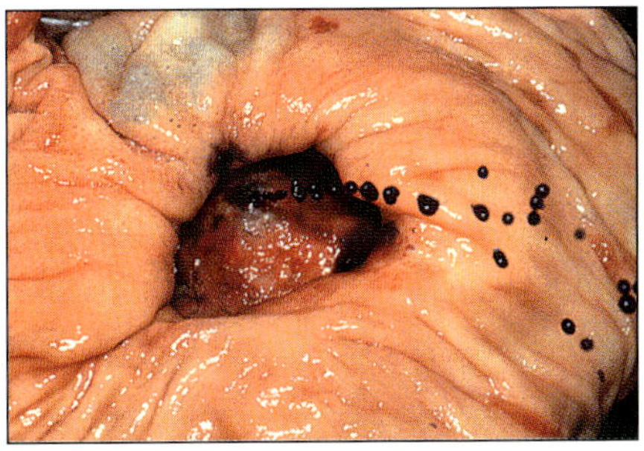

Upper gastrointestinal tract bleeding, page 448.

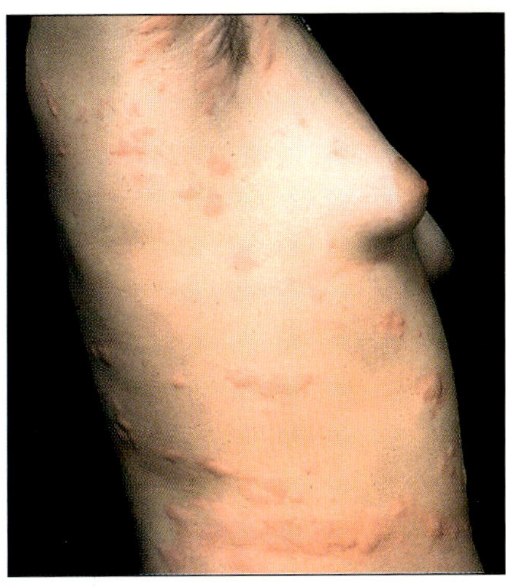

Urticaria, page 454.

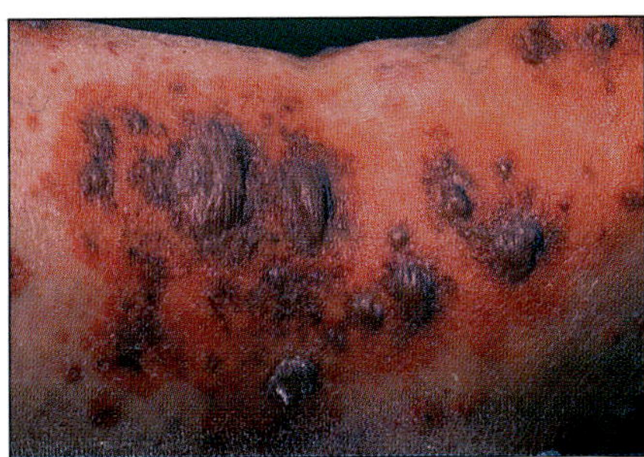

Vasculitis, skin manifestations; page 458.

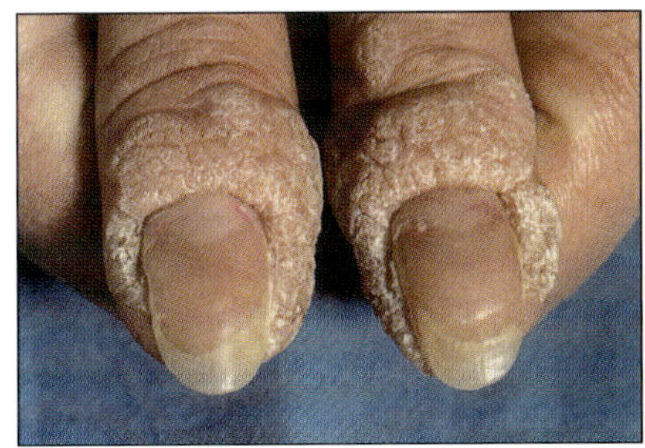

Viral warts, page 462.

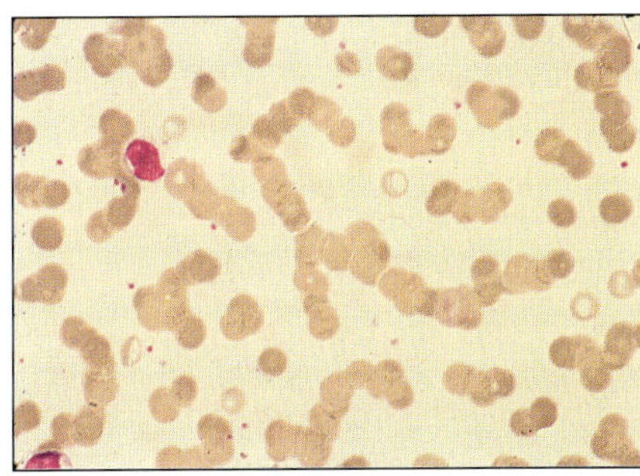

Waldenström's macroglobulinemia, page 464.

DATE DUE